Nursing Staff in Hospitals and Nursing Homes

in Hospitals and Nursing Homes

Is It Adequate?

Gooloo S. Wunderlich, Frank A. Sloan, and Carolyne K. Davis, *Editors*

Committee on the Adequacy of Nurse Staffing
in Hospitals and Nursing Homes

Division of Health Care Services

INSTITUTE OF MEDICINE

NATIONAL ACADEMY PRESS
Washington, D.C. 1996

National Academy Press • 2101 Constitution Avenue, N.W. • Washington, D.C. 20418

NOTICE: The project that is the subject of this report was approved by the Governing Board of the National Research Council, whose members are drawn from the councils of the National Academy of Sciences, the National Academy of Engineering, and the Institute of Medicine. The members of the committee responsible for the report were chosen for their special competences and with regard for appropriate balance.

This report has been reviewed by a group other than the authors according to procedures approved by a Report Review Committee consisting of members of the National Academy of Sciences, the National Academy of Engineering, and the Institute of Medicine.

The Institute of Medicine was chartered in 1970 by the National Academy of Sciences to enlist distinguished members of the appropriate professions in the examination of policy matters pertaining to the health of the public. In this, the Institute acts under both the Academy's 1863 congressional charter responsibility to be an adviser to the federal government and its own initiative in identifying issues of medical care, research, and education. Dr. Kenneth I. Shine is president of the Institute of Medicine.

Support for this project was provided by the National Institute for Nursing Research through an interagency agreement with the Bureau of Health Professions of the Health Resources and Services Administration, U.S. Department of Health and Human Services. The views presented are those of the Institute of Medicine Committee on the Adequacy of Nurse Staffing in Hospitals and Nursing Homes and are not necessarily those of the funding organization.

Library of Congress Cataloging-in-Publication Data

Nursing staff in hospitals and nursing homes : is it adequate? /
    Gooloo S. Wunderlich, Frank A. Sloan, and Carolyne K. Davis,
    editors.
        p. cm.
      "Division of Health Care Services, Institute of Medicine."
      Includes bibliographical references and index.
      ISBN 0-309-05398-6
      1. Nurses—Supply and Demand—United States. 2. Nurses' aides—
Supply and demand—United States. 3. Hospital care—United States.
4. Nursing home care—United States. I. Wunderlich, Gooloo S.
II. Sloan, Frank A. III. Davis, Carolyne K.
      [DNLM: 1. Nursing Staff—supply & distribution. 2. Nursing Staff,
Hospital. 3. Nursing Homes. WY 125 N9748 1996]
    RT86.73.N886   1996
    331.12′91362173′0973—dc20
    DNLM/DLC   96-117
    for Library of Congress   CIP

Printed in the United States of America

The serpent has been a symbol of long life, healing, and knowledge among almost all cultures and religions since the beginning of recorded history. The image adopted as a logotype by the Institute of Medicine is based on a relief carving from ancient Greece, now held by the Staatlichemuseen in Berlin.

COMMITTEE ON THE ADEQUACY OF NURSE STAFFING IN HOSPITALS AND NURSING HOMES

CAROLYNE K. DAVIS,* *(Chair)*, National and International Health Care Advisor, Ernst and Young, Washington, D.C.

FRANK A. SLOAN,* *(Cochair)* J. Alexander McMahon Professor of Health Policy and Management and Professor of Economics, Center for Health Policy Research, Duke University, Durham, North Carolina

DYANNE D. AFFONSO,* Dean and Professor, Nell Hodgson Woodruff School of Nursing, Emory University, Atlanta, Georgia

JAMES F. BLUMSTEIN,* Professor, Vanderbilt University School of Law, Nashville, Tennessee

DONALD L. CHENSVOLD, President, Healthcare of Iowa, Inc., Cedar Rapids, Iowa

LINDA HAWES CLEVER,* Chair, Department of Occupational Health, California Pacific Medical Center, San Francisco, California

JOYCE C. CLIFFORD, Vice President for Nursing and Nurse in Chief, Beth Israel Hospital, Boston, Massachusetts

EDWARD J. CONNORS,* President Emeritus, Mercy Health Services, Morrisville, Vermont

ARTHUR COOPER, Chief of Pediatric Surgical Critical Care, Division of Pediatric Critical Surgery, Harlem Hospital Center, New York City, New York

ALLYSON ROSS DAVIES, Health Consultant, Newton, Massachusetts

ERIKA SIVARAJAN FROELICHER, Professor, Department of Physiological Nursing and Adjunct Professor, Department of Epidemiology and Biostatistics, University of California, San Francisco, California

CHARLENE A. HARRINGTON, Professor and Chair, Department of Social and Behavioral Sciences, School of Nursing, University of California, San Francisco, California

MARK C. HORNBROOK, Program Director, Center for Health Research, Kaiser Permanente, Portland, Oregon

RONALD E. KUTSCHER, Associate Commissioner, Bureau of Labor Statistics, U.S. Department of Labor, Washington, D.C.

SUE LONGHENRY, Surveyor, Joint Commission on Accreditation of Hospitals, Columbus, Ohio

ELLIOTT C. ROBERTS, SR., Professor, Louisiana State University Medical School, New Orleans, Louisiana

---

*Member, Institute of Medicine

Division of Health Care Services

Study Staff:
Gooloo S. Wunderlich, Study Director
Holly Dawkins, Research Assistant
Annice Hirt, Senior Project Assistant

Kathleen N. Lohr, Division Director
H. Don Tiller, Division Administrative Assistant

Acknowledgments

The Institute of Medicine (IOM) Committee on the Adequacy of Nurse Staffing in Hospitals and Nursing Homes acknowledges with appreciation the many persons and organizations, not all of whom can be individually identified, who contributed to the success of this study.

Support for this study was provided by the Division of Nursing, Health Resources and Services Administration of the U.S. Department of Health and Human Services. We particularly wish to thank Evelyn Moses, Division of Nursing, who served as the government project officer for this study. She was always available for participating in all the committee meetings open to the public and the public hearings, and providing guidance and data to the committee throughout the period of its deliberations. We would like to thank Patricia Moritz, National Institute of Nursing Research, where the original request for the study was directed by Congress, for organizing a special session for the committee in conjunction with the 1994 annual meetings of the Gerontological Society of America where she brought together researchers to discuss completed and ongoing research on staffing and quality of care issues in nursing homes. We recognize with gratitude Janet Heinrich, director of the American Academy of Nursing, for organizing with Patricia Moritz a workshop to discuss completed and ongoing research on the relationship between quality of care and nurse staffing and organizational variables in hospitals. This workshop was held in conjunction with the annual meeting of the American Academy of Nursing. Dr. Heinrich's assistance to staff throughout the period of the study is appreciated.

In addition we would like to acknowledge the help provided by many other federal government officials. In particular the committee appreciates the time and efforts of staff of the Health Care Financing Administration for providing the committee and staff with relevant information and participating in committee meetings. We thank the staff of the Bureau of Labor Statistics for providing the committee and staff with special tabulations and other information on employment statistics in the health industry, and on injuries in the workplace.

An important part of the committee's work was analysis of national databases and extensive review of literature. The committee wishes to thank the Health Statistics Group of the American Hospital Association and Marjorie Beyers, executive director, American Organization of Nurse Executives, for making available special detailed tabulations for the committee's use. We recognize with gratitude Scott Bates and Peter Kralovec of that office for preparing the tabulations, some on very short notice, and for patiently answering the many questions for clarification.

Many individuals shared unselfishly with the committee the results of their work, and some carried out special focused projects on behalf of the committee. The committee particularly wishes to thank its Liaison Panel, which comprised representatives of professional associations of nurses, related professional groups, hospitals and nursing homes, unions, and organizations that serve as advocates for nursing home residents (see Appendix B). Several members of the panel also provided the committee with results of special surveys, informational material, and other background information from their organizations throughout the period of the study.

The committee also wishes to thank the staff of various interested organizations, including Margaret Peisert and Arvid Muller of the Service Employees International Union and Karen Worthington and David Keepnews of the American Nurses Association, who were responsive to many committee requests; Sarah Burger of the National Citizens' Coalition for Nursing Home Reform, who organized meetings and provided information that helped the committee understand the specific concerns of nursing home residents and the elderly; Martha Mohler of the National Committee to Preserve Social Security and Medicare, who ably served a double duty as both the Liaison Panel member and the staff contact; and Marcia Richards of the American Health Care Association (AHCA), who organized a meeting with the AHCA long-term care nurse council and was always available to answer questions and provide data.

Although we agreed not to identify these individuals and organizations, we want to express our gratitude to the many site visit hosts who welcomed the committee graciously and shared their thoughts, experiences, insights, and time. The committee also appreciates the efforts of the large number of persons who submitted written testimonies and letters to share their views and experiences, as well as several individuals who provided oral testimony at the public hearings held by the committee. Organizations and individuals who presented oral statements at the public hearings are listed in the Study Activities in Part II of this report.

We are grateful to the authors of commissioned papers prepared for this study. These papers were used extensively by staff and committee in drafting the report. They are included in Part II of the report. In addition the committee had access to a preliminary draft of a paper on "Utilization of Unlicensed Assistive Personnel in Nursing Care Delivery: Examination, Evaluation, and Recommendations for the Future," which was prepared for the committee's use by Greta Krapohl and Elaine Larson, Georgetown University School of Nursing, in fulfillment of a graduate student assignment with the IOM committee. The committee expresses its appreciation to Ms. Krapohl and Dr. Larson, her advisor for the scholarly project.

During the first year of its work, the committee held meetings at which experts made thoughtful presentations on various aspects of the committee's mandate. The presenters and the topics of their talks are listed in Appendix A; their contribution of time and knowledge is appreciated.

We acknowledge with gratitude the contributions of the committee's staff, to whom an important debt of gratitude is owed. The committee is aware of the enormous commitment and effort of our study director, Gooloo Wunderlich. Her organizational skills, as well as her sense of humor assisted the committee throughout its deliberations. Her professionalism and expertise in health care policy development coupled with her excellent writing skills advanced the progress of this report throughout its many reviews and revisions. Coordinating the research and assimilating disparate views was a major undertaking. A disproportionate share of any credit due this report is because of her perseverance, skill, knowledge, and the incredible amount of time she devoted to organizing and writing the report. Holly Dawkins, who served as research assistant, worked closely with the study director on various aspects of the study. She took primary responsibility for organizing the various site visits, guiding committee members through each site visit, and drafting the site visit reports. We recognize and appreciate the substantial staff effort that went into organizing the site visits. Annice Hirt served ably as the senior project assistant. She efficiently managed the logistical and administrative arrangements for the many committee meetings and orchestrated the smooth operation of two public hearings involving large numbers of people. She organized the voluminous research material that committee and staff generated over the course of the study, handled the large volume of correspondence and inquiries, and cheerfully and competently coped with the various drafts of the report under very tight deadlines.

Other IOM staff made valuable contributions to the success of the committee's efforts. Kathleen N. Lohr, director, Division of Health Care Services, was always available to answer questions, provide assistance to committee and staff, and explain to members of the committee the operations of the IOM and the National Research Council. Nina Spruill helped keep our budget in order. Claudia Carl managed the logistics of an extensive report review process, and

Mike Edington shepherded the report through the editing and production process. Sally Stanfield at the National Academy Press was supportive as always.

Finally, we would like to thank the members of the committee for their generous contribution of time and effort in the preparation of the report.

Carolyne K. Davis, *Chair*
Frank A. Sloan, *Cochair*

Contents

SUMMARY   1

PART I: REVIEW AND RECOMMENDATIONS

1   INTRODUCTION   19
     Immediate Origins of the Institute of Medicine Study, 20
     Committee Charge, 21
     Definitions, 22
     Study Approach, 25
     Underlying Assumptions and Values, 27
     Organization of the Report, 28

2   IMPLICATIONS OF POPULATION CHANGE   31
     Introduction, 31
     Growth of the Population, 32
     Diversity of the Population, 34
     Health Status and Disabling Conditions, 38
     Conclusion, 41

3   EVOLVING HEALTH CARE SCENE   42
     Overview, 42
     Private Insurance and Public Payers for Health Care, 46
     Managed Care, 47

Ownership Structure, 50
Hospitals, 51
Nursing Homes, 58
Implications for Nursing Services, 66

4   NURSING PERSONNEL IN A TIME OF CHANGE   68
Supply of Nursing Personnel, 69
Changing Demand for Nursing Personnel, 79
Is Supply Adequate for the Demands of the Next Century?, 87
Summary, 91

5   STAFFING AND QUALITY OF CARE IN HOSPITALS   92
Restructuring in the Hospitals, 94
Measuring Quality of Care in Hospitals, 106
Relationship of Nursing Staff to Quality of Patient Care, 116
Legislative and Regulatory Requirements, 124
Summary, 126

6   STAFFING AND QUALITY OF CARE IN NURSING HOMES   128
Measurement of Quality, 129
Status of Quality of Care in Nursing Facilities, 132
Has Quality of Care Improved Since OBRA 87?, 136
Relationships Among Nursing Staff, Management, and
  Quality of Care, 146
Effects of Reimbursement and Other Factors on Nursing Staff, 162
Residents, Families, Volunteers, and Ombudsmen, 165
Conclusion, 167

7   STAFFING AND WORK-RELATED INJURIES AND STRESS   169
Overview, 169
Incidence of Work-Related Injuries and Illness, 170
Violence, Abuse, and Conflict, 177
Work-Related Stress, 183
Summary, 187

8   EPILOGUE   189

APPENDIXES
A Presentations Made to the Committee, 195
B Liaison Panel, 197
C Separate Statement, *James F. Blumstein*, 199
   Responses by Committee Members, 202
D Acronyms, 205

REFERENCES   209

BIOGRAPHICAL SKETCHES OF COMMITTEE MEMBERS   230

PART II: RESOURCES FOR THE STUDY

1   STUDY ACTIVITIES
    Written and Oral Testimony Submitted to the Committee, 241
    Site Visits Conducted by the Committee, 259

2   STATISTICAL RESOURCES   277

3   COMMISSIONED PAPERS
    Quality of Care, Organizational Variables, and Nurse Staffing, 308
        Joyce A. Verran
    Professional Nursing Education—Today and Tomorrow, 333
        Angela Barron McBride
    Nursing Staff and Quality of Care in Nursing Homes, 361
        Meridean Maas, Kathleen Buckwalter, and Janet Specht
    Quality of Care and Nursing Staff in Nursing Homes, 426
        Jean Johnson, C. McKeen Cowles, and Samuel J. Simmens
    Nursing Facility Quality, Staffing, and Economic Issues, 453
        Charlene A. Harrington
    Nursing Injury, Stress, and Nursing Care, 503
        Bonnie Rogers

INDEX   533

TABLES AND FIGURES

Tables

3.1 Inpatient Activity in Community Hospitals, Total Patients and Patients 65 Years of Age or Older, United States, Selected Years, 1983–1993, 54

3.2 Percent Change in Inpatient Community Hospital Utilization, Untited States, 1994–1995, 55

3.3 Trends in Outpatient Visits and Other Selected Services Offered in Community Hospitals, United States, Selected Years, 1983–1993, 56

3.4 Percent Change in Outpatient Community Hospital Utilization, United States, 1994–1995, 57

3.5 Number of Licensed Nursing Home Beds per 1,000 Population Aged 85 and Older, by Region, Selected Years, United States, 1978–1993, 59

3.6 Number of States by Medicaid Nursing Facility Reimbursement Method and by Number Using Case-Mix Reimbursement, United States, 1979 and 1993, 62

3.7 Number of Licensed Long-Term Care Facilities, United States, 1992 and 1993, 64

4.1 Number of Full-Time and Part-Time Employees in Nursing Occupations, United States, Selected Years, 1983–1993, 72

4.2 Unemployment Rates, Nursing and Other Selected Occupations, United States, Selected Years, 1983–1994, 73

4.3 Number of Full-Time and Part-Time Employees in Hospitals and Nursing Homes, United States, Selected Years, 1988–1994, 78

4.4 Percent Change in Nurse Staffing in Community Hospitals, United States, 1994–1995, 81

5.1 Illustrative Measures of Quality of Care in Inpatient Hospital Settings, with Specific Attention to Nursing Care, 110

6.1 Illustrative Measures of Quality of Care in Nursing Homes, 130

6.2 Deficiencies in Certified Nursing Facilities from the Federal On-Line Survey Certification and Reporting System, United States, 1993, 137

6.3 Resident Characteristics in Nursing Facilities from the Federal On-Line Survey Certification and Reporting System, United States, 1993, 139

6.4 Nurse Staffing Levels for All Certified Nursing Facilities from the Federal On-Line Survey Certification and Reporting System, United States, 1991–1993, 143

6.5 Average Turnover Rates in Nursing Facilities by Staff Category, United States, 1990–1994, 160

6.6 Nursing Facility Hourly Wages by Staff Category, United States, 1990–1993, 161

7.1 Trends in Occupational Injury and Illness Incidence, United States, 1980–1993, 171

7.2 Percent Distribution of Nonfatal Occupational Injuries and Illnesses Involving Days Away from Work, for Selected Occupations and Worker Characteristics, United States, 1993, 172

Figures

2.1 Average annual percent change in population 65 years and older, United States, 1900–2040 (middle series projections), 33

2.2 Number of people 85 years and older, United States, 1900–2050 (middle series projections), 33

2.3 Percent of population 65 years and older by race and hispanic origin, United States, 1900 and 2050, 35

2.4 Parent support ratio, United States, 1950–2050 (number of people 85 years and older per 100 persons 50–64 years old, middle series projections), 37

3.1 Employment in hospitals, United States, 1969–1994, 44

3.2 Nurses as a percent of total full-time-equivalent (FTE) personnel in community hospitals, United States, 1979–1993, 45

3.3 Sources of funds for medical care expenditures, United States, 1993, 46

3.4 Number of people receiving care in HMOs, United States, 1976–1995, 48

4.1 Estimated active supply of registered nurses (RN) per 100,000 population, United States, 1960–1993, 71

4.2 Age distribution of employed registered nurses (RN), United States, 1988, 1993, and 2000, 74

4.3 Highest educational preparation of registered nurses (RN), United States, 1992, 75

4.4 Percent of registered nurse graduates by type of educational program, United States, 1958–1993, 76

4.5 Number of licensed practical nurse (LPN) graduations, United States, 1983–1993, 77

4.6 Ratio of registered nurse full-time-equivalents (FTE) to adjusted patient days, United States, 1983–1993, 80

4.7 Percent change in registered nurse employment in selected areas, United States, 1988–1992, 82

4.8 Median weekly earnings of nursing occupations, United States, 1983–1994, 86

Part I

REVIEW AND RECOMMENDATIONS

Summary

The nation's health care system is in a transition of potentially historic proportions driven by the need for cost-effectiveness under pressures of cost containment and competition, but also made possible by scientific and technological breakthroughs. These forces have led to major changes in the structure, organization, financing, and delivery of health care since the early 1980s.

Managed care organizations have developed rapidly, changing the nature of private health insurance and increasing price competition. These evolving care delivery and payment systems have in turn affected the structure of the health care system by limiting service and directing when and where patients receive care.

Historically the hospital has been at the core of the U.S. health care system, and nursing services are central to the provision of hospital care. However, the changes in payment systems, combined with scientific and technological advances, have permitted shifts from the traditional inpatient care settings to ambulatory, community, home, and nursing home care.[1] Inpatient use of hospitals, length of hospital stay, inpatient days, and the number of beds staffed have all declined. As a consequence, hospitals are changing in ways not considered possible a few years ago. To maintain economic viability, they are rapidly restructuring, merging, and consolidating. They are also redesigning and reconfiguring staffing patterns and, increasingly, moving toward interdiscipli-

---

[1]Throughout the report, the terms "nursing home" and "nursing facility" are used interchangeably.

nary teams of care givers including registered nurses (RN), licensed practical nurses (LPN),[2] and nurse assistants (NA) and other ancillary nursing personnel.[3] They are also downsizing staff to accommodate the reduced volume of inpatient care and to remain economically viable.

The lines between the hospital and the nursing home are beginning to blur. New developments in hospital organization combined with economic and other forces are changing the characteristics of the persons entering nursing homes and are creating new demands for beds and for provision of nursing care in these facilities.

The aging and increasing diversity of the U.S. population and the projected growth of the oldest-old age group will have a major effect on the demand and supply of health services and on the level and type of resources needed to provide those services. These trends are likely to increase inpatient hospital admissions as well as admissions to nursing homes. When combined with the rising severity of illness of patients in both hospitals and nursing homes, these patterns can be expected to exacerbate the long-standing problems in these institutions involving staffing issues, including the paucity of appropriately educated and trained professional nursing personnel.

The implications of these changes in the health care environment for the nursing workforce are profound in terms of numbers, adequate distribution of skills, and educational preparation. Nursing personnel are an integral component of the health care delivery system; therefore, they are affected directly by these changes. It is not surprising that concerns about the fate of patients and health care givers have grown as reported in the media. Within the nursing profession and its supporting organizations there is a high level of uncertainty and concern about what is happening to nursing staff in terms of their physical, psychological, and economic well-being. Individual care givers, professional and trade associations involved in nursing, and unions have expressed concerns that these changes

---

[2]In two states, California and Texas, these nurses are called licensed vocational nurses. In all other jurisdictions they are known as licensed practical nurses. In this report, licensed practical and vocational nurses are referred to as licensed practical nurses.

[3]Ancillary nursing personnel, nursing support personnel, assistive personnel, nurse extenders, unlicensed nursing personnel, multicompetent workers, nurse assistants, or aides are all generic terms used to refer to the various clinical and nonclinical jobs that augment nursing care. This group of employees includes an array of support nursing personnel including certified nurse assistants, orderlies, operating room technicians, home health aides, and others. They assist the licensed nurse by performing routine duties in caring for patients under the supervision of an RN or an LPN. Although Congress defined "nurse" for the purposes of this study to include RN, LPN, and NA, it has not been possible at all times to disaggregate information on NAs from the remaining support personnel because national statistics are often collected and/or tabulated for the group as a whole. For example, the American Hospital Association does not separate information on nurse assistants from that on other "ancillary nursing personnel." Throughout this report, the term ancillary nursing personnel will be used for this group of staff when nurse assistants cannot be disaggregated.

are endangering the quality of patient care and causing nursing personnel to suffer increased rates of injury, illness, and stress.

In response to these expressed concerns, Congress directed the Secretary of the Department of Health and Human Services (DHHS) to ask the Institute of Medicine (IOM) to undertake a study to determine whether and to what extent there is need for an increase in the number of nurses in hospitals and nursing homes in order to promote the quality of patient care and reduce the incidence among nurses of work-related injuries and stress. For the purposes of this study, Congress defined "nurse" to include RNs, LPNs, and NAs.

To carry out this legislative mandate, in March 1994 the Division of Nursing of the Health Resources and Services Administration requested that the IOM appoint a committee of experts to undertake an independent objective study as stipulated by Congress. In response the study committee explored:

- levels of quality of care in hospitals and nursing homes today;
- the relationship of quality of care (or quality of nursing care, to be more precise) and patient outcomes to nurse staffing levels and mix of different types of nursing personnel;
- the current supply and demand for nurses, including both American- and foreign-trained nurses, and the current and expected levels of workforce participation in that professional group;
- existing ratios of nursing personnel to other measures of demand for health care, such as numbers of patients (in hospitals) or residents (in nursing homes) or numbers of beds, and how those ratios might vary by type of facility, geographic location, or other factors;
- the incidence and prevalence of work-related stress and injuries among nurses in these settings; whether the epidemiology of these problems had been changing in recent years; and whether they differ by type of nursing personnel; undergraduate, graduate, and in-service education and training of different types of nurses; and
- the current and projected patient population of the nation, taking into account the aging of the U.S. population (and the aging of the elderly population itself) and the changing racial and ethnic composition of the population, and the implications of these demographic shifts for the types of health care providers— especially nurses of various kinds—that will be needed in future years.

This report responds to that request. To address its charge in a systematic manner, the committee conducted a complex set of activities. It reviewed and analyzed an extensive body of research and relevant literature, both published and currently under way, and other relevant reports; analyzed published and unpublished data from various sources; heard from a large number of experts; held public hearings and obtained a great deal of written testimony; appointed and convened a liaison panel; conducted several site visits; met with representatives of professional groups, consumer advocacy groups, and trade organizations and others; and commissioned several background papers from experts.

In responding to its charge, the committee decided that although interest in and concern among constituent groups about staffing conditions in hospitals and nursing homes today are intense, the future outlook for the nursing services in the health care system is equally critical for planning and policy formulation. Hence it has attempted to take a long-term view, looking ahead at nurse staffing in the context of a rapidly evolving health care system and an increasingly aging population that will dominate the practice of health care givers at all levels and disciplines as the nation moves into the twenty-first century.

The committee's major findings and conclusions based on this review and its deliberations are summarized below, followed by the text of the recommendations.

FINDINGS AND CONCLUSIONS

Nursing Personnel in a Time of Change

To determine the adequacy of nursing personnel in hospitals and nursing homes, the committee first assessed the overall supply of nursing personnel in the context of the shifting demand for their services and the factors affecting that demand.

More than 3 million health care personnel work in nursing services. Hospitals are the major employers of nursing personnel. RNs are the largest group of health care givers in this country. Their supply in terms of numbers is at an all-time high. In 1992, more than 2.2 million persons held licenses to practice as RNs, and 1.8 million of them were employed in nursing positions. The hospital is the first place of employment for most RNs, where historically two-thirds of them work, and the number of RNs employed by hospitals has continued to grow. This is not the case for LPNs, whose numbers in hospitals have been declining for some time. Many LPNs and NAs also work in nursing homes.

Although the focus of health care is shifting away from nursing at the hospital bedside to nursing at the patient's side in a continuum of care, in absolute terms the largest numbers of nursing personnel are still working in hospital inpatient settings. At the same time, with the emergence of rehabilitative services in nursing homes and the increasingly complex case-mix in these facilities, the need for professional nursing in nursing homes is much greater now than in previous years; and in the years ahead, it will be even greater. Recent data suggest that there might be a small increase of these personnel in nursing homes. Nursing homes accounted for about 7 percent of the RN workforce in 1992, up from 6.6 percent in 1988. The committee concludes that as long as long-term care is almost totally dependent on public and out-of-pocket financing, the current paucity of professional nurses employed in nursing homes will likely continue because of fiscal reasons and because of the pay differential between RNs in hospitals and those in nursing homes.

Continuation of current trends toward reduced inpatient hospitalization rates combined with increased acuity of hospitalized patients and the corresponding shift of employment to ambulatory and community care settings could have important implications for the employment of RNs in inpatient hospital settings and for their education and training. In the future, they may be called upon increasingly to fill roles that require increased professional judgment, management of complex systems that span the traditional boundaries of service settings, and greater clinical autonomy.

Likewise, not all nursing homes today are single-focus settings taking care of chronically ill patients who require mostly custodial care. They increasingly are becoming the "hospital" substitute for much of the subacute care that previously was part of a hospital stay. Because of the reduced length of inpatient hospital stays nursing homes are attempting to provide transitional institutional services that in the past would have been provided in the acute care inpatient setting.

All these factors raise important questions about the adequacy of the RN supply in terms of the educational preparation of future RNs. In addressing this issue, several researchers conclude that the aggregate numbers are adequate to meet national needs, at least for the near future, but that the education mix may not be adequate to meet either current or future demands of a rapidly changing health care system. The need to evaluate workforce adequacy for the future in terms both of numbers and of knowledge and skills is clear.

Staffing and Quality of Care in Hospitals

Nursing services are central to the provision of hospital care. Nursing care in hospitals takes on added importance today because the increase in acuity of patients requires intensive nursing care. At the same time, a rapidly changing health care environment, continuing pressures to contain costs, and the rising levels of severity of illness and comorbidity of inpatients all make it imperative for hospitals to explore innovative ways to redesign delivery of care without compromising quality.

Restructuring in the Hospitals

Redesign and reengineering have become principal strategies of the 1990s for many institutions and systems, and increasing numbers of hospitals are restructuring their organization, staffing, and services. Although redesign initiatives are undertaken for a variety of reasons, more than half of the hospital-based efforts are driven by the need to reduce operating costs and have focused on transforming work processes and rethinking roles and jobs. Staff reductions or changes in labor mix are at times implemented without attention to the organizational changes that might facilitate the possibility of better patient outcomes with fewer, more appropriately trained and used staff. Concurrent with the efforts to restructure hospital services has been the development of total quality management and what is referred to as patient-centered care. These innovative approaches to patient care may also involve case management, the development of critical pathways for managing patients most efficiently during a hospital stay, and other steps that, collectively, lead to restructuring in the hospital. Because of the resource intensity of hospital nursing services, restructuring, work redesign, and cost reduction efforts have a direct impact on the nursing workforce.

Changing Roles and Responsibilities of Nursing Personnel

The challenge today is for care givers and patients to think about the continuum of care needed rather than simply the event of hospitalization. Foremost among these changes is to help RNs and other health care givers to learn how to plan for patient care before the patient is admitted to the hospital, as well as for care needed after discharge from the hospital. It is this challenge, along with the demands for increased efficiency within a standard of good quality of care that, in part, has led many hospitals to implement the concept of patient-centered care teams. As managed care expands, expedient decision making and good judgment will be increasingly more important for all health care providers, and the use of interdisciplinary approaches also will become increasingly the norm in the hospital sector.

This system of organizing care relies on the case manager[4] to integrate in-depth clinical knowledge, community resources, and financial and organizational requirements with patient needs and with institutional goals of providing high quality, cost-effective care. In acute care settings this role is most often performed by a RN, frequently one who has been prepared with education beyond the basic program of nursing education.

Leading and managing the organizational transformations described above require talents or training that not all RNs now have. For the evolving hospital, the committee believes that it will be imperative for these management, leadership, and supervisory skills to be fostered through various educational programs. The committee believes that more advanced, or more broadly trained, RNs will

---

[4]"Case management" includes comprehensive oversight of a patient's entire episode of illness incorporating interdisciplinary resource utilization in order to provide high quality, cost-effective care. The clinical and financial management of care is coordinated by "case managers" who often span the boundaries of inpatient, ambulatory and community settings (Satinsky, 1995). Some people prefer to use the term "care manager" in lieu of case manager. Care management suggests the provision of direct care and, in some instances a case manager may also be a care manager. For example, registered nurses who coordinate care for groups of hospitalized patients with the same diagnosis may also assume responsibility for giving some of these patients direct care.

be needed in the future. Such training is essentially like that now provided for RNs who receive certification as, for example, advanced practice nurses.

Over the past 20 to 25 years, a number of studies have attempted to capture adequately the benefits of the clinical nurse specialist for the patients as well as for economic reasons. In particular, the evidence from several randomized clinical trials indicates that: clinical nurse specialists can foster high quality, cost-effective care especially for patients with complicated or serious clinical conditions care, and improve the cost-effectiveness of health care systems and facilities because changing the mix of personnel involved in caring for patients with complex management problems may yield better outcomes, lower costs, or both.

The committee concluded that the way should be clearer for such advanced practice nurses to be used in both inpatient and outpatient settings and for them to be able to take leadership positions and act independently. One obstacle to this, however, is found in the differing ways in which states recognize advanced practice nurses. Some state boards of nursing have not yet recognized the expanded responsibilities that such personnel can and should discharge. To address this problem, the committee believes that all states should recognize nurses in advanced practice in their nurse practice acts and delineate the qualifications and scope of practice of these nurses.

Today, almost all hospitals in the United States use some kind of ancillary nursing personnel. In recent years the position of the nurse assistant (NA) has been changing. In some institutions they are assuming, under an RN's direction, increasing responsibility for more direct care activities than in the past. This results in rising levels of management and supervisory skills being required of RNs.

By definition, NAs have less formal education and training than RNs or LPNs. Far less information about employment trends is available on this group of the nursing workforce than on the more traditional nursing categories. No national standards exist for minimum training or certification of ancillary nursing personnel employed by hospitals. Furthermore, no accepted mechanism exists either to measure competency or to certify in some fashion that ancillary nursing personnel have attained at least a basic or rudimentary mastery of needed skills. The committee is greatly concerned about these lacks and the potential for adverse impact on patient care. It believes that hospitals should take the lead in ensuring that all ancillary nursing personnel employed by them have documented evidence of competency and appropriate training.

Culturally sensitive care will also become increasingly important in the years ahead. The population is not only aging but also is becoming more racially and ethnically diverse. Thus, increasingly, care givers and care receivers may come from different cultural backgrounds. The imperative for cultural sensitivity in training and practice is obvious.

The changes briefly described above are appealing conceptually, and time will tell if they are effective and practical as the hospital sector reinvents itself. In the short term, however, these shifts in the way hospitals do business and the way they organize themselves to conduct that business, are causing notable disruptions and misgivings among the nursing staff. From the frequency and intensity of the commentaries that the committee heard during this study, RNs are concerned about the employment ramifications and, more importantly, the professional implications of the organizational changes that are occurring; they believe that these changes may lead to undesirable and unanticipated effects on quality of care. In the committee's view, the harmful and demoralizing effects of these changes on the nursing staff can be mitigated, if not forestalled altogether, with more recognition on the part of the hospital industry that involvement of nursing personnel from the outset in the redesign efforts is critical.

Rapid changes in the health care delivery system and the resultant unstable situation fuel the concern among the nursing community that large decreases in RN staffing in hospitals are both occurring and leading to decrements in patient care and to threats to the health and well-being of nursing personnel. The committee finds that lack of reliable and valid data on the magnitude and distribution of temporary or permanent unemployment, reassignments of existing nursing staff, and similar changes in the structure of nursing employment opportunities greatly hampers efforts at understanding the problem and planning for the future.

Furthermore, answers to such questions are needed for all levels of nursing personnel. Therefore, hospitals should not concentrate their monitoring and evaluation solely on the relationships between RN staffing and quality of care or on work-related illness and injury. Rather, hospitals should focus their efforts in monitoring and evaluating the redesign of staffing on the entire spectrum of their nursing personnel. The committee also supports productive collaboration between federal agencies and private organizations to develop databases containing information that will shed light on workforce issues and on the relationships of staffing, care processes, and patient outcomes.

Measuring Quality of Care in Hospitals

The committee first looked at quality in terms of the overall quality of care received by the patient in the hospital and examined the relationship between structural variables and both processes and outcomes of care. Recent years have seen important advances in measuring quality of patient care at the individual patient and population levels, involving both process and outcome measures. Existing work, however, has not typically focused on isolating the contribution of nursing care to overall hospital quality.

Ensuring the quality of patient care is central to the mission of health care services in hospitals. During the study, the committee heard considerable concern expressed by RNs that increasing numbers of hospitals are restructuring and re-engineering, resulting in smaller proportions of RNs to total nursing personnel and in a probable negative impact on quality of patient care in those hospitals.

This committee investigated the question of whether the quality of care in hospitals has deteriorated and whether empirical evidence exists of a link between the number and skill mix of nursing personnel and the quality of care.

The committee found that little empirical evidence is available to support the anecdotal and other informal information that hospital quality of care is being adversely affected by hospital restructuring and changes in the staffing patterns of nursing personnel. At the same time, it noted a lack of systematic and ongoing monitoring and evaluating of the effects of organizational redesign and reconfiguration of staffing on patient outcomes. Unfortunately, few recent and objective national data are available that either describe the quality of care in hospitals or that show whether quality has been affected in any way by changes in the system of delivery of care. Indeed, the committee was shocked by the lack of current data relating to the status of hospital quality of care on a national basis, apart from information on indicators such as hospital-specific mortality rates. Because of this lack, the committee is unable to draw any definitive conclusions or inferences about the levels of quality of care across the nation's hospitals today.

The committee does conclude, however, on the basis of the few available studies, that the quality of hospital care in general has not suffered, and may even have improved in some areas, after implementation of the Medicare prospective payment system (PPS). Although quality of hospital care did not suffer after PPS implementation, more patients were discharged too soon and in unstable condition and patients discharged in unstable condition had significantly higher mortality rates. This research suggests that there may be problem areas with the quality of hospital care, but that the extent of these problems today is not known because of the lack of objective current data.

The committee is convinced that investigation of hospital quality of care warrants increasing and immediate attention. Research needs to move beyond hospital mortality as an outcome measure and to focus as well on process-of-care problems that occur during short hospital stays and on outcomes over an episode of care.

Relationship of Nursing Staff to Quality of Care

One of the research challenges in determining the relationship between staffing and quality of care has been the difficulty of isolating the factors (and the relative importance of these factors) that are involved in producing improved patient outcomes. Literature about the effect of RNs on mortality and about variables that affect the retention of RNs is available; differences in mortality rates across hospitals are well documented by several researchers and the literature on RNs' impact on hospital mortality rates is considerable. There is, however, a serious paucity of recent research on the definitive effects of structural measures, such as specific staffing ratios, on the quality of patient care in terms of outcomes when controlling for all other likely explanatory or confounding variables.

Part of the problem lies in the area of severity of illness and risk adjustment, where patient acuity is a significant factor. Across-the-board staffing ratios tend to assume that in some measure all patients are "alike" and can be cared for with the same level and type of resources. Equally difficult is the task of establishing ratios that will be appropriate for all settings and situations. Staffing levels need to be specific to different types of acute care units and facilities.

RN-rich staffing ratios are sometimes associated with improved patient outcomes, such as lower mortality rates among Medicare patients. Such staffing ratios are essentially proxy measures for other organizational attributes of hospitals that grant nurses autonomy over their own practice and control of the resources necessary to deliver patient care and create good relationships with physicians. That is, when nurses have more autonomy, status, and control, their behaviors on behalf of patients result in better outcomes. Despite this type of information on organizational and related factors, the committee was unable to isolate a number-of-RNs effect.

The committee concludes, therefore, that high priority should be given to obtaining empirical evidence that permits one to draw conclusions about the relationships of quality of inpatient care and staffing levels and mix. Such data should focus on nursing care and quality of care across institutions and within given institutions, and across departments and services. The committee is convinced that more rigorous research on the relationship between nursing variables, broadly defined, and quality of care would have significant payoffs for policymakers, nursing educators, hospital administrators.

The committee also is concerned about the paucity of objective research on the relationships among restructuring, staffing, and quality. The committee concludes that a clear need exists for some system of monitoring and evaluating the impact of the rapidly changing delivery system on the quality of patient care and the well-being of nursing staff. For this reason, it has advanced several recommendations intended to provide better information on hospital restructuring and to help in delineating those factors that affect patient outcomes. It also calls for the development of a research agenda in this area and for the articulation of reliable, valid, and practical measures of structure, process, and outcome to be used in quality-of-care research as well as quality assurance and improvement programs. A systematic effort is needed at the national level to collect data and develop a research and evaluation agenda so that informed policy development, implementation, and evaluation are undertaken in a timely manner.

A major part of any such research agenda might call for elaboration of the actual variables—in terms of structure, process, and outcome—that warrant high priority attention in studies of the relationship of nursing care, staffing patterns for nursing, to patient outcomes. The American Nurses Association (ANA), for example, has been developing quality indicators that warrant further investigation. The committee commends the ANA for its exploratory efforts to develop a set of nursing care quality indicators. This research can set an important precedent and standard for the development of meaningful quality standards relating to nursing. This research offers promise for further evolution of external regulatory quality assurance mechanisms (e.g., those of the Joint Commission on Accreditation of Healthcare Organizations [JCAHO]) and for improved public information efforts. Nevertheless, the committee judged that in the future, a broader set of inputs from the nursing community and other affected parties would be desirable. It also believed that efforts based solely in the private sector, with little or no public sector involvement, might be less useful than if federal and state perspectives were taken into account.

The committee supports the current federal requirements and accreditation standards for nursing services in hospitals and emphasizes the need for hospitals to maintain the highest possible standards for nursing care. Moreover, the committee agrees that hospitals should develop improved methods for matching patient needs (severity-of-illness or acuity measures) with the level and type of nurse staffing. The committee endorses efforts to improve systems for planning appropriate nursing care as well as monitoring the outcomes of that care.

Regulation of hospitals is a long-standing part of government responsibility and can take many forms, including certification, licensure, and accreditation. Under the Social Security Act, one pathway to hospital certification is through accreditation by the JCAHO; this is the route to certification used by most hospitals. Hospitals found to have met the JCAHO accreditation standards are deemed automatically to have met the federal Conditions of Participation for the Medicare program and are in effect considered certified to receive Medicare (and Medicaid) reimbursement. Among the key requirements of JCAHO certification are that: nursing care be provided on a 24-hour-a-day, 7-day-a-week basis; nursing services show evidence that each patient's status is monitored and that nursing care is coordinated with the care provided by other professionals; and specific patient care plans be in place and in use for each patient.

Given the continued reliance of the federal government on JCAHO accreditation for hospital reimbursement by federal health programs, the committee was encouraged by the evolution of JCAHO's methods and standards in the past few years and by the more sophisticated attention being paid to the role of nursing care within those standards. The committee endorses the current federal requirements for hospitals to participate in Medicare, which incorporate the use of voluntary accreditation, to assure the quality of hospital care, and it is particularly supportive of requirements that call for matching nursing resources with patient needs. The committee believes that Congress ought to continue to support this element of assuring the quality of care in hospitals.

Some broader issues of changes in nursing services, such as the enhanced responsibilities of advanced practice nurses and the use of ancillary nursing personnel and their competency, cut across the straightforward issue of the relationship between nurse staffing and quality of hospital care. In reflecting on the role of nursing personnel in the future, therefore, the committee has also proposed recommendations about these specific types of nursing personnel.

Staffing and Quality of Care in Nursing Homes

The nursing home market is being stressed by an increasing demand for services combined with a constrained growth rate. To gain insights on issues surrounding the relationship of staffing patterns of nursing personnel to quality of resident care, the committee examined statutory requirements and information gathered during site visits and public testimony; it also reviewed an extensive body of research literature and empirical evidence on the relationships between staffing patterns and quality.

Status of Quality of Care in Nursing Homes

Quality of care in nursing homes is a complex concept, and defining it has been a difficult process. Some facilities provide high quality of care even in the face of fiscal constraint, but the quality of care provided in nursing facilities has for years been a matter of great concern to consumers, health care professionals, and policymakers. Since enactment of the Omnibus Budget Reconciliation Act of 1987 (OBRA 87), some improvement has been reported as a result of increased efforts by the federal government to regulate the quality of nursing homes. Many facilities have increasingly focused on reducing negative outcomes and improving the process of care; in many others, however, quality-of-care problems continue to be reported. Several studies have identified negative outcomes in nursing facilities.

Relationships Among Nursing Staff, Management, and Quality of Care

The committee sought to determine if staffing as a measure of quality of care in nursing homes has improved since the implementation of OBRA 87. A slight but noticeable increase in staffing was evident, attributable partly to the requirements of the 1987 legislation and partly to the staffing needs created by the increased complexity of care required for subacute and other special care residents. The committee strongly endorses the intent of OBRA 87 and supports efforts by facilities and states to improve professional nurse staffing in nursing homes consistent with the intent of the statute.

Many factors, both internal and external, influence staff performance and the quality of care provided to residents. Internal factors include staffing and staff characteristics such as education and training levels, patient characteristics such as acuity levels, job satisfaction and turnover of staff, salaries and benefits, and management and organizational climate. External factors include regulations, reimbursement policies, incentives, excess demand for services, and type and ownership of facility. The committee examined all of these factors through review of the research literature, information from administrative databases, information gathered during site visits and from testimony, review of regulatory requirements, and other relevant reports and reached several conclusions.

During site visits the committee heard complaints from some nursing home staff about the paperwork involved in completing the Minimum Data Set (MDS), which is a crucial part of resident assessment procedures. Although the committee is sympathetic about the time-consuming nature of the forms, it strongly endorses the concept of an individualized care plan for each resident, which requires the use of tools such as the MDS. The committee also endorses current efforts by the Health Care Financing Administration (HCFA) to improve the MDS and to require all facilities to computerize MDS data and provide them to state and federal agencies, thus providing a mechanism for a national database.

The research literature generally agrees on the strong relationship among resident characteristics, nurse staffing time requirements, and nursing costs in nursing homes. It shows that facilities need to adjust their staffing levels to take into account the condition of the residents so that they can ensure sufficient staff to provide for residents' basic needs. The preponderance of evidence, from a number of studies using different types of quality measures, shows a positive relationship between nursing staff levels and quality of nursing home care, which in turn indicates a strong need to increase the overall level of nursing staff in nursing homes.

The research literature does not, however, answer questions about what particular ratio of staff to residents is optimal. Varying circumstances among nursing homes, case-mix differentials, and other external factors affect the type and level of staff needed. The committee thus endorses the HCFA staffing standards but is not inclined to recommend a specific minimum staffing ratio across all types of facilities to meet the needs of all types of patients. The committee affirms that nursing facilities should ensure adequate nursing services to meet the acuity needs of their residents.

The committee recognizes the differences in nurse staffing and quality of patient care in nursing homes, on the one hand, and in hospitals, on the other. Hospitals and nursing homes may operate on very different segments of a staffing–quality relationship curve. Hospitals could be operating in the segment of the curve where returns from increases in staffing are low because they already have relatively high staffing levels; by contrast, nursing homes are operating at the low end of the staffing scale where positive returns from increases in staffing are observable.

Extensive research literature exists on the effect on quality of care of the presence of professional nursing (RNs) to provide hands-on training and guidance to NAs. Given the level of NAs' direct care responsibilities and the minimal training for resident care required of them, professional nurse oversight and availability for close supervision of NAs and LPNs is critical—more so today than in previous years because of the changing characteristics of the residents. Based on the empirical evidence amassed, the committee concludes that a strong relationship between RN-to-resident staffing in nursing facilities and various dimensions of quality, especially resident outcomes, has been established. The committee, therefore, underscores the need to increase the presence of professional nurses in nursing homes on all shifts. Given the findings on the beneficial effects of continuous RN presence on various dimensions of quality, especially resident outcomes, the committee recommends an RN presence on all shifts in nursing homes as an enhancement of the currently required 8-hour RN presence.

The committee of course recognizes that issues of staffing enhancement in nursing facilities cannot be viewed separately from costs. Ultimately, the committee was of the opinion that the public interest and the need for acceptable quality of care must be considered in addition to cost if we as a society are going to maintain a sense of values and responsibility for the care of the elderly, disabled, and disadvantaged. The committee, however, is reluctant to impose uncompensated costs on nursing facilities, and it concludes, therefore, that Medicaid and Medicare payment levels need to be adjusted accordingly. The committee further believes that waivers to this requirement could be granted by states only under exceptional circumstances. All but one of the committee members were in agreement with these positions.

Based on its review of a number of studies, the committee concludes that there is sufficient evidence to show that the presence of geriatric nurse specialists and practitioners enhances quality of care in nursing homes. Moreover, research has shown that cost savings in the long run accrue, particularly due to reduced rehospitalizations and visits to emergency rooms.

Nurse assistants constitute 70 to 90 percent of the nursing staff in nursing facilities. They provide most of the direct care and spend the most time with residents, but as stated earlier, they are the least trained. On the basis of experience and information gathered from the testimonies received, the committee came to the view that the organization, use, and education of NA staff make a substantial difference in the humane care, comfort, and health of nursing home residents and in the job satisfaction and health of the staff. The committee concludes that the training received by NAs should be enriched and that research is needed on the relationship of NA and LPN staff levels and training to quality of care.

The changing focus of services and the increasingly complex nature of the care provided in nursing facilities create new demands for skill, judgment, supervision, and the management of nursing services, Most directors of nursing (DON) in nursing facilities are not academically prepared for their positions. Furthermore, turnover among DONs is high, their salaries are low in comparison with hospitals, and they have limited opportunities for advancement. None of these factors is conducive to strong leadership. In view of the number of employees, budgets, and complexity of care in nursing facilities today, strong leadership from DONs is required if high quality, cost-effective care is to be provided. The committee concludes that nursing facilities should place greater weight on educational preparation when employing new DONs.

In the area of reimbursement policies, the committee notes the existence of several experiments designed to look at outcome-based incentives for improved quality of care. The committee concludes that additional research and demonstration projects on the use of financial and other incentives are needed to improve the quality of care and outcomes in nursing homes.

Staffing and Work-Related Injuries and Stress

Nursing is a hazardous occupation. Whereas the injury and illness rate in private industry as a whole has been stable or declining slightly since 1980, the rates for hospitals and nursing homes during the same period have increased by about 52 percent and 62 percent, respectively. Recent statistics and other information suggest that these institutions are becoming increasingly hazardous places to work, exposing workers to a wide range of risks.

The committee reviewed the literature on work-related injuries, in particular back injuries and needlestick puncture wounds, that affect nursing personnel in hospitals and nursing homes. It also reviewed available research to assess the factors that contribute to work-related stress. The committee was struck by the high rate of injuries to nursing personnel in both hospitals and nursing homes, but except for back injuries the committee is unable to substantiate conclusively any linkages among staffing numbers, skill mix, and work-related problems. The committee is impressed, however, with the apparent effects of leadership from management, good employee training, and existing technologies on reducing the probabilities of injuries among nursing personnel.

The committee concludes that considerable levels of injuries and risk of injury may exist at the level of NAs and other ancillary personnel, especially in long-term-care facilities, who may be subject to great stress and probability of injury (especially back injury) and who may be newly employed and comparatively thinly trained. The committee thus found an important need, especially among new employees, for more aggressive training related to the use of lifting devices, lifting teams, and ergonomic training in lifting techniques to prevent back injuries. The committee concludes that all personnel giving direct care (especially in nursing homes) should receive annual training in lifting and transferring patients. Such efforts would improve the quality of life for health care workers and could represent a significant savings to the health care industry. The committee also concludes that hospitals and nursing homes should develop effective programs to reduce work-related injuries.

Violence toward health care workers appears to be on the rise. Increased violence in the general population, greater use of mind-altering drugs and alcohol abuse, and easier availability of weapons may all contribute to the problem of violence in health care settings. In examining available information on violence and abuse, the committee realized the intricate problems of work situations and of violence and abuse directed at patients, especially residents in nursing homes. Clearly many NAs are not abusive. A certain proportion, however, do verbally or physically abuse, steal from, or otherwise take advantage of nursing home residents. Unfortunately, even a small proportion of abusive staff can affect the health, quality of care, and peace of mind of thousands of nursing home residents. In the committee's view, therefore, nursing facilities should be required to ensure a safe and protective environment for residents by employing personnel who protect and care for residents and do not abuse and steal from them.

The committee believes that much of the incidence of violence in hospitals and nursing homes are preventable and that prevention is a shared responsibility among employers and employees. The committee concludes, therefore, that health care institutions should implement a variety of strategies to prevent assaults against workers and residents and that they should screen applicants for patient care positions for past histories of abuse. Abuse prevention measures should ultimately apply to all who work in nursing homes and, for that matter, in all health care institutions.

RECOMMENDATIONS

On the basis of its findings and conclusions the committee has provided three categories of recommendations: (1) the level and staffing patterns of nursing personnel to promote quality of care in hospitals; (2) the level and skill mix of nursing personnel in nursing homes to promote quality of care in these facilities; and (3) strategies to reduce work-related injuries and stress. The text of the panel's recommendations, grouped according to these categories, follows, keyed to the chapter in which they appear in the body of the report The sequence in which the recommendations are presented does not reflect a priority order.

RECOMMENDATIONS ON STAFFING AND QUALITY IN HOSPITALS

Recommendation 5-1: The committee recommends that hospitals expand the use of registered nurses with advance practice preparation and skills to provide clinical leadership and cost-effective patient care, particularly for patients with complex management problems.

Recommendation 5-2: The committee recommends that hospitals have documented evidence that ancillary nursing personnel are competent and that such personnel are tested and certified by an appropriate entity for this competence. The committee further recommends that the training for ancillary nursing personnel working in hospitals be structured and enriched by including training of the following types: appropriate clinical care of the aged and disabled; occupational health and safety measures; culturally sensitive care; and appropriate management of conflict.

Recommendation 5-3: The committee recommends that hospital leaders involve nursing personnel (RNs, LPNs, and NAs) who are directly affected by organizational redesign and staffing reconfiguration in the process of planning and implementing such changes.

Recommendation 5-4: The committee recommends that hospital management monitor and evaluate the effects of changes in organizational redesign and reconfiguration of nursing personnel on patient outcomes, on patient satisfaction, and on nursing personnel themselves.

Recommendation 5-5: The committee recommends that the National Institute of Nursing Research (NINR) and other appropriate agencies fund scientifically sound research on the relationships between quality of care and nurse staffing levels and mix, taking into account organizational variables. The committee further recommends that NINR, along with the Agency for Health Care Policy and Research (AHCPR) and private organizations, develop a research agenda on quality of care.

Recommendation 5-6: The committee recommends that an interdisciplinary public–private partnership be organized to develop performance and outcome measures that are sensitive to nursing interventions and care, with uniform definitions that are measurable in a uniform manner across all hospitals.

RECOMMENDATIONS ON STAFFING AND QUALITY IN NURSING HOMES

Recommendation 6-1: The committee recommends that Congress require by the year 2000 a 24-hour presence of registered nurse coverage in nursing facilities as an enhancement of the current 8-hour requirement specified under OBRA 87. It further recommends that payment levels for Medicare and Medicaid be adjusted to enable such staffing to be achieved.

Recommendation 6-2: The committee recommends that nursing facilities use geriatric nurse specialists and geriatric nurse practitioners in both leadership and direct care positions.

Recommendation 6-3: The committee recommends that the training for nurse assistants in nursing homes be structured and enriched by including training of the following types: appropriate clinical care of the aged and disabled; occupational health and safety measures; culturally sensitive care; and appropriate management of conflict.

Recommendation 6-4: The committee recommends that research efforts on staffing levels and skill mix specifically address the relationship of licensed practical nurses and nurse assistants to quality of care.

Recommendation 6-5: The committee recommends that, in view of the increasing case-mix acuity of residents and the consequent complexity of the care provided, nursing facilities place greater weight on educational preparation in the employment of new directors of nursing.

Recommendation 6-6: The committee recommends that the Secretary of Health and Human Services fund additional research and demonstration projects on the use of financial and other incentives to improve quality of care and outcomes in nursing homes.

RECOMMENDATIONS ON WORK-RELATED INJURY AND STRESS

Recommendation 7-1: The committee recommends that hospitals and nursing homes develop effective programs to reduce work-related injuries by providing strong leadership, instituting effective training programs for new and continuing workers, and ensuring appropriate use of existing and emerging technology, including lifting and moving devices and needleless medication delivery systems.

Recommendation 7-2: The committee recommends that all hospitals and nursing homes screen applicants for patient care positions filled by nurse assistants for past history of abuse of patients and residents, and criminal records.

1

Introduction

Rapid and unpredictable change throughout society is the hallmark of the twentieth century. Change has become a constant in today's environment in every employment sector, from small businesses to large corporations, from government agencies to non-governmental organizations. The health care sector is no exception, and notable advances are occurring in molecular biology, biomedical technology, data and information systems, and health care delivery.

The U.S. health care system has undergone major restructuring since the early 1980s as a result of scientific and technological breakthroughs, market forces, cost containment efforts, and radically different payment policies for Medicare patients. These forces, combined with the growth of managed care in more recent years, have had a major impact on the organization, financing, and delivery of health care and on the clinicians, technicians, and facilities (both acute care and long-term care) that deliver care.

Steady pressures for cost containment combined with competition, and the rapid escalation of restructuring and mergers, consolidations, and closures of hospitals, have led to work redesign, reconfiguration of staffing patterns, and downsizing. Market competition in an environment of economic constraints has led to a rapid growth of outpatient services and departments, home- and community-based services, and subacute care units. At the same time, inpatient use of hospitals, lengths of hospital stay, numbers of inpatient admissions, and the number of beds staffed have all declined. As a consequence, patients in hospitals have a higher level of acuity (i.e., are on average far sicker) and are in need of more professional, highly skilled nursing care than in earlier years. Professional nurses not only have sicker patients but the boundaries between medicine and nursing have shifted with the advance of science and technology, leaving them with an ever increasing work jurisdiction. The changes in the hospital sector combined with economic and other forces are changing the characteristics of persons entering nursing homes and are placing new demands for beds and for provision of nursing care on these facilities.

The U.S. population is aging. The growing population of the elderly, especially the older elderly, will increase admissions to inpatient hospitals and nursing homes. This situation, combined with the rising acuity of patients in both hospitals and nursing homes, will exacerbate the long-standing problems of staffing, including the paucity of appropriately educated and trained professional nursing personnel.

The emphasis on economic efficiency encourages a balance of costs and benefits. In securing these benefits, however, analysts and decisionmakers should not lose sight of the ultimate goal—the sensitive and compassionate care of patients. Hospitals are responding to the changing health care system by taking several measures, including modifying their staffing levels and their mix of nursing personnel. Individual care givers, professional and trade associations involved with nursing, and unions have expressed concerns that these changes are endangering the quality of patient care and causing nursing staff to suffer increased rates of injury, illness, and stress.

IMMEDIATE ORIGINS OF
THE INSTITUTE OF MEDICINE STUDY

In February 1993 the Subcommittee on Health and the Environment of the House Energy and Commerce Committee held a hearing on the conditions of nursing and nursing care in the United States. A member of the Service Employees International Union (SEIU) described the adverse effects of poor or inadequate staffing on patients and nursing staff.[1] The subcommittee felt that it needed independent assessment of the stated problems. Thus, as part of the National Institutes of Health Revitalization Act of 1993 (P.L. 103-43, Subtitle B, section 1512), Congress directed the Secretary of the Department of Health and Human Services (DHHS) to sponsor a study *to determine whether and to what extent there is need for an increase in the number of nurses in hospitals and nursing homes to promote the quality of patient care and to reduce the incidence among nurses of work-related injuries and stress. For purposes of this study Congress defined "nurse" to include registered nurse (RN), licensed*

---

[1] In response to concerns among its members, in early 1992 SEIU mailed questionnaires to 47,000 registered nurse and licensed practical nurse members inquiring about their perception of the quality of patient care and the quality of work life for the nursing staff. The report on this inquiry received much publicity (SEIU, 1993).

practical nurse or licensed vocational nurse[2] *(LPN), and nurse assistant (NA).* It further directed the Secretary to ask the Institute of Medicine (IOM) to conduct the study.

COMMITTEE CHARGE

To carry out this legislative mandate, in March 1994 the Division of Nursing, Health Resources and Services Administration requested that the IOM appoint a committee of experts to undertake an independent objective study as stipulated by Congress. In response the study committee explored:

- levels of quality of care in hospitals and nursing homes today;
- the relationship of quality of care (or quality of nursing care, to be more precise) and patient outcomes to nurse staffing levels and mix of different types of nursing personnel;
- the current supply and demand for nurses, including both American- and foreign-trained nurses, and the current and expected levels of workforce participation in that professional group;
- existing ratios of nursing personnel to other measures of demand for health care, such as numbers of patients (in hospitals) or residents (in nursing homes) or numbers of beds, and how those ratios might vary by type of facility, geographic location, or other factors;
- the incidence and prevalence of work-related stress and injuries among nurses in these settings; whether the epidemiology of these problems had been changing in recent years; and whether they differ by type of nursing personnel;
- undergraduate, graduate, and in-service education and training of different types of nurses; and
- the current and projected patient population of the nation, taking into account the aging of the U.S. population (and the aging of the elderly population itself) and the changing racial and ethnic composition of the population, and the implications of these demographic shifts for the types of health care providers— especially nurses of various kinds—that will be needed in future years.

The IOM appointed a committee consisting of 16 members representing a range of expertise related to the scope of the study.

---

[2]In two states, California and Texas, these nurses are called licensed vocational nurses. In all other jurisdictions they are known as licensed practical nurses. In this report, licensed practical and vocational nurses will be referred to as licensed practical nurses.

DEFINITIONS

Before responding to Congress' charge to assess the needs for nursing personnel, the committee had to resolve issues of definition, approach, and scope of its inquiry. How is the committee to determine the need to increase staffing? What constitutes an adequate number or type of staff, how does one measure adequacy, and relative to which goals? In mandating this study, Congress specified two goals: (1) to promote the quality of patient care and (2) to reduce the incidence of work-related injuries and stress among nursing staff.

Congress defined nurse broadly. The committee's charge, therefore, is not limited to examining the adequacy of the number of RNs in this country's hospitals and nursing homes; rather, it includes all nursing personnel (RNs, LPNs, NAs).

To provide an operational context for the language of congressional charge, the committee had to develop working definitions of need and adequacy. These concepts are discussed briefly below.

Need

Hospitals

The committee, in defining need in hospitals, adopted the approach taken in a previous IOM study that assessed the needs, availability, and requirements for allied health personnel (IOM, 1989). The committee distinguished between the two different approaches implied by the term need. Need, as used in the context of health resource planning, refers to a normative idea of the number and type of personnel required to provide therapeutic and preventive services to a defined population, independently of ability and willingness to pay. Demand, by contrast, refers to the number and type of personnel that employers are willing to hire and that consumers are willing and able to pay. The demand concept recognizes that nursing services are not free and that, if all else remains the same, the quantity of nursing services demanded will increase (decrease) as the price for the service decreases (increases).

The committee has construed "need" in the congressional mandate to mean "effective demand" for nursing personnel in hospitals. This decision was based on the committee's judgment that this approach is the most useful and responsible guide for hospital-based resource planning.

Nursing Homes

In defining need for nursing home settings, again following the principles laid out in previous IOM reports on the subject (IOM, 1986b, 1989), the committee took a patient-oriented approach in examining nursing care staffing needs; it focused on characteristics of the residents' needs and the corresponding staffing required to provide adequate nursing care. The approach places greater emphasis on the nature of the nursing services required by nursing home populations. In other words, the issue is more about "what" and less about just "how much."

Nursing homes[3] differ from hospitals in several respects. First, the resident in a nursing home typically lacks the power usually ascribed to consumers (even more so than patients in hospitals who are there generally for a very short time), to some extent because of the relatively long-term nature of functional and cognitive impairments. Second, as distinct from hospitals, many residents live in nursing homes for many years. Third, because any private insurance coverage for long-term nursing home care is rare, Medicaid is the principal public payer. Thus, given Medicaid's major role as payer, the government's involvement to ensure that public monies are well spent has been considerable.

While identifying accurately the needed changes in the quality of staffing in a long-term care environment, one must recognize the cost in money, time, and resources required to achieve desired outcomes. These quality improvements mean providing the number, quality, and skills of the health care providers, and the organizing and delivering of services to enhance the quality of life for residents in nursing homes.

Adequacy

One written testimony submitted to IOM aptly described adequate staffing: "Adequacy is not just a number, it is a capability. It is critical that there be not only enough staff, but that they are properly trained and appropriately supervised in their assigned tasks, and they are motivated to care for the elderly and disabled people." That is to say, adequacy of nurse staffing means enough nursing services to provide high quality of care in hospital and nursing home settings and to ensure a safe environment for patients and staff. Further, adequacy to achieve the nursing tasks implies an understanding of the nature and scope of those tasks and a view of how those tasks can be accomplished.

In the case of nursing staff, the nature and scope of the tasks reflect the contribution of nursing to a patient's overall level of quality care. In this regard, the product is an outcome—quality of patient care—that results from a number of inputs. Nursing care is one, but only one, of the important inputs in the achievement of quality patient care.

Quality of care relates to a successful outcome to the illness episode, where success is defined in patient-oriented terms related to functioning, perceived health, and satisfaction. In the case of chronic disease and frailty, however, the episode of illness needs to be decomposed into subphases related to progression,

---

[3]Throughout the report, the terms "nursing home" and "nursing facility" are used interchangeably.

arrest, and palliation of disease. Outcome, therefore, for any particular patient is multidimensional, an array of attributes, and not just whether one recovers or not.

Thus, an assessment of the adequacy of nursing staff must be contextual. Increased nursing staff levels (or a richer skill mix in the nursing staff) may or may not result in an overall increase in quality of patient care, depending on what other inputs would produce in terms quality of patient care. Briefly, adequacy of nursing staff cannot be viewed independently of the availability of other resources with which nurses combine their skills and knowledge to produce quality patient care.

The committee believes that no single model, in all contexts and all circumstances, necessarily leads to an optimal outcome. Many different quantitative and qualitative staffing patterns for nursing care could lead to quality patient care. Thus, adequacy of nurse staffing should be considered not in terms of numbers or ratios alone. Needs for nursing services are affected by other variables such as severity of illness and organization of nursing care. Management and leadership, a culture of caring and compassion, a sense of staff teamwork, availability of facilities conducive to human care, experience, education, and support systems—all are necessary considerations in assessing whether a staffing pattern for nursing care is adequate to contribute to quality patient care. Focusing on nurse staffing inputs without consideration of the totality of circumstances and inputs can lead to a distorted view and appraisal of the conditions affecting patient care.

The committee had to consider another fundamental question: What level of quality is desired by those paying for the services? In health care particularly, quality is a multifaceted concept. The structure of the health care system is not necessarily monolithic; levels of resources committed to the purchase of health care by different private-employer purchasers and by public purchasers (Medicare and Medicaid) differ across states. One cannot determine the adequacy of nurse staffing without making some assumptions regarding the level of demand or willingness to pay on the part of payers. Ultimately, the appropriate level of adequacy is an economic and political decision.

The committee viewed as its first responsibility to provide Congress information on the nature and status of knowledge about the relationship of staffing and quality of patient care and work-related injuries and stress. The committee believes that it has made a substantial contribution in this report by providing insights into the following questions: (1) Is quality of care adequate or deficient? (2) Is staffing related to quality of care? If so, how is it related? (3) Has the incidence of work-related injuries and stress increased? If yes, is this related to staffing levels? and (4) What should be done?

Furthermore, in responding to its charge, the committee decided that although current interest and concern among constituent groups about the staffing conditions in hospitals and nursing homes are intense, the future of nursing services in a health care system is equally critical for planning and policy. Hence, the committee addressed today's needs, and also attempted to take a somewhat long-term view, looking ahead at nursing staff in the context of the health care delivery system evolving into the next century. By the beginning of the next century, the types of care delivered at various sites will undoubtedly differ from the care boundaries that existed only two decades ago.

STUDY APPROACH

The committee addressed its charge with several activities. Mainly, it relied on the use of existing information from a variety of sources to focus on important issues. It reviewed and analyzed an extensive body of research literature, published and currently under way. It also consulted a wide selection of other relevant materials, including various reports, published and unpublished, prepared by unions, nurse and hospital associations and others, based on responses from their members. It assessed comments from their members, reports and other material from nursing home industry groups and nursing home resident advocate groups, analyses of published and unpublished data from the federal statistical systems, trade and professional associations and special detailed tabulations on trends at national and subnational levels obtained from the American Hospital Association; special small surveys conducted by various groups; and research workshops held on behalf of the study committee. The committee did not collect primary survey data or undertake independent inferential analyses of data.

The committee met five times between March 1994 and July 1995 to deliberate on the issues outlined above. Experts were invited to speak to the committee on the various issues at four of these meetings. A listing of these presentations can be found in Appendix A.

To avail itself of expert and detailed analysis of some of the key issues beyond the time and resources of its members, the committee commissioned background papers from experts in areas of relationship of staffing to quality of care, work-related injuries and stress, and education and training issues. The specific papers are included in Part II, Section 3 of this report.

The committee also expanded and augmented its perspective and views with deliberations of a liaison panel, testimony, and site visits.

Liaison Panel

Because of the considerable number and array of professional groups and trade organizations concerned with the issues studied, a liaison panel comprising representatives of 20 organizations was appointed. A roster of the liaison panel members and their affiliations can be found in Appendix B. The panel met formally early in the study. It served in a consultative and information exchange capacity. Several members of the panel provided the committee with results of special surveys, specific informational material, and other background information from their organizations throughout the study.

Testimony

Public hearings provided an opportunity for interested and concerned parties to express their views to the committee and for the committee to obtain, firsthand, an extensive range of opinion on the matters under consideration. In the summer of 1994, the committee sent out over 500 announcements to health care givers, industry associations, unions, nurse associations, national and state boards of nursing, nursing home resident advocates, hospital and nursing home associations, and concerned and interested individuals. The committee received more than 100 written statements in response to its request.

Two public hearings were held in conjunction with the committee meetings, one in Washington, D.C., and the other in Irvine, California. Of the persons and organizations who sent in written statements, 44 of them presented oral testimony at these hearings and responded at that time to questions from the committee. These witnesses represented an extensive range of health care givers and provider organizations, consumers and consumer advocates, professional organizations, unions, and others across the country. A summary of the testimony is included in Part II, Section 1 of this report.

Site Visits

Site visits to localities and facilities around the country collectively are intended to offer insights on the issues confronting the study committee and supplement in important ways the research, analysis of data, discussions with experts, and the committee's own experience. The purpose of these visits is to seek understanding of the issues pertinent to the study mandate and the views of concerned and interested parties, and not to evaluate or draw public judgments about local efforts. Those hosting the site visit teams for this study were assured confidentiality about any information or remarks they might provide to the committee. Consequently, no specific material that could identify facilities or individuals is made public without their explicit permission.

During the fall and winter of 1994–1995, the committee conducted site visits in Mississippi, Missouri, New York, and Oregon. During each of these site visits, two or three committee members and IOM staff met with staff of various hospitals, nursing homes and other organizations, members of professional associations, and groups of concerned individuals to hear firsthand about their concerns, what they perceive as problems, how their operations function, and similar topics.

Committee members attempted to observe a broad range of nurse staffing arrangements in a variety of facilities—public, for-profit, not-for-profit and academic hospitals, proprietary and voluntary hospitals, and nursing facilities—in metropolitan and nonmetropolitan locations. Because individual sites are chosen for the insights they can provide, and loosely to represent a few broad categories, the site visits are not intended to result in an objective, quantitative analysis of national or even subnational nurse staffing patterns. Rather, they afford committee members an opportunity to form impressions based on their personal observations and also to benefit from the experiences of individuals involved directly in issues related to the study mandate. A summary report of the site visits is included in Part II, Section 1 of this report.

UNDERLYING ASSUMPTIONS AND VALUES

The present study should be considered a first step toward addressing a major topic of concern in health care policy, namely, the role of nursing services in ensuring the delivery of quality patient care. These issues must be considered in an environment undergoing rapid changes that are themselves influenced by pressures of cost containment and competition. The issues are complex, and all involve difficult choices. The choices will reflect societal values. In the current health care environment, the traditional roles of various individual and institutional participants are undergoing substantial change. Purchasers of health care are becoming more aware of rising costs. They want cost containment without sacrificing quality of care. They are challenging traditional professional autonomy on decisions pertaining to health care. They are pushing health care providers toward more cost-effective methods.

In response to the emerging dominance of payers, health care providers are considering alternative forms of organization. The open-ended financing that has characterized the health care industry in the past is no longer acceptable. Payers are challenging professionals and other providers to justify the effectiveness and efficiency of their services and to compete on price.

Increasingly, providers also are confronting a fixed budget, negotiated in advance, and are expected to make do (or make a profit) within these financial constraints. Institutions are investigating ways to find more efficient means to deliver services and to cut costs. The goal is to retain quality, but the characteristic of market competition is that, at times, the quality of care that some professionals believe is appropriate is not "in sync" with the level of quality that payers are willing or able to pay for. Thus, costly incremental quality enhancements may be reconsidered in light of fiscal realities. Health care providers are actively thinking about issues of institutional structure and staffing levels and mix of personnel.

At the same time, *the committee strongly believes that during these times of rapid change, while weighing legitimate concerns about health care costs and acknowledging past overuse of some services, society must balance against those concerns both the rights of consumers to receive quality care in a digni-*

fied manner and the rights of those providing that care to work in a safe and healthy environment. The twin goals of providing quality health care can be described as (1) meeting individual needs and (2) ensuring an equitable provision of basic care in a cost-effective manner. The challenge is to assure that all persons (poor and minority included) have equal opportunity to quality health care, i.e., nursing services should be adequate for such care and understanding of, and sensitive to, special needs.

The committee further recognizes the fundamental importance of considering the quality of life of patients and residents in hospitals and nursing homes. The goal of long-term care has been defined as the maintenance or restoration of the highest possible level of physical, mental, and social functioning of individuals within the constraints of their illness, disabilities, and environmental settings (IOM, 1989). For residents in nursing facilities, who are there for a sustained period of time, quality of life means provision of a home-like atmosphere, care and caring, dignity, and sustained efforts to maintain or improve living conditions and, for some, to recognize the inevitability of death.

For care delivered in hospitals, the balance between quality of care and quality of life differs somewhat from the qualities of care and life in nursing homes, but is no less important. Most people with acute care needs enter hospitals for short-term medical attention and the attendant nursing care. Quality-of-life considerations (as distinct from quality of patient care) do not affect such patients as much as they do the residents of nursing facilities, because of the comparatively brief length of stay. In hospitals, quality of care has relevance more in terms of the long-term results of medical decisions and actions taken during the current episode of illness.

ORGANIZATION OF THE REPORT

The committee used four criteria for judging the contents of its final report and its specific recommendations. First, the topic should be within the scope and purview of the committee's charge. Second, the topic should be important, relevant, and within the scope of the study. Third, the evidence about the subject should be sufficient to support and justify its findings and recommendations. Fourth, a recommendation should be attainable at reasonable cost.

The report is organized in a manner responsive to the legislative mandate and the contract charge. Part I of the report contains the committee's findings and recommendations. Part II contains the resources obtained and used by the committee to assist in committee deliberations, including the study activities undertaken, statistical information, and background papers on key issues commissioned from experts in the field.

Hospitals and nursing homes represent two separate but related markets; they have different financing sources, and they face different issues with regard to several topics within the purview of this study. For the most part, they are discussed separately in the report.

The next three chapters set the framework and provide the context within which the committee addressed the key issues under study. They briefly describe the changing demographic profile of the nation, and the implication of these changes for the health care system, the changing demand for, and use of, health resources in hospitals and nursing homes, and the implications for the future supply of nursing staff and the type of education and training that will be needed to adequately prepare them to meet the demands of tomorrow's jobs.

The three chapters that follow review the research literature and the analyses of the key issues studied by the committee. Chapters 5 and 6 review and analyze the relationship of staffing issues and their linkage, where it exists, with quality of care in hospitals and nursing homes. Chapter 7 reviews available information on the incidence of work-related injuries and stress to nursing staff in hospitals and nursing homes, and examines the nature and strength of the relationship between work-related injuries and stress and staffing patterns.

Finally, Chapter 8 provides the committee's epilogue to the study.

Although the committee has made a concerted effort to obtain data and objective evidence based on research, some of its conclusions and recommendations are ultimately derived from professional judgment based on the expertise and experience of committee members, anecdotal information, testimony, and information provided by concerned constituencies. The committee consisted of persons with diverse backgrounds and expertise. Extensive discussions of the available evidence were undertaken during committee meetings to achieve consensus.

For a number of reasons the committee did not address every possible issue that might be considered relevant or related to its specific charge. For instance, the issues surrounding foreign-trained nurses is not addressed by the committee in its discussion of nursing personnel. The committee deferred to the Immigration Nursing Relief Advisory Committee (1995) established under Public Law 101-238. That committee was advisory to the Secretary of Labor and issued its report in May 1995. The committee also did not address in depth the growth of long-term care settings other than nursing homes. Although the importance of these settings is growing, their detailed discussion was beyond the scope of the contract charge. The committee did not research issues of access to hospital and nursing home care in order to keep the report focused. There is some evidence that lack of insurance and discrimination may be factors in reduced access to care by minorities.

At first glance the scope of the study—nursing staff in hospitals and nursing homes— may appear to some to be narrow; in reality, however, it is very broad and complex, especially at a time when the U.S. health care system is undergoing rapid and profound changes. The magnitude of the material that needed to be collected, reviewed, and analyzed to address adequately the study topics also demanded that the committee stay within the specific mandate of the contract and not try to cover all possible related topics.

Although the principal intent of the report is to address the specific concerns of Congress as defined in its mandate, the committee believes that the report will provide guidance to a wider audience responsible for organization, delivery, and financing of health care and for federal health care policy.

Finally, when the study originally was requested, the national debate on health reform was under way. Since then many changes have occurred and many others are under consideration. Because the complexity of the various issues are so great and volatile, the committee made a decision not to speculate outcomes but to conduct its study based on objective and scientific evidence available to it.

2

Implications of Population Change

INTRODUCTION

Major changes in the demographic profile of the United States are under way, and these changes are projected to accelerate in the next several decades. Important demographic shifts include the aging of the population and the projected growth of the oldest old (those 85 years of age or more); the changing racial and ethnic composition of the population resulting from immigration and the rapid growth rates of the minority populations, especially those of Hispanic and Asian origin; the shifts in family patterns (particularly the trend toward smaller family size, childlessness, and divorce); and increasing poverty.

The growing elderly population will be a major determining force in the next century for the demand and supply of health services and, therefore, for the type of resources needed to provide those services. The implications for, and challenge of, the increasing number of aged in the years ahead are compounded when the projected racial and ethnic composition of the population is taken into account along with the age distribution of the elderly population.

These shifts take on added importance and urgency in the context of a rapidly changing health care system, placing intense stress on the system as it tries to hold down expenditures and, at the same time, increase access and maintain quality of health care.

Changes in population imply changes in the health care services that will be needed in the years ahead, especially among the elderly population. The growth and diversity of the elderly population, and a sociodemographic profile of the elderly population are described in the following brief overview. The chapter touches on the health status of, and use of health services by, this segment of the population. It concludes with a brief discussion of the implications for society in meeting these needs for health care services in the next century. The main purpose of this chapter is to provide a general perspective for understanding the implications of these population changes on the demands for health care services in hospitals and nursing homes and the supply of an adequate nursing workforce to provide these services.

GROWTH OF THE POPULATION

The population of the United States has increased by 12 million people, or 5.1 percent, since the 1990 census. Recent projections issued by the Bureau of the Census indicate that the population is expected to reach 276 million by the year 2000, and 392 million in 2050, amounting to a more than 50 percent increase since 1990 (Bureau of the Census, 1993a). The high level of immigration is a major factor contributing to the projected growth of the U.S. population.

The U.S. population is aging and the population in the 21st century will be older than it is now. The growth of the older population may be considered as one of the most important developments of the twentieth century. In 1900, there were 3.1 million people 65 years of age and older, or 1 in 25 persons. In 1994 this number was around 33 million or 1 in 8 persons (Bureau of the Census, 1995b). Yet the growth to date is just the beginning of the aging of America. In fact, the population 65 years of age and older is growing more slowly between 1990 and 2010 than at any time in a period of nearly 130 years. This reflects the aging of the low fertility generations of the 1920s and 1930s (see Figure 2.1). The elderly population, however, is projected to continue to increase both in numbers and as a proportion of the total population. It is projected to more than double by the middle of the next century, increasing from nearly 34 million, or 13 percent of the total population, to 80 million in 2050, or nearly 20 percent of the population. Most of the increase is expected to occur between 2010 and 2030, when the "baby-boom" generation enters the elderly years (see Figure 2.1).

While this rate of growth is projected to drop after 2030, there will continue to be a large proportion of elderly persons in the population. About 40 to 50 years from now it is likely that there will be more elderly persons than young persons (under 15 years of age) in the United States. These projections take on added importance when the age distribution and the racial and ethnic composition of the projected elderly population are considered.

The elderly population is growing older. The population aged 85 and older is the fastest growing age group in the U.S., and it is projected to be nearly six times as large by 2050 as this age group was in 1990 (see Figure 2.2). It is also the most rapidly growing age group among the elderly population. Fewer children and increasing life expectancy have contributed to this shift in the population composition. A 65-year-old person can expect to live another 17 years, and

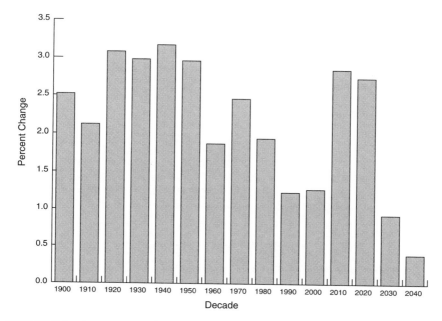

FIGURE 2.1 Average annual percent change in population 65 years and older, United States, 1900–2040 (middle series projections). SOURCE: Bureau of the Census, 1993a.

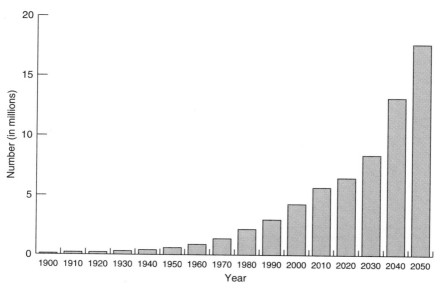

FIGURE 2.2 Number of people 85 years and older, United States, 1900–2050 (middle series projections). SOURCE: Bureau of the Census, 1993c.

those who live to age 85 have an average of 6 more years of life remaining (NCHS, 1993b). This rapid growth of the oldest-old population will have a major effect on the health care system in terms of services needed, education, training and experience of health personnel, knowledge of diseases and treatments for the aged, and demands on resources for the services used by this segment of the population.

DIVERSITY OF THE POPULATION

We speak of "the elderly" as if they were a homogeneous group. Like the rest of the population in the country, they vary widely in terms of their racial composition, ethnic origin, socioeconomic circumstances, family composition, living arrangements, and health care needs.

Racial and Ethnic Composition

An important factor with major implications for the future course of the nation's elderly is the changing racial and ethnic composition of the U.S. population. Since 1980, the growth of minority populations as a whole has been substantially greater than that of the white population. As a result, each of the minority racial and ethnic groups increased during the 1980s as a proportion of the total population, while the non-Hispanic white population declined as a proportion of the total population. Under current assumptions, this trend is projected to accelerate in the years to come, leading to increasing racial and ethnic diversity of the population: by the year 2050, the non-Hispanic white population will account for a little more than half of the nation's people (53 percent). The Hispanic population will experience the largest increase, reaching 21 percent of the total population by 2050. The black population is projected to double its present size by the middle of the next century. Although starting from a much smaller base, and therefore adding fewer people, the Asian and Pacific Islander population is projected to be the fastest growing racial group, with annual growth rates that may exceed 4 percent during the 1990s.[1] By 2050, this population group is projected to be five times its current size (Bureau of the Census, 1993a).

As with the total population, the elderly population today is predominantly white, but more racial and ethnic diversity can be expected in the years ahead (see

---

[1]Although the Hispanic and Asian origin populations are often referred to as aggregate ethnic groups, significant diversity exists within each group. The term "Hispanic," for example, includes many culturally and economically diverse peoples who share a common language. The "Asian and Pacific Islander" population may be the most diverse of America's major minority groups. It comprises diverse groups from more than two dozen countries, differing in language, religion, cultural, and economic background. Treating all these subgroups as a single monolithic population masks the extreme problems faced by some groups as well as the significant progress achieved by other groups and individuals.

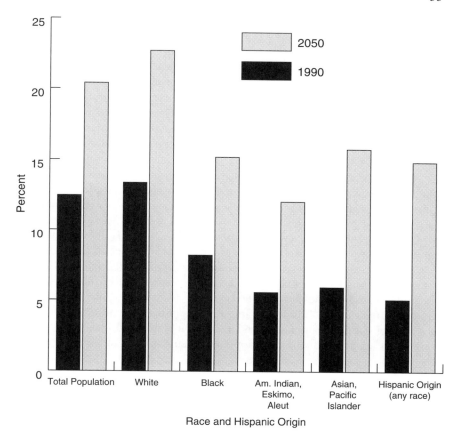

FIGURE 2.3   Percent of population 65 years and older by race and hispanic origin, United States, 1900 and 2050. SOURCE: Bureau of the Census, 1993c.

Figure 2.3). The Hispanic population is projected to account for an increasingly larger proportion of the elderly population as the large numbers of current immigrants begin to age. In 1994, 1 in 10 elderly were of a race other than white. By 2050, this proportion is expected to rise to 2 in 10. The share of the elderly who are of Hispanic or Asian origin is expected to increase rapidly in the coming decades (Bureau of the Census and the National Institute on Aging, 1993b).

In general, minority groups reach old age with fewer economic resources, and they tend to have less education than do non-Hispanic whites. They may also have distinctive health needs, and some—especially immigrant minorities—may follow the diets, health practices, and beliefs of their cultures, which may not always be well understood by some care givers. Thus, as the ranks of the elderly minorities grow, their needs, values, and preferences may necessitate fundamental changes in programs and services for the health care of the elderly.

Access to health care is a function of socioeconomic status, but also to some extent, level of acculturation, ranging from family structure, to education, and facility with the language. Such sociocultural barriers could arise because of differences between receivers and givers of care related to health beliefs and behavior or knowledge about medical services. These differences could make patients reluctant to seek care or comply with prescribed treatments, make care givers insensitive to the needs of patients, and strain relationships between the institutions and their communities.

These barriers often are compounded by inadequate command of the English language. Many elderly immigrants speak little or no English. In 1990, 1 in 7 Americans—nearly 32 million people—spoke a language other than English at home, up from 23 million in 1980. Although fluency in multiple languages is an advantage, speaking a language other than English at home is often a marker for families that are not fluent in English. Among those who speak a language other than English at home, 2 persons in 10 either have very limited English skills or do not speak the language at all. Nearly 1 million persons live in "linguistic isolation," that is, in households where no one aged 14 or older spoke English at all (Bureau of the Census, 1990). The implications of these trends are immense for providing culturally sensitive care and interaction between patients and providers at all levels, and for planning the supply and distribution of nursing personnel.

Sociodemographic Characteristics

Gender Distribution

More women survive to old age than men. In 1994, elderly women outnumbered elderly men by a ratio of 3 to 2, and this difference increases markedly with advancing age. After age 75, most elderly men are married and living with their spouse. Women are more than three times as likely as men to be widowed and living alone. Thus, most elderly men have a spouse for assistance when health fails. The likelihood of living alone increases with age, but much more so for women (Bureau of the Census, 1995b).

Living Arrangements

Changing patterns of family formation and composition (late marriages, smaller families, divorce, childlessness) mean that whereas today's elderly generally have children to turn to when in need, the elderly baby-boomer generation will have far fewer family resources, and specifically fewer younger persons to take care of them. As more persons live longer, issues surrounding the care of the elderly will become more prevalent. Increasingly, those who may be consid-

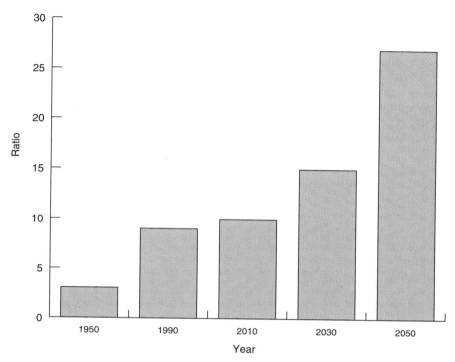

FIGURE 2.4   Parent support ratio, United States, 1950–2050 (number of people 85 years and older per 100 persons 50–64 years old, middle series projections). SOURCE: Bureau of the Census, 1993c.

ered the "young old" (i.e., those in their 50s and 60s) will have surviving older parents and other relatives and may be faced with the prospect and expense of caring for them. According to the Bureau of the Census, the parent support ratio (defined as the number of persons aged 85 and over per 100 persons aged 50 to 64) has tripled from 3 in 1950 to 9 in 1990; this ratio is expected to triple again by the middle of the next century, increasing to 27 (Bureau of the Census, 1993c; Bureau of the Census and the National Institute on Aging, 1993a). (See Figure 2.4.)

The 50- to 65-year age group is often referred to as the "sandwich generation" since they have responsibilities of caring for their children and at the same time of caring for their very old family members. The problem of parent care affects working-age members of the family, especially women who historically have been the informal care givers in the family. With increasing numbers of women in the labor force, the demand for more formal care giver arrangements is increasing.

Income and Poverty

Today's elderly on the average are economically better off and in better health than their counterparts of a few decades ago. Despite the overall improved economic condition of the elderly, significant income differences are observed among various subgroups. In general, minorities, women, the very old, and those who are living alone are all vulnerable to low income and consequent poverty. About 12 percent of the elderly population is poor; the rates are 33 percent for older black persons and 22 percent for elderly Hispanic persons. Elderly women have a higher poverty rate (16 percent) than men (9 percent). Many more of the elderly population are concentrated just above the poverty threshold (Bureau of the Census, 1993b, 1995b).

Living alone is a significant indicator of the likelihood of an elderly person being poor. In 1991, about 18 percent of elderly men and 27 percent of elderly women living alone were poor. As in other characteristics of the elderly population, there were differences among the major racial and Hispanic-origin groups. Nearly 24 percent of elderly white women living alone were poor. One-half of the elderly women of Hispanic origin living alone and 58 percent of the black women living alone were poor (Bureau of the Census and the National Institute on Aging, 1993a).

Social Security and Medicare have contributed in a large way to improve the economic well-being of the elderly. However, Medicare pays for short stays in nursing homes after hospitalization, but does not cover long-term care. Much of the cost of long-term care is borne by the elderly and their families and only when their resources are depleted does Medicaid cover costs. The elderly persons' need for long-term care, at home or in an institution, for example, and the large role played by government programs, make the elderly population economically vulnerable (Treas, 1995a,b).

HEALTH STATUS AND DISABLING CONDITIONS

Today's elderly persons are in better health than their counterparts of some years back. The age-specific rates of disability have begun to decline, particularly among the very old (Manton et al., 1993). Women 85 years of age can expect to live free of disability for two-thirds of their remaining life (Suzman et al., 1992). At the same time, frailty is very common at an advanced age owing to disease, the aging process, disuse of muscles, neglect, or depression.

Although the overall health of elderly persons has improved, many are dependent and frail, with one or more chronic conditions. The risks of chronic conditions and functional impairments increase with age. Most elderly persons report at least one chronic condition such as arthritis, diabetes, hypertension, heart disease, hearing impairments, osteoporosis, and senile dementia. Some of these conditions may be life threatening; others affect the quality of life.

The risk of chronic and disabling conditions increases with age. As more of the elderly live to the oldest ages, increasing numbers will face chronic, limiting illnesses or conditions. The prevalence of these major chronic conditions among the elderly is five times that observed in younger persons. These conditions result in dependence on others for assistance in performing the activities of daily living (ADL), especially among the older elderly, portending a significant increase in the need for health care and social support services.

A person's health declines in older ages because of age-related chronic conditions and disabilities. The proportion of persons needing assistance in everyday activities increases with age. These facts suggest that a large number of elderly will seek hospitalization for serious acute and chronic conditions and they will seek long-term care as part of a continuum of care from independent living to assisted living to institutional care.

Alzheimer's disease is the leading cause of dementia in old age. The risk of the disease rises sharply with advancing age, from less than 4 percent of noninstitutionalized persons 65 to 74 years old to nearly half of those 85 years and older. It afflicted an estimated 3.8 million noninstitutionalized elderly in 1990 (Evans et al., 1990). It is a major reason for older persons' being institutionalized. If no breakthrough occurs in prevention or cure, the prevalence of Alzheimer's disease will increase substantially in the years ahead as the oldest age groups in the elderly population increase. In 2050, the number of persons 65 and older affected by Alzheimer's disease is estimated to be around 7.5 million. Increases in the oldest age groups will account for most of the projected increases over this period if no treatment has been found (Evans et al., 1990). The number in the 65- to 74-year age group is expected to rise only moderately. In contrast, the number affected by this disease in the age group 85 and older will increase almost sevenfold by 2050. These numbers indicate the magnitude of the problem, today and in the future.

Use of Health Services

The aging of the population affects the demand for all health care services, including hospitals, and long-term care. Older persons use more health services than their younger counterparts because they have more health problems. They are also hospitalized more often and have longer lengths of stay than younger persons. The growth of the elderly population is likely to result in increases in inpatient admissions. (Some signs of that happening are reflected in recent statistics as discussed in Chapter 3.)

Thus, hospitals will have to increase their sensitivity and ability to care for the acutely ill aging population. An increase in the number of elderly patients requiring more assistance in all aspects of their care, including ADLs, will impact on staffing requirements for nursing services in hospitals. Moreover, as the length of stay in hospitals declines in general, the emphasis on discharge planning becomes greater than ever. With a shorter length of stay, clinicians have less opportunity to prepare the patient and family for care at home. This becomes more complicated with the aging patient who often exhibits functional decline requiring more intense teaching in preparation for discharge and care at home. The problem is compounded by language barriers.

As the population ages and develops chronic illnesses, the demand for long-term care services including nursing home services will increase. The number of dependent elders (especially those over age 75) is expected to grow as the proportion of total elderly in the population increases (Griffin et al., 1989; Strumpf and Knibbe, 1990). Dependence for assistance ranges from instrumental activities of daily living (IADL), such as cooking, shopping, and cleaning, to personal care ADLs, such as toileting, dressing, bathing, transfer and ambulation, and eating.

With increasing age and disabilities of the residents, shortened hospital stays, and early discharges from hospitals, the demand for nursing facilities to provide more complex services is growing (AHCA, 1995). The degree of medical instability, impairment, and severity of illness in nursing home residents is increasing (Hing, 1989; Shaughnessy et al., 1990; Kanda and Mezey, 1991; Schultz et al., 1994). Medical technology, such as the use of intravenous feedings and therapy, suctioning, rehabilitative services, respiratory care, ventilators, oxygen, special prosthetic equipment and devices, formerly used only in the hospital, has been extended to nursing facilities. These services require more professional nursing care, judgment, supervision, evaluation, and resources than in the past (Shaughnessy et al., 1990).

Only about 5 percent of elderly persons live in nursing homes. However, the total number of elderly persons living in nursing homes has increased in a manner consistent with the increase in the elderly population. Nursing home use increases with advancing age. Whereas 1 percent of those 65 to 74 years lived in a nursing home in 1990, nearly 1 in 4 aged 85 or older did (Schneider and Guralnik, 1990; Bureau of the Census and the National Institute on Aging, 1993a). If current use patterns continue, more than one-half of the women and about one-third of the men who turned 65 years of age in 1990 can be expected to enter a nursing home at least once in their lifetime (Murtaugh et al., 1990). About 43 percent of persons who were 65 years old in 1990 are projected to enter a nursing home some time before they die; more than half of them will spend at least 1 year of their life in a nursing home, and about 21 percent will spend at least 5 years there (Kemper and Murtaugh, 1991). This proportion increases with age. The growth of alternative long-term care settings appears to be having some impact on reducing the demand for nursing home care. Nevertheless, the need and demand for nursing home care is expected to continue. With the growing elderly population and the concomitant increase in the number of persons with multiple chronic conditions and disabilities, these facts have major implications for both medical and nursing practice and for the financing of long-term care.

CONCLUSION

The projected changes in the composition of the U.S. population and the growth of the elderly, especially the older elderly, pose a serious challenge for public policies as they relate to the health and social well-being of that segment of the population. Because a person's risk of being institutionalized is unpredictable and the potential economic consequences are devastating, protecting older Americans from the costs of nursing home care is an important and much debated policy issue. The aged population also will be a major force to be contended with in shaping the health care delivery and financing systems that promote high quality of care, and in developing a nursing and other health care workforce that is knowledgeable and sensitive to the special problems and concerns of the diverse elderly population. While planning today in an environment of budget cuts and cost pressures at all levels, innovative and creative ways must be developed and tried to ensure access and equity in meeting the increasing demands of tomorrow for health care services that will result from these shifts.

The challenge of planning for an aging society will be to recognize and address the differences that already exist within today's generation of elders, as well as those likely to shape the needs of future generations. "The unprecedented increase in the number of older people and the rapidity of the growth in their share of the total population is a new social phenomenon offering both problems and opportunities" (Soldo and Agree, 1988, p. 42).

3

Evolving Health Care Scene

OVERVIEW

The nation's health care system is in a historic transformation driven by rising prices, pressures on public and private budgets, and scientific and technological change. These forces are prompting major changes in the structure, organization, financing, and delivery of health care. The health care delivery system today is not what it was yesterday, and not what it will be tomorrow. Hospitals are changing in ways not considered possible a few years ago. A combination of changes in payment policies and technological and scientific advances has permitted shifts from the traditional inpatient hospital setting to ambulatory care settings, the community, home, and nursing homes. Hospitals increasingly are offering nontraditional services including hospital-based ambulatory care, home health care, and skilled nursing services units (AHA, 1994a). Shortell and coauthors have aptly likened the turbulence in the health care system to "an earthquake in its relative unpredictability, lack of a sense of control, and resulting anxiety. At the epicenter of this earthquake is the American hospital" (Shortell et al., 1995, p. 131).

The boundaries between hospitals and nursing facilities are beginning to blur, and the walls around them are moving outward into the community where community-based home health services and other alternatives to nursing facilities are developing (Shortell et al., 1995). The typical nursing home of the past provided primarily custodial care for the elderly needing assistance; persons with acute conditions were treated in hospitals. Today, the demand for nursing home care is shifting from the traditional custodial care model toward one that often has a rehabilitative component (Johnson et al., Part II of this report[1]). Nursing facilities are beginning to provide a wide array of services to individuals who are disabled with an increasing number of unstable chronic conditions (Morrisey et al., 1988; Shaughnessey and Kramer, 1990). The type of care provided is also changing with the increasing severity of illness and disability of some of the residents; it includes rehabilitative care, ventilator assistance, care for residents with an emerging acute care crisis, and respite care. Special care beds in nursing facilities have expanded rapidly in recent years for patients with Alzheimer's disease or other dementia in general. Subacute care is offered in many nursing facilities for patients discharged from the hospital to the nursing facility (AHCA, 1995).

Impetus for Cost Containment

Enactment of Medicare and Medicaid in 1965 began a period of tremendous growth in health care services, especially hospital services. The combination of (a) increased demand for services stimulated by increased public and private insurance and (b) reimbursement on a retrospective basis has stimulated a rapid rise in use, costs, and expenditures. The need for cost containment policies became evident as the cost of health care reached unprecedented levels and comprised a steadily increasing share of the nation's output.

In 1993, personal health care expenditures (PHCE) reached $783 billion. Although the rate of growth in very recent years is slower than it has been in more than three decades, spending for health care continues to increase faster than the overall economy. While the share of private funds shows a slight decline, public funds as a share of the total PHCE continued to increase, accounting for 43 percent of the PHCE in 1993. Medicare and Medicaid accounted for one-third of all PHCE (Levit et al., 1994). Moreover, the federal government's share of health care costs has been steadily increasing.

Growing concerns about the continuing increases in health spending led to the development of a series of cost containment measures beginning in the mid-1970s. These included the Certificate of Need program (1974–1986); stimulation of competition through support of health maintenance organizations (HMO) starting in 1974; and various constraints on reimbursement in the 1980s. A key step was the enactment of the Tax Equity and Fiscal Responsibility Act (TEFRA) in 1982, which placed a cap on annual operating revenues per inpatient Medicare case at each hospital; it was followed in 1983 by Medicare's Prospective Payment System (PPS), under which hospitals are paid a predetermined amount per

---

[1]The Institute of Medicine (IOM) committee commissioned this paper from Jean Johnson and colleagues. The committee appreciates their contributions. The full text of the paper can be found in Part II of this report.

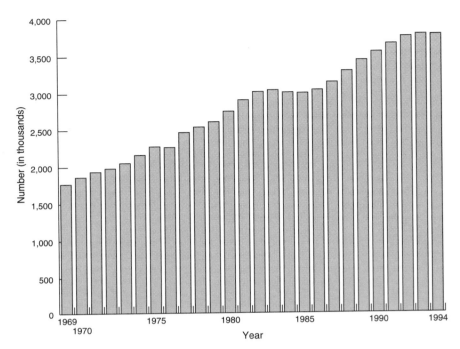

FIGURE 3.1   Employment in hospitals, United States, 1969–1994. NOTE: Monthly employment through October 1995 is higher than comparable employment for 1994. SOURCE: Bureau of Labor Statistics, Current Employment Statistics Program.

Medicare discharge using national rates based on flat rates per admission calculated for each of the approximately 470 (in 1995) diagnosis-related groups (DRG).

Both of these measures have led to major changes in the financing and delivery of health care and have forced hospitals to change the way they staff their facilities and to integrate vertically (with payers) and horizontally (with each other) (ProPAC, 1995). In the years immediately following TEFRA and PPS, the use of inpatient services and hospital employment declined briefly. However, hospital staffing levels began to rise again in 1986 (see Figure 3.1).

A possible explanation for the staffing increase is a combination of scientific and technological advances and an increasing proportion of hospitalized patients tending to be more critically ill requiring more intensive inpatient hospital care and skilled and specialty services, including nursing services (HRSA, 1993). This situation explains to some extent the continuing increases in registered nurse (RN) employment in hospitals even when other employment was declining (see Figure 3.2).

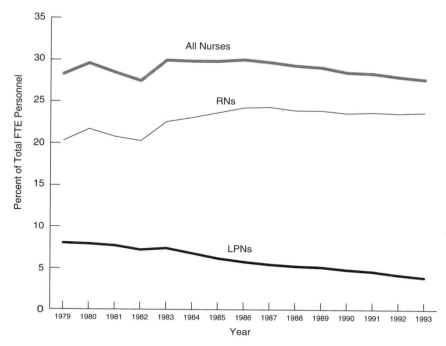

FIGURE 3.2   Nurses as a percent of total full-time-equivalent (FTE) personnel in community hospitals, United States, 1979–1993. NOTE: LPN = licensed practical nurse; RN = registered nurse. SOURCE: American Hospital Association, Annual Surveys, 1979–1993, special tabulations.

Managed care organizations[2] such as HMOs and preferred provider organizations (PPO) developed rapidly, changing the nature of private health insurance and increasing price competition. These evolving payment systems have in turn affected the structure of the health care delivery system by limiting service and directing when and where patients receive their care.

Focus of the Chapter

This chapter presents a brief overview of the major changes occurring on the health care scene, with a focus on the hospital and nursing home sectors, and what these shifts mean for the organization and delivery of nursing services to

---

[2]The term "managed care" as used in this report is broadly understood to encompass organized efforts by third parties, such as health plans, to influence the access, use, and cost of services provided to patients by care givers.

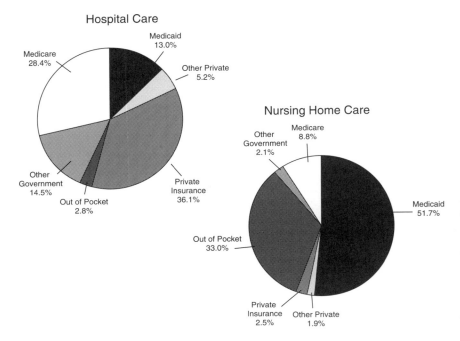

FIGURE 3.3 Sources of funds for medical care expenditures, United States, 1993.
SOURCE: Levit et al., 1994.

patients.[3]   As stated in Chapter 1, hospitals and nursing homes represent two
separate but related health care markets. Hospitals are a part of the basic acute
health care system, and inpatient services are paid for largely by private insurance, Medicare, and Medicaid. The reimbursement for nursing home care, by
contrast, is usually through Medicaid or out of pocket; almost no private insurance for long-term care is being purchased (see Figure 3.3). Also, hospitals
historically have been not-for-profit institutions whereas nursing homes have
been predominantly investor-owned companies. The committee believes that the
issues resulting from the evolving health care environment that the nation is
witnessing are related and yet different in many ways for the two sectors.

PRIVATE INSURANCE AND PUBLIC PAYERS FOR HEALTH CARE

Health care in the United States is financed primarily through a combination
of private health insurance and public coverage, and historically has been pro-

---

[3]For a detailed discussion of the changing health care delivery environment and the evolution of
managed care, see ProPAC (1994), Chapter 3; Shortell et al., 1995; Shortell and Hull, in press.

vided through a fee-for-service (FFS) system. Although public efforts at reforming health insurance have not progressed, the private health insurance sector continues to experience rapid change as it responds to cost pressures from employers. This has led to greater competition in the market and shifts by employers and other purchasers of health care from some insurance companies to other companies, leading to some instabilities in the market. These shifts are reflected in major changes in the organization of the health industry including rapid consolidation into larger corporations through mergers; consolidations and integrated networks; diversification of products; corporate restructuring; and changes in ownership. The most important of the changes is the growth of managed care organizations.

MANAGED CARE

A combination of rising costs of care, dissatisfaction of payers, lackluster growth in personal income, and pressures on public and private budgets has led to the rapid growth of managed care. The emerging health care system is increasingly dominated by managed care organizations that are securing significant discounts from hospitals and physicians while attempting to reduce excess capacity and reduce the demand for high-cost services and procedures. Although HMOs have existed for half a century, their growth especially since 1980 has been phenomenal. The number of persons enrolled in HMOs has risen from about 6 million in 1970 to an estimated 50 million by the end of 1994 (see Figure 3.4). The 20 largest HMO companies have 59 percent of the total national enrollment. Nationally, the net increase in HMO enrollment rate from 1988 to 1993 was 38 percent; New England showed the highest regional level of penetration (26 percent). HMO penetration in Massachusetts reached 34 percent in 1993 and 40 percent by midyear 1994 (GHAA, 1995).

Compared to a typical FFS indemnity plan, HMOs reduce the use of health services. One Congressional Budget Office analysis (CBO, 1995) found that most of the reduction in use of health services is generated by group- or staff-model HMOs, which reduced services by nearly 20 percent. On average, independent practice associations (IPA) do little better than indemnity plans, reducing the use of services by about 1 percent. When these findings are combined using 1992 year-end enrollment patterns for HMOs and IPAs, the estimated average effect of HMOs is to decrease the use of health services by about 8 percent compared to indemnity plans. Approximately 37 percent of HMO enrollment was in group- or staff-model HMOs compared to 63 percent in IPAs and network plans at the end of 1992.

Although cost control has been the dominant force behind the rapid growth of managed care, in recent years the demand for value and accountability has emerged. Purchasers of health care, especially employers, have sought more

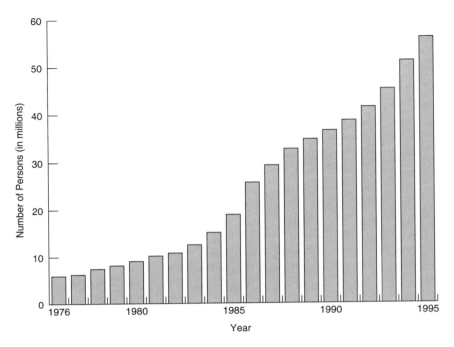

FIGURE 3.4   Number of people receiving care in HMOs, United States, 1976–1995.
SOURCE: Adapted from GHAA, 1995, p. 3.

hard evidence on the quality, effectiveness, and appropriateness of the care they are buying (Shortell and Hull, in press).

A literature analysis of several peer-reviewed studies (Miller and Luft, 1994) found that in comparison to FFS indemnity plans, HMOs had generally lower hospital admission rates, shorter lengths of hospital stay, and fewer uses of hospital services. The studies also showed an average of 22 percent lower use of expensive procedures, tests, and treatments for which less costly alternative interventions were available. For most health conditions, HMOs appear to provide health care roughly comparable to that available through indemnity plans. Compared to FFS indemnity plans, HMO enrollees were less satisfied with service and patient–physician interaction, but more satisfied with the financing aspects of the plans. The authors found that the evidence comparing costs in HMOs and FFS indemnity plans was limited, with inconclusive results. Moreover, not much information is available on the impact of managed care on lowering overall health spending, and there is no persuasive evidence of lower growth rates for costs under managed care. The authors caution against generalizing across all managed care plans because of the rapid growth and diversity of plans in recent years. They express the urgency of additional research on managed care performance on outcomes that goes beyond reducing costs, before the nation moves much further in this direction. At present almost no research has been conducted on whether the savings come from increased efficiency or reduced access and/or quality.

Davis and colleagues (1995) found that FFS enrollees were more satisfied with their plan's access and quality of care; managed care enrollees were more satisfied with their plan's cost, paperwork, and coverage of preventive care. The survey also found a high rate of involuntary plan changing, limited choice of physicians, and low levels of satisfaction among low income managed care enrollees. These findings are based on a population-based survey conducted by the Commonwealth Fund in 1994 of about 3,000 adults insured in FFS plans and managed care organizations.

Critics of managed care contend that the cost containment incentives of managed care may result in underservice and less than optimal care, especially for patients with chronic illness and those of lower socioeconomic status. Little evidence is available with which to evaluate the quality of primary care delivered by managed care plans or to show that the successes of managed care in relatively healthy populations can be replicated among sicker patients (Safran et al., 1994). To help fill that gap, the Medical Outcomes Study (MOS), a longitudinal study of patients' health care use and health outcomes was begun in the mid-1980s.[4] Safran and colleagues found that relative to patients in an FFS plan, those in prepaid plans rated several aspects of an outpatient medical visit less favorably. The investigators compared the extent to which each of the five indicators of primary care quality (accessibility, continuity, comprehensiveness, coordination, and accountability) was rated over a 2-year period by a cohort of chronically ill patients in each of the three insurance plans—FFS indemnity plan, prepaid care through IPA, and group- or staff-model HMO. The investigators found that financial access was highest in prepaid plans; organizational access, continuity, and accountability were highest in the FFS plans; and coordination and comprehensiveness was lowest in HMOs. The authors conclude that these results raise questions regarding the associated cost inefficiencies and outcomes of care. It is an open question whether the magnitude of cost savings will continue after managed care has saturated the health care market.

On the other hand, Lurie and colleagues (1992) in their study of Medicaid patients in Minnesota found no difference in quality of care of chronically mentally ill patients between capitation plans and fee-for-service plans.

---

[4]For further information on the MOS and analyses of the data, see Stewart et al., 1989; Tarlov et al., 1989; Wells et al., 1989a,b; Greenfield et al., 1992; Kravitz et al., 1992; Rubin et al., 1993.

OWNERSHIP STRUCTURE

Several shifts are taking place in the ownership, control, and configuration of health care organizations. One shift is toward proprietary or investor-owned health organization chains (IOM, 1986a). Health organizations are often classified according to ownership because the corporate goals, tax status, and financing structures differ somewhat by ownership categories. Although nonprofit facilities generally have charitable goals, many facilities may seek to maximize revenues. Proprietary facilities generally are oriented to achieving profits, and an increasing number of these health organizations are publicly-traded corporations and multifacility organizations or chains.

The formation of not-for-profit independent hospitals predates that of investor-owned enterprises, although for-profit hospitals have been in existence for some time. For the past several years, a steady shift has been occurring from the traditional independent not-for-profit hospitals to for-profit consolidated enterprises and investor ownership, and not-for-profit hospitals have established for-profit subsidiaries and other arrangements (IOM, 1986a).

The largest proportion of new managed care organizations are proprietary; some traditionally nonprofit corporations are converting to proprietary status.

The majority of nursing facilities are proprietary, and facilities are increasingly owned by investors. Of the total nursing facilities in 1991, 71 percent were reported as proprietary, 24 percent were nonprofit, and 5 percent were government owned (NCHS, 1994). Nursing facilities, like other segments of the health industry, are consolidating into large health care organizations, with the largest chain reporting more than 90,000 beds in 1991.

Profit margins reported for the health care industry have generally been good (Burns, 1992; Abelson, 1993; Rudder, 1994). Forbes reported that in 1994, the all-industry median for return on equity was 12.6 percent for 1 year and 11.4 percent for 5 years (Kichen, 1995). The health care industry ranked first of 21 industry groups for its 5-year return on equity (HCIA and Arthur Andersen, 1994; Kichen, 1995).

Profit-making issues, however, are complex, and detailed discussion of the issues is beyond the scope of this study.[5] The issues of profits on investment and excessive administrative and capital expenditures, however, need to be more fully understood. Few studies of the industry have been conducted, especially those that determine appropriate levels of expenditures for profits, administrative costs, and capital.

---

[5]For a more in-depth discussion of issues surrounding for-profit enterprises in health care, see IOM (1986a) and the literature cited there.

HOSPITALS

As indicated earlier, technology, reimbursement policies, and continuing concern over rising health care costs have combined to stimulate competition in the health care industry. This competition in turn is prompting fundamental restructuring of the organization, financing, and delivery of health care in hospitals.

Hospital care expenditures accounted for 42 percent of personal health care expenditures in 1993. Growth in hospital spending decreased in 1993 for the third consecutive year, mostly because of reduced admissions and lengths of stay. As shown in Figure 3.3, nearly all hospital care is financed by third parties, with only 3 percent paid out-of-pocket. Private health insurance accounted for 36 percent; public funding financed 56 percent of the total PHCE, with the primary payers, Medicare and Medicaid, accounting for more than 41 percent share. Medicare's share of funding for all hospital expenditures was 28 percent in 1993, the highest since the mid-1980s. In 1993, 61 percent of Medicare benefits were for hospital care (including inpatient, outpatient, and hospital-based home health care), reaching $92.7 billion in 1993, an increase of 10.1 percent in just 1 year (Levit et al., 1994).

Hospitals are responding in various ways to the need to reduce costs and to adapt to managed care and other payment arrangements that fix in advance the reimbursements received for patient care. Among the responses are efforts to reengineer care and staffing for that care in innovative ways. These actions and their implications for hospitals and inpatient care are discussed briefly below.

Restructuring of Hospital Services

Integrated Systems

In response to the emerging dominance of payers, providers have engaged in various forms of reorganization and reevaluation. Searching self-examination is part of the current transition in the medical care arena. Physicians are organizing in some communities to negotiate with payers so that they can contract with other providers for the delivery of services to patients. Physicians in this role compete with traditional insurers—HMOs and other managed care organizations. Hospitals are organizing integrated delivery systems in which they purchase physician practices. Thus, hospitals are now competing with physicians and insurance companies in some markets.

Hospitals are developing integrated systems of care through networks, mergers, and consolidations. These structures seek to incorporate the concept of continuum of care, providing services ranging from ambulatory to long-term care in a "seamless" care system for the consumer. Hospitals also are competing for physician referrals and physician loyalty by teaming up with physicians in various types of integrative arrangements. These include physician–hospital organizations, IPAs, and management service organizations. The growth of managed care has largely contributed to this trend toward the development of integrated systems.

The increased number of integrated service delivery networks is one of the more significant structural changes occurring today (ProPAC, 1995). Financing and delivery systems are combining into provider networks and managed care entities. Hospitals are joining together to form systems in which multiple hospitals are owned, leased, managed, or sponsored by a central organization. Between 1984 and 1990, the number of multihospital systems increased from 250 to 311, declining somewhat to 283 systems by 1993, probably as a result of mergers among systems (Shortell and Hull, in press). Groups of hospitals, physicians, other providers, insurers, and/or community agencies are also integrating to form more comprehensive delivery systems to market jointly a comprehensive set of services to plans, insurers, or purchasers in their communities.

These changes are having a major influence on what services are offered and where they are provided and, consequently, on hospital capacity and use. Vertically integrated entities are growing in importance, with increasing emphasis being placed on outpatient and community care in place of heavy inpatient orientation. About 11 percent of community hospitals reported in 1993 that they were already participating in health networks, working together with other hospitals, physicians, and insurers to coordinate a wide range of services for the community (AHA, 1994c). Many others reported working toward such collaborative formations.

Closures and Mergers

Hospitals are closing and entering into mergers and joint ventures at an unprecedented pace in order to strengthen their market share and realize economies of scale (ProPAC, 1995). Hospital closures reduce excess beds and lead to cost savings by allowing the remaining hospitals to spread their costs over a wider patient base. The American Hospital Association (AHA) reported closures of 675 community hospitals between 1980 and 1993.[6]   Thirty-four of the closures occurred in 1993 (AHA, 1994b). As might be expected, rural community hospitals have been particularly vulnerable to closures, outnumbering closures of urban hospitals, while representing slightly less than half of the total number of hospitals (Bogue et al., 1995).

---

[6]AHA defines community hospitals to include institutions that are non-federal, short term, and general or other special hospitals whose facilities are open to the public. Not included are hospital units of institutions, long-term hospitals, psychiatric hospitals, and alcoholism and chemical dependency facilities.

Mergers involve the dissolution of one or more similar organizations and their assimilation by another. Mergers are undertaken either to eliminate direct acute care competitors or to expand acute care networks. They frequently convert inpatient capacity to other functions; only rarely does the acquired hospital continue acute care services after a merger (Bogue et al., 1995). Between 1980 and 1992, AHA reported 215 mergers involving 445 hospitals or health care systems (AHA, 1992).[7] The AHA recorded another 18 completed mergers in 1993 (AHA, 1994c). More than 650 hospitals were involved in mergers or acquisitions in 1994, affecting more than 10 percent of the nation's hospitals. This number includes 219 investor-owned hospitals that were merged into other investor-owned chains and 154 investor-owned hospitals whose mergers into other chains were expected to be completed in 1995. In addition, 301 other hospitals were involved in 176 such arrangements during 1994 (Lutz, 1994).

As a result of closures, mergers, networking, and acquisitions, the number of independent community hospitals has been declining since the late 1970s. After declining rapidly between 1985 and 1990, the rate of decline during the 1990s has slowed. The number of community hospitals declined from 6,193 in 1970 to 5,829 in 1980, and 5261 in 1993. Between 1983 and 1993, admissions to these hospitals declined 15 percent, from 36 million to nearly 31 million (AHA, 1994a). The magnitude of decline varies by region, hospital size, and metropolitan status. (See Table 2.1 in Part II of the report.)

Mergers and integration of institutions, in the context of increasing restructuring of the delivery of health services, may provide an opportunity to rethink the way services are offered in many institutions and offer an approach to structural change. The possibility exists for avoiding duplication and reducing costs. For example, in addition to collapsing centralized services such as human resources, financing, and information services, clinical programs may be consolidated, potentially shifting nursing and other health personnel from their accustomed site of work.

Inpatient Activities

In the years immediately following the establishment of the PPS, noticeable reductions were observed in hospital inpatient admissions and inpatient days of care. Although this trend continued in the 1990s, the rate of the decline has slowed. Declining hospital admissions combined with shorter lengths of stay resulted in a 21 percent decline in inpatient days between 1983 and 1993 (AHA, 1994a). This drop, in turn, has led to a reduction in the number of beds staffed for use (see Table 3.1).

---

[7]The 1992 component of this total was derived from AHA summary of registered hospitals from annual survey data tapes.

TABLE 3.1   Inpatient Activity in Community Hospitals, Total Patients and Patients 65 Years of Age or Older, United States, Selected Years, 1983–1993

Inpatient Activity	Year				Percent Change 1983–1993
	1983	1987	1990	1993	
All patients					
	Number (in millions)				
Admissions	36.152	36.601	31.181	30.748	−14.9
Beds	1.020	0.955	0.928	0.916	−10.2
Inpatient Days	273.200	227.000	226.000	215.900	−21.0
Length of Stay	7.550	7.180	7.240	7.030	−6.9
Persons 65 years or older					
Discharges	11.562	10.295	10.693	11.354	−1.8
Inpatient Days	115.100	92.100	97.200	95.700	−16.9
Length of Stay	9.960	8.950	9.090	8.430	−15.4

SOURCE: American Hospital Association, Annual Surveys, 1983–1993, special tabulations.

For persons 65 years of age and older, however, after a decline of 5.4 percent in admissions and 18 percent in inpatient days between 1983 and 1986, inpatient hospital use has been increasing. The annual number of admissions for this age group grew by 7 percent between 1990 and 1993, whereas admissions for persons under 65 years of age declined by 5.5 percent (HRSA, 1993).

More recent data from the AHA indicate that inpatient admissions are increasing. A comparison of hospital data for the first quarter of 1995 and the first quarter of 1994 shows a 3.2 percent increase in total admissions. This rate of increase in admissions is the highest since 1976. The growth in admissions of persons 65 years and older accounts for a large part of this increase. While admissions show an increase, length of stay continues to decline, marked by a sharp decline of 7.8 percent among patients 65 years of age and older (AHA, 1995a). The drop in length of stay resulted in a decrease in inpatient days (see Table 3.2). Several factors in addition to cost containment influence inpatient length of stay, including reimbursement incentives, technological advances, and increased availability of home health care. The number of staffed beds in U.S. community hospitals has continued to decline since 1983. Between 1983 and 1993, the total number of staffed beds had dropped by more than 104,000 beds (AHA, 1995b (see Table 2.3 in Part II of this report). As seen in Table 3.2, this trend has continued in 1994 and 1995 (AHA, 1994c, 1995a).

Inpatient case mix also has changed in recent years, along with a strong trend toward higher levels of acuity (ProPAC, 1995). This increase in acuity can be attributed to several factors, including movement of less complex services out of

TABLE 3.2 Percent Change in Inpatient
Community Hospital Utilization, United States,
1994–1995

Utilization	Percent Change Quarter Ending March 1994–1995
Beds	−1.5
Inpatient admissions	3.2
Patients ≥ 65 years	5.2
Adjusted admissions	5.9
Inpatient days	−2.6
Length of stay	−6.5

SOURCE: American Hospital Association, National Hospital
Panel Surveys, March Panel, 1994, 1995.

the hospital or into outpatient services, and the pressures to reduce the length of
stay stimulated by changes in reimbursement. The increased acuity of patients
and the consequent complexity of inpatient hospital care and services require
more specialized and intense nursing care than before. This is reflected in the
increased use of special care units such as the intensive care units (ICU) in
hospitals. The number of staffed beds in ICUs in community hospitals increased
by 29 percent between 1983 and 1993. The percentage of total staffed beds that
are ICU beds also rose during this period from 7.5 percent to nearly 11 percent in
1993. During the same period acute care beds dropped from nearly 82 percent to
64 percent (see Table 2.4 in Part II of this report).

Continuum of Care

Historically, the primary function of hospitals has been to treat acute illness
and injury; prevention of disease and promotion of health have been the domain
of the public health system and individual care givers. In the emerging health
care system there are incentives to merge these two roles and to organize the
entire continuum of care (Shortell et al., 1995). In an effort to maintain patient
base as well as to capture market share, hospitals have extended the scope and
type of services offered beyond the traditional acute inpatient services. They now
emphasize prevention, health promotion, and primary care to a much greater
degree than previously.

In responding to the need to reduce costs, hospitals have to some extent
shifted the site of care and consequently some of the costs (Table 3.3). Changes
in payment policies, incentives to treat patients in less costly sites, and technological advances have contributed to the shift for a growing number of services to

TABLE 3.3 Trends in Outpatient Visits and Other Selected Services Offered in Community Hospitals, United States, Selected Years, 1983–1993

	Year			
Total	1983	1987	1990	1993
Number of hospitals offering:				
Home Health Care	795	1,843	1,801	2,047
Hospice Program	513	764	817	964
Skilled Nursing Facilities	752	861	1,073	1,354
Outpatient visits (in millions)	210.0	245.5	301.3	366.9

SOURCE: American Hospital Association, Annual Surveys, 1983–1993, special tabulations.

ambulatory care settings, to post-acute service settings such as skilled nursing facilities, or to home health care and rehabilitation services. This shift has resulted in substantial growth in the use of, and spending on, those areas. Hospital outpatient spending rose 290 percent between 1984 and 1993, while hospital inpatient expenditures went up only 82 percent (ProPAC, 1995). Spending for home health care also has grown rapidly. By 1993 expenditures for hospital-based home health care had reached about $4 billion (Levit et al., 1994).

Outpatient Care

While inpatient hospital use has been declining over the past decade, outpatient care, in terms of both the number of visits and the number of outpatient departments, has risen dramatically (Table 3.4). In 1993, approximately 88 percent of community hospitals reported having an outpatient department, compared to 54 percent in 1985. Furthermore, in 1993, community hospitals reported 367 million outpatient visits, an increase of about 5 percent from 1992 and 75 percent from the number reported in the early 1980s. The increase of outpatient surgeries accounts for much of the growth in outpatient visits. In 1993, more than half of all surgical procedures in community hospitals were performed on an outpatient basis, compared to 24 percent 10 years earlier (AHA, 1994a). Technological advances and cost-cutting efforts by payers have contributed to this growth.

Recently released data from the AHA National Hospital Panel Survey show a substantial increase in outpatient visits (AHA, 1995a). The percentage increase between 1994 and 1995 was 13 percent, the highest rate since 1970. (See Table 2.7 in Part II of this report.)

TABLE 3.4   Percent Change in Outpatient
Community Hospital Utilization, United States,
1994–1995

Utilization	Percent Change Quarter Ending March 1994–1995
Total visits	13.0
Emergency visits	6.5
Clinic visits	16.5
Other visits	14.0

SOURCE: American Hospital Association, National Hospital
Panel Surveys, March Panel, 1994, 1995.

In addition to the growth in outpatient services delivered on hospital premises, many hospitals are developing more hospital-based services to care for patients beyond the acute inpatient hospital care. They are also expanding their long-term care services. The principal factors prompting these changes include the growing numbers of elderly persons, children, and disabled adults requiring long-term, post-acute care; the shift away from long stays in the hospital; technological advances; and payer pressures to reduce hospital stays and to gain market share of the services.

Hospital-sponsored Home Health Services

The number of hospitals providing hospital-sponsored home health services increased from 29.7 percent in 1985 to 38.0 percent in 1992 and 42.2 percent in 1993 (AHA, 1994a). The growth in home health agencies was spurred by the inclusion of these benefits in Medicare. Home health services prior to that time were provided predominantly by public health departments and not-for-profit visiting nurse associations. Since that time, the growth of investor-owned chains and of hospital-sponsored or joint venture agencies has been substantial.

In recent years, the growth in the development of high-technology services such as ventilator care, enteral and parenteral nutrition, antibiotic therapy, and chemotherapy has also been rapid. Increasing use of these high-technology services in home health care has been stimulated by changes in hospital reimbursement.

Hospital-Based Skilled Nursing Units

Unoccupied hospital beds are being converted in some hospitals into post-acute skilled nursing units, hospice units, and special care centers. Patients are "discharged" from the acute care inpatient hospital bed and admitted to the skilled nursing care or hospice unit or to their homes with provision of hospital-sponsored home health services.

Between 1983 and 1993 the number of hospitals reporting use of hospital-based skilled nursing services units more than doubled from 600 to 1,350. Areas with high AIDS caseloads have established special AIDS units. Other special care centers include cancer centers, transplant centers, designated high-level trauma centers, and neonatal intensive care units.

NURSING HOMES

Although the nursing home sector of the U.S. health care system is not undergoing the rapid and intense turbulence occurring in the hospital sector, it is the recipient of seismic fallout from the epicenter of the earthquake (to continue Shortell's [1995] analogy). Fallout from the evolving patterns of reimbursement and delivery of care in hospitals, and other economic and demographic factors, are changing the characteristics of persons entering nursing homes and, therefore, the demand for nursing home beds. At the same time, persons needing primarily custodial care increasingly are looking for alternative long-term care settings. Hence, the sicker patients tend to concentrate in nursing homes. The increased acuity and disability of individuals needing long-term care are placing new types of demands on providers of care. This situation is exacerbated by the aging of the population.

The capacity of nursing homes to meet the increasing demand for services has been strained during the past decade. The demand for nursing home services and other long-term care services is growing with the increasing number of persons who are aged and chronically ill. The total number of licensed nursing facilities was about 16,600 in 1994 (AHCA, 1995). These nursing facilities had 1.67 million beds in 1994. Overall, the supply of beds in nursing facilities has not kept pace with the demand, especially in relation to the growth in the oldest-old population, those persons age 85 years and older (see Table 3.5). This demand will increase in the years ahead as the elderly represent an increasing proportion of the total population.

Occupancy measures the demand for nursing facility services and is often used as an indicator of an undersupply of beds. The occupancy rate in nursing facilities has remained high. The median occupancy rate nationwide was 93 percent in 1994. Wide variations are observed among states, from a high of 98 percent in Georgia, to 79 percent in Texas, to a low of 52 percent in Alaska (AHCA, 1995). Thus, some areas and states may have shortages of nursing home services and others may have an adequate or oversupply of nursing home beds (Swan and Harrington, 1986; Wallace, 1986; Harrington et al., 1992a, 1994a; Swan et al., 1993a; DuNah et al., 1995). In some states, such as Oregon, occupancy is down even when the supply is ratcheted down. Areas with shortages are

TABLE 3.5 Number of Licensed Nursing Home Beds per 1,000 Population Aged 85 and Older, by Region, Selected Years, United States, 1978–1993

Regions	Beds per 1,000 Persons 85 and Older					Percent Change 1978–1993
	1978	1982	1986	1990	1993	
Total U.S.	610.3	559.5	537.0	520.3	479.7	−21.4
North central	729.5	679.9	659.9	636.8	597.4	−18.1
Northeast	516.8	477.7	475.5	470.3	453.6	−12.2
South	594.5	552.9	520.7	504.2	455.1	−23.5
West	571.7	488.9	454.8	436.5	383.6	−32.9

SOURCE: DuNah et al., 1995.

of concern because they may limit access for those in need of services. This overall high occupancy rate reflects both the shortage of beds discussed above and the increase in patients discharged from hospitals needing subacute care and rehabilitative care (HCIA and Arthur Andersen, 1994).

The likely consequence of this shortage is that nursing facilities can be somewhat selective in their admission practices, and some have limited the access of individuals who may have the greatest need for services (Nyman, 1989a).

Forces Affecting Demand for Nursing Home Services

As the population ages and develops multiple chronic conditions, the need for long-term care (LTC) services, including nursing home care, will increase. The demand for nursing facilities to provide more complex services is growing in response to several trends, including increased age and disability of residents, medical technology, cost containment pressures, and government policies (Hing, 1989; Shaughnessy et al., 1990; Kanda and Mezey, 1991; Schultz et al., 1994).

The magnitude of the potential growth in demand is illustrated by the projected growth of the older population discussed in the previous chapter. Medical technology, formerly used only in the hospital, is being transferred to nursing facilities. The use of intravenous feedings and medication, ventilators, oxygen, special prosthetic equipment and devices, and other complex technologies has made nursing home care more difficult and challenging (Harrington and Estes, 1989; Shaughnessy et al., 1990). The kinds of services that are increasingly being provided in some nursing facilities are also creating a greater need for skilled nursing care, in particular, greater professional nursing involvement in the direct care of patients and in supervision, more clinical evaluation, and more financial and human resources.

Several federal government policy changes in the 1980s have contributed to an increase in nursing home demand and government expenditures for nursing home services. As noted earlier in the chapter, the adoption of PPS led to early discharges from acute care hospitals and more referrals and admissions to nursing facilities (Guterman et al., 1988; Neu and Harrison, 1988; Latta and Keene, 1989; U.S. House of Representatives, 1990). Legislation in 1988 established a minimum level of asset and income protection for spouses when determining Medicaid nursing home eligibility, and this too contributed to an increase in Medicaid program costs (Letsch et al., 1992). These policy changes have all encouraged the demand for nursing home services and, thereby, increased Medicaid and Medicare outlays for this type of care.

Some states have also adopted policies to control Medicaid nursing home demand, including Medicaid eligibility policies and preadmission screening programs (Ellwood and Burwell, 1990; HCFA, 1992a,b; Harrington et al., 1994c). These policies may have had a constraining effect on demand and, consequently, on the growth of nursing home capacity.

Expenditures and Payments Policies

Expenditures for nursing home care reached about $70 billion in 1993 (Levit et al., 1994). As seen in Figure 3.1, unlike the hospital market, nursing home care is financed mainly by the government (63 percent in 1993) and out-of-pocket payments (33 percent in 1993). The Medicaid program paid 52 percent of the total bill in 1993; only 9 percent of nursing home care was financed by Medicare and 2 percent by private insurance.

Nearly 69 percent of the residents of nursing homes are recipients of Medicaid for at least some of their costs (AHCA, 1995). The limited role of private insurance and Medicare in paying for LTC distinguishes the long-term care market from the hospital market. Individuals who need nursing home care generally must pay for their own care out-of-pocket. The high cost of long-term care in nursing homes (about $30,000 to $50,000 per year) leads many individuals and families to spend down their resources, often to poverty levels. Those who exhaust their own resources before dying usually become eligible for Medicaid, which will then pay for their care over and above their complete social security and other retirement incomes.

Recent analysis by Spillman and Kemper (1995) shows that 44 percent of persons who use nursing homes after age 65 start as private payers, 27 start and end as Medicaid recipients, and 14 percent spend down assets to become eligible for Medicaid benefits. Of all persons 65 years of age, 17 percent can expect to spend some time using a nursing home and receiving Medicaid benefits; 3 in 5 of this group will have entered the nursing home already eligible for Medicaid.

As a consequence, a number of states have developed initiatives to reduce the strain on the state's budget. These efforts vary from state to state.

Cost Containment Policies

State Medicaid programs have undertaken a number of policy initiatives to control supply and reduce spending on nursing home care. This process began in the early 1980s, when federal budget cuts to state Medicaid programs became standard features of the budget process (Bishop, 1988).

Certificate of Need The most important policy affecting the supply of long-term care beds is the state's certificate-of-need (CON) program. The health planning and CON program established in 1974 (P.L. 94-641) gave states considerable authority and discretion to plan and control the capital expenditures for nursing facilities and other health facilities (Kosciesza, 1987). The effectiveness of CON policies in controlling bed supply has been widely debated (Cohodes, 1982; Friedman, 1982; Swan and Harrington, 1990; Mendelson and Arnold, 1993).

These controversies resulted in the repeal of the program in 1986. Even so, 44 states continued to use CON and/or moratorium policies to regulate the growth in nursing facilities in 1993 (Harrington et al., 1994a). Because of the cost pressures on states, we can expect most states to continue their efforts to limit the supply of nursing home beds even though their bed supply is not keeping pace with the aging of the population.

Medicaid Because Medicaid dominates the LTC market, Medicaid eligibility policies and reimbursement rates are of critical importance to both consumers and providers of nursing home care. The rapidly rising cost of care in a nursing facility, which is consuming an increasingly larger portion of the state Medicaid budget, has been a major concern to state policymakers. States have considerable discretion in developing Medicaid reimbursement methods and rates. Many states have undertaken initiatives to control the growth in nursing home reimbursement rates (Holahan and Cohen, 1987; Bishop, 1988; Nyman, 1988a; Holahan et al., 1993; Swan et al., 1993a,b).

Until 1980, states were required to pay for Medicaid nursing home services on the basis of "reasonable costs"; many states used retrospective reimbursement systems to pay the costs of care (GAO, 1986). The Omnibus Budget Reconciliation Act of 1980 (OBRA 80) gave states greater flexibility in developing reimbursement systems. This provision, known as the Boren Amendment, allowed states to pay nursing facilities based upon what was "reasonable and adequate to meet the costs incurred by efficiently and economically operated nursing facilities in providing care."

Since 1980, there has been a pronounced shift away from retrospective reimbursement to prospective facility-specific methods (Swan et al., 1993a,b; 1994). In addition, the number of states with case-mix reimbursement has increased substantially (see Table 3.6). By 1996, about one-half of all state Medicaid

TABLE 3.6   Number of States by Medicaid Nursing
Facility Reimbursement Method and by Number
Using Case-Mix Reimbursement, United States, 1979
and 1993

	Year	
	1979	1993
Total number of states[a]	50	51
Reimbursement method[b]		
Retrospective	13	1
Prospective, facility-specific	16	17
Prospective, class	4	3
Prospective, combination	17	30
States using case-mix reimbursement	3	19
Average Medicaid per diem rate	$28	$76

[a]The total number of states includes the District of Columbia.
[b]The total number of states for 1979 does not add up to 50 states
as Arizona did not have a Medicaid program in 1979.

SOURCE: Swan et al., 1994.

programs are expected to be using case-mix reimbursement. Medicaid nursing
home reimbursement methods are primarily prospective and vary substantially
across states. These methods create wide variations in rates and have dramatic
impact on nursing home expenditures and staffing (described in chapter 6).

Medicare   Medicare accounts for 9 percent of nursing home expenditures. Medicare retrospective payment methods based on reasonable costs have been widely
criticized as inflationary (Schieber et al., 1986; Holahan and Sulvetta, 1989).
Because prospective reimbursement systems have been shown to reduce costs in
the hospital sector, the Health Care Financing Administration (HCFA) is considering this approach. Congress in OBRA 93 has mandated that Medicare study
prospective reimbursement as a means of controlling nursing facility costs. In
response, HCFA is conducting a demonstration project to study prospective case-
mix reimbursement for Medicare and for participating state Medicaid programs.

The challenge is for Medicare to control its share of the costs while ensuring
access, appropriate care for resource-intensive residents, and high quality of care
(Holahan and Sulvetta, 1989; Weissert and Musliner, 1992a,b).

Alternative Sites of LTC Care

Federal Medicare policies have dramatically expanded coverage for alternatives to care in nursing facilities during the past 5 years. This expanded coverage encouraged the rapid growth in home health care agencies and in the volume of such services (Letsch et al., 1992; NAHC, 1993). Federal and state policies have also expanded alternatives to institutional care under the Medicaid home and community-based waiver programs (Justice, 1988; Lipson and Laudicina, 1991; Gurny et al., 1992; HCFA, 1992b; Miller, 1992; Folkemer, 1994). The net effect of all these programs is not clear; these types of programs may be reducing the demand for nursing facility care in some areas or the programs themselves may be growing as a response to the limited supply of nursing home beds in some areas.[8]

As seen in Table 3.7, growth in the nursing home industry is slower than that observed in alternative types of LTC facilities. The total number of licensed nursing facilities in 1993 was 16,959 (DuNah et al., 1995). These facilities had 1.74 million beds. While the growth in licensed nursing facilities has hovered around 2 percent per year for the past several years, and only 1 percent between 1992 and 1993, the increase in residential care facilities, including board and care, personal care, foster care, and/or assisted living facilities, has been rapid. In 1993, there were 39,080 licensed residential care facilities for the aged with about 642,600 beds (Harrington et al., 1994b). According to the National Health Provider Inventory, in 1991, there were nearly 13,170 board and care facilities with 120,636 beds for the mentally retarded (NCHS, 1994). These facilities do not have skilled nursing care and are not eligible for Medicaid and Medicare payments. During the period 1983–1993, the growth in residential care beds for the aged has been about 11 to 12 percent annually (Harrington et al., 1994c).

In 1993, home health care was provided to about 1.4 million persons per day by 7,000 home health agencies (NCHS, 1993a). Three-quarters of home health patients were 65 years of age and over, and almost 20 percent were 85 years and older. Two-thirds of home health patients were women. Among the home health patients in 1993, about one-half of the admission diagnoses were for the following six conditions: diseases of the heart and hypertension (17 percent); injury and poisoning (9 percent); diabetes (7 percent); and cerebrovascular diseases, malignant neoplasms, and respiratory diseases (6 percent each).

The number of licensed home health care agencies increased by 24 percent just between 1992 and 1993, and licensed adult day care agencies increased by 41

---

[8]A full discussion of the growth of alternative LTC facilities and services is beyond the scope of this study. The reader is referred to another IOM study that defines issues relating to quality of LTC services in home and community-based settings (IOM, 1996). A larger study currently is in the planning stages.

TABLE 3.7   Number of Licensed Long-Term Care Facilities, United States, 1992 and 1993

Type of Facility	Year 1992	1993	Percent Change 1992–1993
Nursing facilities	16,800	16,959	0.9
Intermediate care facilities for the mentally retarded	5,894	6,296	6.8
Residential care facilities[a]	34,871	39,080	12.1
Home care agencies	8,117	10,084	24.2
Adult day care agencies	1,517	2,131	40.5

[a]Includes board and care, personal care, assisted living, and other categories of residential care for the aged that are licensed by states. Categories vary by state.

SOURCE: Harrington et al., in press.

percent in the same period. This growth can be expected to continue, but the growth in this sector generally does not involve skilled nursing personnel. In 1993, expenditures for home health care reached nearly $21 billion, (not including the $4 billion spent for care provided by hospital based home health care). Public financing accounted for nearly one-half of the expenditures for home health care (Levit et al., 1994).

Restructuring of the Nursing Home Industry

Nursing facilities, like other sectors of the health industry, are consolidating into larger health care organizations. Although not as rapidly and widespread as the hospital industry, the nursing homes are diversifying in the services they offer. HCIA and Arthur Andersen (1994) report that 23 of the 25 largest nursing home chains were involved in acquisitions in 1993. Nursing homes and chains are also forming integrated networks of services with hospitals, physicians, subacute care providers, home health care, and other relevant providers. Despite the recent movement toward consolidation within the industry, nursing home chains control only about 35 percent of the market and the 20 largest chains operate only 18 percent of the nursing home industry (HCIA and Arthur Andersen, 1994).

Many providers are developing their own home- and community-based divisions or affiliating with existing providers of those services. Approximately 4 percent of nursing facilities were offering these services in 1992. Nursing facilities are also expanding to cover services such as specialty care, rehabilitation, adult day care, assisted living, and respite care. Approximately 22 percent of all nursing facilities currently offer assisted living services. Some nursing homes are shifting from being primarily a place for custodial care to being facilities with residents receiving short-term rehabilitative care and other complex care requiring high technology such as ventilator-dependent patients discharged from the hospital who need subacute care skilled nursing services (AHCA, 1995).

Special Care Units

In the 1980s, special care units (SCU) emerged as an important intervention for care of persons with special needs, ranging from care requiring high technology to care for dementia. Increasing numbers of nursing facilities are shifting from traditional custodial long-term care to a more specialized level of care (AHCA, 1995). Today more than 1 in 10 nursing facilities have a special unit or program for people with dementia, with more than 1,500 SCUs.

By 1994, nearly 90,000 beds were dedicated to special care. Most of these beds are dedicated to residents with Alzheimer's disease or those needing special rehabilitation services. The most dramatic increase has been in ventilator care beds, from 3,162 in 1993 to 13,291 in 1994. Beds dedicated to special rehabilitative patients increased by 2000 and beds dedicated to AIDS patients grew by 2,300 between 1993 and 1994. Although there is much diversity among SCUs, most incorporate some type of physical modification, including security measures to limit egress, specialized activity programming for residents, and special training for staff, who are often permanently assigned to the unit. These units do not focus only on older adults in the later stages of life, but their development is fueled by Medicare's hospital PPS and other payers of health care (Lyles, 1986; Ganroth, 1988; Swan et al., 1990; AHCA, 1995).

Subacute Care Units

Nursing homes are also expanding to cover subacute care. Subacute care is increasingly becoming acceptable as an alternative to cost-effective health care delivery model. Subacute care units of nursing facilities are emerging in response to the need to provide care to patients who suffer from medical conditions or are recovering from surgical procedures and require a broad range of medical and rehabilitative services. More than 50 percent of nursing home admissions today come from hospitals, and most patients need care for unstable medical conditions. The subacute care option is favored by payers because nursing facilities generally can provide such care at lower cost than hospitals. Many subacute care programs are clinically and therapeutically comparable to the medical, surgical, and rehabilitation units of an acute care hospital, yet the cost of care in a subacute care unit is about 40 to 60 percent less than comparable care in an acute care setting. The higher reimbursement rate for subacute care is also attractive to nursing facilities. Although hospitals are ahead of nursing facilities in establishing subacute care units, several major nursing home chains are rapidly moving into this area. At the present time, more than 10 percent of nursing facilities offer some type of subacute care. Many more skilled nursing facilities and hospital-based skilled nursing units are developing and implementing subacute care programs. Today, more than 15,000 beds are dedicated for subacute care. Growth in subacute care is projected from $1 billion today to $10 billion by year 2000. (Stahl, 1995b).

Rules related to quality assessment and quality improvement, personnel requirements, and admissions practices have been set forth by the Joint Commission on Accreditation of Healthcare Organizations (JCAHO), which has recently incorporated subacute care into its survey process. Outcomes, physical plant, and physician credentials are three major areas addressed in JCAHO Accreditation Standards for Subacute Units (Stahl, 1995a).

IMPLICATIONS FOR NURSING SERVICES

The above narration is a brief overview of the rapid and perhaps fundamental changes occurring in the health care system and the movement toward a continuum of care. Redesign and reengineering have become principal strategies of the 1990s for many health care organizations. Institutional care—hospitals and nursing homes—and the personnel who provide the care are particularly affected.

Although the issues affecting the nursing home industry are somewhat different in kind and intensity from those in hospitals, they have not escaped the effects of the health care transition. Under sustained cost pressures, most states are expected to continue their efforts to limit the supply of nursing home beds, even though the bed supply in many states may not be keeping pace with the aging population. The challenge is to match staffing levels and skills to the changing characteristics of the residents.

The focus of care is shifting. The emphasis is no longer on inpatient hospital care; rather, hospitalization is viewed as one event in a patient-based continuum of care. Health care providers, physicians, and nursing staff are increasingly called upon to change the way they deliver patient care. The model has changed to care delivered across a continuum, not focused on a particular episode of hospitalization, through the use of teams, case managers, and protocols. All these efforts have led to changes in the nursing delivery patterns developed mostly over the last two decades for organizing the delivery of nursing care in hospitals. Such a major transformation of the health care environment cannot be accomplished successfully without support of the nursing professions and without changes in management and governance structures (Shortell et al., 1995; VHA, 1995).

Changes that affect any single part of the health care sector will have implications for the work of nursing personnel and the outcomes expected from their respective contributions. Clearly, given that there are more than 3 million nursing personnel, the number of interactions they have with others in the system is potentially limitless and, therefore, of great relevance.

The transformation of hospitals, nursing homes, and other health care organizations will continue to grow as organizations expand their search for solutions to issues brought about by reform and change in an environment that is increasingly drawn toward delivery of less costly and noninstitutional care. Just as the hospital of the future will serve only very sick patients requiring highly complex care, the nursing home of tomorrow will also serve patients with serious disabilities and with rehabilitative and other subacute care needs. The rest of the population will increasingly receive care in outpatient units, home- and community-based settings, assisted living facilities, and similar settings.

4

Nursing Personnel in a Time of Change

The previous chapter has portrayed an evolving health care system, driven by the need for cost-effectiveness under continued pressures of cost containment and competition. The aging and increasing diversity of the U.S. population and the projected growth of the oldest old will have a major impact in the years ahead on the demand and supply of health services and the level and type of resources needed to provide those services. Nursing personnel are an integral component of the health care delivery system and, therefore, they are most directly affected by these changes.

As discussed in Chapter 3, the structure, organization, and financing of health care is rapidly changing, leading to a shift in the delivery of health care from the inpatient hospital setting to communities and outpatient care. These changes have led to redesign of staffing patterns, and the organization of care in hospitals. They also are downsizing and engaging in various patterns of substitution of personnel to accommodate the reduced volume of inpatient care and to stay economically competitive and viable. Although the volume of inpatient care has declined, patients entering the hospital are sicker than in previous years and, as a consequence, the intensity of care required has increased.

Staffing in nursing homes has improved slightly since the passage of the Nursing Home Reform Act of 1987 (see Chapter 6 for an elaboration of this subject). Nevertheless, the chronic problems of the limited presence of professional nursing at the bedside in nursing homes continue and take on added importance in the current state of transition in the health care system. Most of the direct care in nursing homes has been, and continues to be, provided by nurse assistants.

The implications of the trends identified above for the nursing workforce are profound, both in terms of numbers and in terms of adequate distribution of the skills and educational preparation of the workforce. Determination of the adequacy of the nursing workforce (registered nurses, licensed practical nurses, and nurse assistants) in the institutional health service settings that are within the scope of this inquiry calls for an assessment of the overall supply of nursing personnel in the context of the shifting demand for their services and the factors affecting such demand.

This chapter provides a brief overview of the supply of nursing personnel and their employment trends. It examines the adequacy of the quantity and comments on the educational preparation of the supply, given the changing demands for nursing services. The chapter concludes by briefly commenting on the implications for nursing personnel as the nation approaches the next century, and offers a commentary on the kinds of knowledge and skills needed in the nursing workforce to provide effective nursing care in the future.

SUPPLY OF NURSING PERSONNEL

Nursing personnel for purposes of this study include registered nurses (RN), licensed practical nurses, (LPN), and nurse assistants (NA).[1] Approximately 3 million health care personnel in the United States work in nursing (HRSA, 1992).

RNs and LPNs are subject to state licensing requirements. Although all RNs take the same licensing examination to qualify for practice, they are prepared through 1 of 3 educational pathways that can take 2, 3, or 4 years of training. This diversity in training requirements is a matter of considerable controversy within the nursing profession. All RNs are not alike in terms of basic and advanced clinical education and skills; their responsibilities may range from the provision of direct patient care at the staff level, to management and direction of complex nursing care systems in the institutional and community settings, as well as to teaching and other academic functions.

LPNs primarily provide direct patient care in institutional settings under the direction of a physician or an RN. Nurse assistants and other ancillary nursing

---

[1]Ancillary nursing personnel, nursing support personnel, assistive personnel, nurse extenders, unlicensed nursing personnel, multi-competent workers, nurse assistants, or aides are all generic terms used to refer to the various clinical and nonclinical jobs that augment nursing care. This group of employees includes an array of support nursing personnel including certified nurse assistants, orderlies, operating room technicians, home health aides, and others. They assist the licensed nurse by performing routine duties in caring for patients under the supervision of an RN or an LPN. Although Congress defined "nurse" for the purposes of this study to include RN, LPN, and NA, it has not been possible at all times to disaggregate information on NAs from the remaining support personnel since national statistics are often collected and/or tabulated for the group as a whole. For example, the American Hospital Association does not separate information on nurse assistants from that on other "ancillary nursing personnel." Throughout this report, the term ancillary nursing personnel will be used for this group of staff when nurse assistants cannot be disaggregated.

personnel assist licensed nurses in the provision of basic care to patients, and they work under the supervision of licensed nursing personnel (ICONS, 1993).

At this time, no uniform standards exist for training, competency evaluation, and certification for nurse assistants to qualify for work in all health care settings. Since the implementation of the 1987 Nursing Home Reform Act, nurse assistants employed in nursing facilities, who provide most of the direct care to residents, have to be certified and are required to take a minimum of 75 hours of training within 4 months of employment and be tested for competency in order to be certified to work in nursing facilities. No comparable standard exists for work in hospitals. There appears to be wide variations among hospitals in the level of training provided to this group of nursing staff. For example, in a study of California hospitals, Barter and colleagues (1994) found that the average ancillary personnel in a hospital may receive less than a month of combined classroom and on-the-job training, ranging from less than 1 week to 3 weeks. (See Chapters 5 and 6 for further discussion of NA training.)

Hospitals are the major employers of nursing personnel (RNs, LPNs, and NAs). Many LPNs and nurse assistants also work in nursing homes and other long-term care (LTC) settings, as well as in ambulatory care settings and home health care service. With the exception of hospitals, detailed national data are not readily available on the employment patterns of nursing personnel. Most of the national databases focus on RNs.[2]   The last comprehensive national sample survey of LPNs, comparable to the periodic National Sample Survey of Registered Nurses, was conducted by the U.S. Public Health Service in 1983. Some information on LPNs, however, can be gleaned from data available from the Bureau of the Census of the U.S. Department of Commerce, the Bureau of Labor Statistics (BLS) of the Department of Labor, the National League for Nursing (NLN), and individual LPN programs. Data on nurse assistants are limited to basic employment-related statistics specific to the employment setting and some aggregate data from the employment statistics published by the BLS. Hence, the discussion in this chapter unavoidably is heavily weighted toward supply and demand issues affecting RNs.

Registered Nurses

RNs are the largest group of health care providers in the United States. For several decades, their numbers have been continually increasing in absolute num-

---

[2]National databases available for nursing workforce supply and demand include the National Sample Survey of Registered Nurses, data from the National Center for Health Statistics, the American Hospital Association (AHA) Annual Surveys of Hospitals, AHA Nursing Personnel Surveys, monthly employment statistics compiled by the Bureau of Labor Statistics, and national data on nursing school enrollment and graduations collected by the National League for Nursing.

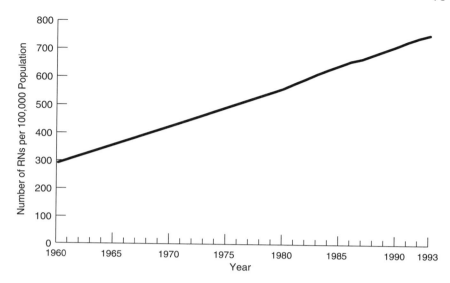

FIGURE 4.1   Estimated active supply of registered nurses (RN) per 100,000 population, United States, 1960–1993. SOURCE: OASH, 1994.

bers and in relation to the population being served, suggesting that the periodic shortages of nurses that the nation has experienced are driven more by increases in demand than by a reduction in quantity. Public policies to alleviate the perceived shortages have focused almost exclusively on developing and funding programs for rapid increases in the supply of nurses, rather than addressing and understanding the issues leading to the recurring shortages, the reasons for the increased demand, and the types and educational mix of the nursing workforce needed and available to meet the changing demand (Aiken, 1995).

In 1992, more than 2.2 million persons held licenses to practice as RNs (Moses, 1994). This number represents an increase of 35 percent since 1980 and a growth of nearly 50,000 per year from 1984 to 1992 (OASH, 1994). In 1960, the nurse-to-population ratio was 292 per 100,000 population, increasing to 560 by 1980, and going up to 755 per 100,000 population by 1993[3] (unpublished estimates from HRSA) (see Figure 4.1).

Between 1983 and 1993, employment of RNs grew more than twice as fast as employment in the economy as a whole (BLS, 1995c) (see Table 4.1).   An estimated 1.8 million of the 2.2 million RNs were employed in nursing positions

---

[3]In the early years almost all care in hospitals was rendered by students of nursing. During the 1960s the hospitals began to gradually phase out their dependence on student nurses for direct care services, which may explain the increase in RN hospital employment in the early 1960s.

TABLE 4.1 Number of Full-Time and Part-Time Employees in Nursing Occupations, United States, Selected Years, 1983–1993

Occupation	Year					Percent Change 1983–1993
	1983	1990	1991	1992	1993	
Total, all occupations	92,586	111,509	110,340	110,746	112,312	21.3
Registered nurse	1,287	1,700	1,756	1,820	1,887	46.6
Licensed practical nurse	576	635	629	654	679	17.9
Nurse assistant	1,116	1,234	1,227	1,308	1,343	20.3

SOURCE: Bureau of Labor Statistics, Industry-Occupation Matrix.

in 1992, an employment rate of nearly 83 percent (Moses, 1994). This compares with about 66 percent for the total U.S. labor force and almost 59 percent for the female labor force (Bureau of the Census, 1995a). Most RNs are women; in 1992 only about 4 percent of the employed RNs were men. Although very small in numbers, the rate of growth since 1988 among men has been faster than among women (Moses, 1994).

Of the 17 percent of RNs who were not working in nursing in 1992, slightly more than 1 percent were actively seeking employment in nursing. The largest portion of those not employed in nursing was not actively looking for jobs in nursing and had not worked in nursing for at least 5 years. Moreover, more than half of those not employed in nursing were 60 years of age and older (Moses, 1994).[4]

Unemployment rates for RNs were slightly higher in 1994 than they had been for a number of years. Nevertheless, the rates have been consistently lower than the average of 2.5 percent for all professional occupations and 2.9 percent for teachers. Table 4.2 shows trends in unemployment rates for nursing personnel.

Characteristics of RNs

Age Composition of RNs   The average age of RNs in 1992 was 43.1 years, representing a continuing increase in average age since 1980. Although some of this increase is to be expected because of the overall aging of the U.S. labor force,

---

[4]Most of the data on nurse supply presented here are from the 1992 National Sample Survey of Registered Nurses and its predecessor surveys. For a detailed description of the registered nurse supply, the reader is referred to the reports of these surveys. These surveys are conducted periodically by the Division of Nursing of the U. S. Public Health Service under Section 951 of P.L. 94-63. The last comprehensive national sample survey of registered nurses was conducted in March 1992.

TABLE 4.2 Unemployment Rates, Nursing and Other Selected Occupations, United States, Selected Years, 1983–1994

Occupation	Year					
	1983	1990	1991	1992	1993	1994
Total, all occupations	8.6	5.0	6.0	6.7	6.1	5.7
Licensed practical nurses[a]	5.3	1.7	1.8	2.0	2.2	3.3
Nurse aides[a]	10.8	6.8	6.7	8.0	7.8	8.0
Registered nurses[a]	1.6	1.1	1.2	1.1	1.3	1.5
Professional workers	3.0	1.9	2.4	2.6	2.6	2.5
Teachers[b]	2.9	1.9	1.9	2.1	2.1	2.3

[a]Does not include labor force participants who were actively seeking work but had no previous work experience in that occupation.
[b]Does not include college and university teachers.

SOURCE: Current Population Survey, special tabulations.

the proportion of RNs who are 35 years of age and older increased more than the proportion of workers in all occupations who were 35 and older. Only 11 percent of the RNs were under 30 years of age in 1992, compared with 15 percent in 1980. If current trends continue, by the year 2000 only about 7 percent will be under 30 years. As can be seen from Figure 4.2, by the year 2000 the nursing workforce will be older than it is today; nearly 70 percent of the RNs will be 40 years of age or older and 34 percent will be 50 years or older.[5] This aging of the RN workforce can have serious implications for an increasingly demanding hospital nursing practice. It also reduces the ability of the RN to perform certain physical tasks. By starting later in life, lifetime years of service also are truncated.

The age at which persons enter nursing, the characteristics of persons taking the basic education preparation for nursing, and other personal factors, can all factor into the rising age of RNs. The average age at which persons enter nursing practice (that is, the age at graduation) has been increasing for each type of RN entry program. The average age at graduations was 30 years in 1992 compared to 23 years in 1988. In 1992, many of the RNs had worked as LPNs or NAs or had worked in a health care occupation immediately prior to entering a basic nurse education program. Twenty-nine percent of RNs in 1992 had worked in a health care occupation immediately prior to entering a nursing education program. The

[5]These projections are routinely developed by the Division of Nursing of the U.S. Public Health Service and currently are being revised, taking into account assumptions based on the most recent data available.

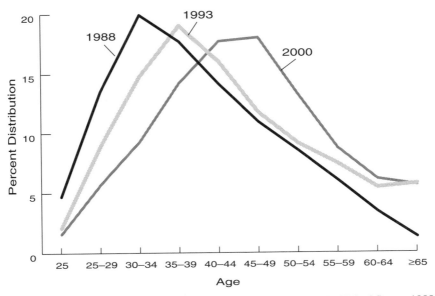

FIGURE 4.2   Age distribution of employed registered nurses (RN), United States, 1988, 1993, and 2000. SOURCE: Moses, 1990, 1994.

majority of this group, 63 percent, had worked as NAs, and nearly 29 percent had worked as LPNs. This group of persons, particularly those who had worked as LPNs, tends to take the educational path of the 2-year associate degree (AD) program (Moses, 1994).

A number of persons are entering professional nursing practice for the first time who have a post-high school degree, and sometimes work experience, in a different field. This number has increased in recent years. The implications of this increase in the number of second-career nurses in the workforce is yet to be fully experienced.

Educational Preparation of RNs

According to the 1992 National Sample Survey of Registered Nurses, 31 percent of employed nurses in all health care settings had a baccalaureate degree in nursing, 31 percent had an AD in nursing, and 30 percent were graduates of diploma programs. Between 1980 and 1992, RNs with ADs in nursing showed the greatest increase; RNs with baccalaureates also showed a substantial growth. Two-thirds of all employed nurses were in staff positions in hospitals. The majority of employed RNs providing direct patient care in noninstitutional settings had less than a baccalaureate degree. For all health care settings taken together, in 1992 half of the top managers and 60 percent of the midlevel manag-

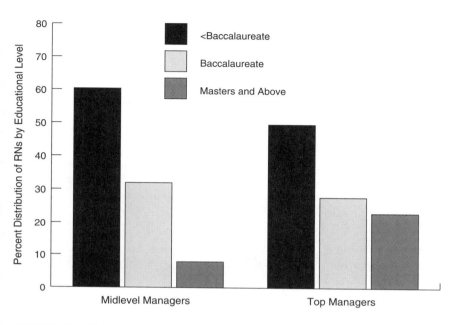

FIGURE 4.3   Highest educational preparation of registered nurses (RN), United States, 1992. SOURCE: OASH, 1994.

ers in nursing had less than a baccalaureate degree (Moses, 1994; OASH, 1994) (see Figure 4.3). Many experts have expressed concern that the continuing trend toward associate degrees may result in a nursing workforce that does not have the knowledge and skills necessary to meet the demand for broad-based skills that will occur in a restructured health care system.

The total number of nursing education programs that prepare RNs has remained around 1,493 during the past decade. In 1993, there were 507 baccalaureate programs, 857 associate degree programs, and 129 diploma programs. Enrollment has been increasing in the basic nursing programs since its low point in 1987, especially in the AD and the basic baccalaureate programs. The number of students who graduate is also increasing. Between 1992 and 1993 the rate of increase was 9.0 percent. This rate is down from nearly 12 percent between 1991 and 1993. In terms of absolute numbers, AD programs are graduating almost twice the number of baccalaureate and diploma graduating students combined (OASH, 1994). However, the rate of growth in graduations from AD programs from 1992 to 1993 is slightly lower than the rate for 1991 to 1992 (See Table 2.12 in Part II of this report). Figure 4.4 shows the trend in graduations by type of basic nursing education programs. The number of new graduates represents the potential increase in nurse supply. With the current increase in basic baccalaureate enrollment, graduations from these programs should increase in the future.

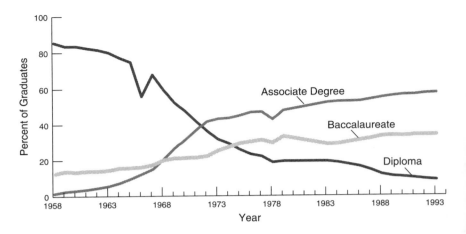

FIGURE 4.4   Percent of registered nurse graduates by type of educational program, United States, 1958–1993. SOURCE: National League for Nursing, Nursing Datasource: Trends in Contemporary Nursing Education, 1981–1994.

Data from NLN for 1994 indicate that graduates from basic nursing educational programs in the academic year 1993-1994 totaled 94,870, an increase of 7.6 percent over the 88,149 graduates in 1992-1993. While increases over the previous year were noted for all three types of programs, the baccalaureate programs showed a far larger increase than associate degree and diploma programs— 18.3 percent. Total first-time enrollments for the academic year 1993-1994 also showed some increase over the prior academic year. The total first-time enrollments were 129,897, 2.4 percent more than the 126,837 in 1992-1993 (NLN, 1995).

Total enrollment for the fall of 1994, however, decreased. As of October 1, 1994, 268,350 students were enrolled in basic nursing educational programs, compared to 270,228 in 1993. Baccalaureate program enrollments showed a 1.8 percent increase, from 110,693 in the fall of 1993 to 112,659 in 1994. Total enrollment in both AD and diploma programs declined.

Licensed Practical Nurses

In the health care delivery system, the LPN provides a level of service between the NA and the RN. Their scope of practice does not allow LPNs to assess and formally plan for care. The 12- to 18-month preparation period focuses primarily on skills such as basic bedside nursing in order to provide direct care under the supervision of an RN.

About 1,100 programs prepare students for licensing as LPNs. The vast

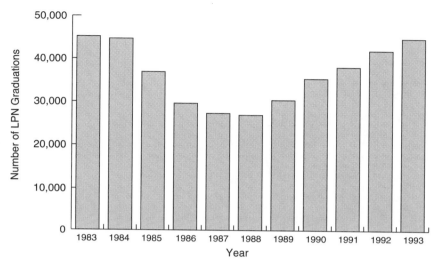

FIGURE 4.5   Number of licensed practical nurse (LPN) graduations, United States, 1983–1993. SOURCE: NLN, 1994b.

majority of these programs are supported by public funding. This funding is very similar to that for AD programs, where 88 percent were publicly funded, compared to 51 percent of basic baccalaureate programs for RNs and 23 percent of diploma programs. Most of the LPN programs are administered by technical or vocational schools. More than two-thirds of the programs in the West were found in junior or community colleges. These are typically 12 months in length (NLN, 1994b).

Annual admissions reached 60,749 in 1993, an increase of 4.3 percent from 1992, and the highest number of admissions in 10 years. Again, LPN admissions were second only to admissions to AD programs. The data also reflect an increase in number of graduations for the fifth consecutive year (see Figure 4.5).

LPNs are the second-largest group of licensed health caregivers in the United States; only RNs are greater in number. They work in hospitals, nursing facilities, home health care, public health and school health clinics, the military, and prisons. Approximately 679,000 LPNs are employed throughout the health care industry, with 262,000 employed in hospitals and 182,110 in nursing facilities (BLS, 1995c). (See Table 4.3 and Table 2.15 in Part II of this report.)   In the hospital setting, the LPN functions primarily under the direct supervision of an RN. The LPN employed in the nursing home setting often serves in the capacity of charge nurse.   Primary responsibilities include supervising the care being provided by NAs, passing medications and doing treatments, and directly monitoring resident conditions.   In either case, the LPN functions under the direction

TABLE 4.3 Number of Full-Time and Part-Time Employees in Hospitals and Nursing Homes, United States, Selected Years, 1988–1994

Health Care Setting	Year				Percent Change 1988–1994
	1988	1990	1992	1994	
Hospital					
Registered nurse	1,039,901	1,114,220	1,201,650	1,203,161	15.70
Licensed practical nurse	290,780	279,775	261,909	262,238	−9.82
Nurse assistant	290,070	300,590	305,624	306,009	5.49
Nursing home					
Registered nurse	86,735	93,121	96,740	109,146	25.84
Licensed practical nurse	136,662	147,667	160,663	182,116	33.26
Nurse assistant	553,420	595,018	639,161	643,080	16.20

SOURCE: Bureau of Labor Statistics, Industry-Occupation Matrix.

of an RN responsible for assessment. The LPN may also serve as the person implementing care as directed in the patient's care plan. According to a survey of newly licensed LPNs, 39 percent work in hospitals and 49 percent work in long-term care facilities. This is in contrast to newly licensed RNs whose first place of employment is overwhelmingly the hospital (NLN, 1994a).

As seen in Table 4.3, LPN employment in hospitals has been declining. At the same time, LPN employment grew slightly in other industries, particularly in long-term care and home health care settings (BLS, 1995c).

Nurse Assistants

The Bureau of Labor Statistics estimates that in 1994, there were approximately 1,259,100 persons working as nurse assistants or aides in the United States. Of these, 306,000 were employed in hospitals and 643,080 in nursing homes. Unemployment rates for nurse assistants were much higher than for LPNs and RNs. Tables 4.1, 4.2 and 4.3 show trends in the employment of NAs in hospitals and nursing homes from 1983 to 1994.

About 17 percent of the nurse assistants are less than 25 years of age and 44 percent are 35 to 54 years old. The proportion of NAs who are black has not changed much over the years; 29 percent of NAs are black compared to 10 percent of RNs and 19 percent of LPNs. Nearly 18 percent of the NAs had not graduated from high school, and about one-half (46 percent) had a high school diploma. The educational level of NAs working in nursing homes is lower than that of NAs working in hospitals (BLS, 1995c).

CHANGING DEMAND FOR NURSING PERSONNEL

Employment Settings

Hospitals

The hospital has been, and still is, the first place of employment for the majority of RNs. Most of the increases in RN supply over the years have been absorbed by hospitals, where historically about two-thirds of the RNs have worked. Hospitals employed 874,000 RNs in 1993 compared with 698,000 in 1983[6] (see Table 2.9 in Part II of this report). As stated earlier, the number of RNs employed in hospitals began to increase rapidly following the advent of Medicare in the 1960s and the consequent expansion of the hospital sector. It has continued to grow ever since. As mentioned in Chapter 3, after implementation of the Prospective Payment System (PPS) for Medicare patients, hospital employment levels in the initial years declined along with associated declines in inpatient occupancy rates and discharge rates and a reduction in the average length of stay (HRSA, 1993).

By 1986, however, despite continued decline in inpatient use, hospital staffing began to rise, especially for more highly trained workers. At the same time that hospitals were reducing their nonnursing staff, RN employment continued to increase (HRSA, 1993) (see Figure 4.6). Hospitals began to restructure the composition of the nursing workforce, often substituting RNs for LPNs and other patient care personnel. The increased demand for RNs in large part resulted from a substitution of RNs for LPNs, NAs, and other patient services personnel. Several factors contributed to this continued demand for RNs while other hospital employment was decreasing. Some have suggested that more RNs were needed because of the changing inpatient case-mix after PPS was implemented. Patients who entered the hospital were sicker than in previous years and the average length of stay was shorter, increasing the need for more highly trained workers to administer the procedures, treatments, and care needed. Since 1980, hospitals have increased staffed beds in intensive care units to allow for the increased acuity of the patients. However, Aiken and Hadley (1988), using regression analysis, found that the additional requirement for RNs resulting from more patients in ICUs was offset by the reduced inpatient caseload.

The changing case-mix of inpatients was not the only factor affecting increased employment of RNs, given the magnitude of the increase in RN employ-

---

[6]The number of RNs employed in hospitals does not include those RNs more appropriately reported in other occupational categories, such as nurse administrators. The AHA data are not disaggregated according to inpatient, outpatient, and other departments.

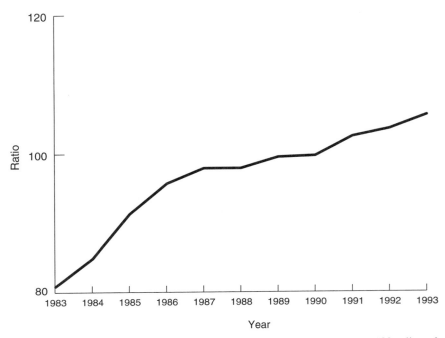

FIGURE 4.6   Ratio of registered nurse full-time-equivalents (FTE) per 100 adjusted average daily census, United States, 1983–1993. SOURCE: American Hospital Association, Annual Surveys, 1983–1993, special tabulations.

ment relative to the patient caseload. The RNs' relative wages during the 1970s and early 1980s also explains the hospitals moving toward a reduced workforce with a richer nursing mix. The widespread substitution of RNs was feasible because the wage difference between LPNs and RNs during the 1970s had narrowed and by the 1980s the average LPN salary was 73 percent of the RN salary (Aiken and Hadley, 1988). This difference was not large enough to be a disincentive for the substitution of RNs, considering that the LPN's scope of practice is more limited and they need supervision by RNs.

Hospitals have increased the aggregate numbers of RNs employed as well as the ratio of RNs to patients. By 1993, around 874,000 RNs were employed in community hospitals throughout the country. Although this number reflects a continuing increase over previous years in the total number of RNs employed and in the number of RNs as a percentage of the total nursing staff (67.5 percent), the rate of increase between 1992 and 1993 was lower than in previous years. (Wide variations reflecting local conditions are noted in the rate of growth across the country.) The annual rate of growth between 1992 and 1993 in the aggregate

TABLE 4.4 Percent Change in Nurse Staffing in Community Hospitals, United States, 1994–1995

	Percent Change Quarter Ending March 1994–1995
Total FTE personnel	−1.6
Total FTE nursing personnel	2.7
FTE RNs	3.5
FTE LPNs	−1.2

NOTE: FTE = full-time-equivalent.

SOURCE: American Hospital Association, National Hospital Panel Surveys, March Panel, 1994, 1995, preliminary, unpublished data.

numbers of RNs employed as well as the ratio of RNs to patients showed some signs of slowing down (see Table 2.9 in Part II of this report).

However, preliminary unpublished data from AHA's National Hospital Panel Surveys comparing the first quarters of 1994 and 1995 show a substantial percentage increase between 1994 and 1995 in the employment of RNs in hospitals, along with an increase in inpatient admissions (see Table 4.4).

Shift in Service Settings

Although the majority of nurses continue to work in hospitals, major shifts in nursing are taking place as a result of continuing cost pressures, the growth of managed care, and scientific and technological advances. As discussed in Chapter 3, the focus of health care is shifting away from nursing at the hospital bedside to nursing at the patient's side in a continuum of care (see Figure 4.7). The 1992 National Sample Survey of Registered Nurses found a greater number and proportion of RNs working in a variety of settings, notably ambulatory care, than in previous years. The largest increase in the rate of growth between 1988 and 1992 was in the outpatient areas. The rate of growth was about 15 percent for RNs working in community and public health settings. The growth in this service sector is largely due to the growth in home health care. Ambulatory care accounted for an 8 percent increase in the RN workforce. Even within the hospital setting, nurse employment in outpatient departments grew much faster than in inpatient units (Moses, 1994). The increase in employment in outpatient departments of hospitals is not surprising because outpatient admissions show a substantial growth. Despite this increase, however, in absolute terms the largest numbers of RNs by far are still working in inpatient settings of hospitals.

Although opportunities for the employment of RNs in settings other than the

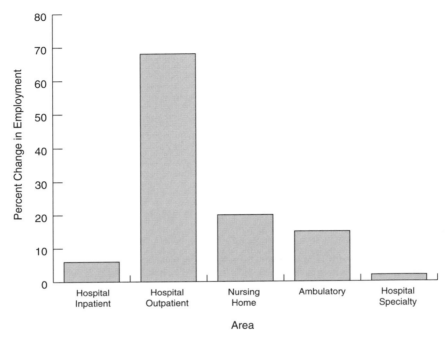

FIGURE 4.7   Percent change in registered nurse employment in selected areas, United States, 1988–1992. SOURCE: OASH, 1994.

hospital have grown in recent years, the absolute number of RNs employed in hospitals has continued to increase. Despite reports of layoffs and downsizing in hospitals and increases in other service settings, hospitals continue to be the first place of employment for a majority of nurses. Over the years the majority of newly licensed nurses have worked in hospitals. This trend continued in 1994, although there was a decline compared to previous years. A national survey of over 61,000 newly licensed RNs conducted in the spring of 1994 by the NLN found that 81 percent of newly licensed nurses were employed in staff positions in hospitals compared to over 90 percent in 1992, and 92 percent in 1990. The 1994 NLN survey also showed that the proportion of newly licensed RNs employed in nursing facilities was rising—11 percent compared to 5 percent in 1992. These results indicate a shift in the first place of employment for RNs, but they have little impact on the total supply of employed RNs; newly licensed nurses represent about 4 percent of the total employed RN workforce (NLN, 1994c; personal communications with E. Moses, Division of Nursing, Public Health Service).

Nursing Homes

Recent data suggest that there might be a slight increase in RNs in nursing facilities. In 1992, nursing homes accounted for about 7 percent of the RN workforce, up from 6.6 percent in 1988 (Moses, 1990; 1994). This increase may be a result of several factors, including the 1987 Nursing Home Reform Act, which requires 24-hour coverage by licensed nursing personnel; the growth of subacute care and special care; and more recently possibly, the reported down-sizing and layoffs of RNs in hospitals. Most of these relatively small numbers of RNs working full time in nursing homes do not provide direct nursing care. More than 87 percent of RNs working full time in nursing homes serve as head nurse, assistant head nurse, director of nursing, or assistant director of nursing. Yet most RNs in nursing homes were prepared in a diploma or AD program. The highest nursing-related education for the majority of RNs working in nursing homes was a 3-year diploma program. Less than 3 percent of the RNs working in nursing homes had their master's degree in 1992. RNs working with the elderly tend to be older than the average RN, with a median age of 45 years, and the majority had been working in the profession for 10 years or more (Moses, 1994).

Given the projected growth of the elderly population, long-term care would appear to be an area for growth in RN employment. With the emergence of rehabilitative services in nursing homes and an increasingly complex case-mix, the need for professional nursing is much greater now, and will be in the years ahead, than ever before. It is unlikely, however, that the country will witness any major movement of experienced RNs from hospitals to nursing facilities. As long as long-term care is almost totally dependent on public and out-of-pocket financing, the current paucity of RNs employed in nursing homes will likely continue for fiscal reasons and because of pay differentials between the RNs employed in hospitals and nursing homes.

Implications of Current Trends

The trends in RN employment discussed above suggest that a continuation of the current trend toward reductions in inpatient hospitalization rates and hospital occupancy rates could have important implications for the employment of RNs in inpatient hospital settings. The full impact of these and of further changes that will be brought about by the continued rapid restructuring of the health care system and the growth of managed care may not have been fully felt yet. The relatively small proportion of the total number of RNs employed in settings other than hospitals, even with the recent dramatic growth in those other settings, also means that very large proportional increases in these employment opportunities would have to take place in order to absorb even a modest decline in hospital employment (Yordy, in press). Moreover, some groups of RNs are likely to be disproportionately affected. Researchers in the field have questioned whether the educational preparation, experience, and skills of many hospital-based staff nurses can be applied in other settings without substantial retraining (Aiken, 1994; McBride, Part II of this report[7]).

As stated earlier in this chapter, a consequence of the reductions in inpatient admissions and lengths of stay is the increasing complexity of care of inpatients. Such changes have implications for nursing resource requirements. The increased acuity of patients, combined with shortened lengths of stay and technologically driven services, would suggest a need for high ratio of RNs per patient, and this appears to have been the trend until now (AHA, 1995a,b). At the same time, hospitals will not be able to continue to absorb ever-increasing numbers of RNs.

Although hospital employment has continued to grow, some have expressed concern that in recent years most of the growth has been in the nonclinical areas. Anderson and Kohn (in press) examined trends in hospital employment in the period 1981 to 1993. The authors define clinical staff to include all professional staff, nursing staff, technicians, and trainees. Nonclinical staff includes all administrative staff, including administrators, assistant administrators, and medical records administrators, and other personnel who do not fit into the clinical category. Using the Medicare case-mix index as a proxy for adjusting for changing case-mix, they found that employment growth in hospitals during the period of the study increased more rapidly in the nonclinical areas than in the clinical areas. They found no statistically significant difference in the employment growth in states with high and low penetration by health maintenance organization, nor in states with and without all-payer ratesetting programs.

Anderson and Kohn (in press) state that the results must be viewed with caution as the data are not adjusted for the differences in hospital output. The hospital product has changed during the study period, and some of the expansion of the administrative staff may have resulted from responses to the changing health care environment, such as marketing for managed care contracts and developing networks and staff needed for new technology. However, the precise extent of changes in nursing and nonnursing resource requirements cannot be reliably estimated from available data. Likewise, the cumulative effect of such changes may differ when compared across all diagnosis-related groups (DRG) and for non-Medicare patients. Medicare case-mix is only an approximation of the change and it is not clear how much of the annual change in the index is due to real case-mix complexity and how much is a result of increased sensitivity of these measures. Moreover, ProPAC (1995), in its analysis of the annual case-mix change, reported that the total real case-mix and the within-DRG case com-

---

[7]The Institute of Medicine (IOM) committee commissioned this paper from Angela McBride. The committee appreciates her contributions. The full text of the paper can be found in Part II of this report.

plexity change for PPS admissions has been decreasing over time (from 1.8 percent in 1987 to 1.0 percent in 1995 and from 0.5 percent in 1987 to 0.2 percent in 1995, respectively). In addition, the shift of less complex cases to the outpatient setting has slowed, reducing increases in the complexity of hospitalized patients.

Salaries

"Nursing has long ignored the obvious point made by economists that high salaries and continued high growth in new jobs are not compatible trends over the long run" (Aiken and Salmon, 1994, p. 319). After a period of low wages in the 1970s and early 1980s, RN salaries have been increasing in recent years. Under continuing pressures to reduce costs, the demand is showing some signs of a slow down. RN salaries rose an average of 33 percent (adjusted for inflation) from 1980 to 1992 (OASH, 1994).[8] Earnings of RNs grew faster than overall earnings in the economy from 1987 through 1992 (see Figure 4.8).

In 1992, the average annual salary for RNs employed on a full-time basis was $37,738. This increase occurred at a time when growth in real incomes for many Americans had stagnated or declined. Nurses in staff-level positions earned an annual average salary of $35,212. Wide variations were noted across geographic areas, ranging from more than $41,000 on the Pacific area, to about $31,500 in the Midwest. Nurses with specialized training earn substantially more than the average. Nurse anesthetists earned on average more than $76,000 in 1992, and nurse practitioners and nurse midwives earned $44,000 a year (Moses, 1994). These increases in salary levels may have also attracted more people to the field of nursing in recent years.

Labor costs account for a major proportion of hospital costs. When hospitals face pressures to cut costs, the usual target is labor. Increasing salary levels, combined with the increasing size of the RN workforce, have made RN employment a large and expensive cost center in the health care system. It would not be surprising then, in the current environment of cost containment, if RNs have become a target for cost cutting. Hospitals are reported to have restructured patient services and staffing, reducing RNs as a proportion of total nursing personnel and increasing the employment of ancillary nursing personnel (SEIU, 1993; ANA, 1995a). The committee heard from many RNs and received testimony suggesting that cost reductions are being achieved through RN layoffs, attrition, productivity increases with fewer staff doing more, substitution of lower-cost personnel, or a combination of the above.

Yordy (in press) suggests that under these circumstances, RNs may have to

---

[8]These figures are averages across all settings. Nursing home salaries are lower than the average and lower than the salaries for hospitals. See Chapter 6 for elaboration of the issue.

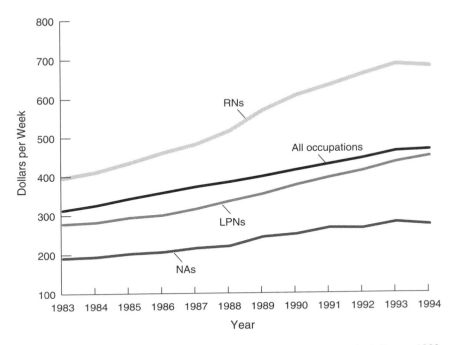

FIGURE 4.8   Median weekly earnings of nursing occupations, United States, 1983–1994. NOTE: LPN = licensed practical nurse; NA = nurse assistant; RN = registered nurse. Earnings are for wage and salaried workers who usually work year-round full time. There was a change in the survey beginning in 1994. SOURCE: Bureau of Labor Statistics, Current Population Surveys.

make choices and trade-offs with regard to future salary demands and job security. They may have to choose lower salaries or increased productivity with fewer jobs. The committee, however, heard many complaints from RNs employed in hospitals that they are already stressed by overwork because of reduced staff. If that is an accurate portrayal of the situation in hospitals, then one of the choices mentioned above disappears, at least for RNs employed in inpatient hospital service.

A major determining factor in hiring a worker is the cost of hiring that worker compared to the alternatives. In a cost-competitive system, persons with the lowest level of training who can do the job are employed, under the assumption that higher training leads to greater compensation. This could mean that nurses with less training are losing positions in the inpatient hospital sector to nurse assistants and other ancillary nursing personnel, while those with advanced training may be able to find new opportunities.

IS THE SUPPLY ADEQUATE FOR THE
DEMANDS OF THE NEXT CENTURY?

As discussed in Chapter 5, in the years ahead RNs will be called upon to fill roles that will require increased professional judgment, supervision and direction of work of others, management of complex systems that span the traditional boundaries of service settings, and clinical autonomy. Clearly a strong education base will be required to provide RNs with the needed preparation for their expected future roles in various settings.

In the future, the RN's role will likely involve greater responsibility for patient care and the management of complex systems of care that span the boundaries of institutions. Career opportunities will open in health promotion and clinical decision making as nursing moves toward community-centered practice.

Hospitals are no longer bastions of acute care, with only inpatient units devoted singularly to the care of the ill. They are increasingly a part of a larger network of services. Thinking, acting, and planning for the continuum of services are critical in today's hospital environment, calling for a workforce that is prepared to provide services in a proactive, highly competent, and holistic manner.

Continuation of the trend toward reductions in hospital inpatient admissions and the corresponding shift of employment to ambulatory and community care settings raise questions about the adequacy of educational preparation of future RNs. The baccalaureate degree curriculum has included the necessary training for practice in ambulatory and public health and other community settings as well as clinical experience. Hence, it has long been held as the standard credential for practice in those settings (Aiken, 1994; see McBride, Part II of this report). Demand for RNs to practice in ambulatory care and community-based settings will increase.

Likewise, not all nursing homes today are single-focus settings taking care of chronically ill patients who require mostly custodial care. These settings, once nearly forgotten in most serious discussions about health care, are now becoming the hospital substitute for much of the traditional acute care patient population. With an increased emphasis on providing subacute care as well as rehabilitative care, nursing homes are attempting to provide transitional institutional services that, in the past, would have been provided in the acute care inpatient setting.

Thus, in each of these care settings, consideration needs to be given to the effectiveness of the current workforce for the future. Changes such as those described above and elsewhere in this report require a full examination of the education and skills needed by those delivering care and services. This is not simply an issue of redeploying workers from one setting to another; the required knowledge and skills differ.

These scenarios raise serious concerns about the growing community college nursing programs designed to prepare nurses primarily for inpatient staff positions. In the future, RNs' roles will require that they exercise more professional judgment and clinical autonomy. In order for RNs to function effectively in a boundary-spanning, interdisciplinary health care system, they will require a new approach to the basic educational preparation of future RNs and some fundamental retraining of those adversely affected by hospital downsizing.

There is general agreement in the nursing community, and within health care in general, that workforce needs and projections for the future must be evaluated. Two questions are central to the deliberations: (1) Do we have an adequate number of nursing staff? and (2) What knowledge and skills should these nurses have?

In assessing the adequacy of the supply of registered nurses to meet the anticipated needs for health care in the twenty-first century, several researchers have conclude that *the aggregate quantity of registered nurses in the United States is adequate to meet national needs, at least for the near future, but their educational mix may not be adequate to meet either current or future demands in a rapidly changing health care system* (Aiken and Salmon, 1994; see McBride, Part II of this report). Workplace settings are changing rapidly and dramatically. This situation calls for continuous review of the education, training, and retraining needed by those in direct and indirect care giving functions. The committee also notes that with a changing health care system, and the consequent changes needed in the education and training of nursing personnel, a thorough evaluation of the current funding of training may be necessary to determine if any redirection is needed.

Nursing Education and Training for the Future

The findings of the Pew Health Professions Commission, related to practitioners needed for the year 2005 and their education, provide a framework for the development of a strategic direction for the future workforce. The issues of formal educational needs are well articulated in numerous publications of this commission beginning with *Healthy America: Practitioners for 2005* and *Health Professions Education for the Future: Schools in Service to the Nation*, and in the abundance of professional literature that has surfaced over the last few years (McBride, Part II of this report).

The knowledge and skills of all health care professionals require advancement in this rapidly changing health care delivery system. The following general areas are discussed in relation to basic professional nursing education: interdisciplinary education and team approaches to care; management of care, including attention to health care costs, professional accountability, and patient outcomes; new modes of care delivery, including community-based care, managed care, and home care. Lastly, some of the changes needed in advanced practice nursing programs are described.

Interdisciplinary Team Care

At this time, the interdisciplinary education of health care workers from different disciplines is the exception rather than the norm. Yet interdisciplinary team approaches to patient care could potentially lead to better patient outcomes (see Chapter 5 for further discussion of interdisciplinary teams). Although the value of interdisciplinary education for RNs and physicians has been espoused for the past three decades, examples of highly effective programs are rare. Changes in the delivery of health care will require nurses prepared to function effectively as members of the health care team. Necessary changes in the educational programs include a need for educational content on collaborative practice, shared decision making, team building, and team practice. In designing such collaborative educational programs, it will be important to transcend the barriers that currently exist. The literature is rich with descriptions of the obstacles to interdisciplinary education, including, for example, differences in the educational levels of learners and difficulties in coordinating schedules. Collaborative clinical experiences with preceptors who are supportive of interdisciplinary team care are just as important as shared classroom teaching and learning.

Management of Care

Professional nurses have long been taught to be managers of their individual patient's care and, to a lesser extent, managers of a team caring for the patient. Future demands will require a greater emphasis on professional productivity and accountability for the care of groups of patients, with particular attention to the relationships between quality and cost of care. Health care students will benefit from courses in information management, health care finance, and system design and functioning. As patient outcomes have assumed a prominent role in research, health care practitioners will be expected to understand the research and base their therapeutic approaches on the most effective interventions.

New Modes of Care Delivery

As the health care delivery system continues its transformation toward community-based care, with managed care as a prominent organizational mode, professional nurses must be prepared to assume leadership roles in delivering care delivery within these new settings. Although the majority of clinical experiences that are part of nursing education currently take place in the inpatient hospital setting, a major shift in the primary site for clinical education is expected. In fact, there is evidence that many schools are changing their curricula and clinical learning experiences to match the pace of changes in the design of delivery systems. Home care, managed care, and community-based care models have received renewed attention, although public health nursing has always been a required component of baccalaureate nursing education.

At the core of the needs for future preparation of professional nurses is the requirement to continue to strengthen clinical decision making and clinical judgment skills. RNs will be called on to provide comprehensive care to a larger numbers of patients with more complex health situations. It is imperative that they be prepared for the complexities of patient care that they will confront.

Advanced Practice Nurses

Prepared as specialists in a clinical content area or generalists for primary care, advanced practice nurses (APN), including nurse practitioners, clinical nurse specialists, nurse midwives, and nurse anesthetists, require a firm foundation in the content areas identified above. Further, there may be some knowledge and skills of particular relevance to their specialty practice that would require even more depth in a particular area. The program content for APNs is currently being reviewed by specific accrediting bodies.

In summary, while there may not be total agreement on the adequate number and mix of type of nurses, there is general agreement that the preparation of both the current and the future nursing workforce must be enhanced.

Differentiated Practice

McBride (Part II of this report) has delineated the current and future issues of professional nursing education, indicating several major challenges that clearly need to be addressed if we are to see an appropriate use of professional nursing services in a restructured health care environment. Her call for differentiation of the RN workforce is supported by the work of Aiken (1994, 1995) and others (Koerner, 1992; Larson et al., 1994; Oermann, 1994a,b).

Differentiated practice using "care partners" appears to be the major restructuring activity that has occurred in 1994 and 1995. According to McBride (Part II of this report), the RN skill mix (that is, the proportion of RNs to other nursing staff) appears to be dropping in many settings, from a range of 76-100 percent to a range of 52-79 percent: "Cost effective care requires all health care providers to avoid duplication of effort and to make full use of the best, least expensive caregivers according to need." While these changes lead to uncertainties and concerns about job security for some, multiple career opportunities will continue to abound for those RNs skilled in health promotion and clinical decision making, and knowledgeable about community resources and the integrated delivery of care.

Throughout the site visits and in oral testimony, the committee heard of the need for more assessment of the capabilities of other care givers, along with the need for training in delegation and supervisory skills, which some RNs believed were currently inadequate for their evolving roles. Many RNs admitted to feeling unsure of their skills and ability to function effectively in these areas. On site visits where successful care partner programs were in place, the committee was informed that in preparation for this type of restructuring considerable time needs to be spent on assessment, delegation, and supervision.

Education must move to an interconnected system of distinct educational levels with differentiated outcomes and a model of differentiated nursing practice should be adopted (McBride, Part II of this report). Aiken (1995) stated that nursing as a profession was producing too many AD graduates and too few baccalaureate and higher-degree nurses to meet future needs. Clifford (1990) has noted that with the health care delivery system being increasingly primary care oriented and boundary spanning, the roles in which nurses will be needed will require more professional judgment and clinical autonomy.

SUMMARY

This chapter has addressed critical issues affecting the nursing workforce, its supply, and the forces affecting its demand. The committee has grappled with the implications of the nature of the current supply of nursing personnel, not just in terms of numbers of RNs, LPNs, and NAs, but also in terms of the distribution of its educational preparations and of the knowledge and skills required in a restructured health care system.

Rapid changes in the health care sector are creating an environment of uncertainty leading to concerns about job security. At the same time, new opportunities for nursing are being created, often away from the traditional inpatient hospital setting. These opportunities will work to the benefit of some and will adversely affect those who do not have the skills and training to move into new types of work. These are major issues of great relevance for the delivery of health care in the twenty-first century. Achievements in scientific and technological advances have made our health care system one of the best in the world and the quality of the health workforce is closely related to the success of the health care system. The committee recognizes that these issues are beyond the scope of its study and cannot be addressed adequately here. It therefore strongly urges the profession of nursing, policymakers, and leaders in the field of health care professions to address these issues comprehensively and decisively so that the country has an adequate nursing workforce in terms of numbers, distribution, and educational mix to provide care in a restructured health care system. The committee also notes that with a changing health care system, and the consequent changes needed in the education and training of nursing personnel, a thorough evaluation of the current funding of training may be necessary to determine if any redirection is needed. For a detailed discusson of federal funding support of nursing education, see Aiken and Gwyther, 1995.

5

Staffing and Quality of Care in Hospitals

Nursing is a critical factor in determining the quality of care in hospitals and the nature of patient outcomes. Twenty-four hour nursing care is one of the distinctive hallmarks of inpatient care in hospitals. Historically, hospitals have been at the core of the U.S. health care system, and nursing services are central to the provision of hospital care. They have also functioned as the traditional place of work for nursing personnel and especially for registered nurses (RN). Nursing personnel comprise the largest proportion of patient care givers in a hospital. Nursing care in hospitals takes on added importance today because increase in acuity of patients requires intensive nursing care.

In recent years, the nursing profession has been especially concerned about the nature of the transformation taking place in the health care sector. Reports of hiring freezes and layoffs of RNs in hospitals have led to increasing apprehension among them and their supporting organizations about the potential threat to the quality of patient care in hospitals as well as their physical and economic well-being. RNs have expressed concerns that hospitals are implementing a variety of nursing care delivery systems involving major staff substitutions, reducing the proportion of RNs to other nursing personnel by replacing them with lesser-trained (and at times untrained), and lower-salaried, personnel at a time when the increasing complexity of hospital inpatient caseloads calls for more skilled nursing care.

At the same time, the aggregate quantity of RNs is at a high level, creating uncertainties about job security. Much health care is moving to ambulatory settings, the community, and the home through home health services. The nursing profession also has concerns about the training needs to accommodate these shifts in work settings. With respect to the hospital setting, a rapidly changing health care environment, continuing pressures to contain costs, and the rising levels of severity of illness and comorbidity of inpatients all make it imperative for hospitals to explore innovative ways to redesign delivery of care without compromising quality.

Throughout the decade of the 1980s, hospital expansion, scientific advances, and technological development led to the use of an increasing number of nursing personnel, particularly the RN. As discussed in Chapter 4, employment of RNs in hospitals has increased steadily for the past several decades. In 1993, RN employment in hospitals continued to increase, but the rate of growth over the previous year showed a slight decline for the first time in many years (AHA, 1995b). However, a comparison of first-quarter 1994 data with preliminary data for the first quarter of 1995, shows that while total hospital employment was down; RN employment increased by 3.5 percent, and licensed practical nurse (LPN) employment declined by 1.2 percent (see Table 4.3). These figures may represent a 1-year artifact or an indication of an underlying shift in the health care delivery system.

Information about trends in employment levels of RNs and other nursing personnel needs to be understood in the context of the changing health care system, as elaborated in Chapters 3 and 4. In particular, hospital inpatient lengths of stay continued to decline, along with inpatient days; admissions increased in 1995 after remaining relatively level in 1994. The increasing acuity of patients requiring intense nursing care, the large increase in hospital outpatient services, and the relative increase in beds dedicated to intensive care units also may account for at least part of the continued increase in hospital employment of RNs.

In sum, although the committee heard reports of widespread layoffs of RNs and other nursing personnel, national statistics suggest that in the aggregate these employment losses appear to have been more than offset by hires. (This generalization does not hold for licensed practical nurses [LPN], whose employment by hospitals has been declining for some years.) The continued growth in RN employment appears to run counter to many assertions the committee heard from nurses during site visits, testimony and numerous written and oral communications throughout the study. Aggregate trends, of course, obscure local and regional variations that respond to local market conditions and other factors, and anecdotal information cannot be discounted totally as it often is a warning indicator of changes that are not yet reflected in national statistics.

This chapter examines the relationship of staffing patterns of nursing personnel in hospitals and quality of patient care. The chapter begins with a discussion of the restructuring of hospital care and the changing roles of nursing personnel in hospitals. It then provides a brief overview of the elements of quality of care, measurement issues, and the status of quality in hospitals. Next, it proceeds to assess whether there is any reliable evidence linking nurse staffing to the quality of patient care in hospitals. The chapter ends with a brief overview of legislative and regulatory requirements for hospital quality assurance.

RESTRUCTURING IN THE HOSPITALS

As the average length of stay for patients decreased and subsequently as the number of staffed beds also declined, hospitals began redesigning their systems of care, scheduling practices, and approaches to the care of hospitalized patients, in order to accommodate this decreased need.

Increasing numbers of hospitals are restructuring their organization, staffing, and services. Redesign and reengineering have become principal strategies of the 1990s for many institutions and systems. Although redesign initiatives are undertaken for a variety of reasons, more than half of the efforts are driven by the need to reduce operating costs, and have focused on the transformation of work processes and the redesign of roles and jobs. Staff reductions or changes in labor mix are at times implemented without attention to the organizational changes that might facilitate the possibility of better outcomes with fewer, more appropriately trained and used staff, while at the same time focusing on improved patient outcomes (VHA, 1995).

The labor intensity of nursing services in hospitals cannot be disputed when one considers the fact that the average nursing department's full-time-equivalent (FTE) personnel represent around 40 percent of the overall hospital FTE personnel and around 30 percent of the average annual hospital budget (Witt Associates, 1990). This means that the nursing department represents the largest single department within the institution. In light of the efforts by hospitals to meet the multiple demands that are reshaping their future and requiring them to reduce costs, the nursing department can be a major area for cost reduction efforts simply because of the size of the budget. Brannon (1994, p. 3) notes that in "response to greater market competition and pressures to contain cost, community hospitals not only transformed themselves into diversified health care organizations, [but] corporate managers reorganized the work of hospital workers to contain labor costs and increase productivity. Nursing was at the center of these changes." However, because it is assumed that the changing health care system needs to balance costs with maintaining or improving quality of care, assuring that both the right number and the right kind of nursing resources are available becomes essential for a coordinated and cost-effective health care system.

Concurrent with the efforts to restructure hospital services has been the development of total quality management and what is often referred to as patient-centered and patient-focused care. The typical patient in a traditionally-organized hospital may interact with as many as 60 staff in one 4-day hospital stay (Lathrop, 1992). Hence, efforts for redesigning hospital care have been focused on the integration of many hospital services in an effort to provide more patient-centered or -focused care. Both these efforts—total or continuous quality management and patient-centered care have led to major work design and organizational change in several hospitals. These innovative, team approaches may also involve case managers,[1] the development of critical pathways for managing patients most efficiently during a hospital stay, and other steps that, collectively, lead to restructuring in the hospital.

The restructuring of hospital inpatient services is but one part of the larger restructuring efforts of the care delivery system related in large part to managed care and the development of integrated delivery systems. While much anecdotal information is available about these changes, objective data are not available to determine how widespread these changes are and whether or not this redesign accomplishes its dual goals of increasing patient-centered care and cost reductions.

Because of the resource intensity of hospital nursing services, restructuring, work redesign, and cost reduction efforts have a direct impact on the nursing workforce. It is not surprising, therefore, that the restructuring of hospitals and redesign of nursing services are among the most pressing issues for the nursing profession and ultimately for the future of health care delivery in hospitals. Staffing to provide safe, effective, and therapeutic patient care is a challenge for nurse administrators under any circumstances, and substantial changes are occurring in the organization and delivery of hospital care.

Changing Roles and Responsibilities of RNs

While the RN in the hospital remains in the pivotal position for coordinating care in hospitals, sometimes as a case manager, the position of the nurse assistant (NA) has been changing. In some institutions it is being upgraded, with NAs assuming, under the direction of the RN, increasing responsibility for more direct care activities than in the past. This results in an increasing level of management and supervisory skills being required of RNs. In some hospitals the redesign of the nurse assistant role has occurred in conjunction with the redesign of other support activities such as dietary, housekeeping, and transportation services. The integration of these functions is viewed as one way to have fewer people interacting with the patient, while also providing the potential for cost savings.

These redesign efforts have led to changes in the patterns developed over the

---

[1] "Case management" includes comprehensive oversight of a patient's entire episode of illness incorporating interdisciplinary resource utilization in order to provide high quality, cost-effective care. The clinical and financial management of care is coordinated by "case managers" who often span the boundaries of inpatient, ambulatory and community settings (Satinsky, 1995). Some people prefer to use the term "care manager" in lieu of case manager. Care management suggests the provision of direct care and, in some instances a case manager may also be a care manager. For example, registered nurses who coordinate care for groups of hospitalized patients with the same diagnosis may also assume responsibility for giving some of these patients direct care.

past two decades for organizing the delivery of nursing care in hospitals. The challenge today is for care givers and patients to think about the continuum of care needed rather than simply the event of hospitalization. The emphasis is no longer on the inpatient hospital care of a patient, but rather to view the event of hospitalization as one event in the illness continuum. Changing the emphasis to a continuum of care requires hospital nursing services to develop new structures and practices. Foremost among these changes is to help nursing and other health care givers to learn how to plan for patient care before the patient is admitted to the hospital, as well as for care needed after discharge from the hospital.

This change also calls for more flexibility in staffing patterns and time schedules that will focus on the needs of the patient. Flexibility in scheduling was a major issue of the late 1980s when hospitals had nursing shortages. A change to 12-hour schedules with fewer days worked by nursing staff became a standard in many hospitals in an effort to increase nurse satisfaction and thereby decreasing the turnover of nursing staff. Today's work redesign appears to be changing some of those schedules back to the more traditional 8-hour day and 40-hour week, reducing some costs in doing so and providing the potential for more stability in staffing systems that provide opportunity for some nursing staff to practice across the boundaries of inpatient and ambulatory or community nursing care.

It is this latter challenge, along with the demands for increased efficiency within a standard of good quality of care that, in part, has led many hospitals to implement the concept of care teams. These care teams are generally interdisciplinary in nature, bringing members of the appropriate disciplines together from all areas, ambulatory, inpatient, and community for example, to collectively develop a plan of care that will optimally benefit the patient, meet a pre-established set of standards, and use as few resources as possible in carrying out the plan of care. Such care teams often use practice guidelines, sometimes referred to as care maps or critical pathways, to determine the plan of care and progress of the patient along a time line established for the continuum of care. These guidelines are similar to decision trees and require a team of care givers who engage in high levels of effective communication and have the knowledge and skills required to enter into collaborative planning and evaluation. As managed care becomes more the norm, expedient decision making and good judgment will be increasingly more important for all health care providers and the use of interdisciplinary approaches such as care teams also will become increasingly the norm in the hospital sector (Sovie, 1995).

In order to accomplish the work of care teams effectively and efficiently, case managers are often used. This system of organizing care relies on this manager to integrate in-depth clinical knowledge, community resources, and financial and organizational requirements with patient needs and the institutional goals of providing high quality, cost effective care. While the needs of the patient should determine who will be the case manager, in acute care settings this role is most often performed by an RN, frequently one who has been prepared with education beyond the basic program of nursing. In most hospitals the nursing case manager is the person who spans the boundaries of inpatient, ambulatory, and community nursing (Girard, 1994).

In summary, the dynamics of staffing and scheduling in hospitals, always more complex than one would expect, have taken on even greater complexities as care giving becomes much more interdisciplinary in nature and care givers are required to consider more than the event of illness presented, that is, the current hospitalization or the current outpatient visit. The continuum of care, sharing of information across the system, and the increasing involvement of patients and families in their own care giving requires that staffing be considered in its broadest definition.

Evolving Roles in Advanced Practice Nursing

The committee takes note of the growing trend toward complexity of illness and sophisticated care management of patients in an illness episode that includes the event of hospitalization but is not limited to it. The care planning and managing begins before the patient is admitted to the hospital and continues beyond the hospitalization to discharge planning and management of care needed after discharge from the hospital. Leading and managing the organizational transformations described above require talents or training that not all RNs now have. For the evolving hospital, the committee believes that it will be imperative for these management and leadership skills to be fostered through various educational programs. The committee believes that more advanced, or more broadly trained, RNs will be needed in the future. Such training is essentially like that now provided for RNs who receive certification as, for example, advanced practice nurses (i.e., clinical nurse specialists, nurse practitioners, nurse midwives, and nurse anesthetists).

Clinical nurse specialists can be found in every specialty area of nursing. In each of these areas clinical nurse specialists function as practitioners, educators, case managers, consultants, researchers, and administrators; in the mental health arena, they may also serve as psychotherapists. They play a critical role in the ongoing clinical management of caseloads of patients. Nurse practitioners manage patients with acute and chronic conditions. They frequently have responsibility for managing patients with illness such as diabetes or hypertension. They also are responsible for the ongoing primary care of a group of healthy individuals.

The value of such clinical nurse specialists, in terms of both patient care and economic factors have been studied over the past 20 to 25 years. In particular, a number of randomized clinical trials have been conducted.

One set of studies was directed at testing the effectiveness of programs conducted by clinical nurse specialists in caring for hospitalized elderly patients, especially in comprehensive discharge planning. Outcomes such as length of stay, number of, or length of time before rehospitalization, and costs, as well as functional status, were all better among those patients whose care was coordinated and implemented by clinical nurse specialists. Neidlinger and colleagues (1987) found the use of a comprehensive discharge planning protocol implemented by a clinical nurse specialist saved an average of $60 per patient day more than their control group. In a follow-up to this study Kennedy and colleagues (1987) found that for the same control and experimental groups the experimental treatment group's average length of stay was reduced by 2 days, and the length of time before hospital readmission increased by 11 days.

A pilot study by Naylor (1990) had similar results. She found that there was a significant difference between the two groups in frequency of hospital readmissions. Later, in a randomized clinical trial, Naylor and colleagues (1994) found that from initial discharge to 6 weeks after discharge, patients in the intervention group managed by clinical nurse specialists had fewer number of hospital readmissions, fewer total days of rehospitalization, lower readmission charges, and lower charges for health care after discharge. Functional status was the focus of a study by Wanich and colleagues (1992). These researchers found that in their clinical trial patients in the intervention group (those whose care was coordinated by the clinical nurse specialist) were more likely to improve in functional status than those who did not who did not receive such care. These same patients were less likely to deteriorate on measures of functional status during their hospital stay. These outcomes may also help to reduce length of hospital stay and decrease costs, although cost was not measured as an outcome in this study.

Oncology clinical nurse specialists have also been shown to improve patient outcomes. McCorkle and colleagues (1989), for example, conducted a randomized clinical trial of lung cancer patients. The study demonstrated that lung cancer patients receiving care from specialized oncology clinical nurse specialists experienced less distress, less dependence, fewer rehospitalizations, and shorter lengths of stay than did patients cared for without intervention from these advanced trained personnel. According to Russell (1989) the cost of care for patients undergoing a modified radical mastectomy who were followed by an oncology clinical nurse specialist was significantly lower than for those not so followed. Their average length of stay was 3.4 days, while that of the control group was 6.7 days. The costs of hospitalization averaged a difference of $1,668.43 per patient.

Another set of studies involved low birthweight infants and families who received care and consultation from clinical nurse specialists. Outcomes such as length of stay were better and costs were lower among study participants who were in the group using such specialist nurses (Brooten et al., 1986; 1988; Damato et al., 1993).

The ability of clinical nurse specialists to function in a number of different roles and their ability to work independently to solve problems and be patient advocates as well as integral members of a health care team have been cited as a reason for improved outcomes and cost savings that they help to bring about. Nurses in this role are an important part of the total patient care picture across settings and as such are essential to improved patient outcomes.

Although the discussion to this point has drawn on the use of advanced practice nurses in discharge planning and working with patients in the home after hospitalization, the place of such personnel in the entire continuum of care for which hospitals are responsible needs to be understood. For one thing, all but the smallest hospitals operate outpatient clinics of various sorts (including those that deal with non-urgent problems of patients who present to emergency departments). Moreover, as the U.S. health care system restructures itself, many larger hospitals and academic health centers are becoming the center of integrated health delivery systems that vertically integrate providers from small physician office practices through multispecialty groups through a variety of other aspects of health care. With this trend, plus the growing phenomenon of delegation and substitution of responsibilities from physicians to nurses (i.e., nurse practitioners or other types of advanced practice nurses), it is clear that the role of advanced practice nurses is now and will continue to expand.

Based on this type of information, combined with what was learned from testimony, site visits, and the professional expertise and experience of its members, the committee concludes that high-quality, cost-effective care for certain types of patients, particularly those with complicated or serious clinical conditions, will be fostered by the use of such advanced nurse specialists. The committee believes that increased use of advanced practice nurses would improve the cost-effectiveness of our health care systems and facilities. That is to say, changing the mix of nursing personnel involved in caring for patients with increasingly complex management problems may yield both improved outcomes and lower costs.

RECOMMENDATION 5-1: The committee recommends that hospitals expand the use of registered nurses with advanced practice preparation and skills to provide clinical leadership and cost-effective patient care, particularly for patients with complex management problems.

Advanced practice nurses are typically classified in at least one of four ways, and their educational training and duties differ accordingly. *Clinical nurse specialists* typically are master's degree-trained RNs; some may also have PhDs. Their clinical specialties can include oncology, neonatology and, or, pediatrics, mental health, adult health, women's health, geriatrics, and AIDS. They commonly work in clinical settings and provide primary care; case management services; psychotherapy; and a variety of organizational, administrative, and leadership services as well. *Nurse practitioners* are usually prepared at the master's degree level and also certified in a specialty area of practice, such as pediatrics, family practice, or primary care. Their usual responsibilities include managing clinical care; they conduct physical examinations, track medical histories, make diagnoses, treat minor illnesses and injuries, and perform an array of counseling and educational tasks. Nurse practitioners may also, in some circumstances, order and interpret diagnosis tests and prescribe medications. *Certified nurse midwives* are RNs who have graduated from a nurse midwifery program accredited by the American College of Nurse-Midwives (ACNM) and are certified as a nurse-midwife by the ACNM; some may have taken a master's program offered by a school of nursing or a school of public health. They provide prenatal and gynecological care, deliver babies in a variety of settings (hospitals, birthing centers, or homes), and render postpartum care. Finally, *certified RN anesthetists* have a bachelor of science in nursing and 2 to 3 years of additional education and training in anesthesiology, often at the master's level. They, too, have a rigorous certification process, managed through programs approved by the American Association of Nurse Anesthetists. Particularly in rural areas, these nurse specialists may administer the majority of anesthesia or anesthetics in health care settings today.

Clearly, well-trained advanced practice nurses can function in a number of different roles. They can work independently to solve patient care problems, serve as patient advocates, and be integral members of a health care team. Advanced practice nurses can improve the cost-effectiveness of health care systems and facilities because changing the mix of personnel involved in caring for patients with complex management problems may yield better outcomes, lower costs, or both. The committee concludes that the way should be clearer for such personnel to be used in both inpatient and outpatient settings and for them to be able to take up leadership positions and act independently.

One obstacle, however, to accomplishing the changes advocated in this section lies in the differing ways in which states recognize advanced practice nurses, chiefly in terms of the breadth of independent authority (e.g., diagnosing, prescribing, and dispensing of medical therapeutic agents or controlled substances) (Pearson, 1995; Ray and Hardin, 1995). Some state boards of nursing have not yet recognized the expanded responsibilities that such personnel can and should discharge. *To address this problem, the committee believes that all states should recognize nurses in advanced practice in their nurse-practice acts and delineate the qualifications and scope of practice of these nurses.*

Ancillary Nursing Personnel

Today, almost all hospitals in the United States use some kind of ancillary nursing personnel. As stated in Chapter 4, this group of personnel includes nurses aides or assistants (NA), some of whom may be certified, as well as a variety of other ancillary personnel. By definition, they have less formal education and training than RNs or LPNs; on average, when hired they may also have less exposure to, and time or experience in, the inpatient setting. Their education, however, does not stop after the basic training. Many serve for several years and learn from physicians, RNs, and LPNs to perform tasks that once were not done by NAs and to be responsible for specific aspects of clinical care.[2]

As already noted, far less information about employment trends is available on this group of the nursing workforce than on the more traditional nursing categories. However, the transformation of the hospital care delivery system is clearly going to involve these types of personnel at least in the near future. The use of NAs and other ancillary nursing personnel to assist RNs with patient care is reported to have increased in recent years. In most instances, NAs and other ancillary nursing personnel are used in simple bedside care or as unit assistants (e.g., changing dressings, taking vital signs such as blood pressure and temperature); in some instances, they are being used to assist RNs in total bedside care or in other duties such as telemonitoring, lifting teams, electrocardiography, or physical therapy (Barter et al., 1994). In other cases, tasks performed by these types of personnel may overlap with those of other support units, such as dietary, housekeeping, or transportation services.

Krapohl and Larson (1995) describe the evolution of nursing delivery systems in hospitals, from team nursing (with all the variations such as clinical, nonclinical, and integrated nursing models) to primary nursing models. The various "patient-focused" team models that some hospitals are implementing incorporate less skilled nursing personnel to varying extent; the models themselves vary according to the specific needs of different hospitals (or hospital systems). The authors also reviewed the literature regarding the use and evaluation of ancillary nursing personnel in hospitals and found no strong evidence to confirm that these nursing personnel improve (or reduce) quality or increase (or decrease) nurse or patient satisfaction. A review of studies of primary nursing also do not conclusively show the superiority of primary nursing models over various team nursing models. They conclude, basically, that although nursing care has been provided in hospitals since the hospital's beginning, no single delivery system has emerged as ideal. The authors also note the methodological and design weaknesses of the studies reviewed.

Nevertheless, some informal information about these new team approaches is encouraging. The committee learned, for instance, about variations of the "partners-in-practice" program pioneered in the 1980s, which linked NAs and other ancillary nursing personnel with an RN (Manthey, 1988, 1992). At the site visit in Oregon, committee members and staff were able to observe and interact

---

[2]This phenomenon may have a parallel to the RN's role. RNs trained some years back were not instructed to perform duties such as utilization review, case management, long-term discharge planning, or cost containment, or to be involved in managed care, capitation, or contractual agreements for reimbursement. They have been learning the new concepts necessary to function today.

with care teams in which RNs assumed a very close working relationship with the other care partners. Nursing personnel at all levels worked together at all times; thus, RNs were able to assess the knowledge and clinical capabilities of each member of the team and, where necessary, step in to supervise, and then teach, the less-well-prepared nursing personnel. Other hospitals have implemented similar systems, according to information made available to the committee.

The underlying message of the literature review and the observational information gathered by the committee is that, in the hospital sector, issues of training and competency of non-RN staff remain critical. No national standards exist for minimum training or certification of ancillary nursing personnel employed by hospitals (unlike, as discussed in Chapter 6, for NAs in the nursing home sector); thus, they vary widely in educational attainments and in their training for simple nursing or quasi-nursing tasks. Furthermore, no accepted mechanism exists either to measure competency or to certify in some fashion that ancillary nursing personnel have attained at least a basic or rudimentary mastery of needed skills. Hospitals vary widely in the levels of training they provide to these personnel. Barter and colleagues (1994) found that 99 percent of the hospitals in California reported less than 120 hours of on-the-job training for newly hired ancillary nursing personnel. Only 20 percent of the hospitals required a high school diploma. The majority of hospitals (59 percent) provided less than 20 hours of classroom instruction and 88 percent provided 40 hours or less of instruction time. RNs and their supporting organizations have expressed much concern that NAs and other ancillary nursing personnel are being given various nursing-related tasks in hospitals in the absence of competency requirements. The committee is greatly concerned about this lack and the potential for adverse impact on patient care.

> **RECOMMENDATION 5-2: The committee recommends that hospitals have documented evidence that ancillary nursing personnel are competent and that such personnel are tested and certified by an appropriate entity for this competence. The committee further recommends that the training for ancillary nursing personnel working in hospitals be structured and enriched by including training of the following types: appropriate clinical care of the aged and disabled; occupational health and safety measures; culturally sensitive care; and appropriate management of conflict.**

The committee believes that hospitals should take the lead in ensuring the competence of, and provision of appropriate training to, all direct care personnel employed by them, including ancillary nursing personnel. The committee does not believe that the first course of action should be enforcement by law or regulation at the federal, state, or municipal level. It does caution however, that if real quality-of-care problems were to emerge in hospitals that could be related to negligence by hospitals in ensuring competence, then the public might be expected to clamor for the enactment and enforcement of more stringent, external, regulation. Such rules would then protect the public from problems that hospitals themselves should have guarded against.

Hospitals are in a better position than nursing homes to assure the competence of NAs because NAs are not the predominant care givers in hospitals that they are in nursing homes. Hospital NAs are more likely to work in teams with other care givers and to have more direct supervision from the RN, who is more immediately available than is usually the case in nursing homes.

Finally, culturally sensitive care will become increasingly important in the years ahead. As noted in Chapter 2, the population, and therefore the patient population, is not only aging but also is becoming more racially and ethnically diverse. Thus, increasingly, care givers and care receivers may come from different cultural backgrounds. The imperative for cultural sensitivity is obvious.

Involving Personnel in Planning for Change

The changes briefly described above are appealing conceptually, and time will tell if they are effective and practical as the hospital sector reinvents itself. In the short term, however, these shifts in the way hospitals do business, and the way they organize to conduct their business, are causing notable disruptions and misgivings among the nursing staff. From the frequency and intensity of the commentaries that the committee heard during this study, RNs are concerned about both the employment ramifications and more importantly the professional implications of the organizational changes that are occurring; they believe that these changes may lead to undesirable and unanticipated effects on quality of care.

In response to pressures to contain costs and improve quality of care, which may or may not be related to the downward trend in inpatient hospital use, hospitals are restructuring services, units, and activities. These efforts are generally oriented toward increasing productivity or efficiency and/or reducing operating costs. As stated above, redesign efforts often involve the integration and coordination of work across departmental lines, which may also lead to elimination of positions, layoffs, redefinition of positions, and realignment of supervisory lines.

Restructuring of inpatient services in hospitals, accompanied by a changing mix of nursing personnel, is an inevitable consequence of the demands by society, through the payers of care, to control the costs of health services. Downsizing of the patient care workforce in inpatient hospital settings will continue, at least in the near future. Nursing personnel will not be immune from such downsizing. "Reengineering" of patient care processes, including changes in skill mix, will also continue, at least for the short term.

Overall, the sense of disquiet about the future, especially among RNs, was palpable, in part because of the unpredictability of the effects of these changes and in part because of the seeming lack of input and control that many nurses felt about the changes being made. The committee heard from nurses who had lost their positions in hospitals about management decisions for downsizing that had been made without any staff involvement—a phenomenon that adds to the feelings of threat and uncertainty for many hospital-based RNs. At the same time, the committee had the benefit of learning about other hospitals where management involved staff in substantial ways in reaching solutions about how the necessary staff restructuring ought to take place. At one of its public hearings, for instance, the committee heard from witnesses about the beneficial results of using free federal mediating services. On site visits, committee members visited some hospitals where change had been successfully implemented through well-conceived planning and implementation processes that involved both nursing administrators and staff nurses.

In the committee's view, the harmful and demoralizing effects of these changes on the nursing staff can be mitigated, if not forestalled altogether, with more recognition on the part of the hospital industry that involvement of nursing personnel from the outset in the redesign efforts is critical.

> **RECOMMENDATION 5-3: The committee recommends that hospital leaders involve nursing personnel (RNs, LPNs, and NAs) who are directly affected by organizational redesign and staffing reconfiguration in the process of planning and implementing such changes.**

The committee found impressive the testimonies and descriptions of these collaborative "redesign" efforts that involved all levels of nursing personnel in the restructuring process as illustrated above. The rationale for inclusion of nursing personnel in hospital restructuring efforts relates to several factors: such involvement brings to the table the professional knowledge and experience needed in developing such changes, staff commitment to the decisions made, and may affect the likelihood of success and of improvement in the quality of care. It is not simply to make the affected nursing staff feel better. Change is likely to fail if a top-down approach is imposed on hospital nursing staff.

Furthermore, the health care sector is moving rapidly to adopt principles of continuous quality improvement and total quality management as means for addressing issues in quality of care, for advancing the state of the art of quality measurement and management, and for promoting continuous progress in health care processes and patient outcomes. These newer quality assurance and improvement techniques rely heavily on input from multiple segments of a health organization's personnel and departments; that is, they do not deal with quality issues that relate to only a single department, in part because most problems in health institutions and facilities are systemic rather than traceable to single events, people, or units. Logic alone would dictate, therefore, that as an organization wishes to reinvent its structure and systems, it ought to adopt these same principles of involving individuals from across the departmental and personnel spectrum.

Tracking the Effects of Change

Although available national statistics on hospital employment do not show reductions in levels of nursing staff at the national level, the media frequently report on staff layoffs in hospitals. Anecdotal information abounds, and ad hoc inquiries are conducted by unions, nurse associations, magazines (of their membership and subscribers), and other organizations. Unfortunately, the very low response rates of many of these inquiries and the deficiencies in the design of surveys and of questions do not permit consumers or policymakers to derive objective measures of the links between staffing patterns and processes and outcomes of care, and to draw valid conclusions.

As a consequence of declining trends in inpatient hospital use, some hospitals have been reducing the number of operating beds and reducing nursing positions by attrition or layoffs. Other hospitals are closing, and some are converting beds to long-term care and other services. Some RNs, LPNs, and NAs have been laid off or redeployed from acute care units to other services, programs, or settings. These types of downsizing and consequent restructuring efforts necessarily affect employment of nursing personnel and will continue as long as hospitals face low-use patterns. This turbulence in the health care delivery system and the resultant unstable situation fuel the concern that large decreases in RN staffing in hospitals are both occurring and leading to decrements in patient care and to threats to the health and well-being of nursing personnel.

As stated earlier, throughout the period of the committee's study changes were occurring in hospitals in the use of RNs and in the ratio of RNs to other nursing personnel in the organization of the delivery of patient care. Many of them intimated that such changes potentially will diminish the quality of care provided but the committee was unable to find evidence of a decline in the quality of hospital care because of any changes in staffing. Lacking reliable measures and data, no one is in a position to draw valid conclusions. The amount of testimony provided, however, and the depth of concern cited, was sufficient to lead the committee to believe that this is an area that requires on-going monitoring and research in order to ensure that the responsibility for providing safe, effective, quality, and cost effective care is fulfilled within the health care system.

The committee finds that lack of reliable and valid data on the magnitude and distribution of temporary or permanent unemployment, reassignments of existing nursing staff, and similar changes in the structure of nursing employment opportunities greatly hampers efforts at understanding the problem and planning for the future. Answers are needed to numerous questions, such as: What happens to nursing staff after they are laid off? Are they employed in another hospital or reemployed at the same hospital? Do they move to outpatient, community, or long-term care settings? Do they return to school for retraining or for more advanced nurse training? Do they leave nursing altogether for another occupation?

Information on RN employment patterns is necessary. Research is needed on whether career paths of RNs will change markedly over the next 5 to 10 years. These changes can have implications for career choices, curriculum design, structure of occupational ladders, and perhaps, quality of care. Among the many questions that warrant attention are the implications of restructuring for career choices, the structure of occupational ladders, and both entry and midcareer curriculum design.

> **RECOMMENDATION 5-4: The committee recommends that hospital management monitor and evaluate the effects of changes in organizational redesign and reconfiguration of nursing personnel on patient outcomes, on patient satisfaction, and on nursing personnel themselves.**

More detailed data also are needed on the employment patterns of NAs and LPNs over time. Throughout its deliberations the committee focused largely on RNs not only because they form the largest proportion of nursing personnel in this country and because their professional associations are the most well organized, but also because of the paucity of comparably detailed data on NAs and LPNs. For that reason, hospitals should not concentrate their monitoring and evaluation solely on the relationships between RN staffing and quality of care or on work-related illness and injury. Rather, *hospitals should focus their monitoring and evaluation efforts of the restructuring and redesign of staffing on the entire spectrum of their nursing personnel.*

The federal agencies concerned with health workforce data and research have a major role to play. Thus, in this regard the committee supports the missions of agencies such as the Division of Nursing of the Bureau of Health Professions (in the Health Resources and Services Administration), the National Institute of Nursing Research (in the National Institutes of Health), and the National Center for Health Statistics (in the Centers for Disease Control and Prevention) all in the Department of Health and Human Services. The need for timely and relevant data that is amenable to integration across systems is urgent. In the committee's view, these agencies should work productively together and in collaboration with private organizations to develop databases containing information that will shed light on workforce issues and on the relationships of staffing of nursing personnel and care processes and patient outcomes.

MEASURING QUALITY OF CARE IN HOSPITALS

The legislative mandate to this Institute of Medicine (IOM) committee asks it to examine structural issues—the number of nurses and the mix of types of nurses—but it also asks the committee to focus on outcome issues in terms of nurses themselves as well as the quality of patient care that could involve either processes, or patient outcomes, or both.

The committee looked at quality broadly beyond nursing inputs in terms of the overall quality of care received by the patient in the hospital, and examined the relationship between structural variables and both processes and outcomes of care. In this effort, it was guided by the IOM's definition of quality of care: ". . . the degree to which health services for individuals and populations increase the likelihood of desired health outcomes and are consistent with current professional knowledge" (IOM, 1990, vol. I, p. 21).

The IOM definition does not contend that quality can or should be defined in terms of available resources. Excluding resource constraints in the definition provides the opportunity for Quality assurance (QA) and Quality Improvement (QI) systems to distinguish quality-of-care problems from problems arising from resource availability. Quality measurement methods and QA/QI approaches should be able to (1) identify how and to what degree resource constraints affect structure, process, and outcome elements of health care; (2) identify the agent(s) that are responsible for the constraints and have the authority to address the problems they may be causing; and (3) perhaps conduct corrective actions and monitor progress in improving care.

How one measures or improves the quality of health care is linked closely to the assumptions made about what constitutes quality of care in the first place. This multidimensional definition of quality of care is compatible with the perspective that patients, consumers, providers, payers, and public entities all have interests in the quality of care rendered by health care institutions and personnel. Having an understanding of the important dimensions of quality of care is a key initial step toward developing measurement and intervention approaches and implementing QA/QI strategies. Standards and indicators of performance must be closely linked to the operational concepts used in defining quality. Care is then assessed or measured against criteria or benchmarks to determine whether standards are met and where lie opportunities for improvement, regardless of whether specific standards have been met or exceeded.

Elements of Quality of Care

The most fundamental conceptual framework in the area of quality of care was articulated three decades ago by Avedis Donabedian (1966); his formulation is based on a triad of structural factors, process-of-care variables, and outcomes or end results of that care. These elements are briefly discussed below to provide some context for discussions in this and the next chapter.

Structural Variables

Structural criteria are, in effect, proxy measures of quality of care—for an entire organization such as a health plan, hospital, or nursing home, or for an individual health care clinician such as a nurse or physician. Structural criteria may involve variables such as the numbers of various kinds of staff (such as RNs or LPNs or NAs), staff-to-patient or staff-to-bed ratios, the training and supervision expected of or given to staff, the patient record system, the procedures for infection control, building code requirements, and the quality of the physical plant and equipment. These elements may all reasonably be thought to affect the processes of care and, hence, the subsequent health and functional outcomes of patients in hospitals or residents in nursing homes.

Structural measures focus on the presumed capacity of people and entities to deliver adequate or high quality care, but they do not measure the care itself. Accordingly, deficiencies in structural measures cannot be confidently used as direct evidence either of poor care or poor outcomes, but failings in this area, whether perceived or real, certainly can be considered indicative of problems until proven otherwise.

The principal problem with structural variables is that little empirical evidence has been generated linking structural variables directly with good (or bad) processes or (especially) outcomes of care. Thus, the question of whether problems with the levels of nurse staffing or the mix of competencies within a nursing staff may be associated with poor care and risk of patient harms is a reasonable one, but the probable lack of explicit information on any association between such structural variables and the larger issues of interest must be clearly understood from the outset.

Process of Care

The process of care encompasses what is done to, with, and for the patient or health care consumer. Process criteria pertain to the appropriate and correct performance of specific "technical" procedures and services; they also involve interpersonal skills and attitudes, such as those of compassionate communication. Process indicators are very broad, and over the years they have constituted the most widely used set of measures of quality of care. They can include such elements of good quality care as promoting the participation of the patient or resident in the selection of care management strategies and honoring privacy of information and personal space.

Outcomes of Care

Outcome measures are typically considered to be the end results of health care in terms of biologic, psychologic, and functioning variables. They may include various health indicators such as death rates, rates of illness, or rates of specific complications of illness, as well as physiologic measures such as blood pressure, serum glucose, or cholesterol levels—that is, the kinds of clinical measures that appear to matter more to physicians and other clinicians. More broadly, however, health outcomes encompass functional abilities (both physical and cognitive), pain or discomfort, energy and vitality, and mental and emotional well-being—in short, aspects of health status that matter most to patients and their families. This committee embraces the broad view of outcome measures taken by prior IOM committees (IOM, 1990), that is, health-related quality-of-life variables regarding physical, social, and emotional heath, cognitive and physiologic functioning, and overall well-being.

Table 5.1 shows an illustrative list of measures pertinent to nursing quality in the inpatient hospital setting. Although the items in the table are selective and illustrative only of major areas of interest, the committee is cognizant of the fact that data would not be easy to acquire for many of these measures.

Measurement of Quality

In the current health care environment, the attention to, and importance placed on, quality of care are increasing at a notable rate. This is predicated on several factors: the belief that institutions and plans in a competition- or market-oriented health care sector will have to compete on more than price; the vastly greater ability than before of those in the health sector to measure both processes and patient outcomes reliably; and the markedly improved understanding of how to implement effective programs for improving quality. More effort is also being directed at understanding the effectiveness of services and outcomes for both individuals and populations.

Recent years have seen important advances in measuring quality of patient care at the individual patient and population levels,[3] involving both process and outcome measures. From the vantage point of this study, however, existing work has not typically focused on isolating the contribution of nursing care in measuring the quality of patient care in hospitals. Hegyvary (1991), for instance, notes that the literature about productivity in nursing services does not address results in patient care and almost without exception does not raise the question of quality of care.

A fairly wide array of quality indicators has been developed including mortality, unanticipated hospital readmission, hospital-acquired complications, and nosocomial infections. Hospital-specific mortality rates have received particular

---

[3]Concerns about hospital quality of care date to the pioneering nurse Florence Nightingale and British battlefield hospitals in the Crimean War, and to the surgeon E.A. Codman and his concerns about the end results of care in Boston hospitals at the turn of the century. Without question, hospital care left much to be desired then.

TABLE 5.1 Illustrative Measures of Quality of Care in Inpatient Hospital Settings, with Specific Attention to Nursing Care

Structural Measures of Quality

Hospital-specific characteristics
- Governance and ownership
- Size
- Teaching status
- Presence of specialized units and services
- History of accreditation, licensure status
- Payer mix (e.g., proportion Medicare, Medicaid, private insurance, private pay)
- Extent of computer-based patient record systems
- Census (e.g., numbers of patients per year, per department)
- Presence of an active quality assurance or quality improvement program

Staff characteristics
- Staffing levels of full-time physicians, attending physicians, residents, etc.
- Staffing levels of nurses (e.g., numbers, proportions of types of nurses)
  - Registered nurses
  - Licensed practical nurses
  - Nurse aides/assistants
  - Other ancillary nursing personnel
- Educational and other qualifications of nurse staff
- Other nurse staffing factors
  - Use of agency personnel, float personnel
  - Ratio of full-time to part-time nurses
  - Staff turnover rates
  - Types of nursing shifts used
  - Existence of care teams in nursing
- Staffing levels of other types of clinical personnel (physical therapists, occupational therapists)
- Use of volunteers

Process-of-Care Measures

- Diagnostic and monitoring services
  - "Nursing history"
  - Monitoring vital signs
- Nursing services
  - Medications
  - Bathing, toileting, feeding

- Care Planning
  — Developing a nursing care plan upon admission
  — Developing or assisting in devising plans for discharge and postadmission care
  — Preventive steps, such as planning for appropriate use of fall prevention techniques
  — Pain management
  — Patient and family reassurance and communication
  — Response to patient needs and requests (e.g., for liquids, lotion for dry skin, position change)
- Responding to emergencies
- Communication with other clinical staff (e.g., physicians, therapists, social workers)
- Patient charting and documentation of care given
- Counseling and patient education services

Outcome Measures

- Adverse events during admission
  — Unanticipated complications, iatrogenic events or nosocomial infections
  — Medication errors
  — Return to surgery
  — Falls and other patient injuries
- Status at discharge (dead, alive)
- Physiologic characteristics at discharge (e.g., vital signs upon discharge)
- Functional outcomes at discharge (e.g., health status measures such as mobility)
- Mental and emotional status at discharge
- Patient and family satisfaction with care
- Compliance with discharge plan
  — Patient and family understanding of discharge instructions, care plan
- Postdischarge events
  — Return to hospital for emergency care
  — Return to hospital for unplanned readmission
  — Unexpected death, unplanned entry into nursing home, shortly after discharge

attention in the past few years, beginning with the release of such information by the Health Care Financing Administration (HCFA) in the late 1980s and subsequent efforts by various states to do the same (at least for selected types of admissions or operating procedures such as coronary artery bypass graft surgery). Many of these efforts have been carried out using large administrative databases. In general, major questions remain about the reliability, validity, and generalizability of the information from these types of mortality rate studies.

For example, Thomas and colleagues (1993) reviewed the seminal work on risk-adjusted mortality rates and conducted detailed validity studies for three conditions (cardiac disease, acute myocardial infarction [AIM], and septicemia) to determine whether death rates appear to relate to quality of care as evaluated by an experienced physician peer reviewer. They report that of 9,721 cases involving angina and cardiac surgery, 1,103 (11 percent) were considered poor quality; the figures for AMI were 776 of 6,004 cases (13 percent), and for septicemia, 285 of 1,709 cases (17 percent) (Thomas et al., 1993, Tables 3, 4, and 5). With respect to the question of using risk-adjusted mortality rates derived from large administrative databases, however, the investigators concluded that this strategy may be inappropriate unless the quality–outcome relationship is explicitly validated.

Especially complex are questions of (a) whether information on hospital performance as measured by death rates or complication rates will be correlated for different clinical services and (b) whether death rates are correlated with complication rates. Recent work (e.g., Iezzoni et al., 1994; Silber et al., 1995) suggests, in particular, that complication rates will not be related significantly to mortality rates. Those problems notwithstanding, it should be clear that for the purposes of this study, such information tells little, if anything, about the precise role of nurse staffing levels or mix in promoting higher-quality patient care. In fact, one study presents data that link mortality with length of stay (and with other resource-use variables) but that do not demonstrate any relationship between mortality and staffing, such as personnel measured in FTEs, total staff per admission, or RN-to-LPN ratio (Bradbury et al., 1994).

In addition, for many years, "generic screens" have been core quality measures for hospital inpatient care.[4] Usually based on actual review of patient records or discharge abstracts, these involved items such as adequacy of discharge planning, medical stability of the patient at discharge, unscheduled return to surgery, or trauma suffered in hospital in addition to the broader measures noted. Depending on the level of detail in such quality screens, more information

---

[4]"Generic screens" are measures of various aspects of care, typically in hospitals for inpatient care, that are used by quality assurance or risk management staff to identify potential problems with quality of care. Commonly used are the adequacy of discharge planning, medical stability of the patient at discharge, deaths, nosocomial infections, unscheduled returns to surgery, and trauma suffered in the hospital (IOM, 1990). They are generic in the sense that they are not condition or diagnosis specific and, thus, they can be applied to the care of every type of patient in the facility.

on the role of nursing staff in producing high (or low) quality of care could be obtained or at least inferred. However, this type of data collection can be very time-consuming and costly for the amount of useful information gained that might point to quality-of-care problems; the federal Peer Review Organization (PRO) program for Medicare, at least, has in recent years turned away from use of record review for generic screens as a basic tactic for quality assessment.

The use of computerized algorithms to screen for possible quality problems, by applying them to hospital discharge abstract data (e.g., large-scale hospital databases), has been a more recent development. Some methodological research (Iezzoni et al., 1992) suggests that computerized indicators show some promise in terms of identifying hospitals that warrant more intensive review for quality-of-care reasons (e.g., untoward complications of care), because they do a reasonably good job of identifying quality problems, although they may also incorrectly point to problems in a rather large number of cases.[5]   Thus, more work is required to demonstrate the reliability and validity of computerized screens for targeting hospitals for more in-depth quality review. Moreover, as with the earlier generic screen approach, these types of measures tell little about nursing care per se.

Status of Hospital Quality of Care

Quality of patient care is central to the delivery of health care services in hospitals. A major factor precipitating this study were reports, emanating chiefly from nursing groups, that the quality of hospital care is declining, brought about by restructuring and reengineering, and consequent reductions in the proportion of nursing personnel trained as RNs. During the study, the committee heard considerable concern expressed by RNs that hospitals are restructuring and reengineering in increasing numbers that are resulting in smaller proportions of RNs to total nursing personnel, and about the probable negative impact on quality of patient care in those hospitals. Unfortunately, very little recent objective, national data are available that describe the status of quality of care in hospitals and assess if it has been affected in any way by changes in the system of delivery of care. There is virtually no research on the effects of ratios of RNs per bed on patient outcomes. Unlike staffing based on patient acuity, across-the-board staffing ratios assume that all patients can be cared for with the same level and type of resources.   The difficulty in establishing staffing ratios appropriate for all settings and situations across the country is obvious. Given the variation that exists in patient acuity and the total patient care environment, the committee believes

---

[5]In this study, of the 100 discharge abstracts reviewed by a panel of 24 physicians for quality problems, 30 were considered to reflect some kind of problems but the number of problematic abstracts varied from about 15 to 45 among the reviewing physicians.

that it is neither practical nor desirable to establish specific ratios of nursing personnel enforceable by regulation or law. The committee is not discounting what it heard at the public testimony and site visits that unequivocally expressed concerns about trends in quality, both present and future. However, based on studies conducted in the 1980s, there are indirect indicators that in general quality of hospital care has not declined.

Similar concerns were expressed at the time the Medicare Prospective Payment System (PPS) was implemented in the early 1980s. Many observers predicted major quality problems in the hospital sector. The main reason was simply that the diagnosis-related groups (DRG)-based PPS system turned financial incentives for hospitals completely around (compared to the incentives under traditional cost reimbursement schemes), leading many to believe that hospitals would be forced to scrimp on patient services. An in-depth before-and-after evaluation of the effects of DRG-based PPS was conducted by a team of investigators from the RAND Corporation (Draper et al., 1990; Kahn et al., 1990a,b,c; Keeler et al., 1990, 1992; Kosecoff et al., 1990; Rogers et al., 1990; Rubenstein et al., 1990). The researchers found that in general quality of hospital care did not suffer as a result of PPS implementation, and indeed may have even improved in some areas.[6] The researchers found that where the process-of-care and the documentation were improved, the outcomes were improved. The study revealed consistent results between outcome as measured by mortality and the process of care variables (Keeler et al., 1992). Severity-adjusted mortality decreased after PPS.

The RAND researchers also found wide variations in quality among hospitals. Differences between types of hospitals were large, with the lowest group estimated to have four percentage points higher mortality than major teaching hospitals in a cohort of patients with an average mortality rate of 16 percent (Keeler et al., 1990).

Moreover, although quality of care did not suffer after PPS, the RAND study confirmed that more patients were discharged too soon and in unstable condition. Those who were discharged in unstable conditions had significantly higher mor-

---

[6]The RAND research team sampled hospital records of about 17,000 patients in a total of six DRGs from 300 hospitals in five states before and after implementation of the Medicare PPS. The goal was to determine the effect of DRG-based PPS on quality of hospital care. Quality was measured by both outcome measures—30- and 180-day mortality rates after admission and an indicator of whether the patient was discharged from the hospital in an unstable condition—and measures of implicit and explicit process. The implicit process indicators were summary measures of process of care giving the physician reviewers' overall assessment of the quality of the care process for a particular hospitalization. The explicit measures consisted of five standardized disease-specific process scales; these included physician cognitive diagnostic processes, nurse cognitive diagnostic processes, technical diagnostic processes, technical therapeutic processes, and intensive care unit/telemetry monitoring. Nursing was reflected in most of the explicit process measures. Detailed severity-of-illness data were recorded and used to control for severity of illness in the empirical analysis.

tality rates. Kosecoff and colleagues (1990) analyzed the data on the level of patient's medical instability at the time of hospital discharge. Using data about five medical conditions—congestive heart failure, acute myocardial infarction, pneumonia, cerebrovascular accident, and hip fracture—the authors established the following measures of medical instability: fever, new incontinence, new chest pain, new shortness of breath, new confusion, new elevated heart rate, new elevated respiratory rate, high diastolic blood pressure, newly lowered systolic blood pressure, newly lowered heart rate, and new premature ventricular contractions. They found that 17 percent of the patients in the study were discharged with at least one disability; 39 percent were discharged with at least one measure of sickness; 24 percent had an abnormal last laboratory value. The risk of death at 90 days following discharge was 16 percent for patients discharged unstable and 10 percent for patients discharged in stable conditions. Instability at discharge had increased since the introduction of PPS. Pre-PPS, 15 percent of discharged patients were unstable, as compared with 18 percent post-PPS, a 22 percent increase. Most of the increase in instability was concentrated in those patients who were discharged to their homes; after PPS, 43 percent of them were more likely to be unstable than prior to PPS. They comment that given continued reductions in hospital compensation rates, the problem of instability at discharge warrants additional research to answer questions such as, "Are increases in instability caused by inappropriately early discharges, too many tests in a shortened hospital stay, incorrect use of new medications, or by changes in nursing practices (e.g., fewer nurses per patient and less time to talk with the patient or monitor incontinence or disorientation)?" (p. 1982). The study also revealed that one quarter of nursing home patients were admitted from the hospital with an instability. Answers to these questions require new data.

Some of the issues raised by the authors may be responsive to nursing care. Although the quality of nursing care was measured, details about performance of RNs have not been provided in the reports published to date.[7] Inferentially, however, the levels of quality of nursing care must have been well within acceptable limits, given the overall findings of acceptable quality of care and the fact that decisions to discharge patients (unlike the planning for discharge and for care postdischarge) are not made by nurses.

This landmark research illustrates the value of a well-executed and comprehensive study of the effects of an intervention on the quality of hospital care. Unfortunately, such studies are very expensive and can be somewhat dated by the time the data are collected and analyzed, and the results are published. Data from the RAND studies are based on the experience in the late 1980s. Similar studies

---

[7]As this report goes to press, the RAND researchers are further analyzing their data with the goal of publishing analyses concerning nursing processes of care and the quality of care under the DRG-based PPS system.

have not been undertaken since; hence, no comparable recent data are available to examine if quality of hospital care is improving, deteriorating, or remaining unchanged.

Similarly, with some exceptions, studies suggest that quality of care has remained the same or possibly improved under managed care (see Chapter 3). It should be acknowledged that the studies reviewed were conducted in the 1980s, an era when there were comparatively few managed care organizations. Care delivered by some of the more recent entrants into managed care may be more problematic.

The committee is shocked by the lack of current data relating to the status of hospital quality of care on a national basis, apart from information on indicators such as hospital-specific mortality rates (which HCFA no longer makes easily accessible). The committee, therefore, is unable to draw any definitive conclusions or inferences about the levels of quality of care across the nation's hospitals today. Briefly, quality of hospital care in general did not suffer and may have even improved after implementation of PPS, as shown by the few studies available. At the same time, there may be problem areas with quality of hospital care as suggested by these studies, but the extent of the problem today is not known because of the lack of objective current data. The committee is convinced that investigation of hospital quality of care warrants increasing and immediate attention. Research also needs to move beyond hospital mortality and focus also on the process-of-care problems and conditions that occur during short hospital stays and investigate outcomes over an episode of care.

RELATIONSHIP OF NURSING STAFF TO QUALITY OF PATIENT CARE

The issues surrounding the relationship of staffing levels and staffing patterns of nursing personnel and outcomes have taken on added importance since the committee was established. Hospitals are restructuring and redesigning the organization and delivery of patient care, and the committee heard many reports of reduction of nursing staff and its adverse effects on quality of care. Very little current data are available describing the quality of care in hospitals, and assessing if it has been affected in any way by changes in the system of delivery of care in the hospitals.

The precise questions about the relationship of nursing staff to quality of patient care in hospitals must be clear. One inquiry asks: Do simply the total numbers (or FTEs) of RNs, or the ratio of different types of nurses (usually RNs to LPNs, or RNs to NAs and other ancillary staff), make a difference? For example, are higher ratios of RNs to LPNs correlated in some fashion with better outcome measures (such as lower diagnosis-specific or hospital-specific death or complication rates)? The other question asks: What particular nursing tasks, skills, or ways of organizing teams of nurses (and possibly other health care personnel) are related to better processes of care and superior patient outcomes? These issues are examined in the remainder of this section.

Nursing Staff and Quality of Care

Differences in mortality rates across hospitals are well documented by several researchers. Literature on RNs' impact on hospital mortality rates is considerable. Prescott (1993) provides a comprehensive review of empirical evidence of the impact of nursing staff levels and mix on quality of patient care in hospitals. Much of the evidence came from regression analyses that used RNs as a share of total hospital nursing employment as an explanatory variable—essentially, a basic "numbers" variable. Overall, she found "substantial evidence linking RN staffing levels and mix to important mortality, length of stay, cost and morbidity outcomes" (p. 197). While nurse staffing is not the only factor predictive of mortality outcome, it is an important one affecting the quality of hospital care.

Many factors potentially contribute to high quality of care in any setting; Prescott's review appropriately emphasized studies that considered the role of multiple determinants. Because hospitals are very complex organizations, isolating the role of a single input is difficult, and one cannot eliminate the possibility that, even in a well-controlled analysis, variables such as RN share is surrogates for other, unmeasured quality determinants (Hegyvary, 1991). For example, hospitals with a high proportions of RNs to other staff, may also have the attributes of greater status, autonomy, and control by RNs (Aiken, 1994); these attributes, in turn, may be the determining variable for better quality nursing care and thus better patient outcomes. On the other hand, the ratio of RNs to total nursing employment may be high in hospitals with comparatively few total nursing personnel; if the total number of nursing staff is low enough, the high proportion of RNs may not be correlated with particularly good quality levels.

The performance of a system is determined as much by the arrangement and interaction of its parts as by the performance of the individual components (Scott and Shortell, 1983). Isolating the specific contribution of nursing personnel to the quality of patient care may not be feasible because of the way care is delivered in a hospital, involving contributions of a wide array of staff—nurses, therapists, physicians, and other allied health personnel.

Knaus and colleagues (1986) compared predicted and actual mortality rates for treatment in 13 ICUs. Predicted death rates for each ICU were derived from the acute physiology and chronic health evaluation (APACHE) scores of individual patients. The authors found that although RN staffing levels and positive physician–nurse communication were important factors in achieving lower than expected mortality, the difference between predicted and actual mortality rates were more related to the process of care (e.g., the level of coordination and communication among care givers) than to the structural attributes of the ICUs (e.g., therapies offered, teaching versus nonteaching status). Mitchell and colleagues (1989) in a demonstration project to document fiscal costs and patient care effectiveness of critical care nursing in a unit characterized by valued organizational attributes, reported findings similar to those of Knaus and colleagues. Units characterized by a high perceived level of nurse-physician collaboration, highly rated objective nursing performance, and significantly more positive organizational climate were associated with desirable clinical outcomes such as low mortality ratio, no new complications, and high patient satisfaction.

In a later analysis based on the APACHE III study, Zimmerman and colleagues (1993) report on the difficulty of measuring ICU performance with currently available measures. The authors attempted to identify and evaluate those organizational and management factors that might be associated with ICU effectiveness and risk-adjusted mortality rates. Nine ICUs participating in the APACHE III study were identified. These units varied significantly in their risk-adjusted mortality rates. Structural and organizational data were collected, and on-site observations of the nine units were conducted. The authors report that the on-site analysis failed to identify the units with significantly high or low performance levels and that organizational and management practices are not sufficient to identify levels of ICU performance as measured by risk-adjusted patient survival rates. High levels of team orientation among care givers was associated with ICU efficiency, but not with ICU risk-adjusted mortality rates. Furthermore, units with lower levels of performance exhibited some excellent organizational practices and high-performing units exhibited some poor organizational practices.

Hartz and colleagues (1989) analyzed Medicare discharges in 1986 and found that the percentage of nursing personnel who were RNs was one of the five significant predictors of hospital mortality rates. Specifically, hospitals with a higher percentage of RNs and hospitals with a higher staffing levels had lower adjusted mortality rates.

Verran (Part II of this report)[8] prepared for the committee a detailed review of the literature on quality of hospital care, organizational variables, and nurse staffing. On the basis of both published research and research recently reported at an invitational conference, she concluded that (1) the proportion of RNs on a nursing staff has a positive influence on severity-adjusted Medicare mortality rates; (2) a professional practice environment (defined as a unit-level self-management model including participant decision making, use of primary nursing, peer review, and a salaried status for RN staff) has a beneficial influence on severity-adjusted Medicare mortality rates, over and above the influence of staffing mix; and (3) implementation of a professional practice model is cost neutral.

---

[8]The IOM committee commissioned this paper from Joyce Verran. The committee appreciates her contributions. The full text of the paper can be found in Part II of this report.

Verran discussed several methodological problems with existing studies: low sample size, in part reflecting the high cost of data collection, at the unit of the hospital in which nurses practice; the lack of nurse-sensitive patient outcome measures; the fact that many pertinent outcomes occur after the patient leaves the hospital and, relatedly, the lack of longitudinal data on patients postdischarge; and the inconsistency of outcome measures among studies, which makes broad generalizations difficult (Verran, Part II of this report).

She notes that much of the research to date has not addressed the association between nurse staffing skill mixes and numbers and quality of care. The studies reported at the conference, for instance, were conceptualized and funded in response to the nursing shortage of the late 1980s. Consequently, the variables used in those studies are more focused on nurse retention than on the effects of nurse staffing on patient outcomes. Moritz (1995) also gives an exhaustive review of outcomes and effectiveness research that bears on questions of quality of care and the link between nursing processes or outcomes and broader patient outcomes. For example, in reviewing the available information on the importance of organizational models, she draws attention to the growing body of work on clinical outcomes and health status as it applies to nursing research. Her paper does not mitigate the view, however, that at present the evidence of the impact of nurse staffing and mix on quality of hospital care should be viewed as, at best, suggestive of a relationship, but not conclusive.

In investigating the relationship of nursing staff and patient outcomes, hospital organization has received comparatively little attention even though a substantial body of research documents a relationship between organizational attributes of hospitals and nurse satisfaction and turnover. Far less attention has been given to the relationship between nursing organization and patient outcomes (Kramer and Schmalenberg, 1988a,b; Aiken et al., 1994). When institutional attributes or characteristics are the focus of hospital mortality studies, many organizational correlates are examined, of which nursing often is one (Shortell and Hughes, 1988; Hartz et al., 1989). Nurse-to-patient ratios or nurses as a percentage of total nursing personnel are sometimes found to be significant correlates of patient mortality rates, but usually these studies give little consideration to the mechanisms by which staffing ratios might affect patient outcomes.

Several recent studies point to the organization of nursing within hospitals as the operant mechanism by which nurse staffing affects patient outcomes. Shortell and colleagues (1994) studied the role of nurse staffing and managerial factors as determinants of performance of hospital intensive care units (ICU). Although their sample size was small (42 ICUs), this research is important in its attempt to isolate the role of various organizational variables and staffing on hospital performance. In particular, controlling for patient case-mix, the authors found that the availability of state-of-the-art technology was a statistically significant determinant of risk-adjusted mortality. The quality of the care giver interaction affected risk-adjusted ICU length of stay. When these and other factors are held constant, the ICU nurse-to-patient ratio had no effect on any of the outcomes analyzed, giving weight to the suspicion that variables other than nurse staffing per se affect patient outcomes in the hospital context.

In a study examining Medicare mortality rates, Aiken and colleagues (1994) found that magnet hospitals (that is, hospitals with low RN turnover and vacancy rates and high levels of RN satisfaction) have lower patient mortality than control hospitals. In a presentation to the IOM committee (October, 1994), Aiken summarized the study findings. These findings indicate that lower Medicare mortality rates, as well as improved work-related well-being for RNs, are linked to hospital organization characteristics that result in RNs having: (1) more autonomy to provide care in their professional roles and within their areas of expertise; (2) greater control over what other care givers do in the patient care environment and over resources; and (3) well-documented and well-developed professional relationships with physicians.

Aiken and colleagues also conducted a study of specialized AIDS care units. The combined results of these two studies provide interesting information concerning the organization of nursing care. The magnet hospital study indicates that the preferred organizational structure is one in which the hospital management sees its primary responsibility as delivering patient care, and therefore both places a high value on the quality of nursing services and actively supports the professional role of nursing services. The research on specialized AIDS care units demonstrated how, in the absence of the preferred hospital-wide organization of nursing services, unit-level organization of care can help create environments where the RN autonomy and control that promote lower mortality rates can develop. Specifically, Aiken and colleagues found that AIDS care units foster RN autonomy and control through RN specialization (which promotes autonomy and interaction with physicians based on mutual expertise) and the correlation between patients' high care needs and RNs' areas of specialization. Furthermore, these two studies confirm that the same factors that lead hospitals to be identified as effective from the standpoint of the organization of nursing care are associated with lower mortality among Medicare patients.

Aiken and colleagues concluded that although RN-rich staffing ratios are sometimes associated with improved outcomes, the results of their research indicate that such staffing ratios are essentially a proxy measure for other organizational attributes of hospitals that grant nurses autonomy over their own practice and control of the resources necessary to deliver patient care and create good relationships with physicians. The committee concurs with the findings of Aiken and colleagues (1994, p. 783), "that the mortality effect derives from the greater status, autonomy and control afforded nurse in the magnet hospitals, and their resulting impact on nurses' [RNs'] behaviors on behalf of patients—i.e., this is not simply an issue of the number of nurses, or their mix of credentials."

Clearly, one of the research challenges in determining the relationship between staffing and quality of care has been the difficulty of isolating the factors (and the relative importance of these factors) that are involved in producing improved patient outcomes. Aiken and Salmon (1994, p. 324) contend that "[n]urses place considerable importance on having high nurse-to-patient staffing ratios and that, in general, they have been reluctant to think critically about other strategies that could be as, or more, important in achieving good patient outcomes." The issue is not just a matter of staffing ratios. In the authors' view, what RNs do and how they do it are both more important than simply how many RNs there are. These studies suggest that RNs may have overestimated the value of staffing ratios and skill mix in hospitals and underestimated the importance of the organization of nursing. The committee is of the view that more attention to organizational factors can lead to more efficient use of RNs and other nursing personnel and at the same time improve patient outcomes.

In summary, *the committee concludes that literature on the effect of RNs on mortality and on factors affecting the retention of RNs is available. But there is a serious paucity of recent research on the definitive effects of structural measures, such as specific staffing ratios, on the quality of patient care in terms of patient outcomes when controlling for all other likely explanatory or confounding variables.* Part of the problem lies in the area of severity of illness and risk adjustment, where patient acuity is a significant factor. Across-the-board staffing ratios tend to assume that in some measure all patients are "alike" and can be cared for with the same level and type of resources. Equally difficult is the task of establishing ratios that will be appropriate for all settings and situations.

At least one committee member strongly supports mandated minimum staffing levels specific to different types of acute care units and facilities but recognizes that specifying any particular minimum level was beyond the scope and competency of the committee. All committee members support the current federal requirements and accreditation standards for nursing services and support the need for hospitals to maintain the highest possible standards for nursing care. Moreover, the committee agrees that hospitals should develop improved methods for matching patient needs (severity-of-illness or acuity measures) with the level and type of nurse staffing. The committee supports efforts to improve systems for planning appropriate nursing care as well as monitoring the outcomes of that care.

The committee believes that high priority should be given to obtaining empirical evidence that permits one to draw conclusions about the relationships of quality of inpatient care and staffing levels and mix. Such data should focus on nursing care and quality of care across institutions and within given institutions, and across departments and services. Existing work has not typically focused on isolating the contribution of nursing care in measuring the quality of patient care in hospitals.

Thus, the committee is convinced that more rigorous research on the relationship between nursing variables, broadly defined, and quality of care would have significant payoffs for policymakers, nursing educators, and hospital administrators.

> **RECOMMENDATION 5-5: The committee recommends that the National Institute of Nursing Research (NINR) and other appropriate agencies fund scientifically sound research on the relationships between quality of care and nurse staffing levels and mix, taking into account organizational variables. The committee further recommends that NINR, along with the Agency for Health Care Policy and Research (AHCPR) and private organizations, develop a research agenda on staffing and quality of care.**

Several other agencies of the U.S. Department of Health and Human Services also have a major role in health workforce data collection and research, including the Division of Nursing in the Bureau of Health Professions, the Health Resources and Services Administration; the National Center for Health Statistics (the principal health statistics agency of the federal government) in the Centers for Disease Control and Prevention; and the Health Care Financing Administration. Finally, private organizations could be partners in these research programs, for example, hospital associations (e.g., Hospital Research and Education Trust, the American Hospital Association [AHA]; and state hospital associations, some of which [e.g., in Maryland and New York State] conduct work of this sort already) and private philanthropic and research foundations, particularly those with long-standing interests in health personnel, organization of the health care sector, or quality of care.

A major part of any such research agenda might call for elaboration of the actual variables—in terms of structure, process, and outcome—that warrant high priority attention in studies of the relationship of nursing care, staffing patterns for nursing, to patient outcomes. As discussed below, for example, the American Nurses Association (ANA) has been developing quality indicators that warrant further investigation.

Report Cards

During its work, the committee heard a great deal about the need for more information on hospital quality of care to be made available to policymakers and the public. The reasons are several: to improve the workings of a competitive health care market, to enable the public to make better choices about health care plans, and generally to reflect the nation's expanding interest in generating and using information to help improve the quality and cost-effectiveness of health care. One notable indication of this movement is the growing belief in "report cards"—that is, summary collections of indicators or measures of health care providers' performance. Such report cards may serve as conduits of information about the quality of inpatient care in individual institutions and facilities or entire health care systems.[9] Despite the surge of interest and activity in report cards, however, they are still in the early stages of design and implementation. The ultimate feasibility of linking report card use to actual improvements in the quality of care remains to be seen.

One example of a report card approach that relates to the central questions before this committee—the role of nursing in quality of care and patient outcomes—is that being developed by Lewin-VHI for the ANA (ANA, 1995b; Lewin-VHI, 1995). Because very few of the report cards under development document the specific effects of nursing on the quality of care delivered in hospitals, ANA felt the need for quality indicators that would clarify elements of quality of care from a nursing practice perspective. The organization thus commissioned Lewin-VHI, in 1994, to develop performance indicators for nursing care in hospital settings.

In the first phase of the project, the developers identified 21 categories of measures with an apparent conceptual link to nursing. The candidate measures suffered from significant practical limitations, however: lack of a strong research base linking them to nursing outcomes, lack of specificity to nursing, lack of necessary data collection mechanisms, and lack of applicable risk adjustment systems. Thus, considerable empirical validation of the measures was needed.

The committee is informed that work on the second phase of the project is under way. Seven indicators have been identified for further research because the necessary data collection mechanism exists and/or because of their specificity to nursing: (1) patient satisfaction; (2) pain management; (3) skin integrity; (4) total

---

[9]The committee charge did not directly include the topic of report cards for hospitals. However, this is a growing movement, and the committee judged that some observations were relevant for this discussion.

For one thing, most sets of indicators that might be used in hospital-specific report cards fall short of those implied in the IOM definition of quality of care (IOM, 1990). Although they generally include some patient satisfaction indicator, rarely do they include functional status and well-being (i.e., reliable and valid measures of "desired health outcomes") as that concept is meant to be understood. Neither do any of the existing sets of hospital quality indicators apparently include the detailed structural measures that would allow examination of relationships between different staffing patterns or team compositions and the "end results" of care.

Lewin-VHI (1995) identifies two categories of report cards: provider based and plan based. According to this report, most provider-based report cards address the quality of hospital care but tend to focus on a limited number of quality indicators such as mortality rates or length of stay (at best, a proxy measure of quality). As discussed elsewhere in this chapter, this approach presents serious limitations to any effort to examine the effects of nursing care on quality of hospital care for at least two reasons: (1) no measures reflect nursing care as distinct from hospital care, and (2) the information provided by only mortality and length-of-stay data is insufficient to understand the quality of patient care processes or outcomes other than death.

nursing care hours per patient; (5) nosocomial infections (urinary tract infection, pneumonia); (6) patient injury rate; and (7) assessment of patient care requirements (Telephone communications with Janet Heinrich, Director, American Academy of Nursing).

The committee commends the ANA for its exploratory efforts to develop a set of nursing care quality indicators. This research can set an important precedent and standard for the development of meaningful quality standards relating to nursing. It offers promise for further evolution of external regulatory quality assurance mechanisms (like those of the Joint Commission on the Accreditation of Health Care Organizations [JCAHO]) and for improved public information efforts. Nevertheless, the committee judges that in the future, a broader set of inputs from the nursing community and other affected parties is desirable. It also believes that efforts based solely in the private sector, with little or no public sector involvement, might be less useful than if federal and state perspectives were taken into account. Therefore:

> **RECOMMENDATION 5-6:** **The committee recommends that an interdisciplinary public–private partnership be organized to develop performance and outcome measures that are sensitive to nursing interventions and care, with uniform definitions that are measurable in a uniform manner across all hospitals.**

Such a partnership should involve a group comprising the following: various professional associations of nurses (clearly including ANA but not limited to it); leaders in the nursing profession in areas such as quality assessment and improvement, health services research, and nursing education; hospital systems and associations; accrediting bodies that have long experience with setting quality standards and criteria; researchers and experts in administrative databases who are familiar with developing uniform minimum data sets in the health area; and government officials representing the health agencies that pay for care, monitor quality of care, or track education and training curricula, as well as have long experience in developing uniform minimum data sets for national use.

LEGISLATIVE AND REGULATORY REQUIREMENTS

Regulation of hospitals is a long-standing part of government responsibility. States have had their own licensing requirements for hospitals and other facilities since the early part of the century. Regulation has taken many forms, such as certification, licensure, and accreditation.[10]

---

[10]A comprehensive review of hospital accreditation, deemed status, and similar regulatory issues, as well as of quality assurance requirements and programs (e.g., HCFA's Peer Review Organizations) was beyond this committee's charge. Such reviews are available from other sources (e.g., IOM, 1990). Hence the committee did not undertake such a review.

Since Medicare and Medicaid legislation was passed in 1965, the Social Security Act has required that providers be certified as a condition of participation in the program. This is accomplished through mechanisms known as *Conditions of Participation* that are promulgated through specific standards in the Code of Federal Regulations. For hospitals to be so certified for participation, the Social Security Act requires that facilities be licensed and in good standing by the state. In addition, hospitals must meet all federal certification standards, and the federal HCFA is authorized to determine whether hospitals meet these federal requirements. HCFA may conduct on-site inspections to observe care and review records to determine compliance, or it may ask state agencies to carry out these surveys.

Under the Social Security Act, certification may also be based on accreditation, which is in turn based on a concept of *deemed status.* Hospitals found to meet accreditation standards by the JCAHO are deemed automatically to meet the federal Conditions of Participation in the Medicare program—in effect, they are considered to be certified to receive Medicare (and Medicaid) reimbursement. HCFA performs independent validation surveys of individual hospitals on a sample basis as an assurance that the federal government can rely on the JCAHO approach. In addition, accreditation by the JCAHO is a requirement for hospitals approved to conduct graduate medical education residency programs and is frequently a requirement for payment by health maintenance organizations (HMO) and health insurance companies.

Certification by JCAHO requires that (a) nursing care be provided on a 24-hour-a-day, 7-day-a-week basis; (b) nursing services show evidence to the surveyors that each patient's status is monitored; (c) provision of nursing care is coordinated with the provision of care by other professionals; and (d) specific patient care plans be in place and in use for each patient. Furthermore, JCAHO standards for nursing care place a new emphasis on the role, responsibility, qualifications, and accountability of the nurse executive, including the authority and responsibility for ensuring that standards of nursing practice are in place and meet JCAHO's patient care standards (JCAHO, 1994).

The hospital organization must provide "a sufficient number of qualified nursing staff members to assess the patient's nursing care needs; plan and provide nursing care interventions; prevent complications and promote improvement in the patient's comfort and wellness; and alert other care professionals to the patient's condition as appropriate" (JCAHO, 1994, p. 521). The "Care of Patients" chapter of the standards manual (part of the patient-focused section) directs attention to a wide set of elements of good care. These include the following:

- "Formulation, maintenance, and support of a patient-specific plan for care, treatment, and rehabilitation;"
- "Implementation of the planned care, treatment, and rehabilitation;"

- "Monitoring the patient's response to the care, treatment, and rehabilitation provided, the actions or interventions taken, and/or the outcomes of the care provided;"
- "Modification of the planned care, treatment, and rehabilitation . . . based on reassessment, the patient's need for further care, and the achievement of identified goals;" and
- Planning and coordination of the "[c]are, treatment and rehabilitation necessary after the patient's discharge from the organization" (JCAHO, 1994, p. 125).

A large majority of hospitals seek and attain accredited status.[11] The JCAHO renders five types of accreditation decisions, depending on the extent to which hospitals are judged (on the basis of institution-specific survey data) to comply with published standards of performance; the five accreditation levels are (1) accreditation with commendation, (2) accreditation, (3) conditional accreditation, (4) provisional accreditation, and (5) not accredited.

Given the continued reliance of the federal government on this approach to certification for hospital reimbursement through federal health programs, the committee is encouraged by the evolution of JCAHO methods and standards in the past few years and by the more sophisticated attention being paid to the role of nursing care in those standards. It also takes note of a new initiative, the Council on Performance Measurement, which will serve as an advisory body for evaluation of performance measurement systems, especially with respect to considering whether they are suitable for incorporating into future accreditation processes.

All in all, therefore, *the committee endorses the current federal requirements for hospitals to participate in Medicare, which incorporate the use of voluntary accreditation, to assure the quality of hospital care, and it is particularly supportive of requirements that call for matching nursing resources with patient needs. The committee believes that Congress ought to continue to support this element of assuring the quality of care in hospitals.*

SUMMARY

Hospital restructuring and redesign of staffing systems are undertaken for a variety of reasons that include controlling costs and adjusting to the dramatic changes in the delivery of health care. Hospitals are restructuring to maintain their economic viability, but they need to do so without adversely affecting the outcomes of the care they provide. The changes now taking place in the hospital sector involve major rethinking of the use of different types of clinical staff, as

---

[11]Some hospitals are accredited in a similar fashion by the American Osteopathic Association, rather than the JCAHO, but the underlying philosophy of being certified to receive Medicare reimbursement and to conduct graduate training programs is the same.

well as reconfiguration of units, departments, and care teams. The redesign of nursing services also is leading to changes in the roles and responsibilities of RNs and to increased emphasis on interdisciplinary teams. These developments have prompted uncertainty in employment and great concern among RNs about the potential for erosion of quality of hospital care, and about their own well-being.

In this chapter the committee has examined these concerns, specifically whether quality has deteriorated and whether empirical evidence exists of a link between the number and skill mix of nursing personnel and the quality of patient care. The committee has found that little empirical evidence is available to support the anecdotal and other informal information that hospital quality of care is being adversely affected by hospital restructuring and changes in the staffing patterns of nursing personnel. At the same time the committee notes a lack of systematic and ongoing monitoring and evaluating of the effects of changes resulting from organizational redesign and reconfiguration of staffing on patient outcomes.

Researchers have concluded that although RN-rich staffing ratios are sometimes associated with improved outcomes, the results of their research indicate that they are essentially proxy measures for organizational measures. For quality of care changes, the committee was unable to isolate a number-of-RNs effect from the organizational and related factors attending different levels of staffing. The committee concludes that high priority should be given to obtaining empirical evidence that permits one to draw conclusions about the relationships of quality of inpatient care and staffing levels and mix.

The committee, however, is concerned about the paucity of objective research on the relationship between staffing and quality, and the effects of restructuring. The committee concludes that a clear need exists for a system for monitoring and evaluating the impact of the rapidly changing delivery system on the quality of patient care and the well-being of nursing staff. For this reason, it has advanced several recommendations intended to provide better information on hospital restructuring and to help in delineating those factors that affect patient outcomes. It also calls for the development of a research agenda in this area and for the articulation of reliable, valid, and practical measures of structure, process, and outcome to be used in quality-of-care research as well as quality assurance and improvement programs. *A systematic effort is needed at the national level to collect and analyze current and relevant data and develop a research and evaluation agenda so that informed policy development, implementation and evaluation are undertaken in a timely manner.*

Some broader issues of changes in nursing services, such as the enhanced responsibilities of advanced practice nurses, and the use of ancillary nursing personnel and their competency, cut across the straightforward issue of the relationship between nurse staffing and quality of hospital care. In reflecting on the role of nursing personnel in the future, therefore, the committee has also proposed recommendations about these specific types of nursing personnel.

6

Staffing and Quality of Care in Nursing Homes

Nursing homes are an important component of the health care industry that is becoming increasingly complex. As discussed in Chapter 3, the nursing home market is being stressed by an increasing demand for services combined with a constrained growth rate.

The previous chapter explores the relationship of staffing patterns of nursing personnel to quality of patient care in hospitals and examines the structural variables of staffing and their relationship to processes and outcomes of care. This chapter examines the interrelationship of quality of care and staffing in nursing homes. The chapter begins with a discussion of the measurement of quality of care in nursing homes, followed by an overview of the status of quality and the legislative and regulatory efforts to improve quality. The chapter next discusses whether these efforts have achieved their objectives, namely, improvement of the quality of care. It then examines staffing levels and skills as they exist today and their linkages to quality of care. Finally, it examines the determinants of staffing, by taking into consideration the roles of third-party payment and regulation.

To gain insights on these issues, the committee examined the statutory requirements, available empirical evidence, and information gathered during site visits and public testimony. It also reviewed extensive research literature on the relationship between staffing patterns and quality of care. The committee deliberated long and hard on the issues before reaching the conclusions and recommendations put forth in this chapter.

MEASUREMENT OF QUALITY

Quality of care in nursing homes is a complex concept, confounded by regulations, debates about what should be measured to assess quality, case-mix, facility characteristics, and methods of measurement (Mezey, 1989; Mezey and Lynaugh, 1989). "Quality of nursing home care has proven to be one of the most politically volatile—yet societally critical—issues confronting the American public. The issue strikes at the core of individual concern about possible functional impairment and potential loss of impairment and potential loss of independence [, c]omplicated by the likelihood of personal impoverishment . . ." (Wilging, 1992b, p. 13). In short, it is the focus of providers, consumers, regulators, and public policymakers.

Defining quality in nursing facilities has been a difficult process. Quality of care in nursing homes has been defined both as an input measure and as an outcome (Kruzich et al., 1992). The Institute of Medicine (IOM) definition is cited in Chapter 5. As elaborated there, quality can be approached in terms of three concepts: structure, process, and outcome. Table 6.1 presents an illustrative list of the measures of quality of care in nursing homes. These include human, organizational, and material resources.

Elements of Quality of Care

Traditionally, nursing home quality has been measured by *structural* variables. Important among these are (1) inputs, such as the level and mix of staffing; (2) characteristics of facilities, such as ownership, size, accreditation, and teaching status; and (3) characteristics of the facility's residents, such as demographics and payer mix. Staffing is a structural measure that affects the processes and outcomes of care in nursing facilities, but it is considered in part to be determined by facility ownership and payment sources. Case-mix relates to quality in that demands on staff (both numbers and quality) are highly related to the needs of patients. Studies indicate that a low percentage of private-pay patients in a facility is a negative indicator of quality of care (using deficiencies as indicators). It is argued that because private-pay residents pay a higher per diem rate than do Medicaid residents, nursing homes generally compete for private-pay residents on aspects of structure and process associated with quality. This competition may be desirable because it also creates an incentive to provide quality care even in a bed-shortage environment. (Nyman, 1988b; Spector and Takada, 1991).

Although structural measures assess the availability of resources as a necessary precondition for their use, *process* measures examine actual services or activities provided to or on behalf of residents. In the context of nursing homes, the process of care focuses on providing special care and treatment to prevent problems with outcomes such as cognition, hearing and vision, physical functioning, continence, psychosocial functioning, mood and behavior, nutritional and

TABLE 6.1 Illustrative Measures of Quality of Care in Nursing Homes

Structural Measures

- Staffing levels (nurses, PTs, OTs, etc.)
- Staffing mix
- Staff turnover
- Wages/benefits
- Management/leadership structure
- Facility: size, location, ownership
- Availability of private rooms
- Volunteers

- Governance
- Age/condition of plant, equipment (include mobility development)
- Payer mix (percent mix, etc.)
- Case mix
- Accreditation
- Teaching status

Process-of-Care Measures

- Assists with ADL/IADL (includes bathing, skin care)
- Injury (staff and patient)
- Infection control (includes residents and staff)
- Resident services: special care to prevent problems
- Overuse of restraints
- Use of urinary catheters
- Bladder training

- Delivery of "hotel" services (sanitation)
- Assessment (includes care planning), frequency and completeness
- Abuse prevention
- Quality assurance (RA and MDS)
- Access and use of medical care
- Resident rights

Outcome Measures

- Mortality
- Hospitalization
- Facility-acquired pressure sores, skin breakdown
- Functional status change
- Pain control
- Depression
- Injuries
- Urinary incontinence

- Weight loss
- Infectious disease
- Patient satisfaction
- Family satisfaction
- Thefts/abuse
- Staff injuries/illness
- Staff satisfaction

NOTE: ADL = activities of daily living; IADL = instrumental activities of daily living; OT = occupational therapist; PT = physical therapist, RA = resident assessment; MDS = Minimum Data Set.

dental care, skin condition, and medications (Morris et al., 1990). Because many persons tend to stay in nursing facilities for considerable lengths of time, often for months or years, process measures tend to assume greater importance than they do in hospitals, where the average length of stay is 7 days (Kane, 1988; Kane and Kane, 1988).

A number of studies of nursing home quality have examined process measures (Zimmer, 1983, 1989; Zimmer et al., 1986). Some of these measures describe how personal services to residents are provided. These measures include help with activities of daily living (ADL) and provision of special services. At the same time, in high-quality institutions, staff avoid overuse of psychotropic medications (chemical restraints) and physical restraints. Critical to provision of high-quality care is a patient-specific care plan. Finally, residents have basic rights that society accords to other individuals. Thus, these rights also constitute elements of quality captured by the process measures.

The *outcomes* of nursing home care include changes in health status and conditions attributable to the care provided or not provided. Outcomes of long-term care are "most fairly expressed in terms of the relationship between expected and actual outcomes." For some nursing home residents, realistic expectations for the outcomes of care may be maintained levels of health or slower-than-expected rates of decline, rather than improved health (R.L. Kane, 1995, p. 1379). The currently used measures of outcome include global measures such as mortality rates and rehospitalization rates (Lewis et al., 1985; GAO, 1988a,b; Spector and Takada, 1991); summary measures of functional status; and specific indicators such as incidence of facility-acquired pressure sores and urinary incontinence (Nyman, 1989b). Satisfaction of both residents and their families are also quality indicators because nursing home care and professional performance encompass more than the provision of technical services (Hay, 1977). Ultimately, determining the expected and actual outcomes of care for nursing home residents will require sophisticated and increased attention to assessment of individuals' initial health status, quality of life, sociodemographic characteristics, and the nature of treatment provided (e.g., palliative or curative), with the goal of determining the outcomes attributable to treatment after controlling for other variables (R.L. Kane, 1995).

Patient Characteristics

Nursing home residents and the primary missions of nursing homes vary, as well as the way in which variations affect how specific quality-of-care measures should be interpreted. At the risk of oversimplification, there are three types of residents: (1) those who use the facilities for recovery and rehabilitation following an acute hospital stay; (2) the terminally ill; and (3) persons with multiple chronic conditions and cognitive and functional impairments who are expected to stay in nursing facilities for the rest of their lives. The second and third types of patients have been predominant in past years. In the last decade or so, the number of residents in the first category has grown appreciably (Spence and Weiner, 1990).

Patient mix affects staffing and the levels and mix of services provided, but also how various quality-of-care indicators should be interpreted. For example, a resident undergoing rehabilitation should maintain or experience improvements in functional status as the stay progresses. By contrast, for the terminally ill, decline in functional status is to be expected; control of pain and other dimensions of quality of life are paramount. Because indicators have different meanings depending on the resident's circumstances, quality-of-care indicators must be applied and interpreted with due regard for those meanings.

STATUS OF QUALITY OF CARE IN NURSING FACILITIES

Although in many facilities good care has been provided, even in the face of considerable financial constraints, the quality of care in some nursing facilities has long been a matter of great concern to consumers, health care professionals, and policymakers (NCCNHR, 1983).

The IOM Committee on Nursing Home Regulation (IOM, 1986b) reported widespread quality-of-care problems in nursing homes. These findings were confirmed by the U.S. Senate (1986) and the General Accounting Office (GAO, 1987). Using studies from the 1970s and early 1980s, testimony in public meetings conducted by the committee, news reports, state studies of nursing homes, and committee-conducted case studies of state programs, the earlier IOM committee concluded that "problems identified earlier continue to exist in some facilities: neglect and abuse leading to premature death, permanent injury, increased disability, and unnecessary fear and suffering on the part of residents" (IOM, 1986b, p. 3). Although that IOM report noted some indication that these "disturbing practices now occur less frequently" (p. 3), the study also expressed concern about the poor quality of life in many nursing homes. It singled out problems of residents being treated with disrespect and of frequently being denied any choices of food, roommates, the time they rise and go to sleep, their activities, the clothes they wear, and when and where they may visit with family and friends. The committee stated flatly that the quality of medical and nursing care in nursing homes "left much to be desired" (p. 3).

Other studies, many published around the time of the IOM (1986b), U.S. Senate (1986), and GAO (1987) reports, have specifically examined quality of care in nursing homes. A number of clinical practices have been associated with poor patient outcomes.[1] For example, urethral catheterization may place residents at greater risk for urinary infection and hospitalization or other complications such as bladder and renal stones, abscesses, and renal failure (Ouslander et

---

[1]These are clinical problems that are not necessarily unique to nursing home settings.

al., 1982; Ouslander and Kane, 1984; Ribeiro and Smith, 1985). Similarly, tube feedings also increase the risk of complications including lung infection, respiration, misplacement of the tube, and pain (Libow and Starer, 1989). Several studies of nursing facilities have shown the prevalence of a range of negative (or poor) patient outcomes such as urinary incontinence, falls, weight loss, infectious disease (Libow and Starer, 1989). Other poor patient outcomes identified include preventable declines in physical functioning (Linn et al., 1977); mortality and hospital readmissions during the first year of nursing home placement/residency (Lewis et al., 1985; GAO, 1988a,b; Spector and Takada, 1991); behavioral/emotional problems, cognitive problems, psychotropic drugs reactions, and decubitus ulcers (Zinn et al., 1993a,b).

Legislative and Regulatory Efforts to Improve Quality

To participate in the Medicare or Medicaid programs, long-term care facilities are required to meet federal certification requirements established by the Health Care Financing Administration (HCFA) (42 CFR Part 843) under the Social Security Act. Long-term care facilities include skilled nursing facilities (SNF) certified for Medicare, nursing facilities (NF) certified for Medicaid, and dual-certified facilities for both programs. State survey agencies are authorized to determine whether SNFs and NFs meet the federal requirements. Surveyors conduct on-site inspections to observe care, review records, and determine compliance. These surveys are used as the basis for entering into, denying, or terminating a provider agreement with the facility.

In the early 1980s, the federal government proposed deregulation of the nursing home industry. At the same time, Congress was concerned about quality-of-care problems in nursing facilities because of reports and complaints by consumer groups. Problems with the regulatory process had been identified in an evaluation of state survey processes (Zimmerman et al., 1985). Because of the growing concern about nursing home quality, Congress requested a study by the IOM to examine the regulation of nursing facilities. The IOM Committee on Nursing Home Regulation documented quality-of-care problems and recommended revision and strengthening of the federal/state regulatory process (IOM, 1986b). Its recommendations, as well as the active efforts of many consumer advocacy and professional organizations, led Congress to enact a major reform of nursing home regulation in 1987 included in the Omnibus Budget Reconciliation Act of 1987 (OBRA 87). This legislation was refined through subsequent related legislative enactments in 1988, 1989, and 1990.

OBRA 87

OBRA 87 has been characterized as a "watershed"; it provided a definition of quality in long-term care that focused measurement of quality on resident outcomes and resident rights, and it recognized that without appropriate attitude and motivation, quality of care cannot be provided (Wilging, 1992a, p. 22). OBRA 87 specified that a nursing facility "must provide services and activities to attain or maintain the highest practicable physical, mental, and psychosocial well-being of each resident in accordance with a written plan of care . . ." (sec. 1919(b)(2)). This legislation was a "landmark" statute in at least three respects.

First, for the first time, nursing homes receiving federal funds were required to ensure a high quality of life in addition to providing a high quality of care.

Second, the requirement that well-being be maximized implied that *improvements* in health and functional status be achieved, when possible, thereby shifting the focus from provision of custodial to provision of rehabilitative care. To achieve the objective of the highest level of well-being, nursing homes were required to develop individual care plans and a resident assessment process. Under the provisions of OBRA 87 and federal guidelines, nursing homes participating in Medicare and Medicaid programs must use the resident assessment instrument (RAI) to assess residents on admission, annually thereafter, and on any significant change in the resident's status. The RAI consists of the minimum data set (MDS) for resident care assessment and care screening (which is described more fully below) and resident assessment protocols (RAP). The purpose of these assessments is to identify a resident's strengths, preferences, and needs in key areas of functioning and to guide the development of the resident's care plan (Phillips et al., 1994).

Third, OBRA 87 recognized that implementation of its provisions would require additional resources and training. Therefore, it encouraged state Medicaid programs to adjust their rates to reflect the new OBRA standards. This is arguably the first time that Congress explicitly recognized that high-quality care and quality assurance efforts come at a price.

HCFA Regulations

HCFA issued the enabling regulations in October 1990. These regulations mandated a number of changes. First, the regulations eliminated the hierarchy of conditions, standards, and elements that had been in prior regulations to that point.

Second, the 1990 regulations mandated comprehensive assessments of all nursing home residents, using the MDS forms (Morris et al., 1990). Nursing facilities are required to complete the MDS forms for each resident within 14 days of admission, when there are major changes in health status, and at least annually. Facilities also are required to use the assessment in the care planning process. The federal survey procedures (conducted by state agencies) check the accuracy and appropriateness of the assessment and care planning process for a sample of residents.

Third, more specific requirements for nursing, medical, and psychosocial services were designed to attain and maintain the highest practicable mental and physical functional status (Zimmerman, 1990). These requirements were specified in the new regulations, and a detailed set of HCFA interpretive guidelines was developed for use by state surveyors in 1990. The state surveys were redesigned to be more outcomes oriented than had previously been the case. Such outcome measures include residents' behavior, their functional and mental status, and certain physical conditions (such as incontinence, immobility, and decubitus ulcers). For example, the regulations established criteria for and prohibited the use of physical restraints and antipsychotic drugs without a specific indication of need, and they require periodic review and dose reduction unless clinically contraindicated. In addition, regulations detailing and protecting residents' rights were added.

Nursing Home Resident Assessment Tools

An important recent advance stemming from OBRA 87 was the development of the Nursing Home Resident Assessment System by Hawes, Phillips, and their colleagues. This system designed the nursing home minimum data set mentioned above for resident assessment and developed detailed protocols for resident assessment of specific problem areas to guide the care planning process (Morris et al., 1990). The purpose is to assess the functional, cognitive, and affective levels of residents. The MDS items were field-tested in 1990; the final version included 15 domains: cognitive patterns, communication/hearing patterns, vision patterns, physical functioning and structural problems, continence, psychosocial well-being, mood and behavior patterns, activity pursuit patterns, disease diagnoses, health conditions, oral/nutritional status, oral/dental status, skin condition, medication use, and special treatments and procedures (Morris et al., 1990).

Now under development are quality indicators (QI), which use the MDS as a part of the National Nursing Home Case-Mix and Quality Demonstration (NHCMQ) study funded by HCFA. Among them are QIs for accidents, behavioral/emotional problems, cognitive problems, incontinence, psychotropic drugs, decubitus ulcers, physical restraints, weight problems, and infections. The QIs for individual residents and for facilities are compared to national norms, by taking into account predisposing factors and case-mix factors related to each QI. QIs that may indicate poor quality of care are identified and given to state surveyors to examine in the certification survey process (Zimmerman et al., 1995). Using QI data, state surveyors are expected to determine whether or not the identified QIs are the result of or are related to poor care processes.

HCFA has proposed issuing regulations to require all nursing facilities to store and transmit RAI information electronically. Although, as of late 1995, the final rule had not been published, most providers are proceeding on their own. Nearly 62 percent of nursing facilities have begun computerizing resident assessments (AHCA, 1995). When fully computerized, QIs may be a valuable tool for monitoring the quality of nursing home care. Certainly, the QIs will augment the current nursing home survey process.

Survey and Certification

In November 1994, HCFA (1994a) released its final regulations for the survey, certification and enforcement of SNFs and NFs (42 CFR Parts 401–498). The provisions shaped the process of surveying and certifying facilities and specified procedures for enforcement. HCFA is also undertaking efforts to train state surveyors in using the new survey, certification, and enforcement procedures.

Several alternative remedies may be imposed on facilities that do not comply with federal requirements, instead of or in addition to termination. These include civil money penalties of up to $10,000, denial of payment for new admissions, state monitoring, temporary management, immediate termination, and other approaches. The extent and type of enforcement actions depend on the scope of problems (whether deficiencies are isolated, constitute a pattern, or are widespread) and the severity of violations (whether there is harm or jeopardy to residents).

HAS QUALITY OF CARE IMPROVED SINCE OBRA 87?

The committee sought to determine whether quality of care in nursing homes is improving as a result of these increased efforts by the federal government to regulate quality. Consumer groups, staff, and providers report some improvements in nursing home care (Cotton, 1993; Fagin et al., 1995; 1995 IOM public hearings). A number of facilities have successfully focused on reducing the inappropriate use of physical and chemical restraints, and some report that the focus of the federal survey on resident problems represents a substantial improvement in the survey process.

Between 1989 and 1993 the percentage of residents who were restrained dropped from 40 percent to 19 percent. Despite this progress, wide variations among states indicate that further progress is possible (AHCA, 1995). Deficiencies issued to facilities have declined since OBRA 87 was implemented. The average number of deficiencies declined from 8.8 per facility in 1991 to 7.9 in 1993 (Harrington et al., 1995). Survey data also show that the percentage of facilities without any deficiencies has increased slightly to 11.4 percent in 1993.

Nevertheless, a recent analysis of the On-Line Survey and Certification Reporting System (OSCAR) data for 1993 also showed that despite some improvements in quality, state surveyors continue to find deficiencies of varying kinds and seriousness (see Table 6.2). Data compiled on all nursing facilities in the United States surveyed in 1993 were examined. With respect to the process of

TABLE 6.2   Deficiencies in Certified Nursing Facilities from the Federal On-Line Survey Certification and Reporting System, United States, 1993

Types of Deficiencies	Percent of Facilities with Deficiency
Process Deficiencies	
Unsanitary food (The facility must prepare and serve food under sanitary conditions)	30
Inadequate care plan (The facility must develop a comprehensive care plan for each resident)	25
Inadequate sanitary environment (The facility must provide housekeeping/maintenance services for a sanitary environment)	20
Hazards in the environment (The facility must ensure that the resident environment remains free of accident hazards)	20
Improper restraints (Residents have the right to be free of physical restraints used for discipline or facility convenience)	18
No comprehensive assessment (The facility must make a comprehensive assessment of resident needs)	16
Inadequate infection control (The facility must investigate, control, and prevent infections)	15
Inadequate activities (The facility must provide an ongoing program of activities to meet resident needs)	12
No 24-hour nursing (The facility must provide sufficient numbers of personnel on a 24-hour basis)	5
No RN on duty 7 days a week (The facility must have an RN on duty 8 hours a day for 7 days a week)	5
Outcome Deficiencies	
Failure to maintain dignity (The facility must promote care for residents that maintains dignity and respect)	19

continued on next page

TABLE 6.2 Continued

Types of Deficiencies	Percent of Facilities with Deficiency
Outcome Deficiencies (continued)	
Inadequate treatment of incontinence (Incontinent residents must receive appropriate treatment)	12
Failure to prevent pressure sores (The facility must ensure that residents without pressure sores do not develop them)	9
Inadequate treatment of pressure sores (The facility must provide necessary treatment of residents with pressure sores)	9
Poor nutrition (The facility must ensure that residents maintain acceptable levels of nutritional status)	9
Abuse of residents (Residents have the right to be free of verbal, mental, and other abuse)	2

SOURCE: Harrington et al., 1995.

care, nursing facilities were given deficiencies for a range of problems. Frequently cited problems include inadequate care plans, unsanitary and hazardous environments, and unsanitary food (this category is a "catch all" and includes minor problems such as crumbs left under the toaster and dumpster left uncovered to more serious problems such as unclean kitchen, inappropriate food and dishwasher temperatures, and other sanitation issues that could lead to foodborne disease transmission). In the area of outcomes, failure to maintain dignity and respect toward residents was a significant problem.

Restraints have been severely criticized because their use may cause decreased muscle tone and increased likelihood of falls, incontinence, pressure ulcers, depression, confusion, and mental deterioration (Evans and Strumpf, 1989; Libow and Starer, 1989; Burton et al., 1992; Phillips et al., 1993). Although much progress has been made in reducing the use of restraints, Graber and Sloane (1995) found that a number of facilities fail to recognize and promote the independence of residents. They found that despite the implementation of OBRA 87 regulations, nearly one-third of North Carolina nursing home residents remained physically restrained. The characteristics associated with restraint use and with restraint violations can be used to identify facilities most likely to benefit from

TABLE 6.3 Resident Characteristics in Nursing Facilities from the Federal On-Line Survey Certification and Reporting System, United States, 1993

Characteristics	Percent of Residents
Chairbound	48
Bedfast	5
Organic psychiatric conditions	37
Receiving psychoactive medications	33
Bladder incontinence	48
Bowel incontinence	42
Indwelling catheters	8
Contractures	18
Physical restraints	20
Pressure sores	8

SOURCE: Harrington et al., 1995.

assistance and education in reducing use of physical restraints. A recent study by Phillips and colleagues (1993) found that physical restraints continue to be overused but that the use of such restraints actually requires more, rather than less, staff time and care and therefore may increase total nursing home costs. The authors estimated the effects of restraint use on licensed nurse time, nurse assistant time, and total wage-weighted care time, while statistically adjusting for those other resident characteristics that have been shown to affect staffing. As a case in point, residents who are restrained receive more time from nurse assistants than do similarly impaired residents who are not restrained.

The improper use of psychotropic drugs, although reduced in recent years, continues to be identified as a significant issue in several studies (Harrington et al., 1992b). Senate hearings in 1991 focused on problems associated with the misuse and inappropriate use of chemical restraints, which both OBRA 87 and the implementing regulations issued by the Health Care Financing Administration (HCFA) in 1990 were designed to reduce (U.S. Senate, 1991).

Recent reports (SEIU, 1994, 1995a,b; *Consumer Reports*, 1995) continue to point to deficiencies in quality of care and staffing problems in some nursing facilities of large chains. According to these reports, some of these facilities were unable to meet the published quality assurance plans of their parent entities.

Many residents of nursing homes have serious disabilities and problems that need skilled nursing care. Table 6.3 shows that in 1993, 48 percent of all nursing

---

[2]The IOM committee commissioned this paper by Johnson and colleagues. The committee appreciates their contributions. The full text of the paper can be found in its entirety in Part II of this report.

facility residents were chairbound and 5 percent were bedfast. Of the total residents, 37 percent had some severe psychiatric conditions that were not reversible (such as Alzheimer's disease), and another 33 percent were receiving some type of psychoactive medication for such conditions. Nationally in 1993, 48 percent of nursing facility residents were reported to have bladder incontinence and 8 percent had urinary catheters; 42 percent had some bowel incontinence. Some 20 percent of residents had physical restraints, 18 percent had physical contractures (muscle rigidity of the limbs), and 8 percent had pressure sores (decubitus ulcers). These conditions indicate the need for nursing care and careful reviews to determine whether the quality-of-care programs provided to address them are adequate.

In summary, despite the recent improvements in nursing home quality and regulatory compliance, in the committee's judgment the quality of care provided by some nursing facilities still leaves much to be desired. The number and type of deficiencies and complaints reported by state licensing agencies, consumer advocacy groups, families, and residents show poor quality in some facilities. These problems have demonstrated the need for continued research and for the development of public policies that could improve both the processes and the outcomes of care.

Measures relating to deficiency citations need to be carefully interpreted. For one thing, achieving 100 percent compliance with regulatory requirements would be an unrealistic public policy objective. For another, no survey process is perfect.

A report prepared for the American Health Care Association (AHCA) to assess the reliability of the survey process noted specific aspects of the process that needed improvement and identified areas for further educational efforts and assistance for surveyors. The problems identified were often related to unclear guidance regarding operational definitions of scope and severity of resident outcomes in defining deficiencies (Johnson-Pawlson, 1994). A national evaluation of the survey process identified a number of areas in which better procedures are needed (Abt Associates and the Center for Health Policy Research, 1993). However, it is likely that surveyors are reasonably accurate at the extremes in identifying very good facilities and very bad ones (Johnson et al., Part II of this report[2]). A report by the Office of the Inspector General of the Department of Health and Human Services (DHHS) also concluded that most states are doing an adequate job in carrying out survey responsibilities required by the 1987 federal legislation, but work continues to be needed to improve the current survey process (OIG, 1993). The recent release of the final federal enforcement regulations for SNFs and NFs should also improve the regulatory process (U.S. DHHS, 1994).

Finally, the committee notes that although OBRA was enacted in 1987, it is being implemented in an incremental manner. Implementing regulations were first issued in 1990, and final regulations for certification and enforcement of nursing facilities were only issued in November 1994. It is not reasonable, in these circumstances, to expect overnight changes that would drastically reduce deficiencies or improve the performance of nursing homes across the nation.

Status of Staffing

The committee sought to determine if staffing as a measure of quality of care in nursing homes has improved as a result of OBRA 87, subsequent federal legislation, and the responses of state governments. In attempting to answer that question, the committee examined three types of evidence: government standards, empirical evidence, and committee testimony and site visits.

Federal Standards

To the extent that new federal requirements were binding on facilities, some improvement in staffing and the consequent quality might be anticipated. OBRA 87 required nursing facilities to have licensed nurses on duty 24 hours a day; a registered nurse (RN) on duty at least 8 hours a day, 7 days a week; and an RN director of nursing. The statute permits the director of nursing and the RN on staff for 8 hours to be the same individual. In addition, OBRA 87 specifies that facilities have sufficient staff to accomplish the care objectives described above (sec. 1919(4)(C)(i)).

As stated in chapter 4, Staffing ratios have increased slowly in recent years (HCIA and Arthur Andersen, 1994). This slight improvement can be attributed in part to the requirements of OBRA 87 and in part to the staffing need to care for residents who require specialized services (such as subacute care and services for residents with Alzheimer's disease).

Any effect of the nurse coverage requirements may have been mitigated in some circumstances by the waiver provisions of OBRA 87. Because of the nursing shortage at that time, Section 1919(b(4)(C)(ii) of the Social Security Act authorizes any state to waive the requirements for 24-hour licensed nursing service as well as the 8-hour-a-day RN presence if certain criteria are met. The facility is required to demonstrate that, despite diligent efforts, it has been unable to recruit appropriate personnel. The state must also determine that a waiver will not endanger the health and safety of individuals residing in the facility. Waivers must be obtained by facilities annually.

Quite a large number of facilities have obtained waivers. The Secretary of DHHS reported to Congress on initial waivers granted through January 1993. In 1993, governments in 13 states granted waivers to 518 of the 5,302 facilities certified for Medicaid only (HCFA, 1994b). Of these facilities, 66 were waived from the requirement to provide 24-hour licensed nurse services. More prevalent are waivers for the 8-hour RN requirement. As of January 31, 1993, the states had granted such waivers to 490 facilities. Some progress has been made in the intervening period. For example, by May 1995 the number of waivers granted dropped to 157. All of them were for the requirement for RN presence.[3]

The committee is encouraged by the progress made by states in reducing the number of waivers, especially those related to 24-hour licensed nurse presence. Since increasingly sicker and older persons requiring skilled nursing care are being discharged from the hospitals to nursing facilities, more needs to be done by the facilities to ensure an RN presence to provide care for the residents. With the adequacy of the RN supply at the present time and reported layoffs in hospitals, nursing facilities should have less difficulty in meeting this statutory requirement without waivers. *The committee strongly endorses the intent of OBRA 87 and supports efforts made by facilities and states to improve professional nurse staffing in nursing homes consistent with the intent of the statute.* The committee hopes that the states continue the progress made in reducing the waivers granted and that they work diligently toward eliminating them in the foreseeable future.

State Standards

In addition to federal standards, some states have established their own standards, although these may vary widely across states. Mohler (1993) surveyed states regarding their staffing requirements for nursing facilities. She found that the majority of states had specific minimum staffing standards in addition to the federal standards for nursing facilities. Some states specified standards for RNs and others for nurse assistants; still others had standards for both. For example, Minnesota requires a minimum of 2 hours of nursing care per resident day for all licensed nursing facilities, although these hours are not required to be distributed evenly across the evening or night shifts (Chapin and Silloway, 1992). States can also impose state penalties on facilities that have substandard staffing based on state regulations. These data suggest that many states have concluded that they need staffing standards for nursing facilities in addition to those of the federal government.

Empirical Evidence on Staffing

The committee reviewed the available data and research literature that provide empirical evidence of changes in staffing in nursing homes that may have occurred since the enactment of OBRA 87. Comparing data from the 1991 National Health Provider Inventory with corresponding data from the 1985 National Nursing Home Survey (NCHS, 1987; HRSA, 1994), the committee deter-

---

[3]Telephone communication with Steven Pelovitz, Associate Administrator, Health Care Financing Administration.

TABLE 6.4 Nurse Staffing Levels for All Certified Nursing Facilities from the Federal On-Line Survey Certification and Reporting System, 1991–1993

Nurse Staffing Levels	Year		
	1991	1992	1993
Medicaid-Only Facilities			
Number of facilities	9,120	12,463	12,132
Hours per resident day			
RNs	0.3	0.3	0.3
LPNs	0.6	0.6	0.6
NAs	2.0	1.9	2.0
Total nurse hours[a]	2.9	2.8	2.9
Medicare/Medicaid and Medicare-only facilities			
Number of facilities	819	1,110	1,234
Hours per resident day			
RNs	1.0	1.2	1.4
LPNs	1.2	1.4	1.5
NAs	2.4	2.5	2.7
Total nurse hours[a]	4.4	4.8	5.2
Total All Facilities			
Total Number of facilities	9,624	13,133	12,913
Hours per resident day			
RNs	0.4	0.4	0.4
LPNs	0.6	0.6	0.7
NAs	2.0	2.0	2.1
Total nurse hours[a]	3.0	3.0	3.1

NOTE: RN = registered nurse; LPN = licensed practical nurse; NA = nurse assistant.

[a]The columns do no necessarily add to the total nurse hours because the number of facilities is not the same in each category. The number represents the national average for facilities on which data are available.

SOURCE: Harrington et al., 1995.

mined that overall staffing ratios for RN time and total staff time per resident day had increased very slightly over the 18 minutes of RN time and 2 hours of total staff time per resident day reported in 1985 (NCHS, 1988). Moreover, most estimates assume that staff are evenly distributed over 24 hours, which is generally not the situation. Most facilities have fewer staff (both licensed and total staff) on evening and night shifts and on holidays and weekends than during daylight or "regular" hours of operation.

Kane reported that Friedlob's 1993 doctoral dissertation analyzed the results of a large sample of nursing homes and their residents in 6 states (R.A. Kane, 1995). About 39 percent of the sample received no care from an RN during the 24-hour study period; the average RN time per resident was 7.9 minutes; the average licensed practical nurse (LPN) time, 15.5 minutes; the average nurse assistant (NA) time, 76.9 minutes.

Zinn (1993a) found wide variations in nursing home staffing patterns in 10 standard metropolitan statistical areas (SMSA) studies, even after controlling for case-mix.

Current staffing data collected by state surveys are available from the federal OSCAR. As shown in Table 6.4, between 1991 and 1993, RN hours or total nursing hours per resident day in facilities certified as Medicaid-only did not change. RNs continue to report 0.3 hour (or 18 minutes) per resident day, and LPNs 0.6 hour. In Medicare-only and Medicare and Medicaid dual-certified facilities, staffing levels for all categories of nursing increased appreciably over the 3-year period. The committee notes, however, that the vast majority of facilities were *not* Medicare certified during this period, and those not certified by Medicare had a much lower staffing base. Thus, staffing levels improved somewhat for dual-certified facilities but remained essentially unchanged for Medicaid-only facilities. The differences reflect, at least to some extent, differences in acuity and reimbursement levels.

Ratios for the country as a whole obscure substantial variation among states and among facilities within states. OSCAR data show that in 1993, 96 facilities in 20 states reported having no RN staff. It is not known if this was the result of reporting errors or represented a real absence of RN staff. Reporting problems with the current OSCAR data on staffing have been identified. Actual staffing levels in nursing facilities may be lower or higher than the levels reported because of over- or underreporting and other errors. Staffing data are reported by the facilities to state surveyors and are not always reviewed by the surveyors.

Public Hearings and Site Visits

The committee conducted public hearings and site visits to learn about these issues directly from the persons and organizations affected. Many complaints were voiced at the public hearings by resident advocates, licensed nurses, and nurse assistants about inadequate quality of care and staffing shortages at all levels. Representatives of the nursing home industry, however, described improvements in the quality of nursing care indicating that, in their view, staffing was on average adequate. They also described the financial and other constraints under which facilities operate.

The committee cannot generalize from such testimony. Rather it notes the lack of current, nationally representative, and valid data on the characteristics of nursing facilities, their residents, and the staffing in these facilities, as well as on processes and outcomes of care in nursing facilities. The last comprehensive National Nursing Home Survey was conducted in 1985. The data from this survey have been used extensively by researchers, policymakers, industry, and resident groups. The survey provided detailed information on nursing facilities, staffing, discharges, and patient characteristics. Primarily because of budget constraints, this survey was not conducted again until a decade later in July 1995. The committee regrets, however, that because of budgetary problems, the survey instrument has been pared down. The committee understands that critical detailed information on staffing and discharges such as that collected in 1985 will not be collected. Only total numbers of full-time equivalent RNs, LPNs, and NAs will be collected. Current, comprehensive data are needed for research, policy formulation, management of the nursing home industry, and consumer information.

Information derived from administrative databases such as the OSCAR files and similar sources should be made available in a format that is reliable and understandable to the public. Every effort should be made to ensure the quality and accuracy of these administrative files, to adequately train the persons surveying and reporting the information, and to ensure that the information is used appropriately. These issues surrounding the availability of reliable, accurate, valid, and timely data need attention in order to ensure that policies are made and evaluated on a solid factual and analytical basis.

During its site visits, the committee repeatedly heard complaints from nursing home staff about the paperwork imposed by OBRA 87 and the states. In particular, they indicated that a substantial part of the RN's time was spent completing paperwork associated with the MDS, so that staff had insufficient time for direct patient care. The link between the completion of the MDS and the provision of high quality of care was not always apparent in every facility. Data from such assessments are essential to the development of outcome-oriented measures of quality and the implementation of a resident-focused federal certification process. Some viewed the MDS as another intrusion imposed by external sources on their time rather than as a clinical tool for improving the quality of resident care and the management of patient care. Also, committee members noted that at some sites, when the staff complained about the burden of MDS, they did not distinguish between the MDS and other state and local forms that were merged with it. The general belief among some of those interviewed was that they provide quality care and that quality can be better improved with more time devoted to patient care instead of paperwork. Clearly, social engineering is needed to create a different climate and professional nurses should be central to this endeavor.

Although the committee is sympathetic about the time-consuming nature of the forms, it does not conclude that the existing implementation is unnecessarily burdensome. The committee is concerned, however, about the apparent lack of consensus among nursing home staff in recognizing that such clinical tools are needed at the grass-roots level. Some have also questioned the quality of the information entered on the MDS because of an emphasis on meeting regulatory survey requirements. The MDS is supposed to reflect accurately what happens so that appropriate interventions are undertaken in a timely manner. It is meant to be a link among assessment, planning, intervention, and evaluation, but it is seen by many staff in the nursing facilities as a legal requirement that they have to complete. In some instances, the nurse who is required to complete all the care plans based on the MDS may not ever see the patients in question. Some nursing facilities hire consultant nurses for the purpose of completing the MDS and other documentation (Schnelle, 1994).[4] The committee believes that use of consultant nurses for this purpose only is undesirable, and it strongly discourages facilities from continuing the practice.

The committee strongly endorses the concept of an individualized care plan for each resident. Such care planning requires the use of tools like the MDS. A uniform, comprehensive resident assessment system is essential to the development of an individualized care plan for each resident that focuses on improving, maintaining, or minimizing decline in the resident's functional status and quality of life.

The committee endorses HCFA's current efforts at improving the instrument and requiring all facilities to computerize MDS data and provide them to state and federal agencies, thus providing a mechanism for a national database. The committee further encourages the states to adopt use of the MDS without unduly adding additional elements to it.

RELATIONSHIPS AMONG NURSING STAFF, MANAGEMENT, AND QUALITY OF CARE[5]

Many factors influence staff performance and the quality of care provided to residents. Some are internal to the organization, such as staffing and staff characteristics, education and training levels of the staff, job satisfaction and turnover of staff, salaries and benefits, and management and organizational climate. Others are external to the facility itself, such as regulations, reimbursement policies, incentives, excess demand for services, and type of facility. This section exam-

---

[4]Discussion held at the special invitational session on Quality and Staffing in Nursing Homes, sponsored by the National Institute of Nursing Research on behalf of the IOM study, in conjunction with the 1994 annual meeting of the Gerontological Society of America in Atlanta, November, 1994.

[5]Much of the information in this section was taken from the background papers commissioned from Johnson et al., Maas et al., and Harrington, for use by the IOM committee. The committee appreciates their contributions. The full text of the papers can be found in Part II of this report.

ines the internal factors. Factors external to the facility are discussed in the next section.

Nursing Staff Levels and Skill Mix

Staffing and Resident Characteristics

There is universal agreement in the research literature on the strong relationship among resident characteristics, nursing staff time requirements, and nursing costs in nursing facilities. Several studies have examined these relationships and attempted to quantify them (Weissert et al., 1983; Arling et al., 1987). Case-mix is an important factor in examining the relationships between research needs and nursing staff required to meet those needs. Resident characteristics were studied in terms of staffing resources in facilities judged to offer high quality of care in the development of the Resources Utilization Groups (RUGS) (Fries and Cooney, 1985). Additional studies were used to create an updated RUGS II (Schneider et al., 1988). Substantial work has been conducted as part of the Multistate Nursing Home Case-mix and Quality Demonstration Project sponsored by HCFA beginning in 1989 (Fries et al., 1994). The basic principle of the case-mix project is that resources should be allocated based on resident need and that sicker and more debilitated residents need more services both in terms of amount of staff time as well as level of expertise. As a result of research into case-mix, the third iteration of a resource utilization grouping (RUGS III) has been developed (Fries et al., 1994). RUGS III was developed with 44 resident groups, which were defined to explain 56 percent of the resource utilization variance (Fries et al., 1994). Based on the data from the case-mix project, it is evident that the need for nursing time and nursing skills varies significantly depending on the resource classifications. These data show that facilities need to adjust their staffing levels to take into account the condition of the residents. Fries and colleagues' (1994) research has documented that much of staffing is driven by the type of residents.

The use of staffing standards or ratios as a structural indicator of the quality of nursing homes presupposes that higher ratios lead to improved care processes and outcomes. Although it is not clear that any fixed staffing-to-resident ratios can be established across all facilities and all types of residents, facilities should use "acuity indexes" or other case-mix methods for adjusting their staffing levels to ensure sufficient staff to provide for the basic needs of residents.

Staffing and Quality of Care

Considerable attention has been devoted by researchers and policy makers to the issues of how many staff and what type of staff are needed to meet the needs and expectations of nursing home residents as measured by care processes and outcomes. Several studies have been conducted by experts in the field to examine these relationships. They show a strong relationship between both general level of nursing staff and RN staff (or professional nursing staff, in particular) and resident outcomes.

Not surprisingly, higher nursing staff levels (nursing staff hours per resident day) in nursing facilities have been associated with higher quality of care as measured in terms of care processes and various outcomes. Type of nursing staff may be more important than the availability nursing staff hours per se. Nursing care is a major service provided by nursing homes. Some experts believe that nursing facilities that rely predominantly on unskilled nursing staff with minimal presence of licensed nursing staff jeopardize the quality of nursing home care.

The studies reported below examine the relationships between the nursing staff and other nursing home characteristics as independent variables and quality of care as measured in terms of care processes and resident outcomes as the dependent variables. Nursing staff as an independent variable is examined in various ways in these studies. Some researchers have used total numbers of nursing staff or aggregate nursing staff levels, others have examined the number or level of RNs (referred to at times as professional nursing staff), still others have looked at staffing as the ratio of RNs to LPNs or RN to total nursing staff (sometimes referred to as skill mix). Table 6.1 provides an illustrative list of structure, process, and outcome measures used to measure quality of care in nursing homes.

In a landmark study by Linn and colleagues (1977), conducted over a 9-year period, 1,000 men transferred from a general medical hospital into 40 community nursing homes were studied. Information was gathered about the men at the time of discharge from the hospital, 1 week after transfer, and 6 months later. The purpose of the study was to determine the relationship of nursing home characteristics to differential outcomes of patients placed in several homes. Patients' outcomes measured were mortality, functional status, and discharge from the nursing home. The independent variables were nursing home characteristics—an array of structural variables such as facility size, ratios of RN hours per patient, LPN hours per patient, NA hours per patient, total staff hours per patient, professional staff hours per patient, costs per month, medical records, meals, patient appearance, services, policies, physical plant, and safety. Outcomes were related to the nursing home characteristics by multivariate analysis of variance, controlling for expected outcomes—age, and diagnoses of cancer and chronic brain disease. The authors found that a higher ratio of RN hours per patient was consistently and significantly associated with all three outcome measures: patient survival, improved functional status, and discharge from the nursing home. Hours per patient day of the other care givers or the total staff to patient ratio were not related to outcomes. Meal service was related to mortality and functional status; medical records, higher professional staff to patient ratios, and services were related to discharge from the nursing home. Over half of the remaining nursing home variables were never associated significantly with any of the patient outcomes. The authors conclude that increasing RN hours and giving more attention to meal service will have a positive impact on patient outcomes.

Nyman (1988b) examined if quality requires more financial and physical resources using the 1983 Iowa Outcome Oriented Survey. Eight nonhealth quality variables were used, including plant maintenance, room maintenance, room furnishings, care plan, diet plan, Medicare plan, resident care, and quality of life. The independent variables included licensed nurse hours, NA hours, administrative hours, for-profit status, number of beds and other variables. Nurse hours per patient were positively related to seven of the eight quality variables, and significantly related to three. NA hours per patient or any other labor input were not positively or significantly to the quality variables. These findings suggest that simply requiring more staffing in general may not be sufficient to insure quality. None of the quality measures constructed from these data were significantly related to higher average costs.

Using data from reports of 455 Medicare-certified skilled nursing facilities, and controlling for case-mix, Munroe (1990) examined the relationship between facility quality and nursing personnel. The purpose of the study was to determine the extent to which RN staffing patterns influenced nursing home quality. He found a positive significant relationship between nursing home quality as measured by numbers of health-related deficiencies received by the facilities and a higher ratio of RNs to LPNs hours per resident day after controlling for several variables including case-mix. The author concluded that the configuration (or staff mix) of nursing personnel may be more important than total nursing hours.

Based on analysis of 2,500 nursing home residents in 80 nursing facilities in Rhode Island, Spector and Takada (1991) used multivariate models to estimate what structure and process variables are associated with resident outcomes after controlling for resident characteristics. Outcomes measured over a 6-month period included mortality, functional decline, and functional improvement. They found that higher staff levels and lower RN turnover were related to functional improvement and found that low staffing in homes with very dependent residents was associated with reduced likelihood of improvement. High urinary catheter use, low rates of skin care, and low resident participation rates in organized activities were all associated with poor resident outcomes. Overall, few process or structure variables were significantly related to mortality.

Cohen and Spector (in press) found that staffing ratios per residents have a significant impact on resident outcomes. Their analysis of a nationally representative sample of nursing homes and nursing home residents highlights the complex nature of the relationship between RN and LPN staffing and resident outcomes, and shows that staff mix is more important than the overall numbers of staff. Using regression analysis, the authors estimated the relationship between "staff intensity" and resident outcomes to determine if in fact more intensive staffing results in better outcomes. Staff intensity in this study is measured as the number of full-time-equivalent (FTE) staff per 100 residents adjusted for case-mix. Three staffing equations were estimated—RNs, LPNs, and total nursing staff. Three resident outcome equations were estimated. The dependent variables were: mortality within a year, having a bedsore, and functioning defined as ADL status at the end of the year, controlling for health status. Staff intensity effects were found for both mortality and ADL outcomes, but not for bedsores. A higher RN intensity was associated with a lower rate of mortality. The authors calculate that addition of half of an FTE RN (about 10 percent increase in RN on average staffing) would save about 3,000 lives annually. A higher intensity of LPN staffing improved functional status as measured by ADLs, although this impact was relatively small. Having more NAs had no impact on resident outcomes, at least the ones measured in this study. The authors suggest that less variation in NA numbers across nursing homes than in RNs and LPNs may explain to some extent the failure to observe a NA staffing effect on quality.

The finding that RNs affect mortality and LPNs affect functional outcomes is consistent with other research findings. RNs are more trained than LPNs. RNs provide leadership in terms of the organization of the entire nursing care in the facility. They are the ones trained to identify early a potential life threatening situation, and recognize regression of condition in a resident. In a medical emergency an RN deals with the problem until a physician is consulted. LPNs on the other hand are more involved in the day-to-day nursing care than RNs, and they are better trained than NAs in nursing procedures and routines. These results suggest that RNs and LPNs are not substitutes, but have different values for the outcomes of residents.

The authors conclude that since professional nurse staffing intensity has a direct impact on quality, as measured by resident outcomes, quality can be improved by directly influencing the mix of staffing. Efforts to improve quality should be focused more on increasing the intensity of professional nursing staff than only on nonprofessional nursing staff. The authors caution not to interpret the data to mean that the level of NA staffing is unimportant; they do suggest, however, that efforts to improve quality should be focused more on increasing the intensity of the professional than only on the nonprofessional staff.

Zinn (1993b) conducted a study using data on approximately 14,000 nursing facilities from the 1987 Medicare and Medicaid Automated Certification Survey (MMACS). Using a weighted two-stage least square regression model and controlling for case-mix, she found that a lower ratio of RN hours to other nursing staff hours was associated with greater use of urinary catheters, physical restraints, and tube feedings, and with less toileting of residents.

Braun (1991), in a retrospective cohort study of 390 veterans discharged to 11 nursing homes and followed for 6 months investigated the relationship between nursing home quality and patient outcomes of mortality, rehospitalization, and discharge, controlling for severity of illness and case-mix differences. The Multiphasic Environmental Assessment Procedure (MEAP) was used as for quality assessment. Additional quality indices were used as independent variables such as process of nursing care, RN hours, equipment, and Medicaid status. The results of the analysis show that the quality-of-care variable "RN hours" was significantly and inversely related to mortality, while the quality-of-care variable "use of nursing process" was significantly related to probability of discharge.

Using data originally collected by the Missouri Division of Aging during its routine inspection of nursing homes, Cherry (1991) studied 134 Medicaid and Medicare certified nursing homes in Missouri to assess the role of the ombudsman in nursing home quality as measured by the various health related outcomes. In addition to the ombudsmen program, the independent variables included RN hours per resident day, LPN hours per resident day, NA hours per resident day, case-mix, profit, percent of Medicaid residents, and facility size. The only variable contributing significantly to improved quality of care was RN hours per resident day. Increased RN hours were positively associated with improved quality of care measured through a composite of outcome indicators including number of residents developing decubitus ulcers per immobile residents, number of residents catheterized per incontinent residents, number of urinary tract infections per incontinent residents, and rate of antibiotics use per resident. In contrast, hiring more LPNs and in particular more NAs did not necessarily yield similar increases in quality. Adding more NAs also increases the need for supervision and is not in itself a solution to alleviating poor care. The presence of an ombudsman program was found to be significantly associated with quality for skilled nursing homes where there was ample RN staffing.

Gustafson and colleagues (1990) found a significant correlation between nursing staff levels and six measures of quality incorporated into the Quality Assessment Index constructed by them for measuring nursing home quality. A study of nursing homes in Maryland found that higher total staff levels are related to fewer nursing deficiencies (Johnson-Pawlson, 1993).

An anthropological study conducted by Kayser-Jones and colleagues (1989) analyzes the clinical and sociostructural-structural factors contributing to the hospitalization of nursing home residents. Data were collected by participant observation and event analysis. Qualitative analysis of the data found that "insufficient" and "inadequately trained" nursing staff were contributing factors to the deterioration and eventual hospitalization of nursing home residents. A large proportion of the patients could have been treated in the nursing home if the nursing staff had been available and able to administer IV therapy and to monitor the response to treatment and effectively communicate with the physician. Most of the nursing care was provided by a small number of LPNs, but mostly by NAs. The shortage of nursing staff also contributed to nutritional problems. Staffing is an important variable that influences eating behavior. Inadequate staffing results in (1) the feeding of residents in a hurried manner that does not preserve their dignity (e.g., giving residents a large amount of food with each bite, feeding several residents at once, mixing food); and (2) inadequate nutritional intake, resulting in resident weight loss and necessitating the use of liquid supplements and sometimes tube feedings with all its attendant risks. These findings are supported by the research of Blaum and colleagues (1995), which showed poor resident nutrition associated with being dependent on staff for feeding.

Several clinical intervention studies support the need for professional nurse presence to provide the leadership and direction for assisting staff in order to assure that the success of interventions efforts as measured by reductions in physical restraints, presence of bed sores, or falls, continues beyond completion of the study period (see, for example, Evans and Strumpf [1994] and Mezey and Lynaugh [1989] discussed in the next section).

Some researchers (Schnelle, 1990; Schnelle et al., 1990; Hawkins et al., 1992) tested staff management procedures and policies (such as oral and written feedback, professional staff and gerontology specialists working along with the NAs and guiding and training them, and the continuing presence of the supervisory professional nurse even after the intervention period) for assuring that NAs are appropriately trained and motivated to carry out the intervention protocols for decreasing incontinence. Schnelle (1994) reported that during the period of the studies the investigators gave on-site, on the floor training, and walked the floors with the NAs to train staff and to ensure adherence to protocol. These interventions showed significant improvements in resident dryness. However, the interventions only had a positive effect until the controlled conditions were withdrawn; then staff reverted to previous practices. In a multisite study, the staff management system and incontinence protocol were continued in only one of the sites after the controlled conditions ceased. At this site, the director of nursing was particularly interested and involved, and frequently got out on the floor and actually put her hands on the patients to see how often they were wet. Schnelle concluded that it was the knowledge, hands-on interest, and leadership of the RN that resulted in the sustained use of the intervention protocols.

Given the level of NAs' direct care responsibilities and the minimal training for resident care required for them, professional nurse oversight and availability to work closely through constructive supervision of NAs and other licensed nurses is critical (see Johnson et al., Part II of this report). Johnson and colleagues' analysis of OSCAR data indicates a continuing increase in case-mix since 1992. Clinical care gets complicated as residents are likely to have multiple chronic conditions, which require understanding each illness and the interacting effects. Residents are sometimes on complicated medication and treatment regimens requiring pharmacological knowledge. Hence, as the case-mix increases, resident care requires a highly qualified nursing staff present at all times, with the nurse needing a broad base of knowledge covering basic nursing, geriatrics, rehabilitation, and psychiatric skills. Today, an LPN may be the only licensed nurse in a facility in the evenings and night time to attend to resident care; an LPN does not meet the qualification requirements stated above. Increasing the number of RNs becomes very important as the case-mix index of a facility increases. Johnson and colleagues (Part II of this report), in their analysis of "high- and low-quality" facilities, found a positive relationship between the amount of RN time and quality of care. Given this relationship, RN participation in care is very important. They concluded that the current federal requirement of one RN for 8 hours a day, 7 days a week is not sufficient to ensure quality of care for residents.

The preponderance of evidence from a number of studies using different types of quality measures has shown a positive relationship between nursing staff levels and quality of nursing home care, indicating a strong need to increase the overall level of nursing staff in nursing homes. There is a strong need to improve the overall level of nursing staff (RNs, LPNs, and NAs) in nursing homes, but prescribing a staffing ratio across all residents and facilities is inadequate. Research literature does not answer the question of whether a particular ratio of total nursing staff to residents is optimal. Moreover, varying circumstances among nursing homes, case-mix differential within and between facilities, and other factors, including those described in the next section, also affect the type and level of staffing needed. *The committee, therefore, endorses current HCFA staffing standards but is not inclined to recommend a specific minimum staffing ratio across all types of facilities to meet the needs of all types of patients.* Nursing facilities, however, should ensure adequate nursing services to meet the acuity needs of its residents.

Based on the empirical evidence presented above, the committee concludes that a relationship between RN-to-resident staffing and quality of care in nursing facilities has been established. Although the committee did not uncover any research specifically testing 24-hour nursing presence in a controlled experiment, there was sufficient evidence in the literature reviewed that the presence of RN (including geriatric nurse specialists) improved quality of care in nursing homes. Research reviewed above provides abundant evidence that the needs of current residents require highly capable staff, consistent with RN education, and that participation of RNs in direct care giving and providing hands-on guidance and supervision to the NAs and LPNs in caring for the residents is positively associated with quality of care. *The committee, therefore, supports the need to increase professional nurses in nursing homes on all shifts.* Given the findings on the beneficial effects of continuous RN presence on various dimensions of quality, especially on outcomes, and on the use of RNs versus LPNs on the number of health-related deficiencies in nursing homes, the committee supports an increase in the mix of RNs to other nursing staff. Particularly problematic, however, is the lack of any RN presence in many facilities on the evening and night shifts. In light of the data that indicate the fairly low level of education and high turnover rate among NAs in nursing homes, the knowledge and judgment of an RN is critical to recognize a crisis or a regression of a condition. Early detection and intervention related to particular signs and symptoms often forestall the use of more expensive care resources, most notably hospitalization; this is the work of the professional nurse. Based on the above evidence and the committee members' professional experience and expertise, the committee gives priority to mandating improvement in this area of enhancement.

    RECOMMENDATION 6-1: The committee recommends that Congress require by the year 2000 a 24-hour presence of registered nurse coverage in nursing facilities as an enhancement of the current 8-hour requirement specified under OBRA 87. It further recommends that payment levels for Medicare and Medicaid be adjusted to enable such staffing to be achieved.

The committee deliberated hard on this issue, and some committee members are hesitant to impose additional costs on the facilities. The committee recognizes that this recommendation entails additional costs and, therefore, is recommending that Medicare and Medicaid reimbursements be adjusted accordingly, once reliable figures on potential additional costs can be derived. The empirical evidence, however, is convincing, and trends for the future suggest an increasing need for professional nursing presence. *The committee further believes that waivers to this requirement could be granted by states only in exceptional circumstances.* The committee estimates that the cost of the substitution of the additional 16 hours of RN time (over the current 8 hours) for those hours of LPN time across all nursing facilities in the nation could amount to roughly $338 million. This figure is a rough estimate and may be considered an overestimate since most Medicare-certified facilities and some Medicaid-certified facilities already have RNs on 24-hour duty and because of the expectation, based on the geriatric nurse practitioner studies discussed below, that some offsetting cost-savings would be achieved from prevention of complications, higher levels of function, and fewer hospitalization resulting from early detection of signs and symptoms and timely intervention.[6] Ultimately, the committee believes that the public's interests and needs for basic quality of care must be considered in addition to cost if we as a society are going to maintain a sense of values and responsibility for the care of the elderly, disabled, and disadvantaged. At the same time the committee recognizes the possible hardships for a few facilities, such as those in remote rural areas, to recruit and retain 24-hour RN coverage. One committee member dissented from the committee's decision to recommend the 24-hour presence of registered nurses in nursing facilities. His separate statement is included in Appendix C of this report.

---

[6]The source and assumptions used in arriving at the rough estimate are as follows: There are about 16,608 nursing facilities in the United States (AHCA, 1995). The differential between an RN and an LPN salary is $3.98 per hour (AHCA, 1995). Note that RN presence for 8 hours a day is currently required. Then, $3.98 × 16 hours = $64.00 per day; $64.00 × 365 days = $23,260 annually per facility × 16,608 facilities = $338 million. The committee assumes and fully expects that detailed cost calculations will be undertaken by HCFA, states, and other parties involved.

The committee strongly believes that research should continue to further refine the relationships between staffing and resident outcomes, controlling for the relevant intervening factors including structural and organizational variables. The committee also urges continued efforts towards completing the very important case-mix demonstration project under way and going the next step to link the categories being developed of resource needs and measurement of staff time to meet those needs with the quality-of-care measures.

Geriatric Specialists

The IOM Committee on Nursing Home Regulations encouraged nursing homes to employ specialty-trained gerontological nurses and to encourage gerontological nursing (IOM, 1986b).

Studies of gerontological nurse specialists (GNS) and geriatric nurse practitioners (GNP) in nursing homes have shown that they can improve resident outcomes and contribute to quality by changing the focus from custodial to rehabilitative care (Kane et al., 1976, 1988) and by increasing the ability of facilities to care for more complex and acutely ill patients (Mezey and Scanlon, 1988). Employment of GNPs does not adversely affect nursing facility costs or significantly affect profits. There is also some evidence of cost savings, particularly in medical service use by newly admitted patients. GNPs also reduce the use of hospital services (Buchanan et al., 1990).

Evans and Strumpf (1994), investigating the relative effects of two experimental interventions delivered by GNSs on the use of physical restraints and resident and staff outcomes, found that staff mix and resident personal competence were important factors in the occurrence of disturbing behaviors likely to be managed by restraint. These disturbing behaviors occurred more frequently in situations where the availability of licensed nurses was low and resident frailty high. Further, although staff increased their assessment and intervention skills, the investigators noted the need for a "consistent professional presence" of a clinician with geriatric expertise to maintain minimal restraint use in the facility. Findings suggest that quality outcomes (e.g., restraint reduction) do not necessarily require more staff per se, but do require staff who have the requisite knowledge base, gerontological expertise and education, as well as resident-centered assessment, monitoring, care planning, evaluation, and support in their efforts to provide quality individualized care (Evans and Strumpf, 1994; Strumpf, 1994).

A number of demonstrations have provided convincing evidence that GNPs and GNSs are effective in nursing homes. HCFA supported the evaluation of two demonstration projects, the Robert Wood Johnson Foundation Teaching Nursing Home (TNH) Program and the Nursing Home Connection (Massachusetts 1115: Case Managed Medical Care for Nursing Home Patients), while the Kellogg Foundation supported the Mountain States program to place GNPs in nursing homes. These evaluations confirmed that nurses with advanced preparation in care of the elderly decrease unnecessary hospitalization and use of emergency rooms, improve admission and ongoing patient assessments, provide better illness prevention and case finding, decrease incontinence, lower the use of psychotropic drugs and physical restraints, and generally improve the overall management of chronic and acute health problems. These improvements in care occurred without incurring additional costs and in some instances at a reduced cost.

The experience of the TNH program provides further evidence of the need for professional gerontological nurses in nursing homes (Mezey and Lynaugh, 1989, 1991; Mezey, 1994). In comparing the TNH to matched nursing homes in the same state, with the only difference being the presence of an advanced practice nurse in the former, the residents in TNHs had significantly fewer hospitalizations than those in the comparison homes and fewer emergency room visits. There also were notable improvements in a variety of quality indicators such as the management of urinary incontinence; decreased use of psychotropic medications, including long-acting benzodiazepines and other such medications related to poor quality outcomes in nursing homes; and less use of restraints.

Based on the above review of research, the committee concludes that there is sufficient evidence that presence of geriatric nurse specialists/practitioners enhances quality of care in nursing homes. Moreover, research has shown that cost savings in the long run accrue, particularly due to reduced rehospitalizations and visits to hospital emergency rooms.

RECOMMENDATION 6-2: The committee recommends that nursing facilities use geriatric nurse specialists and geriatric nurse practitioners in both leadership and direct care positions.

Nurse Assistants

Nurse assistants constitute 70 to 90 percent of nursing staff in nursing facilities (IOM, 1986b; NCHS, 1987; Maraldo, 1991). They provide most of the direct care and spend the most time with the residents. More than 90 percent of the NAs are women (BLS, 1995c; Crown et al., 1995). Three-fourths of the NAs in nursing homes have not completed high school. They often come from low-income families, earning close to minimum wage; less than half of them have any employer-based health insurance coverage, and even fewer have pension plans. In all these social and economic charactersistics, hospital NAs fare better (Crown et al., 1995).

As stated earlier in this report, because of the Medicare Prospective Payment System (PPS) and advances in medical technology, the acuity level of nursing home residents and the complexity of care provided are increasing. Changes in the characteristics of the residents, low staffing and low wages place added demands on the care givers, especially NAs.

The public hearings and site visits provided information from some nursing home personnel who worked at facilities with low NA staffing. *In some nursing homes there is a clear need for more NAs to provide bedside care.* Such situations were reported to have resulted in consequences such as failure to turn patients as required and decubitus ulcer formation; these may require hospitalization and other costly medical interventions. Furthermore, NAs are responsible for turning the patients in bed at regular intervals. If this is not done, contactures are likely to develop. NAs also feed patients and can be their primary source of companionship and psychological support. Thus, inadequate NA staffing leads to increased risk of medical complications and expense, intermittent discomfort from hunger and thirst, escalated need for even more nursing care, and sensory and psychological deprivation.

On the other hand, the committee also received testimony and saw nursing homes in which NA staffing was exemplary. One person who provided testimony to the committee felt strongly that the role of nurse assistants should be recreated to make it their primary mission to assist the resident rather than to assist other staff. At the facility with which this NA is affiliated, nurse assistants are called "resident assistants," and each is assigned to care for "families" of approximately five residents from the time the residents rise to the time they retire for the night. This witness strongly urged that the focus of NAs' work be shifted in this way and also urged that their titles be changed to "resident assistant" to emphasize this new role. Innovative and successful programs decrease barriers between staff and patients, emphasize meeting residents' needs, increase respect for the work of the NAs, provide continuing education for NAs, experiment with flexible staffing patterns and tasks, and hold teams accountable for all aspects of residents' care. These programs seem to be associated with noteworthy resident, family, and staff satisfaction and with decreased staff turnover or use of sick leave. These remarkable institutions also find decreased medical problems that lead to resident hospitalizations, decreased incontinence, decreased use of restraints, and increased likelihood of residents walking or being able to make easy transfers.

Overall, on the basis of experience and information gathered from the testimonies received, the committee believes that the organization, use, and education of NA staff members make a substantial difference in the humane care, comfort, and health of nursing home residents and in the satisfaction and health of nursing staff.

In general, nurse assistants—who provide the largest portion of direct personal care to residents—receive little training for provision of care in a nursing facility. OBRA 87 requires 75 hours of training and testing for competency for nurse assistants within 4 months of employment and 12 hours of in-service training per year (sec. 1819(b)(5)). Federal regulations require that each state maintain a registry of NAs, but the exact nature of the training, certification, and requirements varies by states. Also, some states include NAs in their registry based on reciprocity with other states. With the increasing acuity of residents in nursing facilities and the complexity of care needed today, some argue that additional training tied to the clinical problems identified in nursing facilities is desirable. The committee heard testimony from certified nurse assistants working in nursing homes about the need for more clinical training and experience as part of their program leading to certification, as well as for the development of career ladders for NAs. There is also a management issue of provision of continuing on-the-job training and one-on-one guidance. Unfortunately, research is lacking on the effect of nurse assistant staffing and training on quality of care in nursing homes. As stated above, in public testimony and on site visits, however, the committee heard support for this relationship.

> **RECOMMENDATION 6-3:** The committee recommends that the training for nurse assistants in nursing homes be structured and enriched by including training of the following types: appropriate clinical care of the aged and disabled; occupational health and safety measures; culturally sensitive care; and appropriate management of conflict.

> **RECOMMENDATION 6-4:** The committee recommends that research efforts on staffing levels and skill mix specifically address the relationship of licensed practical nurses and nurse assistants to quality of care.

Management and Leadership

The changing focus of services and the increasingly complex nature of the care provided in nursing facilities place new demands for skills, judgment, supervision, and management of nursing services. Concern has been expressed by a number of nursing leaders about the training and educational preparation of RNs working in nursing facilities and especially of the directors of nursing (DON). Ballard (1995) indicates that the role of the DON or a nurse administrator ideally involves knowledge of nursing, management, organization theory, finance, marketing and planning, personnel administration, supervision, and government regulations. Most DONs in nursing facilities are not academically prepared for their positions (Bahr, 1991), having little or no specific education about the aging process, gerontological nursing principles, or managerial skills. In contrast to hospitals, where DONs only rarely have less than a bachelor's degree and often have graduate education, those in nursing homes are often graduates of associate degree and diploma programs in which leadership and management are not part of the basic preparation, and they rarely have advanced clinical training in gerontology. Again, this comparison is at the national aggregate level. Wide rural–urban variations can be found in the educational levels of RNs in managerial positions in hospitals.

Turnover among DONs in nursing facilities is high, amounting to more than

36 percent annually (AHCA, 1995), their salaries are low in comparison to hospitals, and they have limited opportunities for advancement. None of these factors is conducive to strong leadership. However, in view of the number of employees, budgets, and complexity of the care in nursing facilities today, strong leadership from the DON is a prerequisite for provision of high-quality, cost-effective care. Therefore:

RECOMMENDATION 6-5: The committee recommends that, in view of the increasing case-mix acuity of residents and the consequent complexity of the care provided, nursing facilities place greater weight on educational preparation in the employment of new directors of nursing.

In this regard, the committee is of the opinion that a bachelor's degree in nursing with special training in management and gerontology should be the preferred credential. In particular DONs need training in the management and administration of nursing facilities. The committee also urges that such facilities ensure a commitment to continuing education.

Job Satisfaction, Turnover, and Compensation

The committee can find no direct evidence of a relationship between job satisfaction and quality of care, although a relationship is widely perceived to exist (Bond and Bond, 1987).

Staff Turnover

Nursing homes with higher NA-to-bed ratios and those that include nursing assistants as part of the care team, value their opinions, and acknowledge their important role in provision of quality care have lower turnover rates (Reagan, 1986; Wagnild and Manning, 1986; Willcocks et al., 1987; Wagnild, 1988; Birkenstock, 1991; Robertson et al., 1994; Mor, 1995). As discussed earlier in this chapter, information gathered from site visits, testimony, and small group meetings with DONs and others suggests that some facilities have reduced turnover by providing free on-site child care, health insurance, and other benefits. High RN and LPN turnover is associated with lower quality of care (Erickson, 1987; Wright, 1988; Munroe, 1990; Spector and Takada, 1991). More specifically, high turnover compromises the continuity of care and supervision of staff. Job turnover is also costly in terms of hiring, training, and facility productivity losses, but most important, high turnover rates adversely affect residents who do not cope well with frequent changes in staff (McDonald, 1994). Excessive turnover of these personnel, heavy use of part-time staff, and the use of floating or agency staff also compromise the quality of care (Erickson, 1987).

Permanent assignment of staff to residents results in more quality outcomes

TABLE 6.5   Average Turnover Rates in Nursing Facilities
by Staff Category, United States, 1990–1994

Type of Staff	July 1990	July 1991	January 1993	January 1994
Administrator	28.5	26.4	21.4	27.2
RN	43.5	51.6	45.3	56.3
LPN	*a*	*a*	44.8	52.5
NA	85.1	94.3	80.1	100.4

[a]Before 1993, data for LPN and RN positions were collected as a
combined category.

SOURCE: AHCA, 1994b, 1995.

for residents and greater satisfaction and feelings of accountability for employees
(Patchner and Patchner, 1993). Evaluation of a primary care model of delivery of
nursing aide care (e.g., permanent aide assignment, a team approach, and enhanced communication) in nursing homes demonstrated increased quality-of-
care indicators such as improved behavior, affect, and social activities among
residents (Teresi et al., 1993).

National data on turnover indicate very high rates for all types of nursing
personnel in nursing homes, especially nurse assistants (see Table 6.5). Moreover, staff turnover rates appear to have increased in recent years.

Compensation

High rates of turnover in nursing homes are attributable to several causes.
The low rate of compensation, compared to hospitals, has been a factor. In 1992,
RNs' annual earnings in nursing homes were 14–17 percent below those in hos-
pitals (Moses, 1994). On the one hand, RNs in nursing homes have, on the
average, less educational preparation than those in hospitals. On the other hand,
RNs in nursing facilities are much more likely to be employed in administrative
positions than are those in hospitals (24 versus 3 percent in 1992) (Moses, 1994).
Wages of nursing assistants are generally near the minimum wage and are comparable to levels offered by fast food chains and retail establishments. As with
RNs, nursing assistants are paid appreciably less in nursing homes than in hospitals (Gold, 1995) (see Table 6.6), and they lag behind NAs in home health care
agencies as well (Hospital and Healthcare Compensation Service, 1994).

Many nursing facilities do not provide their employees with health benefits.
Recently, AHCA (1994a) estimated that if mandatory national health insurance
were adopted by Congress, nursing facility costs passed on to Medicaid would
increase by $1 billion, and similar costs to Medicare would increase by $100

TABLE 6.6 Nursing Facility Hourly Wages by Staff Category, United States, 1990–1993

Type of Staff	Year			
	1990	1991	1992	1993
Administrator	$18.55	$19.43	$20.74	$21.58
DON	15.66	16.75	18.36	19.30
RN	12.81	13.76	14.75	15.49
LPN	9.74	10.31	10.96	11.51
NA	5.19	5.48	5.81	6.06

NOTE: DON = director of nursing; RN = registered nurse; LPN = licensed practical nurse; NA = nurse assistant.

SOURCE: AHCA, 1994b, 1995.

million. The 1994 average health insurance costs for nursing facilites were estimated to be 4 to 6 percent of the payroll. If all employees were provided health benefits, the health insurance costs would increase to almost 8 percent of the payroll (AHCA, 1994a).

Under a number of assumptions about the behavior of nursing facilities, higher levels of RN compensations result in reduced nursing home demand for RNs. Using data from 14,000 nursing facilities in 1987, Zinn (1993b) found that nursing facilities adjust staffing and care practices to local market conditions, as would be expected. In areas where RN wages were higher, nursing facilities employed more nonprofessional nursing staff. Thus, after controlling for resident characteristics, nursing facilities have economic incentives to hire fewer RNs in areas with high RN wages.

Clearly, the combination of low average wages and benefits contributes to high turnover and poor quality of care. During its site visits and in public testimony the committee heard many comments about the low level of wages and fringe benefits in nursing facilities, with the result that recruiting and retaining nurses are major problems for nursing homes. *The committee is sympathetic to the need for increased compensation as a means of improving care. To achieve parity with other providers such as hospitals would increase the cost of care especially to Medicare and Medicaid. Higher compensation can possibly reduce the demand for RNs in nursing homes. It depends, however, on state Medicaid reimbursement methods and the internal resource allocation priorities that are established by nursing homes themselves.* These quality and cost tradeoffs must be considered in addressing this major problem in nursing homes.

Ownership

The relationship of facility ownership to staffing, quality, and costs has been the subject of numerous studies and controversy. One of the key issues debated is whether the proprietary nature of the nursing home industry affects quality. A review of the research on ownership and quality shows a mixed picture in terms of the relationship (Koetting, 1980; Greene and Monahan, 1981; O'Brien et al., 1983; Hawes and Phillips, 1986; Nyman et al., 1990; Davis, 1991). Some researchers have found no relationship between ownership and quality (Cohen and Dubay, 1990); others have found nonprofit nursing facilities to be associated with higher quality of care. Davis (1991) in her review of the literature on ownership and quality concluded that the findings were mixed.

A recent study of nursing facilities using the 1987 MMACS data from 449 free-standing nursing facilities in Pennsylvania found that nonprofit nursing facilities provided significantly higher quality of care to Medicaid beneficiaries and to self-pay residents than for-profit facilities when case-mix is controlled for (Aaronson et al., 1994). The authors found that nonprofit facilities had higher staffing levels and fewer adverse outcomes from pressure sores, controlling for case-mix, but no difference in restraint use.

Johnson and colleagues (Part II of this report) also explored the relationship of ownership and quality by categorizing facilities into high- and low-quality facilities using OSCAR data and examining the characteristics of each set of facilities. They found that for-profit facilities that are not chain owned fell into the high-quality category at as high a rate as nonprofit facilities, while having substantially fewer staff and the highest proportion of Medicaid covered residents. Chain-owned for-profit facilities fell into the poor-quality category at a higher rate than expected. They suggest that this could be because chain-owned facilities do not have a direct accountability or because the management structure of some chain-owned facilities does not provide effective oversight of quality of care. Another interesting finding of their analysis is that rural facilities are more than twice as likely to be in the high-quality category. The authors suggest that a rural facility may be more community sensitive than a facility in urban areas. The community sensitivity may be due to staff knowing the residents they care for and being concerned about the reputation of the facility.

EFFECTS OF REIMBURSEMENT AND OTHER FACTORS ON NURSING STAFF

Reimbursement and Staffing

Method and Level of Reimbursement

As discussed in Chapter 3, nursing homes derive most of their revenue from charges to private-pay patients and from Medicaid. Conceptually, both the level and the method of Medicaid reimbursement are determinants of nurse staffing levels. Traditionally, Medicaid is paid on a retrospective cost basis. Under this form of reimbursement, payment is made on the basis of costs incurred. This approach has been rapidly supplanted by other methods in which some or all of the rate is set prospectively (Swan et al., 1993a,b). Prospective-class (flat-rate) methods set prospective rates for groups of nursing homes within a state. Prospective facility-specific methods set rates by facility, generally using cost reports from earlier periods. Some states set rates prospectively but allow for retroactive adjustments (Swan et al., 1993a,b).

There is limited empirical evidence on the effect of level and method of Medicaid reimbursement on nurse staffing in nursing homes. Cohen and Spector (in press), using data from the 1987 National Medical Expenditure Survey, found that states with higher Medicaid reimbursement had more LPNs per 100 residents, adjusting for case-mix. However, a statistically significant effect was not obtained for RN staffing. They further found that Medicaid cost-based reimbursement led to substitution of RNs for LPNs. Presumably because payment is lower and there is excess demand for care on the part of Medicaid eligibles, facilities with high proportions of residents on Medicaid tend to have a lower quality of care as measured by process indicators (Nyman, 1985, 1989b; Gertler, 1989). Elderly persons who are potentially eligible for Medicaid have experienced access barriers to nursing home care in areas where a high proportion of potential nursing home residents are private (Ettner, 1993). One suggestion has been to tie the Medicaid reimbursement rate to the proportion of private patients in the home (Nyman, 1989b).

Case-Mix Reimbursement

Case-mix reimbursement attempts to tie payment to a facility's case-mix severity. Case-mix reimbursement systems were developed for Medicaid as a means of making closer linkages among resident needs, payments, and costs and as a way of removing access barriers for heavy-care Medicaid patients (Schlenker et al., 1985; Schlenker, 1991a,b). As noted above, 19 states were using case-mix systems in 1993 (Swan et al., 1994). The most commonly used case-mix measure has been functional status (using activities of daily living), although other disability scales have been used (Weissert and Musliner, 1992a,b). As mentioned earlier, one of the best known approaches has been the RUGS methodology developed by Fries and Cooney (1985), which has been updated into RUGS II and RUGS III versions (Fries et al., 1994). Resident characteristics are typically examined for the amount of personnel resources needed to provide care to residents, which can be determined in different ways such as staff time and cost studies (Weissert et al., 1983; Fries and Cooney, 1985; Arling et al., 1987; Fries et al., 1989, 1994). Once costs are determined, they are tied to resident characteristics (Weissert and Musliner, 1992a,b). As Fries and colleagues (1994) point out, the development of classification systems and resource use groups is primarily a technical process, but the development and assignment of reimbursement categories is primarily a political process.

Several studies have been conducted of case-mix (Weissert et al., 1983; Cameron, 1985; Fries and Cooney, 1985; Arling et al., 1987, 1989; Schneider et al., 1988; Fries et al., 1994). Weissert and Musliner (1992a,b) have summarized the results of the many studies of case-mix reimbursement. These studies reported that most states that have used case-mix reimbursement have improved access for some heavy-care residents (Ohio, Illinois, Maryland, and New York). On the other hand, there continued to be problems with access in some case-mix reimbursement states such as West Virginia (Holahan, 1984; Butler and Schlenker, 1988; Weissert and Musliner, 1992a,b). Access problems under case-mix, such as lengthy waiting lists for admissions, have occurred especially in areas where there is a low supply of beds (Nyman, 1988b), where there are Medicaid processing delays (Weissert and Cready, 1988), and where reimbursement rates are low. Access problems occurred for those with low-care needs and where community-based alternatives were not necessarily available (Butler and Schlenker, 1988; Feder and Scanlon, 1989).

Critical to the success of case-mix reimbursement is the adequacy of the case-mix measures themselves. The committee construes analysis of the underlying technical issues to be beyond the scope of its charge. (There is an extensive literature on this subject. See, for example, Fries and Cooney, 1985; Hu et al., 1986; Rohrer et al., 1989; Fries et al., 1994.) However, although attempting to base payment on severity is meritorious in principle, there may be problems in implementation. Classification errors may actually discourage delivery of quality therapeutic care, for example, if the system does not adequately account for comorbidities such as behavioral problems stemming from mental illness (Rohrer et al., 1989).

Case-mix reimbursement generally has not led to increases in nursing staff-to-resident ratios. In Maryland, there was no evidence that extra nursing home payments were used to add more staff (Feder and Scanlon, 1989). New York also did not increase staff even though resident case-mix increased (Butler and Schlenker, 1988). Although West Virginia had some evidence of poor quality (e.g., increased catheterization), nursing resources did increase in 1979–1981 (Holahan and Cohen, 1987; Weissert and Musliner, 1992a,b). In the San Diego experiment, where facilities were given financial incentives to take more heavy-care residents, there was no evidence that extra payments were spent on extra care (Meiners et al., 1985). Of the six state systems reviewed by Weissert and Musliner (1992a,b), only Illinois was rated as having improved quality (Holahan, 1984; Butler and Schlenker, 1988).

HCFA is undertaking a demonstration project to introduce Medicaid case-mix reimbursement in four states in 1994–1995. As Weissert and Musliner

(1992a) have noted, it is not clear whether substantial new advances will be made in designing improved case-mix reimbursement systems in the demonstration project. An evaluation has been planned that will examine the outcomes of the demonstration on access, quality, and costs.

Incentives to Enhance Quality of Care

A conceptually attractive alternative to basing payment on inputs is to reward nursing homes based on *aggregate* outcomes achieved (Willemain, 1980; Kane et al., 1983). There have been several experiments with outcomes-based incentives. A social experiment was conducted in San Diego to test the effectiveness of monetary incentives in improving the health of nursing home residents and reducing Medicaid expenditures. With data from the San Diego project, Norton (1992) used the Markov model to represent the resulting health changes of nursing home residents. He found that offering incentives for improved outcomes had beneficial effects on both the quality and the cost of nursing home care. Furthermore, nursing homes admitted more persons with severe disabilities. The savings came not from more efficient use of nursing homes, but rather from savings from earlier hospital transfers. The experience in other locations has been mixed, however. Although the Illinois quality incentive program appears to have succeeded in increasing the quality of care, the validity of the outcome measures was not established (Geron, 1991). Connecticut's system was discontinued because the program's goals were not reached (Geron, 1991). Maryland's system of paying facilities to turn and position patients to prevent decubitus ulcers and to pay for improvement in ADLs for 2 months has been rated as effective (Weissert and Musliner, 1992a,b). Michigan's effort has not been evaluated (Lewin/ICF, 1991).

The committee finds the concept of reimbursing for improved outcomes intriguing, but recognizes that the implementation issues require further analysis. Also, using outcomes-based incentives may have some practical limits. In such cases, consideration should be given to linking reimbursement to process measures known to be associated with high quality of care.

RECOMMENDATION 6-6: The committee recommends that the Secretary of Health and Human Services fund additional research and demonstration projects on the use of financial and other incentives to improve quality of care and outcomes in nursing homes.

RESIDENTS, FAMILIES, VOLUNTEERS, AND OMBUDSMEN

The role of residents, family members, and other persons external to the nursing home has received limited attention in the context of discussions of quality of care in nursing homes. Family members and others have at least three potential roles: as care givers and as advocates for patients, and as payers. The nursing home industry has become one of the most regulated in the country, not only because of the importance of government funding but also because patients lack power in relationship to nursing homes. They generally lack the ability to leave or to change the facility when they are dissatisfied. Often they are deficient in their ability to communicate their opinions and feelings. To avoid additional regulation, greater reliance needs to be placed on other agents to act in residents' interests.

In particular, the committee notes that information gathered from site visits and testimony supports the use of volunteers in nursing facilities. Volunteers are used by nursing facilities to various degrees and in various roles. Representatives of the two "model" nursing facilities testified to the committee about their successful implementation of innovative approaches to the delivery of care. One received a great deal of help from volunteers, while the other received some, but not a notably large amount of, help. Although volunteers can clearly add to the quality of life for residents, both of these witnesses emphasized the role of the nursing staff in achieving the great improvements in residents' well-being following implementation of the new models. Benefits to residents include improved linkages to the community, multigenerational interactions, human contact, avoidance of isolation, and special errands and services, such as letter writing and craft activities. The committee endorses these practices and urges nursing facilities to develop and strengthen volunteer programs.

The committee found very little research on the role of families in nursing home care. Bowers (1988) proposed a collaborative approach to care that would encourage families to become more involved in technical aspects of care while facilitating staff's emotional involvement with residents.

Kayser-Jones (1990) examined the use of nasogastric (NG) feeding tubes in nursing homes. Two themes of interest emerged from family interviews: (1) there was little or no communication among health care providers, patients, and their families regarding the use of NG tubes; and (2) some families perceived that the tubes were used for the convenience of the staff who did not want to take the time, or did not have the patience, to feed residents (Kayser-Jones, 1990). In a study to evaluate the effects of a special care unit (SCU) for Alzheimer's residents, Maas and colleagues (1991) found that family members were dissatisfied with their lack of involvement in the care of their relatives, with the activities provided for the residents, and with the amount of resources devoted to the provision of care.

Maas and colleagues (1994) are currently testing the effects on family and staff satisfaction and stress, as well as on resident outcomes, of an intervention designed to create a family–staff partnership for the care of institutionalized persons with Alzheimer's disease. Staff and family members need to have the knowledge and skills that best prepare them to understand and recognize quality resident outcomes, to be better able to establish cooperative relationships, and to share decisions so that the optimal resources of both staff and families are used to achieve quality outcomes.

Ombudsman programs and other forms of community presence may improve nursing home quality of care. Long-term care ombudsmen "advocate to protect the health, safety, welfare, and rights of the institutionalized elderly," and a recent IOM study has come out strongly in favor of this program (IOM, 1995, p. 1). The IOM report is an in-depth examination of the strengths and weaknesses of the ombudsman program; it specifically addresses the extent of compliance with the program's federal mandates; the availability of, unmet need for, and effectiveness of the ombudsman program; the adequacy of resources available to operate the program; and the need for and feasibility of providing ombudsman services to older individuals who are not residing in long-term care facilities. Cherry (1991) compared the effects of community presence programs on the quality of nursing care with a random sample of 134 Medicare- or Medicaid-certified long-term care facilities in Missouri. The presence of an ombudsman program was found to be one of the more important factor associated with quality for intermediate-care facilities and also was significantly associated with quality for skilled nursing homes where there was ample staffing of RNs.

CONCLUSION

Ideally, the committee would have found some major source of inefficiency that, when remedied, would release substantial revenues that could be used to enhance the ability of nursing homes to improve staffing. Such staffing increases would then lead to improved quality of care, as the empirical studies have demonstrated can be accomplished. An alternative approach would be to convert "excessive" nursing home profits and overhead to patient care. No rigorous study of profitability in nursing homes, or for that matter in hospitals or managed care systems, has been conducted, but the committee found a widespread perception of an imbalance of compensation between care givers, on the one hand, and executive officers and owners, on the other. Committee members are sympathetic with the notion that such an imbalance exists, but even if such resources were reallocated to patient care, the committee is not certain that this would provide the "magic bullet" for appreciably increasing the number and quality of staff capacity.

Any discussion of staffing needs to take into account the financing of staffing needs. To the extent that additional funds from an outside source are necessary, it becomes a question of from where they will come. A major barrier to increased staffing in nursing facilities concerns the fiscal limits of governmental support. Since government pays for nearly 63 percent of current nursing home expenditures (Levit et al., 1994), Congress has been reluctant to increase staffing requirements to needed levels, even though some members of Congress have been sympathetic to the need for increased staffing. The small staffing increases under OBRA 87 required substantial new resources. These staffing increases were apparently based on the amount legislators and industry leaders considered to be politically and fiscally feasible, because most of the costs for increased staffing would be reflected in increases in federal and state Medicaid budgets.

Since OBRA 87 was passed, federal legislation has been considered by selected congressional representatives for increased staffing beyond the OBRA requirements, but such legislation has not had the political support to proceed. States have the authority to increase their Medicaid payment rates as a means of increasing staffing standards, but the pressures on some states with rapidly growing Medicaid budgets make it unlikely that they will initiate increases in nursing home staffing requirements. The research reviewed has shown that low-quality facilities have a higher proportion of Medicaid residents, and Medicaid rates are usually lower than private-pay rates. Policymakers are faced with difficult choices invoving trade-offs between quality and costs. Since the population of this country is aging and the oldest-old age group is increasing, and there is no cure in sight for chronic diseases such as Alzheimer's, the demand for nursing home care will not abate, even with the growth of alternative long-term care facilities. Funding mechanisms will have to be explored to ensure adequate staffing to care for residents with multiple chronic conditions and with special care or subacute care needs. It is clear that *substantial improvements in the quality of nursing home care are not possible without the allocation of increased financial resources for additional and appropriately qualified staffing.*

7

Staffing and Work-Related Injuries and Stress

OVERVIEW

This Institute of Medicine (IOM) committee was charged by Congress to determine whether and to what extent the need exists to increase the number of nursing personnel in hospitals and nursing homes as a means of reducing the incidence of work-related injury and stress among such health care workers. This mandate is both broad and narrow. It is broad because it does not limit the committee to study specific injuries or illnesses. At the same time, it is narrow in the sense that the committee was not asked to comment on the full range of hazards (infectious biologic, chemical, environmental, physical, and psychosocial) to which nursing staff are exposed in the workplace. Specifically the committee charge was to explore possible linkages between staffing levels and skill mix of nursing personnel and the incidence of work-related injuries and stress among nursing personnel.

Nursing personnel work in a wide range of health services settings including hospitals, nursing homes, and ambulatory and community-based environments. In performing their duties, they encounter a remarkable range of work-related hazards. Some evidence suggests that fatigue related to overwork and staffing patterns, including shift work, can contribute to injuries and stress among staff providing nursing services (Gold et al., 1992; Phillips and Brown, 1992). Factors such as the physical work environment, organizational and institutional characteristics and policies, and personal work habits contribute to exposure to the risk of injury and stress. Exposure to occupational hazards—physical, psychological, biological, chemical, and environmental—could have both short-term and long-term effects on the health and safety of the health care giver and, ultimately, on the safety and quality of patient care (Tan, 1991). A sizable proportion of the victims of nonfatal violence are care givers in hospitals and nursing homes. Evidence also exists of abusive and violent behavior of staff toward patients, at times resulting from stress and overwork and at other times from a breakdown of quality controls and appropriate supervision.

This chapter provides a brief overview of the incidence of work-related injuries in hospitals and nursing homes, violence and abuse of nursing staff, and violence and abuse directed toward residents of homes and stress among nursing personnel in hospitals and nursing homes. It then reviews available national statistics and research literature on occupational hazards to examine the risk factors associated with work-related injuries and stress and the linkages with the structural variables of staffing levels and skill mix.

INCIDENCE OF WORK-RELATED INJURIES AND ILLNESS

The health services industry is one of the largest employers in the United States, employing almost 9 million persons in 1993 (BLS, 1995c). More than half of this workforce is employed in hospitals and nursing homes. Recent statistics and other information suggest that these institutions are becoming increasingly hazardous places of work, exposing workers to a wide range of risks.

In 1993, private industry workplaces reported 6.7 million injuries and illnesses, a rate of 8.5 cases for every 100 full-time workers (BLS, 1994c). Of the 6.7 million cases, nearly 6.3 million were injuries that resulted in time lost from work. As shown in Table 7.1, while the injury and illness rate for private industry as a whole has remained about the same or declined slightly since 1980, the rates for hospitals and for nursing and personal care homes during the same period have increased by about 52 and 62 per 100 full time workers, respectively. During the same period, hospitals reported about 338,000 cases, an incidence rate of nearly 12 per 100 full-time workers, and nursing and personal care facilities reported about 216,000 cases, a rate of 17 percent (see Table 7.1).

Nine industries, each with at least 100,000 injuries annually, accounted for nearly 2 million, or 30 percent, of the 6.7 million injuries in 1993 (BLS, 1994a). Hospitals ranked second, and nursing and personal care facilities ranked fourth, among these industries.

Overexertion, being struck by an object, and falls at the same level[1] are the leading ways in which workers are hurt on the job. These events account for

---

[1]Falls "at the same level," as contrasted with "falls to a lower level" (such as those incurred by construction laborers and roofing or sheet metal workers who fall from a height), is a category of disabling event used to measure varying degrees of disabling work-related injuries. These injuries are reported by employers to the Bureau of Labor Statistics as part of the Annual Survey of Occupational Injuries and Illnesses.

TABLE 7.1 Trends in Occupational Injury and Illness Incidence, United States, 1980–1993

	Incidence of Injuries and Illnesses per 100 Full-Time Workers		
Year	Private Industry, Total	Hospitals	Nursing and Personal Care Homes
1980	8.7	7.9	10.7
1981	8.3	7.2	10.5
1982	7.7	7.3	10.1
1983	7.6	7.4	11.0
1984	8.0	7.3	11.6
1985	7.9	8.1	13.3
1986	7.9	7.6	13.5
1987	8.3	8.5	14.2
1988	8.6	8.7	15.0
1989	8.6	8.5	15.5
1990	8.8	10.6	15.6
1991	8.4	11.5	15.3
1992	8.9	12.0	18.6
1993	8.5	11.8	17.3
Percent Change			
1986–1993	7.6	30.1	45.7
1980–1993	−2.3	52.0	62.0

SOURCE: BLS, Survey of Occupational Injuries and Illnesses, 1980–1993.

more than one-half of the 2.3 million nonfatal injuries and illnesses that resulted in days away from work (BLS, 1995a). Workers in nursing and personal care facilities had the highest rate of injuries among all private industries due to overexertion or falling to the same level (BLS, 1995b).

Not surprisingly, most of the injuries and illnesses involving days away from work that are reported by registered nurses (RN), licensed practical nurses (LPN), nurse assistants (NA), orderlies, and attendants occur among women. Most of the workers in these occupations are women. NAs, who are employed predominantly in hospitals and nursing homes, ranked second only to truck drivers and laborers in the incidence of injuries and illness that involved loss of work days (BLS, 1995a). For persons in all occupations who had worked less than a year, NAs were reported as having the most injuries and illness, primarily strains and sprains mostly involving the back. They cited overexertion related to patient care as the primary cause. The major source of injury reported is the patient or the resident whom the aide was trying to lift or help in other ways (see Table 7.2). The association between job category and injury may be confounded by the nature of the work activities; NAs' work involves a great deal of heavy lifting.

TABLE 7.2 Percent Distribution of Nonfatal Occupational Injuries and Illnesses Involving Days Away from Work, for Selected Occupations and Worker Characteristics, United States, 1993

Characteristics	All Occupations	Registered Nurses	Licensed Practical Nurses	Nurse Assistants, Orderlies, and Attendants
Total number of injuries and illnesses	2,252,591	31,422	15,014	103,944
		Percent of total workers		
Sex				
Men	66.2	8.2	4.6	10.5
Women	32.7	91.0	94.6	88.9
Health services industry				
Nursing and personal care facilities	4.0	10.2	32.4	57.6
Hospitals	5.0	77.5	51.4	20.8
Length of service with employer				
Less than 1 year	30.6	17.8	20.2	38.9
1 to 5 years	33.5	36.4	39.6	38.4
More than 5 years	26.5	35.5	29.7	15.0
Not reported	9.4	10.4	10.5	7.7
Nature of injury, illness				
Sprains, strains	42.6	62.1	64.7	65.5
Back pain	2.6	3.4	3.7	5.0
Part of body affected				
Trunk	38.6	54.6	56.1	60.1
Back	27.3	44.7	41.3	45.6
Source of injury, illness				
Floor, ground surfaces	15.1	14.5	15.0	10.9
Health care patient	4.4	45.4	48.7	61.3
		Days		
Median days away from work	6.0	5.0	5.0	6.0

SOURCE: BLS, Survey of Occupational Injuries and Illnesses, 1993.

Relationship of Staffing and Injuries and Stress[2]

Analysis of literature on injuries and stress experienced by nursing personnel provides valuable information on issues involved in work-related injuries and stress. The studies reviewed suggest that the nature of the work, inadequate staffing patterns, clinical issues, equipment, organizational and institutional characteristics, lack of administrative support, lack of decision making authority, lack of resources, training and education, poor body mechanics, physical environment, and pressure to work in at-risk conditions *all* contribute to the problem of injuries and stress among nursing personnel. Rogers (Part II of this report) observes, however, that the data from these studies are limited because of the lack of replication and because of little evidence of any correlation between staffing and patient outcomes. Sample sizes and sample designs are sometimes questionable in terms of being able to generalize from the findings of individual studies. Many of the studies are descriptive and retrospective in design, and many report only anecdotal findings.

Back Injuries

Back pain is a major problem among the working population of the United States. Most people (about 8 out of 10) experience low back pain at some time in their lives. About 50 percent of the working-age population reports low back pain every year (AHCPR, 1994). Back injuries are among the greatest causes of lost time from work, and they are one of the most expensive workers' compensation problems today (McAbee, 1988). They constitute the greatest number of lost work days and the greatest amount of compensation paid in industry (Owen, 1985; SEIU, 1994).

Nursing staff in hospitals and nursing homes, by the very nature of their work, are particularly vulnerable to the hazards of back injuries and associated pain. These injuries result in time lost from work, disability, reduced productivity, and expense of medical care, and staff turnover. Even so, the extent of low back pain and injury in nursing personnel is thought to be underestimated. Owen (1989) found in a survey of 503 nurses that only 34 percent of respondents with work-related low back pain filed an injury report, and 12 percent contemplated leaving the profession because of back problems. Of all injuries in private industry reported to the Pennsylvania Bureau of Workers' Compensation in 1989, 22 percent were for back injuries. For nursing homes this proportion was 36 percent (SEIU, 1991).

---

[2] Much of the information in this section was taken from papers commissioned by the IOM committee from Bonnie Rogers and Maas and colleagues. The committee appreciates their contributions. The full text of the papers can be found in Part II of this report.

Back injuries are a particularly troubling problem for the staff of nursing homes. They account for a higher percentage of all injuries in nursing homes than in other industries. As stated earlier, the major sources of injuries to nursing home workers are lifting and moving patients and overexertion. Back injuries are the most common injuries among NAs, and their incidence is higher among NAs than among other nursing personnel. Nursing home work is often difficult, stressful, and labor intensive, especially for NAs, who have the most direct contact with residents and do most of the heavy lifting.

Studies also found that recently employed nursing staff are more likely to injure their backs than are more experienced personnel (Greenwood, 1986; Neuberger et al., 1988; Garrett et al., 1992; Feldstein et al., 1993; BLS, 1995a). This fact is noteworthy because high turnover rates of NAs involve frequent additions of new staff who are more prone to injuries than staff with longer tenure or more expertise. *The situation clearly suggests the importance of and need for more aggressive training related to the use of lifting devices and lifting teams especially for new employees, including ergonomic training in lifting techniques to prevent back injuries.*

Staffing levels in nursing homes have not kept pace with the increased demands for more and better-trained nursing personnel. The case mix of nursing home patients is increasing in complexity as hospitals discharge patients early and transfer them to nursing homes. With sicker and more dependent patients than in the past, nursing homes have become more stressful and hazardous in terms of injuries. This situation is reflected in high turnover among NAs who do most of the heavy lifting. Understaffing (both qualitative and quantitative) leads to injuries, which leads to further understaffing, and the needs of patients go unmet. For instance, if the number of NAs on the floor is low, then it is not possible to have two or more of them available to lift a single person. Often NAs are forced to lift residents alone when assistance is not immediately available.

Garg and colleagues (1992) found that the prevalence of low back pain among NAs is high. On average, in their study, an NA had experienced four episodes of low back pain in the past 3 years, and had not reported three of the four episodes; 51 percent of the NAs had visited a health care provider for work-related low back pain. Assistive devices (e.g., hydraulic lift) were used less than 2 percent of the time. Patient safety and comfort, lack of accessibility, physical stresses associated with the devices, lack of skill, increased transfer time, and lack of staffing were some of the reasons cited for not using such assistive devices. The 2-person walking-belt manual method technique, which is used for transfer of residents from one position or location to another, was perceived to be the most comfortable, secure, and least stressful approach. However, adequate numbers of well-trained personnel are needed to carry out this method. In addition, environmental barriers (such as confined workplaces, uneven floor surfaces, beds that are not adjustable, stationary railings around the toilet, and similar obstacles) made resident care in nursing homes more difficult.

Workers in nursing homes are not alone in experiencing these problems. Several studies indicate that care givers in hospitals have reported work-related back pain and injury, and they implicate lifting techniques, poor staffing, ergonomics, inadequate communication, and physical constitution as contributory factors (Harber et al., 1985; Marchette and Marchette, 1985; Arad and Ryan, 1986; Jensen, 1987; Carney, 1993; Jorgensen et al., 1994). Recommended approaches to reduce the incidence of occupational back injury include better mechanical lifting devices, improved staffing, enhanced training and education, and more attention to worker job capabilities.

Kaiser-Permanente Medical Centers in Portland, Oregon, found back injury rates (based on workers' compensation claims) ranging from 10 to 30 percent on hospital units (Feldstein et al., 1993). Nearly two-thirds of the 53 orthopedic staff nurses in one large hospital reported work-related back pain, and 90 percent indicated patient handling as responsible for their most severe pain episodes (Cato et al., 1989). While assistive devices were considered adequate, levels of staff were cited frequently as inadequate for lifting assistance. Better staffing and staffing availability, improved body mechanics, and assistance with transfers were identified as the most helpful risk reduction strategies.

Several studies and anecdotal reports implicate poor staff-to-patient ratios in the high incidence of back pain and injury in both hospitals and nursing homes (Rodgers, 1985; McAbee, 1988; Larese and Fiorito, 1994). Nursing staff are often forced to lift alone when assistance is not immediately available, which suggests a link between injuries and numbers of staff. Other variables identified are poor working conditions and equipment design, all of which affect the quality of care available or provided. The authors identify a role for management in the prevention of injuries and re-injuries to the back.

The linkage suggested by these studies among staffing patterns and levels, work conditions, and back injuries needs to be validated. Research is necessary to examine the correlation between levels and training of nursing personnel (i.e., RNs, LPNs, and NAs) and patient load, on the one hand, and injury, illness, staff retention, and patient care and satisfaction, on the other. *All personnel giving direct care (especially in nursing homes) should have annual training in lifting and transferring patients. Such efforts would improve the quality of life for health care workers and would represent a significant savings to the health care industry.*

Needlestick Injuries

Needlestick incidents put nursing personnel at risk of contracting hepatitis B, hepatitis C, and human immunodeficiency virus (HIV) and are the most frequently reported occupational exposure routes to such viruses (Marcus et al., 1991). Nursing staff are the primary victims of needlestick injuries (McEvoy et al., 1987; Wilkinson, 1987; Henderson et al., 1990; Marcus et al., 1991; Doan-

Johnson, 1992). Conservative estimates place the incidence of more than 800,000 needlestick injuries each year among health care workers in the United States (Jagger, 1990). Of the 42 health care workers known by the Centers for Disease Control and Prevention (CDC) to have been occupationally infected with HIV through December 31, 1994, 13 (31 percent) were nurses (CDC, 1994). This estimate is generally thought to be an underestimate of the actual number of occupationally-acquired infections.

Most occupational HIV infections are caused by deep needlestick injuries or cuts from sharp objects and the resultant deposition of HIV-contaminated blood beneath the skin. Yet a far more common outcome of a deep needlestick injury or a cut from a sharp object is hepatitis B virus infection (Alter et al., 1976; Grady et al., 1978; Seeff et al., 1978); it occurs in 30 percent of all cases following exposure to hepatitis B core antigen as contrasted with the 0.3-percent risk associated with exposure to HIV (Geberding et al., 1987; Marcus, 1988; Henderson et al., 1990). Notwithstanding these facts, the universal precautions promulgated by the CDC (1988) and enforced by the Occupational Safety and Health Administration (OSHA) are not universally observed by health care workers (Courington et al., 1991). Infractions may occur in up to 60 percent of cases, irrespective of health care workers' participation in programs designed specifically to ensure compliance with universal precautions (Shelley and Howard, 1992). The reasons for such behavior are unclear, but certainly deserve further study.

The question of how to reduce needlestick injuries and the related sequelae remains, therefore, a critical one for both patient and worker safety. However, reliance on needleless systems for medication administration and accessing lines for blood in the hospital and scrupulous adherence to proper technique during invasive procedures, particularly those that are exposure prone, would appear to be the most cost-effective approach available at this time for prevention of work-related deep needlestick injuries and cuts from sharp objects among health care workers. The next step should be to decrease the injuries associated with disposal of needles and other sharp objects.

Some researchers have identified improved staffing and equipment and employee education as contributory factors in reducing the incidence of needlestick injuries (Neuberger et al., 1988). Others include instituting appropriate and effective engineering controls, ensuring compliance with regulatory mandates and work practice policies and guidelines, conducting surveillance programs, and providing useful educational instructions. Further research is critical, however, to measure the outcomes and effectiveness of all such interventions.

In summary then, the committee is struck by the high rates of injuries to nursing personnel in both the hospital and the nursing home setting but it only found conclusive evidence of a strong link between nurse staffing per se and injuries for the category of back injuries. The committee is impressed, however, with three trends that emerge from the information cited above and the further information obtained through its site visits and public testimony—namely, (1) the effect that visible concern and leadership from high management levels can have in reducing injuries; (2) the overriding importance of good training, especially for lesser educated nursing staff; and (3) the utility of existing technologies for patient care (in hospitals) and resident services (in nursing homes) in reducing the probability of certain types of injuries.

RECOMMENDATION 7-1: The committee recommends that hospitals and nursing homes develop effective programs to reduce work-related injuries by providing strong leadership, instituting effective training programs for new and continuing workers, and ensuring appropriate use of existing and emerging technology, including lifting and moving devices and needleless medication delivery systems.

Governance, administration, and management structures of any organization should be committed to workers' safety and health in order for strong programs to be established. Unions and other labor groups and professional associations can exert pressure, and federal or state statutes and regulations can provide pressure and sanction, but effective safety programs depend on absolute support from the highest organizational levels. At the same time, supervisors and workers on the front lines must be part of the leadership in safety and health. They know the problems and have ideas about solutions. Shared responsibility and shared resources lead to the best results.

Training in safe procedures, group dynamics, and leadership are important elements in this arena. Incentives and rewards for low injury rates must be judiciously used because in some circumstances they could lead to underreporting of incidents and therefore missed opportunities for prevention. Early intervention can help prevent accidents and injuries and ameliorate stress in the workplace that may, if not dealt with, lead to workers' compensation claims and other undesirable consequences.

VIOLENCE, ABUSE, AND CONFLICT

Violence and Abuse of Health Care Workers and Nursing Staff

In the United States, violent injuries to health care workers in the workplace were reported at least as early as the end of the nineteenth century (Goodman et al., 1994). Violence toward health care workers appears to be on the rise (Lipscomb and Love, 1992). Lack of a standard definition of violence makes it difficult to arrive at accurate estimates of the scope of the problem. Increased violence in the general population as a means of solving problems, greater use of mind-altering drugs, alcohol abuse, and the increased availability of weapons may all contribute to the problem of violence in health care settings (Lipscomb and Love, 1992). Patients carrying hidden weapons are a concern in psychiatric and general emergency departments across the country.

Hospitals

Workplace-related violence has been increasingly recognized as a particular problem for nursing personnel, especially in settings located in inner cities, and particularly in emergency departments and psychiatric facilities. The committee heard many reports during site visits and in testimony about assaults in hospitals, especially those located in inner cities, and particularly in emergency departments. Witnesses who testified before the committee emphasized the crowded nature of emergency rooms, the characteristics of the patients coming in, and the lack of sufficient staff as contributory factors to the risk of violence directed at health care personnel.

The increase in violence in the health care setting reflects to a large extent the increase in violence in the community. In 1992, private industry reported about 22,400 incidents of nonfatal assaults and acts of violence requiring an average of 5 days away from work (BLS, 1994b). Most of the violent acts involved threats, hitting, kicking, beating, biting, stabbing, squeezing, pinching, scratching, twisting, rape, and shooting. Thirty-eight percent of workers subjected to nonfatal violence were health care givers in nursing homes and hospitals (BLS, 1995d). Most of these care givers were female NAs and licensed nurses. Typically they required 3 to 5 days away from work to recuperate from their injuries. Ironically, some of these workers were injured by patients who resisted their assistance or were assaulted by patients who were prone to violence (BLS, 1994b).

Until recently, studies of violence in health care settings have focused mainly on assaults on staff by patients in psychiatric care settings such as mental health hospitals, psychiatric hospitals, or psychiatric units of hospital. Around 70 to 80 percent of staff in mental facilities reported assaults on them by patients (Lanza, 1983; Poster and Ryan, 1989).

In response to its members' concerns, the Emergency Nurses Association conducted a national survey in 1994 of emergency department nurse managers (Emergency Nurse Association, 1994). In this survey, violence was defined to include verbal and physical assaults with or without weapons. Factors contributing to violence toward staff were alcohol abuse, drug abuse, anger and high stress, overcrowding of the department, open access to the emergency department, and psychiatric patients. Other relevant factors included prolonged waiting times, gang-related activities, increasing numbers of patients needing care for injuries resulting from violence, trauma, and staff-to-staff conflicts. Other studies of emergency and psychiatric departments of hospitals also found incidences of physical attacks on medical and nursing staff and carrying hidden weapons to the hospital (McCulloch et al., 1986; Lavoie et al., 1988; Goetz et al., 1991).

Unfortunately, these and other studies revealed that staff are often unable to predict who the weapon carriers are.

Several administrative, organizational, and environmental factors have been associated with violent injuries in the workplace. These include limited training in the management of violent behavior (e.g., containing or restraining an assailant); staffing levels and patterns, including the use of agency nursing staff; and the day shift tour of duty. Hospital administrators and nurse managers must facilitate staff awareness of the potential for violent situations and enhance the capability to deal with them effectively.

Nursing Homes

Nursing staff, particularly NAs in nursing homes, are also subject to abuse by residents. Studies about the incidence of aggressive resident behavior in nursing homes are sparse, but the few studies available suggest that the presence of behavioral problems is a matter of concern (Zimmer et al., 1984; Beck et al., 1991).

Management of aggressive resident behaviors presents difficult care problems for nursing staff. Researchers have documented frequent incidence of aggressive behavior displayed by residents including physical and verbal abuse (Everitt et al., 1991). Sometimes aggressive resident behaviors are violent. In a study of 101 nursing homes and intermediate care facilities, Winger and colleagues (1987) found 84 percent of residents in nursing home and 54 percent of residents in intermediate care facilities displayed behavior that endangered self and others. Meddaugh (1987) reviewed charts and incidence reports on 72 residents in a skilled nursing facility and found 26 (27 percent) residents abused staff 1 to 2 times in a 3-month period. Lusk (1992), in an exploratory study, found a variety of injuries such as black eye or torn shoulder cuff requiring surgical repair from residents' aggressive behaviors as reported by nurse aides. Rudman and colleagues (1993) in their study of two Department of Veterans Affairs nursing facilities found a higher incidence of physically aggressive behavior in facilities with a greater percentage of neurologic and psychiatric patients. In a study of 124 residents in 4 nursing homes, Ryden and colleagues (1991) found that 51 percent of aggressive behavior was physical, 48 percent verbal, and 4 percent sexual.

The committee notes that one feature of Alzheimer's disease and other cognitive and emotional impairments found among older patients is lack of cooperation with efforts to provide personal care. For instance, the behavior could include for some patients violent resistance to undressing and bathing. The issue is that the patients are not so much engaging in unprovoked violence against nursing staff, rather residents may believe they are defending themselves against what they perceive to be unwanted touching and personal assault. The regimentation of institutional life makes many patients uncooperative and some of them manifest their feelings in particularly hostile mannerisms and verbal abuse (Everitt et al., 1991).

Violence toward staff may be to some extent an indicator of poor quality of care. Patients in some instances may be reduced to violence as the only way to gain control over their environment. The problem here may be the lack of recognition of good nursing practice in (1) designing nursing home environments that stimulate residents to take responsibility for their own behavior, and (2) rewarding individual staff initiative as opposed to rewarding conformity to make life easier for staff.

In summary, the evidence to date suggests that violence directed at health care workers in hospitals and nursing homes is a significant and growing issue for worker safety, peace of mind, and ultimately good patient care. *The committee concludes that it is critical that health care institutions implement strategies to prevent such assaults on workers and that they provide adequate security especially in the high-risk departments (such as emergency room areas or psychiatric units). It also concludes that staff training in effective ways to control violent patients is essential as part of a long-term strategy by which health facilities and institutions can prevent or minimize the harms that may stem from violence and abuse directed at health care workers.*

Violence and Abuse Against Patients and Residents

Physical, verbal, and psychological abuse can and does occur in all settings, from hospitals and nursing homes to personal residences, and it can be inflicted by family members as well as health care personnel (including nursing staff). Relatively little has been written about abuse of the elderly in the peer-reviewed medical and health policy literature, although some discussion of this issue of abuse has appeared (Lachs and Pillemer, 1995).

Nursing Homes

What attention has been given to this problem over the years has tended to focus on abuse by NAs working in nursing facilities, and the issue, particularly in nursing homes, is receiving increasing amounts of attention in local and national media. The Gannett News Service, for instance, prepared a series of articles on the topic in February 1994, that were picked up by various newspapers around the country. Requests for further information on the series led Gannett to compile all the articles in an 8-page special investigative report (Eisler, 1994).

Reports of abuse in the press range from neglect, humiliation, and theft to battery and even rape (e.g., Allen, 1994; Bernardi, 1994; Eisler, 1994). Similarly, in the first half of 1995, the *20/20* television news magazine, using hidden cameras, produced a segment documenting abuse. Other investigators have characterized the behavior of NAs as rude, neglectful, uncaring, insulting, and sometimes verbally and physically abusive (Kayser-Jones, 1990). Physical abuse resulting from poor care, such as skin breakdown, rough handling, or inattention to bowel and urinary elimination needs, is another serious problem that occurs in institutions and can be inflicted by health care personnel (Baker, 1977).

Clearly, many NAs in nursing homes are not abusive. A certain proportion, however, do verbally or physically abuse, steal from, or otherwise take advantage of nursing home residents. Unfortunately, even a small proportion of abusive staff can affect the health, quality of care, and peace of mind of thousands of nursing home residents. Pillemer (1988) has developed a theoretical model of maltreatment as an outcome of staff and residents that are influenced by aspects of the nursing home environment and by certain factors exogenous to the facility. According to his model, which is supported by a review of literature, the characteristics of staff who are more likely to be abusive are young age (Penner et al., 1984), lower levels of education (Baltz and Turner, 1977; White, 1977), male (U.S. Department of Justice, 1985; Straus, 1986), least experienced (Penner et al., 1984), and more stressed (Heine, 1986).

Nursing home residents are very vulnerable, given that their average age is around 80 years, that many may be quite frail, and that many may be relatively isolated from family and friends. In the committee's view, therefore, nursing facilities should be required to ensure a safe and protective environment for residents by employing and retaining employees who protect and care for them and do not abuse and steal from them. Some observers suggest that the stressful work role of NAs in these facilities leads to exhaustion and burnout that may in turn precipitate abuse, and they argue that mechanisms are needed to help nonprofessional staff deal with their work-related stress (Foner, 1994).

Moreover, personnel with questionable backgrounds should be barred from employment as care givers to the old and frail. Because of the large numbers of NAs and their mobility resulting from high turnover rates, however, tracking those with histories of abusive or criminal behavior is difficult. Movement from one facility to another, from one state to another, or even from one facility of a chain of facilities to another can be sufficient to hide an abusive staff person.

At present, employers may be reluctant to conduct extensive checks on new employees for fear of litigation. Standard requirements for such background checks, however, would give facilities the authority to refuse employment to those with questionable and criminal backgrounds. Although theft and resident abuse are considered common occurrences in some nursing facilities, some of them may be reluctant to terminate employees with problem behaviors because of legal liabilities. On the other hand, facilities that fail to take action against abusive or problematic employees clearly are subject to receiving deficiencies and open themselves to legal liability.

The Omnibus Budget Reconciliation Act of 1987 (OBRA 87) requires each state to maintain a registry of NAs who have satisfactorily completed NA training and/or a competency program. In addition, OBRA 87 (sec. 1819(e)(2)) mandates that states include in these registries documented findings of a state regarding resident abuse, neglect, or misappropriation of resident property by any individual on the registry as well as any statement by the individual disputing the findings.

To date, however, these registries have had limited effect, in part because of difficulties in verifying the accusations of abuse and delays in posting the information. A major limitation of the registries is that at best they only make it possible to prevent abuse from happening again. Registries cannot prevent abuse from happening initially, nor do they prevent abusive individuals from moving to a less regulated state or work environment. Fear of litigation also prevents prior employers from saying anything about past abusive behavior during a reference check. At the present time a person does not get on the state registry unless convicted or "documented."

The committee is not satisfied with this state of affairs insofar as protection of vulnerable patient and resident populations is concerned. Although it recognizes that the main difficulties probably lie in the nursing home arena, it also takes note of the fact that employment of NAs and other types of ancillary nursing personnel in hospitals is increasing. In the end, the committee came to consensus on a broad recommendation concerning the responsibilities of health facilities in not employing problematic staff.

> **RECOMMENDATION 7-2: The committee recommends that all hospitals and nursing homes screen applicants for patient care positions filled by nurse assistants for past history of abuse of patients and residents, and criminal records.**

Issues for review in the screening process should include arrest record, behavioral problems, substance abuse, and unsatisfactory work habits. Some states currently require reporting and background checking for new employees. When state licensure departments maintain records on individuals who have disciplinary and behavioral problems, this recommendation would apply only if the information did not include all the areas of inquiry mentioned by this committee. Hospitals and nursing homes should consider engaging the services of consulting firms to assist them in the screening process for potential new hires. To mitigate the issue of invasion of privacy, facility personnel offices should post appropriate notices announcing that all applicants must pass a complete and satisfactory background check before an employment decision is final.

Responsibility for neglect and abuse is by no means confined to NAs or similar ancillary personnel. Failure of the system because of poor management practices of facilities can also lead to an NA ending up on the registry. *Thus, the abuse prevention system should ultimately be applicable to all who work in nursing facilities and, for that matter, all health care institutions.*

The vulnerability of patients and residents, as well as health care personnel, to abuse, violence, and injury is becoming better documented. To protect these groups, basic and continuing education programs need to be developed that prepare nursing personnel to intervene in situations involving conflict and violence. Necessary skills include early recognition, assessment, conflict resolution, and emergency management.

Conflict Resolution

Although most health care facilities are diligent in observing residents' rights, none can guarantee that every right of every individual will be respected. Problems and conflicts are bound to occur, and complaints often can be equitably and amicably resolved within the facility or institution. In nursing homes, when a problem cannot be resolved internally, however, a resident or family member may contact the local office of the state long-term care (LTC) ombudsman program. Examples of problems and conflict between a resident or his or her family member(s) and staff that may be settled through various conflict resolution mechanisms include feelings of being deprecated or belittled; perceptions that a loved one is not receiving all available services or treatments; concerns about financial matters that are not fully explained or accounted for; feelings of discrimination; and concerns that the facility staff does not adequately discuss treatment, transfer, or discharge options.

Citing the dearth of research regarding maltreatment of residents of nursing homes, Pillemer (1988) suggests that staff behaviors are influenced by aspects of the nursing home environment and by certain factors exogenous to the facility. More recently, Pillemer and Hudson (1993) reported on an evaluation of a model abuse prevention curriculum for nursing assistants. According to the authors, those involved showed high satisfaction with the program, which reduced conflict and abuse of residents. The committee expresses strong support of all these efforts to develop innovative conflict resolution and similar programs and curricula.

WORK-RELATED STRESS

Extensive information documents that nursing work is stressful and that it can lead to a variety of work-related problems such as absenteeism, staff conflict, staff turnover, morale problems, and decreased worker effectiveness (Doering, 1990; Hiscott and Connop, 1990; Rees and Cooper, 1992; Fielding and Weaver, 1994). Exacerbated stress can lead to burnout and turnover of nursing personnel. Both the causes and correlates of work-related stress, and the outcomes and sequelae for nurses as well as patients or residents, are of concern to this committee.

Sources and Consequences of Stress

Several research studies focusing on nursing staff in acute care settings have attempted to identify a wide range of factors associated with stress. They include overwhelming workload, limited facilities and space, inadequate help, too much responsibility, too little continuing education, poor organization, excessive paperwork, inadequate communication with physicians, intrastaff tensions, and many other variables. Lack of recognition and lack of administrative support and leadership also can lead to stress. Although RNs frequently reported in testimony and during the committee's site visits that low staffing levels cause stress, empirical evidence does not corroborate their perception, although it clearly can exacerbate other stressful circumstances, as discussed below.

Some early studies of stress found that critical care nurses and intensive care nurses experience more stress than do staff in other units, but research has not consistently validated this finding (MacNeil and Weisz, 1987; Yu et al., 1989; Foxall et al., 1990). A survey of emergency room RNs, identified inadequate staffing and other resources, too many nonnursing tasks, changing trends in emergency department use, and patient transfer problems as causes of stress. They also described shortages of nursing staff during busy periods and at night, and the use of untrained relief staff, as other important factors in stress (Hawley, 1992).

One specific source of stress among health care workers is shift work. According to a 1991 review of 16 studies conducted by the Office of Technology Assessment (OTA, 1991), rotating nurses reported higher levels of stress, had more sleep disturbances, had significantly higher personal health problems, and suffered more injuries and accidents related to lack of sleep than fixed-shift nurses. Other research studies on shift work also reported adverse effects on performance, workers' health, performance, and mental and physical fitness (Gold et al., 1992).

Nursing personnel who work with the elderly confront many complex and potentially stressful situations in nursing homes where the work is highly demanding and labor intensive. Nursing personnel who work with patients with Alzheimer's disease are especially vulnerable to the effects of stress and burnout. These patients present many difficult care and management problems because of their progressive cognitive, functional, and psychosocial deterioration, which can result in bizarre and combative behaviors, emotional outbursts, and wandering. Moreover, nursing home staff are often poorly trained to cope with the disruptive behaviors of residents and are, therefore, repeatedly frustrated by their inability to manage recurrent problems (Stolley et al., 1991). Many nursing homes are also not equipped with environmental structures or the support and service systems required to care appropriately for the person with Alzheimer's disease (Peppard, 1984).

One recent study, using a quasi-experimental design with repeated measures, examined whether staff who cared for patients with Alzheimer's disease on a special care unit (SCU) experienced less stress and burnout than staff who cared for such patients on traditional (integrated) units (Mobily et al., 1992). The principal area of stress reduction for nursing personnel working on the SCU involved staff knowledge, abilities, and resources. Similarly, subscale analysis indicated significantly less stress for staff who worked in the SCU with respect to residents' verbal and physical behavior. The SCU was designed specifically to provide the special environmental structures and support and service systems that are required to enhance functioning and decrease associated behavioral problems of patients. These may be important factors in reducing stress and burnout for staff caring for residents suffering from Alzheimer's disease (Mobily et al., 1992). The investigators also recommended that, whenever possible, staff who work with such residents be screened carefully and selected for their ability to be sensitive to their needs, their flexibility, their imagination, and their ability to respond to persons with impaired communication and ever-changing moods (Coons, 1991). Specialized training in the care of residents with Alzheimer's disease is also a critical factor.

High stress at work can create morale problems that ultimately detract from the staff member's job performance (Sheridan et al., 1990). The causal model developed from research on work-related stress and morale among nursing home employees highlights both antecedents and outcomes of work-related stress (Weiler et al., 1990). The outcomes of work-related stress are linked to adverse physical and psychological consequences (LaRocco et al., 1980). According to Weiler and colleagues (1990), these outcomes can include: (1) burnout, defined as a syndrome of emotional exhaustion, depersonalization, and lack of personal accomplishment; (2) depression, which is the degree of negative affect experienced by nursing personnel; (3) poor or low job satisfaction, which involves effective orientation of nursing personnel toward the work situation; and (4) work involvement, defined as the degree to which nursing personnel identify with their job.

Although *burnout* has been the focus of many studies (see, e.g., Pines and Maslach, 1978; Dolan, 1987; Husted et al., 1989; Berland, 1990; Oehler et al., 1991; Johnson, 1992; Kandolin, 1993; Duquette et al., 1994), a uniform definition of burnout has not been established. Proposed definitions range from a simple equation of burnout with staff turnover to effectively including all four of the outcomes identified above by Weiler and colleagues. Nevertheless, most definitions found by the committee tend to describe burnout as having psychological, physical, and behavioral components. Pines and Maslach (1978, p. 236) define burnout as "a syndrome of physical and emotional exhaustion involving the development of a negative self-concept, negative job attitude and loss of concern and feeling for clients." In the long-term care setting, Heine (1986) characterizes burnout as a loss of concern for residents and physical, emotional and spiritual exhaustion that may lead to indifference or negative feelings toward elderly residents, overuse of chemical or physical restraints, and heightened potential for abuse. Because of the variety of definitions of burnout, the committee chooses simply to use the term for a state in which stress has resulted in persistent lower job satisfaction and potentially reduced work performance and effectiveness. At extreme levels of burnout, measurable problems such as increased staff turnover may occur. Goldin (1985), for instance, found that burnout results in such administrative difficulties as high rates of tardiness, absenteeism, and attrition.

Dolan and colleagues (1992) discuss issues surrounding the propensity of nursing staff to quit, which has been acknowledged as the best predictor of turnover. Behaviors related to stress, burnout, and depression are notable and can have a subsequent impact on quality of care and turnover. The investigators surveyed 1,237 staff who worked in 30 Quebec hospital emergency rooms and intensive care units about 14 job demands (the response rate was 84 percent). Results indicated that lack of professional latitude (which included restricted autonomy, skill underutilization, and lack of participation in clinical decision making), clinical demands, role difficulties, and workload problems all contributed to the propensity to quit. The authors suggested that interventions aimed at improving the quality of work and the general work-related quality of life should be implemented to enhance employee mental health, reduce rates of turnover, and curb costs.

The work conditions of RNs are repeatedly cited as being a source of stress. Some authors indicate that the quality of nursing care is seriously jeopardized and that RNs often leave nursing as a result of stress or burnout (Anonymous, 1986; Masterson-Allen et al., 1987; Lucas et al., 1993).

Many organizational factors have been cited that influence nursing stress, burnout, and productivity in nursing care, and that may result in short-term or long-term absenteeism. Research by Hare and Pratt (1988) has shown that higher levels of nursing burnout in both acute and LTC settings may be related to the nature of the physically and emotionally strenuous work tasks, low status in comparison to other positions in the health care system, limited training, low wages and benefits, and, of interest to this report, poor staff-to-patient ratios. Duquette and colleagues (1994) indicate that organizational stressors influence the development of burnout, particularly role ambiguity, staffing, and workload; age, with younger RNs being more susceptible to seeing their role as more ambiguous and their workload heavier; and buffering factors including hardiness, social support, and coping. Weiler and colleagues' (1990) causal model, developed from research on work-related stress and morale among nursing home employees, highlights both the antecedents and consequences of stress. The investigators suggest a variety of interventions to address organizational responses to stress. They include improved in-service training, increased variety in job tasks, improved supervision, clear and realistic objectives for resident care, higher wages and better benefits for staff, and adequate staffing levels. They note that higher compensation and richer staffing levels may be considered nonnegotiable by some administrators because of the cost implications associated with their implementation, but that the costs related to staff burnout, absenteeism, and turnover, can far outweigh the costs associated with adequate staffing and compensation. Health care administrators must address the issues of the impact of organizational stressors on nurses if there is to be any hope of resolving the problem (Whitley and Putzier, 1994). New approaches to staff selection and recruitment, flexibility in staffing, increased resources, and increased decision making by nurses is essential.

Changes in the physical environment and structural factors may also be critical elements in preventing or alleviating stress and work-related tension and pressures. Lyman (1987) suggests that physical and architectural features, such as adequate space, separate activity rooms, staff offices and toilet facilities, resident care facilities, barrier-free hallways, visible exits with amenities such as wide entry doors and ramps, and emergency exits, may decrease care giver burden and stress.

Enhancing social support networks is another important strategy that can serve as a buffer against the stresses inherent in working with the elderly. Problems with support in the work environment, especially from peers and supervisors, have repeatedly been shown to be a primary source of stress among nurses (Cronin-Stubbs and Rooks, 1985). Further, compelling evidence exists that social support serves to mitigate the adverse effects of stress and to reduce burnout among nursing staff (Constable and Russell, 1986).

SUMMARY

The committee has reviewed the literature on work-related injuries, violence and abuse, and stress afflicting nursing personnel in hospitals and nursing homes. Nursing is a hazardous occupation, and nursing personnel are exposed to a wide variety of health and safety hazards—biologic, chemical, environmental, mechanical, physical, and psychosocial. The committee has also reviewed available research to assess the factors that contribute to work-related injuries and to stress and burnout. *Except for back injuries, the committee is unable to substantiate conclusively the linkages among staffing numbers, skill mix, and work-related problems.*

In examining available information on violence and abuse, the committee became aware of the intricate problems of pressure-filled work situations and of violence and abuse directed at patients, especially the residents of nursing homes. It concludes that considerable problems may exist at the level of NAs and other ancillary nursing personnel especially in nursing facilities, who may be subject to great stress and probability of injury (especially back injury) and who may be newly employed and comparatively thinly trained.

The committee believes that many injuries and much of the violence toward staff in hospitals and nursing homes are preventable and that prevention is a shared responsibility of employers and employees. The committee urges hospitals and nursing homes to assess the effectiveness of prevention training and other models of organizational and nurse leadership described in contemporary research studies on the subject. It also urges hospitals and nursing homes to develop and implement strategies to prevent or reduce the incidence of injuries, violence and abuse, and stress and burnout in these health care workplaces.

8

Epilogue

During the nearly 2 years in which this Institute of Medicine (IOM) committee met, it learned much about health care delivery and the role of nursing personnel in the health care system that did not relate directly to its formal charge. The committee acknowledges that many issues relating to nursing and health extend beyond the scope of this report. Some of those issues should at least be mentioned. Committee members believe these observations provide a richer context in which their specific views of the future and recommended next steps should be understood. At its last meeting, the committee listed a number of points noted here.

Issues surrounding the adequacy of nursing staff proved inextricable from broader issues of health care access, quality, workforce, and costs. The committee believes that its findings and conclusions will inform current dialogues concerning the organization and delivery of health care, quality of patient care, safety and work experience of all nursing personnel, and suggest increased flexibility of the nation's nursing community for meeting tomorrow's health care challenges. It also believes that the changes now taking place in health care organization and financing, and in other parts of the health care workforce, will have important consequences for nursing. Because of the manner and extent to which health systems are being reconfigured, job security to registered nurses (RN) is declining in favor of new boundary spanning career opportunities.

The committee also recognizes the centrality of nursing care to the provision of health care services in an immensely broad array of health care settings, from institutional to community-based to home-based care. Large numbers of people, day in and day out, are directly touched by nursing personnel.

The committee understands that a number of the workforce issues it was asked to address should be examined in the context of emerging forms of practice, such as patient-centered teams, networks, and independent practice. The evolution in duties and responsibilities of a wide array of health care workers might be characterized as a revolution. The nursing community, including RNs, nurses in advanced clinical practice, licensed practical nurses (LPN), and nurses assistants (NA) and other ancillary nursing personnel, lies absolutely at the center of this revolution. Clinical practice, management, education and training, and research are a few of the different roles RNs undertake. Anecdotal information suggests that increasing numbers of NAs are being employed in hospitals, and at times are assigned tasks that have not been clearly delineated and for which they may not have been trained. The rapid rate of change in these and other areas requires more research and, doubtless, changes in education and training programs for the future.

The committee found itself deliberating on many issues involving RNs, LPNs, and ancillary nursing personnel such as nurse assistants, in terms of the roles they play in the delivery of care in hospitals and nursing homes, respectively. Supply and demand information about LPNs is not as rich as the information available about RNs. Even less is known, and few data are available, about NAs; yet they are a large proportion of the total nurse workforce. To the extent that these nursing personnel remain a significant, but comparatively invisible, part of the nursing community, this paucity of information about their actual roles in health care delivery, their training, and their career paths complicates sensible policy-making about education, reimbursement, and similar matters.

The committee observed the need for: (1) greater investment in the nursing workforce; (2) improved leadership, organizational, and management skills within the ranks of the nursing community; and (3) the need for better coordination with other care givers. Nursing should not be viewed in isolation from other professions and training should reflect the relation to those other professions. At the same time, there is a need for a clear nursing identity reflecting new skills and new roles within the health care system. Recent reorganizations of hospitals sometimes result in a diminution of the old nursing identity. If adjustments are not forthcoming such changes could ultimately impact negatively on patient care.

The committee stands firmly behind the proposition that the relationship between nurse staffing and quality of patient care has been clearly established for the nation's nursing homes. In other words, the value added to resident health and well-being by an adequate number and educational mix of nurses is clear. The committee recognizes the differences in nurse staffing and quality of patient care in nursing homes on the one hand, and in hospitals on the other. Hospitals and nursing homes may operate on very different segments of a staffing–quality relationship curve. Hospitals could be operating in the segment of the curve where returns from increases in staffing are low because they already have relatively high staffing levels. By contrast, nursing homes are operating at the very low end of the staffing scale, so positive returns from increases in staffing are observable.

The committee recognizes that the relationships between quality and costs are complex and difficult to disaggregate. Analysis of the mechanisms underlying these relationships merits a high priority. The committee thus underscores the importance of conveying to the public the need for much better mechanisms by which policymakers can analyze these factors.

The level of external interest in this project and the implied level of expectations on the part of several interested constituencies were extraordinarily high. The committee welcomed all input and appreciated the many individuals and organizations who provided information or otherwise helped the committee to meet its charge.

Several committee members were aware of the fact that many analyses of the nursing workforce, as well as several related IOM studies, have appeared in recent years. Some (such as the 1986 IOM study on improving the quality of nursing home care) have had instant impact; in other cases, however, recommendations not unlike those appearing in this report have required a longer time to exert an appreciable influence. The committee reflected on the question of what differences have arisen since the previous studies were conducted. It concluded that one major difference is the ability of researchers, policymakers, and others to use better measures of patient outcomes and nursing processes of care, and thus to determine and document how the proposed changes will bring about meaningful improvements in the health care system and in the well-being of patients and the nation's population in general.

In settings where patients and residents cannot receive all necessary services from paid staff members, volunteers can be a distinct asset. Volunteers can never fully replace staff, but they can provide companionship, contact, comforts (such as letter writing and craft materials) and assistance (such as help with eating), and can even be part of an informal quality assurance mechanism. The committee was impressed with the devotion of nursing personnel, families, volunteers, and other care givers. The committee noted that it is critical that the public—and not just investors and policymakers—have a participatory role in the major decisions ahead on health care.

This study was mandated at a time that, in retrospect, seems rather calm. In the intervening months, press and media reports on the issues studied by the committee increased, and unstructured and unpredictable changes driven by continuing cost containment pressures, private sector interests, and market forces are swiftly and unmistakably altering the health care landscape. This turbulence has made the work of the committee markedly more challenging, and also more difficult; in particular, it has complicated the task of issuing recommendations that will be timely and pertinent beyond today. In the committee's view, policymakers and the public need to understand, far more deeply than they may at this moment, how rapid change is affecting the nation's ability to make reasoned decisions about the health of the nation into the next century. While markets will adjust to supply and demand conditions over the long term, it is possible for policy to influence these demand and supply conditions. Incentives to invest in new technologies, for example, may result in an increased demand for new technical skills by nurses or, possibly, a substitute for those skills. Policies can range from *laissez faire* (do nothing) to active intervention in demand and supply conditions such as education, research, regulation, taxation, and information. Then it is important to ask the question what the effect will likely be on the quality of patient care and on the nursing staff providing the care. This then leads to the question of appropriate policy responses.

Finally, the committee's work on several of the issues it was asked to examine was impeded by the spotty availability of timely, reliable, and valid data with uniform definitions and classification. Thus, committee members expressed a common concern about the lack of sufficient data to address the questions they were charged to address. Insights gleaned from public testimony, site visits, and similar activities cumulatively added to the understanding of today's health care system, nursing services, and the quality of patient care. These issues will continue to represent major concerns in the years ahead. Adequate funding is essential for research and evaluation to help ensure that efforts to constrain the costs of nursing do not, in fact, result in serious consequences for the health of our citizens.

APPENDIXES

Presentations Made to the Committee

Expectations and hopes for the study
  Marla Salmon, Director, Division of Nursing, Health Resources and
    Services Administration; and
  Ada Sue Hinshaw, Director, National Institute of Nursing Research

Nurse staffing and quality of care in nursing homes
  Jean Johnson, Assistant Professor and Dean for Health Sciences Programs,
    George Washington University Medical Center

Federal/national databases: Availability for analysis
  Evelyn Moses, Chief Nursing Data and Analysis Staff, Division of
    Nursing, Bureau of Health Professions, Health Resources and Services
    Administration

Influence of availability of nurses on quality of care
  Patricia Moritz, Nursing Systems Branch Chief, Extramural Programs
    Division, National Institute of Nursing Research

Nursing: An important component of hospital survival under a reformed health
care system
  Patricia Prescott, Professor, University of Maryland, Baltimore, School of
    Nursing

Nurse burnout, patient outcomes: Staffing ratios versus organization of nursing
  Linda Aiken, Trustee Professor of Nursing and Sociology, and Director,
    Center for Health Services and Policy Research, University of
    Pennsylvania

Forces affecting employment and work environment of nursing staff in hospitals
  Peter Buerhaus, Director, Harvard Nursing Research Institute, Harvard
    School of Public Health

Study of nursing home staffing ratios: Overview
  Marvin Feuerberg, Analyst, Health Standards and Quality Bureau, Health
    Care Financing Administration and Edward Mortimore, Analyst, Health
    Standards and Quality Bureau, Health Care Financing Administration

Developing and utilizing a nursing quality report card for acute care: Report of a
study conducted for the American Nurses Association by Lewin-VHI
  Mary Walker, Chairperson, Congress for Nursing Practice, American
    Nurses Association, and Associate Professor, University of Kentucky
    College of Nursing

Results of ongoing and completed research relating to nurse staffing, organizational variables, and quality outcomes in acute care settings: Report of a workshop
  Joyce Verran, Professor and Division Director of the Adult Health Nursing
    Unit, College of Nursing, University of Arizona at Tucson

Nursing in hospitals, looking at the future: A case study in restructuring
  Helen Ripple, Director of Nursing, University of California, San Francisco,
    Medical Center, and Associate Clinical Director, University of
    California, San Francisco, School of Nursing

Purpose and plans for the minimum data set (Version 2.0)
  Susan Nonemaker, Senior Program Analyst, Division of Long Term Care
    Services, Health Standards and Quality Bureau, Health Care Financing
    Administration

The long-range nursing manpower demand project of the Greater Cleveland Hos-
pital Association
  Scott Sutorius, Vice President and Principal Investigator; Leah Shaikh,
    Project Manager; and
  Patricia Prescott, Professor, University of Maryland, Baltimore, School of
    Nursing

B

Liaison Panel

Institute of Medicine (IOM) studies frequently rely on liaison panels to broaden the expertise of the committee, to inform interested and concerned parties about the study and its activities, and to provide a forum for discussion of the issues. In some studies, liaison panels may be given specific charges and asked to provide the committee with specific products. Other studies may never formally convene a meeting of the liaison panel, per se, but may work with the members of the panel informally and individually. Organizations nominate members of a liaison panel to speak on their behalf and to provide advice and assistance about the issues under consideration; because liaison panel members serve in an advisory capacity to the IOM formal committee, they may have known biases and conflicts of interest.

The IOM convened a liaison panel, comprising representatives of professional associations of nurses, related professional groups, hospitals and nursing homes, unions, and organizations that serve as advocates for nursing home residents. The panel met formally for a one-day meeting on August 1, 1994. It served in a consultative and information exchange capacity. Several members of the panel provided the committee with results of special surveys, specific informational material, and other background information from their organizations throughout the period of the study. They also helped to identify data sources, potential witnesses for the public hearing, and contacts for the committee's site visits.

Organizations represented on the liaison panel are listed below:

Organization	*Representative*
American Association of Colleges of Nursing	Polly Bednash
American Association of Critical-Care Nurses	Melissa A. Fitzpatrick
American Association of Homes and Services for the Aging	Evelyn F. Munley
American Association of Occupational Health Nurses	Kathleen Bean
American Association of Retired Persons	Alan Buckingham
American Health Care Association	Mary Kay Ousley
American Hospital Association	Marjorie Beyers
American Licensed Practical Nurses Association	Paul M. Tendler
American Medical Directors Association	Rebecca Elon
American Nurses Association	Geraldine Marullo
American Nursing Assistants Association	Steve P. Gorsline
American Organization of Nurse Executives	Diana Weaver
Association for Federal, State and Municipal Employees	Constance Brown
Joint Commission on Accreditation of Healthcare Organizations	Carole H. Patterson
National Association of Directors of Nursing Administration/LTC	Joan C. Warden
National Citizens' Coalition for Nursing Home Reform	Sue Harang
National Committee to Preserve Social Security and Medicare	Martha M. Mohler
National Federation for Specialty Nursing Organizations	Connie Whittington
National League for Nursing	Eloise Balasco
Service Employees International Union	Rhonda Goode

APPENDIX

C

Separate Statement and Responses

Appendix C consists of two parts. Part 1 is a separate statement prepared by committee member James Blumstein. Part 2 is a response to that statement by other committee members.

PART 1: SEPARATE STATEMENT FROM THE REPORT OF THE COMMITTEE

James F. Blumstein

Overall, this report reflects a reasonable statement about the issues the Committee was charged with investigating. Although I and probably most committee members disagree with certain statements or would state certain items in different ways, in general we have agreed to compromise in order to reach consensus. Nevertheless, I feel constrained to comment separately on what was probably the single most contentious issue confronted by the committee, recommendation 6-1, which recommends 24-hour registered nurse (RN) coverage for all nursing homes by the year 2000 along with the appropriation of sufficient funds to pay for this enhanced level of service.

Two provisions—one contained in the Recommendation and the other in the text explaining the Recommendation—warrant highlighting. First, the term "coverage" is used in recommendation 6-1. This suggests that full-time staffing should not be mandated. Presumably, the requirement could be satisfied by having RN services available on an "on-call" basis. This procedure is followed in traditional medical circumstances, and would allow for efficiencies by allowing

RN services to be "on-call" for more than a single facility. For larger facilities, a staff RN might be appropriate and feasible on a 24-hour basis (this staffing is already in existence for many nursing homes, either because it is required or on grounds of good practice), but for smaller facilities and in less wealthy Medicaid jurisdictions, the more economical sharing arrangement might suffice. This recognizes that some increments of quality might have to be traded off in the name of reasonable expenditure constraints and alternative claims on Medicaid and Medicare dollars.

Second, the 24-hour RN coverage mandate contained in recommendation 6-1 is subject to appropriate waiver. No criteria are specified in this waiver provision. Some committee members believed that the waiver should apply only when RN personnel are unavailable; others felt that waivers are appropriate when economic considerations make the requirement unwise in terms of cost–benefit analysis, especially in light of the opportunity costs associated with the 24-hour RN requirement in some foreseeable situations. Further, the "unavailability" standard inherently has an economic dimension, since the unavailability problem would be reduced or eliminated if money were no object and the price were, therefore, right.

Despite the flexibility implied by the term "coverage," I reluctantly state my disagreement with recommendation 6-1 because it is not based on careful consideration of evidence and a balancing of competing claims on public resources; rather, the Recommendation was reached without consideration of alternative uses of public funds or consequences from this proposed new mandate.

My substantive concerns have two components. First, the committee made this recommendation without any hard evidence about the costs involved or about the value of the benefit to be derived. Second, inadequate consideration was given to the desirability of allowing states freedom to set priorities and allocate public funds.

(a) There were few data presented or discussed regarding the cost of recommendation 6-1. There was an estimate provided by the nursing home industry that each additional hour of mandated nursing service would result in an increased nursing home cost for Medicare and Medicaid of $3.4 billion per year.

One cannot just multiply $3.4 billion per year by the additional 16 hours proposed in recommendation 6-1 to calculate the incremental cost of the proposal above existing expenditures. Many nursing facilities satisfy the proposed standard, but that number was not presented to the committee during its deliberations regarding recommendation 6-1. Further, the Recommendation does not necessarily call for additional hours of nursing service but only for upgrading the quality of nursing service. Thus, the industry's estimate does not provide an appropriate measure of the incremental cost of the committee's proposal. The problem is that the committee had no evidence to determine how many facilities would be affected and to what extent. Estimation of cost in such circumstances is back-of-the-envelope guesswork at best. In response to this criticism, a subsequently developed ballpark estimate has been included in the report, but the committee had no opportunity to discuss the estimate or consider it in terms of putative benefits or alternative expenditures.

In addition, although the committee could assert that staffing levels in general have a positive correlation with quality of care in nursing homes, it could not pin down those benefits in causal terms with any precision. Just what precisely is the benefit that will come from the proposed Recommendation? This is hard to identify or measure with specificity.

Further, the committee made no effort—because the literature would not sustain such an effort—to evaluate the benefits that might accrue. To support recommendation 6-1, it is not enough to recite a relationship between overall staffing intensity and aggregate quality outcomes. More precision is needed, and some mechanism for evaluating the purported benefits is necessary in order to conduct sensible policy discussions and to establish priorities for public spending responsibly. Why 24-hour coverage and not 16 hours? Why only one RN in even larger facilities? With this gap in data, the Recommendation takes on the air not of professional or scientific judgment but of politics.

Implicitly, the committee acknowledges this. See Chapter 6, page 167: ("The small staffing increases under OBRA 87 required substantial new resources. These staffing increases were apparently based on the amount legislators and industry leaders considered to be politically and fiscally feasible, . . ."), and on that score, an IOM committee has no special wisdom.

(b)   Recommendation 6-1 is another proposed federal mandate at a time when these mandates are being called into question. The committee was conscious of this concern and, responsibly, included a funding element to the Recommendation. Nevertheless, at least for Medicaid, state participation in financing is currently a requirement; thus, this is the kind of mandate that Congress has recently disavowed.

Beyond a basic requirement, which is satisfied by current rules, local priorities should generally be respected. This is particularly true when the costs are unknown and the nature and value of the benefits are also uncertain. Since Medicaid accounts for such a large proportion of nursing home services, public dollars are at issue, and in the absence of some overriding federal interest (such as assurance of civil rights), local political tastes should prevail. States may differ politically with respect to evaluating alternative claims on public resources. This could mean that some states would prioritize other needs in health care, or it could mean that states would elect non-health care expenditures such as schools or prisons as higher spending priorities. Beyond the basic requirement, states should be allowed to choose how to allocate public dollars on the basis of their own political priorities and on the basis of their self-perceived financial capacity.

PART 2: COMMITTEE MEMBERS' RESPONSES TO THE SEPARATE STATEMENT OF JAMES F. BLUMSTEIN

We are compelled to respond to the statements of Mr. Blumstein because we disagree with the position that he has stated in his response to the report, especially the statement that the recommendations were made without careful consideration of the evidence. On the contrary, these decisions were made carefully with great deliberation and with consideration of the financial costs.

Recommendation 6–1, as stated by the committee, was that every nursing facility should be required to have direct care by at least one registered nurse on a 24-hour-a-day basis as a minimum mandate. This recommendation to strengthen current standards grew out of strong research findings that facilities with more registered nurses have a higher quality of resident outcomes. The data from nursing facilities showed that some had inadequate numbers of registered nurses, which we considered showed the need for stronger minimum standards.

Based on the research findings, some members of the committee supported even stronger minimum mandated staffing levels for registered nurses and other nursing personnel, including nursing assistants. The primary reason that many experts have been unwilling to support even higher staffing standards is the high cost to the Medicaid program, which pays for a majority of nursing facility days of care in the United States. Thus, the concern is strictly one of political and economic feasibility—not a dispute among nursing professionals over the need for more nursing personnel.

Not only are high professional standards for nursing facility care advocated by professionals who are knowledgeable about the needs of residents, but such standards have been demonstrated to make a difference in terms of resident outcomes. Research conducted by economists, sociologists, nurses, and other health services researchers has been carefully detailed and documented in this report, and it is the basis of the recommendations made. The research indicates that if more nursing professionals were added, the outcomes in nursing facilities could be substantially improved.

Although some nursing professionals on this committee argued that the needs were much greater than the modest recommendation made by the committee, even our views were tempered by the poor national economic climate and the perceived financial crisis in the Medicare and Medicaid programs. If the recommendations were based solely on the need for nursing care and professional standards, the recommended standards could have been substantially greater.

The committee debated the current waiver provisions for facilities that cannot meet the staffing standards. The general perspective was that facilities should not be granted waivers and should make every possible effort to meet the minimum federal standards. The current availability of registered nurses in the market argues against the need for waivers, even in rural areas. The committee, however, did not ask for the repeal of these waivers because there may be some extenuating circumstances that it could not foresee. The committee did not propose the exact criteria for waivers specifically because such criterion development was beyond both the scope and the expertise of its members.

The committee did consider the costs of recommendation 6–1 and found that it would be approximately $338 million dollars. The committee has specific data on the cost difference between a licensed practical nurse (LPN) and an RN salary from the Department of Labor, which show that the differential was about $4 per hour in 1994. If every nursing home in the United States needed to convert one LPN to one RN on the evening and night shifts (which is an overestimate since many facilities already meet the minimum standard), the cost of the recommendation would be approximately $338 million. This seemed a rather small investment in a $74-billion-dollar industry in 1994 (less than 1 percent of total expenditures) to improve the quality of care for the most vulnerable individuals in our society.

Mr. Blumstein raises the issue that the cost of each additional hour of nursing service is estimated to be $3.4 billion. This cost is not applicable to the recommendation, because facilities already have at a minimum at least one licensed practical nurse on the evening and night shifts, as required under current law. Since the recommendation is not adding new nursing hours but rather upgrading the educational requirements for nursing personnel already present in facilities, Mr. Blumstein's estimates are not correct.

Those who dislike regulations should understand that adding more nursing care could save on regulatory efforts in the long run. It should reduce the high admission rates from the nursing home to hospitals and lower the total costs of hospital care under both the Medicare and Medicaid programs. In the long run, increasing professional nurse staffing in nursing homes could result in substantial savings to both the Medicaid and the Medicare budgets.

Current research data on nursing facilities, like other health services research data, do not have the precision that we would like. However, although we may lament that the real world of nursing facility and hospital care is too complex to calculate the exact cost–benefit in adopting improved staffing standards, we must make our best judgments based on the information available. This brings us to the recommendations that were made for a small increase in minimum staffing standards and continued research to improve the quality of care delivery in the most efficient way.

Dyanne Affonso
Linda Hawes Clever
Joyce Clifford
Edward Connors
Carolyne K. Davis

Erika Froelicher
Charlene A. Harrington
Sue Longhenry
Elliott C. Roberts, Sr.

Personal Response to the Separate Statement of James F. Blumstein

First, I find Mr. Blumstein's statement extremely difficult to follow; therefore, I will not try to respond to all aspects of it. However, I personally object to the inclusiveness of the language in the second sentence of this statement that says ". . . most all committee members disagree with certain statements. . . ." It is my belief that the committee worked very hard to have consensus in this important report. Any compromises I may have made related to what I might have desired to *add* to the report, not with what is *in* the report.

I do not believe that a dissenting statement of one member of the committee should suggest that there was disagreement by other members as well, and I strongly urge that this statement be limited to the author and not include any reference to the opinions of other committee members.

It also concerns me that the statement suggests that recommendation 6-1 was made without "careful consideration of evidence. . . ." This recommendation was not made lightly, and it was not made without recognition of the financial burden that it might incur. Mr. Blumstein suggests that registered nurses could be on-call rather than on the premises of a facility. This suggestion is totally unacceptable as a means of providing minimum professional protection and care for very ill and disabled individuals, who frequently have complex nursing and medical care needs, as well as medical emergencies, that require immediate skilled nursing attention.

I voted for this recommendation because it was the right thing to do in light of the increasing acuity of care needs in nursing homes, the knowledge that we do have about the relationship of quality and staffing, and my own 30 years of experience in developing, implementing, and evaluating nurse staffing in hospitals.

Joyce C. Clifford, RN, MSN, FAAN
Vice President, Nursing and Nurse-in-Chief
Beth Israel Hospital
Boston, MA 02215

APPENDIX
D

Acronyms

The list below includes agencies, organizations, health personnel, surveys and programs.

AACN	American Association of Colleges of Nursing
ACNW	American College of Nurse Midwives
AAHSA	American Association of Homes and Services for the Aging
AD	associate degree in nursing
ADL	activities of daily living
AHA	American Hospital Association
AHCA	American Health Care Association
AHCPR	Agency for Health Care Policy and Research
AIDS	acquired immunodeficiency syndrome
AMI	acute myocardial infarction
ANA	American Nurses Association
APN	advance practice nurse
BLS	Bureau of Labor Statistics
BSN	bachelor's-of-science degree in nursing
CAHF	California Association of Health Facilities
CBO	Congressional Budget Office
CCU	critical care unit
CDC	Centers for Disease Control and Prevention
CNA	certified nurse assistant

CNAP	Career Nurse Assistants Program
CON	certificate of need
CQI	continuous quality improvement
DHHS	Department of Health and Human Services
DON	director of nursing
DRG	diagnosis-related group
ER	emergency room
FANEL	Federation for Accessible Nursing Education and Licensure
FFS	fee-for-service
FTE	full-time-equivalent employee
GAO	General Accounting Office
GHAA	Group Health Association of America
GI	gastrointestinal
GNP	geriatric nurse practitioner
GNS	gerontological nurse specialist
HCFA	Health Care Financing Administration
HIV	human immunodeficiency virus
HMO	health maintenance organization
HRSA	Health Resources and Services Administration
IADL	instrumental activities of daily living
ICU	intensive care unit
IOM	Institute of Medicine
IPA	independent practice association
IV	intravenous
JCAHO	Joint Commission on Accreditation of Healthcare Organizations
KP	Kaiser Permanente
LPN	licensed practical nurse
LTC	long-term care
LVN	licensed vocational nurse
MDS	minimum data set
MMACS	Medicare and Medicaid Automated Certification Survey
MOS	Medical Outcomes Study
MRI	magnetic resonance imaging

NA	nurse assistant
NADONA	National Association of Directors of Nursing Administration/Long-Term Care
NAPNES	National Association for Practical Nurse Education and Service
NCCNHR	National Citizens' Coalition for Nursing Home Reform
NCHS	National Center for Health Statistics
NCSBN	National Council of State Boards of Nursing
NF	nursing facility
NG	nasogastric
NHCMQ	National Nursing Home Casemix and Quality Demonstration
NICHD	National Institute of Child Health and Human Development
NIH	National Institutes of Health
NINR	National Institute of Nursing Research
NLN	National League for Nursing
OBN	Ohio Board of Nursing
OBRA	Omnibus Budget Reconciliation Act
OSCAR	On-Line Survey Certification and Reporting System
OSHA	Occupational Safety and Health Administration
OT	occupational therapist
OTA	Office of Technology Assessment
PHCE	personal health care expenditures
PHS	Public Health Service
PPO	preferred provider organization
PPS	Prospective Payment System
PRB	Population Reference Bureau
PRO	peer review organization
ProPAC	Prospective Payment Assessment Commission
PSRO	professional standards review organization
PT	physical therapist
QA	quality assurance
QI	quality indicators
RAI	resident assessment instrument
RAP	resident assessment protocols
RN	registered nurse
RUG	resource utilization group
SCU	special care unit
SEIU	Service Employees International Union
SMSA	standard metropolitan statistical area
SNF	skilled nursing facility

TQM   total quality management
TEFRA   Tax Equity and Fiscal Responsibility Act
TNH   teaching nursing home

UAP   unlicensed assistive personnel
UHF   Unicare Health Facilities

VA   Department of Veterans Affairs

References

Aaronson, W., Zinn, J.S., and Rosko, M.D. Do For-Profit and Not-For-Profit Nursing Homes Behave Differently? *The Gerontologist* 34:775–786, 1994.

Abelson, R. Health. *Forbes,* pp. 162–167, January 4, 1993.

Abt Associates and the Center for Health Policy Research. Briefing Points on Preliminary Evaluation Results. Briefing for the HCFA Leadership Conference. Bethesda, Md.: Abt Associates, July 27, 1993.

AHA (American Hospital Association). *Hospital Mergers and Consolidations: 1980–1991.* Chicago: AHA Section for Health Care Systems, 1992.

AHA. *AHA Hospital Statistics: The AHA Profile of United States Hospitals 94/95. 1994–95 Edition. Data Compiled from the American Hospital Association 1993 Annual Survey of Hospitals.* Chicago: AHA, 1994a.

AHA. *Hospital Closures 1980–1993: A Statistical Profile.* Prepared by the AHA Health Care Information Resources Group. Chicago: AHA, 1994b.

AHA. News Release: New Health Care Trends Unveiled in Latest AHA Statistics Book. Washington, D.C.: AHA Washington Office, 1994c.

AHA. *Economic Trends. Key Trends in Calendar Year 1995.* (AHA National Hospital Panel Survey, March panel.) Vol. 11, no. 2. Chicago: AHA Health Statistics Group, 1995a.

AHA. Special tabulations from AHA annual surveys, 1983–1993, prepared for the Institute of Medicine Committee on the Adequacy of Nurse Staffing in Hospitals and Nursing Homes. Chicago: AHA, 1995b.

AHCA (American Health Care Association). Costs of an Employer Health Care Mandate. *Provider: The Magazine for Long Term Care Professionals* 20(5):8, 1994a.

AHCA. *Facts and Trends: The Nursing Facility Sourcebook.* Washington, D.C.: AHCA, 1994b.

AHCA. *Facts and Trends: The Nursing Facility Sourcebook.* Washington, D.C.: AHCA, 1995.

AHCPR (Agency for Health Care Policy and Research). *Acute Low Back Problems in Adults. Clinical Practice Guideline No. 14.* S. Bigos, O. Bowyer, G. Braen, et al., eds. Pub. no. 95–0642. Rockville, Md.: AHCPR, 1994.

Aiken, L.H. The Hospital Nursing Shortage: A Paradox of Increasing Supply and Increasing Vacancy Rates. In: C. Harrington and C.L. Estes, eds. *Health Policy and Nursing.* Boston: Jones and Bartlett, 1994.

Aiken, L.H. Transformation of the Nursing Workforce. *Nursing Outlook* 43:201–209, 1995.

Aiken, L.H., and Gwyther, M.E. Medicare Funding of Nurse Education: The Case for Policy Change. *Journal of the American Medical Association,* 273:1528–1532, 1995.

Aiken, L.H., and Hadley, J. Factors Affecting the Hospital Employment of Registered Nurses. In: *The Secretary's Commission on Nursing. Final Report, vol. 2.* Washington, D.C.: U.S. Department of Health and Human Services, 1988.

Aiken, L.H., and Salmon, M.E. Health Care Workforce Priorities: What Nursing Should Do Now. *Inquiry* 31:318–329, 1994.

Aiken, L.H., Smith, H.L., and Lake, E.T. Lower Medicare Mortality Among a Set of Hospitals Known for Good Nursing Care. *Medical Care* 32:771–787, 1994.

Allen, J. Two Charged with Battery at Long Grove Nursing Home. *Daily Herald* (Ill.), p. 1–News 11, August 17, 1994.

Alter, H.J., Seef, L.B., Kaplan, P.M., et al. Type B Hepatitis: The Infectivity of Blood Positive for E Antigen and DNA Polymerase After Accidental Needlestick Exposure. *New England Journal of Medicine* 295:909–913, 1976.

ANA (American Nurses Association). The Report of Survey Results: The 1994 ANA Layoffs Survey. *The American Nurse* (March):1,7, 1995a.

ANA. Summary of the Lewin-VHI, Inc., Report: Nursing Report Card for Acute Care Settings (photocopy). Washington, D.C.: ANA, 1995b.

Anderson, G.F., and Kohn, L.T. Employment Trends in Hospitals Between 1981 and 1993. *Inquiry,* in press.

Anonymous. What Really Makes Nurses Angry. *RN* 49(1):55–60, 1986.

Arad, D., and Ryan, M. The Incidence and Prevalence in Nurses of Low Back Pain: A Definitive Survey Exposes the Hazards. *Australian Nurse Journal* 16:44–48, 1986.

Arling, G., Nordquist, R.H., Brant, B.A., and Capitman, J.A. Nursing Home Case Mix. *Medical Care* 25:9–19, 1987.

Arling, G., Zimmerman, D., and Updike, L. Nursing Home Case Mix in Wisconsin. *Medical Care* 27:164–181, 1989.

Bahr, R.T. Reaction to the Invitational Conference "Mechanisms of Quality in Long Term Care: Service and Clinical Outcomes." Pp. 103–109 in: *Mechanisms of Quality in Long Term Care: Service and Clinical Outcomes.* Pub. no. 41–2382. New York: National League for Nursing Press, 1991.

Baker, A. Granny Battering. *Nursing Mirror* 144:65–66, 1977.

Ballard, T.M. The Need for Well-Prepared Nurse Administrators in Long-term Care. *Image: Journal of Nursing Scholarship* 27(2):153–160, 1995.

Baltz, T.M., and Turner, J.G. Development and Analysis of a Nursing Home Aide Screening Device. *The Gerontologist* 17:66–69, 1977.

Barter, M., McLaughlin, F.E., and Thomas, S.A. Use of Unlicensed Assistive Personnel by Hospitals. *Nursing Economic$* 12(2):82–87, 1994.

Beck, C., Rossby, L., and Baldwin, B. Correlates of Disruptive Behavior in Cognitively Impaired Elderly Nursing Home Residents. *Archives of Psychiatric Nursing* 5(5):281–291, 1991.

Berland, A. Controlling Workload. *Canadian Nurse* 86(5):36–38, 1990.

Bernardi, N. Patient Sues Nursing Home over '93 Rape. *Courier-News* (Ill.), pp. A1, A7, August 16, 1994.

Birkenstock, M. From Turnover to Turnaround. *Geriatric Nursing* 12(4):194–196, 1991.

Bishop, C.E. Competition in the Market for Nursing Home Care. *Journal of Health Politics, Policy and Law* 13(2):341–361, 1988.

Blaum, C.S., Fries, B.E., and Fiatarone, M.A. Factors Associated with Low Body Mass Index and Weight Loss in Nursing Home Residents. *Journals of Gerontology: Medical Sciences*, 50A(3):M162–M168, 1995.

BLS (Bureau of Labor Statistics). Shifting Workforce Spawns New Set of Hazardous Occupations. *Issues in Labor Statistics*. Summary 94-8. Washington, D.C.: U.S. Department of Labor, 1994a.

BLS. Violence in the Workplace Comes Under Closer Scrutiny. *Issues in Labor Statistics*. Summary 94-10. Washington, D.C.: U.S. Department of Labor, 1994b.

BLS. Workplace Injuries and Illnesses in 1993. *Issues in Labor Statistics*. Summary 94-600. Washington, D.C.: U.S. Department of Labor, 1994c.

BLS. *Survey of Occupational Health and Injuries*. Summary 95-5. Washington, D.C.: U.S. Department of Labor, 1995a.

BLS. *Work Injuries and Illnesses by Selected Characteristics, 1993*. Summary 95-142. Washington, D.C.: U.S. Department of Labor, 1995b.

BLS. Special tabulations prepared for the Institute of Medicine Committee on the Adequacy of Nurse Staffing in Hospitals and Nursing Homes. Washington, D.C.: U.S. Department of Labor, 1995c.

BLS. Violence in the Workplace. Prepared by G. Toscano and W. Weber. *Compensation and Working Conditions*. Washington, D.C.: U.S. Department of Labor, 1995d.

Bogue, R.J., Shortell, S.M., Sohn, M.-W., et al. Hospital Reorganization After Merger. *Medical Care* 33:676–686, 1995.

Bowers, B. Family Perceptions of Care in a Nursing Home. *The Gerontologist* 28:361–368, 1988.

Bradbury, R.C., Golec, J.H., and Steen, P.M. Relating Hospital Health Outcomes and Resource Expenditures. *Inquiry* 31:56–65, 1994.

Brannon, R.L. *Intensifying Care: The Hospital Industry, Professionalization, and the Reorganization of the Nursing Labor Process*. From the series *Critical Approaches in the Health Social Sciences Series*, R.H. Elling, ed. Amityville, N.Y.: Baywood Publishing Company, 1994.

Braun, B.I. The Effect of Nursing Home Quality on Patient Outcome. *Journal of the American Geriatrics Society* 39:329–338, 1991.

Brooten, D., Kumar, S., Brown, L.P., et al. A Randomized Clinical Trial of Early Hospital Discharge and Home Follow-up of Very-Low-Birth-Weight Infants. *New England Journal of Medicine* 31:934–939, 1986.

Brooten, D., Brown, L.P., Munro, B.H., et al. Early Discharge and Specialist Transitional Care. *Image: Journal of Nursing Scholarship* 20(2):64–68, 1988.

Buchanan, J.L., Bell, R.M., Arnold, S.B., et al. Assessing Cost Effects of Nursing-Home-Based Geriatric Nurse Practitioners. *Health Care Financing Review* 11(3):67–78, 1990.

Bureau of the Census. *Language Spoken at Home and Ability to Speak English: United States Regions and States, 1990*. Pub. no. CPH-L-133. Washington, D.C.: U.S. Department of Commerce, 1990.

Bureau of the Census. *Race and Hispanic Origin. 1990 Census Profile, No. 2*. Washington, D.C.: U.S. Department of Commerce, 1991b.

Bureau of the Census. *Population Projections of the United States, by Age, Sex, Race, and Hispanic Origin: 1993 to 2050. Current Population Reports*. Prepared by J.C. Day. Pub. no. P25-1104. Washington, D.C.: U.S. Department of Commerce, 1993a.

Bureau of the Census. *Poverty in the United States: 1992. Current Population Reports, Consumer Income*. Series P60-185. Washington, D.C.: U.S. Department of Commerce, 1993b.

Bureau of the Census. *We the American. . . Elderly*. Pub. no. WE-9. Washington, D.C.: U.S. Department of Commerce, 1993c.

Bureau of the Census. *Statistical Abstract of the United States: 1994*. 114th ed. Washington, D.C.: U.S. Department of Commerce, 1995a.

Bureau of the Census. *Statistical Brief. Sixty-Five Plus in the United States.* Pub. no. SB/95-8. Washington, D.C.: U.S. Department of Commerce, 1995b.

Bureau of the Census and the National Institute on Aging. *Profiles of America's Elderly. Living Arrangements of the Elderly.* Pub. no. POP/93-2. Washington, D.C.: U.S. Department of Commerce and the National Institutes of Health, 1993a.

Bureau of the Census and the National Institute on Aging. *Profiles of America's Elderly. Racial and Ethnic Diversity of America's Elderly Population.* Pub. no. POP/93-1. Washington, D.C.: U.S. Department of Commerce and the National Institutes of Health, 1993b.

Burns, J. Long-Term-Care Chains Show Slight Growth. *Modern Healthcare* (May 18):81–94, 1992.

Burton, L.C., German, P.S., Rovner, B.W., et al. Mental Illness and the Use of Restraints in Nursing Homes. *The Gerontologist* 32:164–170, 1992.

Butler, P.A., and Schlenker, R.E. *Administering Nursing Home Case Mix Reimbursement Systems: Issues of Assessment, Quality, Access, Equity, and Cost: An Analysis of Long-term Care Payment Systems.* Final Report. Denver: Center for Health Services Research, University of Colorado Health Sciences Center, 1988.

Cameron, J.M. Case-mix and Resource Use in Long Term Care. *Medical Care* 23:296–309, 1985.

Carney, R.M. Protect Your Nursing Athletes! *Nursing Management* 24(3):69–71, 1993.

Cato, C., Olson, K., and Studer, M. Incidence, Prevalence and Variables Associated with Low Back Pain in Staff Nurses. *AAOHN (American Association of Occupational Health Nursing) Journal* 321–327, 1989.

CBO (Congressional Budget Office). *The Effects of Managed Care and Managed Competition.* A CBO Memorandum. Washington, D.C.: CBO, February 1995.

CDC (Centers for Disease Control). Universal Precautions for Prevention of Human Immunodeficiency Virus, Hepatitis B Virus, and Other Blood-Borne Pathogens in Health-Care Settings. *MMWR (Morbidity and Mortality Weekly Report)* 37:377–382, 1988.

CDC (Centers for Disease Control and Prevention). *HIV/AIDS Surveillance Report* 6(2):21, 1994.

Chapin, R., and Silloway, G. Incentive Payments to Nursing Homes Based on Quality-of-Care Outcomes. *Journal of Applied Gerontology* 11(2):131–145, 1992.

Cherry, R.L. Agents of Nursing Home Quality of Care: Ombudsmen and Staff Ratios Revisited. *The Gerontologist* 31:302–308, 1991.

Clifford, J.C. The Future of Nursing Practice. Pp. 617–623 in: N. Chaska, ed. *The Nursing Profession—Turning Points.* St. Louis, Mo.: Mosby, 1990.

Cohen, J.W., and Dubay, L.C. The Effects of Medicaid Reimbursement Method and Ownership on Nursing Home Costs, Case Mix, and Staffing. *Inquiry* 27:183–200, 1990.

Cohen, J.W., and Spector, W.D. The Effect of Medicaid on Quality of Care in Nursing Homes. *Journal of Health Economics*, in press.

Cohodes, D.R. What to Do About Capital? *Hospital & Health Services Administration* 27(5):67–89, 1982.

Constable, J.F., and Russell, D.W. The Effect of Social Support and the Work Environment upon Burnout Among Nurses. *Journal of Human Stress* 12:21–26, 1986.

Consumer Reports. Nursing Homes: When a Loved One Needs Care. August:518–528, 1995.

Coons, D. Training Direct Service Staff Members to Work in Dementia Care Units. Pp. 126–143 in: D. Coons, ed. *Specialized Dementia Care Units.* Baltimore, Md.: The Johns Hopkins University Press, 1991.

Cotton, P. Nursing Home Research Focus on Outcomes May Mean Playing Catch-up with Regulation. *Journal of the American Medical Association* 269:2337–2338, 1993.

Courington, K.R., Patterson, S.L., and Howard, R.J. Universal Precautions Are not Universally Followed. *Archives of Surgery* 126:93–96, 1991.

Cronin-Stubbs, D., and Rooks, C. The Stress, Social Support, and Burnout of Critical Care Nurses: The Results of Research. *Heart and Lung: The Journal of Critical Care* 14:31–39, 1985.

Crown, W.H., Ahlburg, D.A., and MacAdam, M. The Demographic and Employment Characteristics of Home Care Aides: A Comparison with Nursing Home Aides, Hospital Aides, and Other Workers. *The Gerontologist* 35:162–170, 1995.

Damato, E.G., Dill, P.Z., Gennaro, S., et al. The Association Between CNS Direct Care Time and Total Time and Very Low Birth Weight Infant Outcomes. *Clinical Nurse Specialist* 7(2):75–79, 1993.

Davis, K., Collins, K.S., Schoen, C., and C. Morris. Choice Matters: Enrollees' Views of Their Health Plans. *Health Affairs* 14(2):99–112, 1995.

Davis, M.A. On Nursing Home Quality: A Review and Analysis. *Medical Care Review* 48(2)129–166, 1991.

Doan-Johnson, S. Taking a Closer Look at Needle Sticks. *Nursing92* 22(8):24,27, 1992.

Doering, L. Recruitment and Retention: Successful Strategies in Critical Care. *Heart and Lung: The Journal of Critical Care* 19(3):220–224, 1990.

Dolan, N. The Relationship Between Burnout and Job Satisfaction in Nurses. *Journal of Advanced Nursing* 12(1):3–12, 1987.

Dolan, S.L., Van-Ameringen, M.R., Corbin, S., and Arsenault, A. Lack of Professional Latitude and Role Problems as Correlates of Propensity to Quit Amongst Nursing Staff. *Journal of Advanced Nursing* 17(12):1455–1459, 1992.

Donabedian, A. Evaluating the Quality of Medical Care. *Milbank Memorial Fund Quarterly* 44:166–203, July (part 2), 1966.

Draper, D., Kahn, K.L, Reinisch, E.J., et al. Studying the Effects of the DRG-Based Prospective Payment System on Quality of Care: Design, Sampling, and Fieldwork. *Journal of the American Medical Association* 264:1956–1961, 1990.

DuNah, R., Harrington, C., Bedney, B., and Carillo, H. Variations and Trends in Licensed Nursing Home Capacity in the States, 1978–1993. Paper prepared for the Health Care Financing Administration. San Francisco: University of California, 1995.

Duquette, A., Kerouac, S., Sandhu, B.K., and Beaudet, L. Factors Related to Nursing Burnout: A Review of Empirical Knowledge. *Issues in Mental Health Nursing* 15:337–358, 1994.

Eisler, P. *A Special Investigative Report: Criminal Care.* Arlington, Va.: Gannett News Service, 1994.

Ellwood, M.R., and Burwell, B. Access to Medicaid and Medicare by the Low-Income Disabled. *Health Care Financing Review* Annl. Suppl.:133–148, 1990.

Emergency Nurses Association. *Prevalence of Violence in Emergency Departments.* Park Ridge, Ill.: Emergency Nurses Association, 1994.

Erickson, J. Quality and the Nursing Assistant. *Provider: The Magazine for Long Term Care Professionals* 13(4):4–6, 1987.

Ettner, S.L. Do Elderly Medicaid Patients Experience Reduced Access to Nursing Home Care? *Journal of Health Economics* 11:259–280, 1993.

Evans, D.A., Scherr, P.A., and Cook, N.R. Estimated Prevalence of Alzheimer's Disease in the United States. *The Milbank Quarterly* 68(2):267–289, 1990.

Evans, L.K., and Strumpf, N.E. Tying Down the Elderly. *Journal of the American Geriatrics Society* 37:65–74, 1989.

Evans, L.K., and Strumpf, N.E. Reducing Restraints in Nursing Homes: A Clinical Trial. Paper presented at a special invitational session on Quality and Staffing in Nursing Homes sponsored by the National Institute for Nursing Research on behalf of the IOM study, and held in conjunction with the 1994 annual meeting of the Gerontology Society of America in Atlanta, November 1994.

Everitt, D.E., Fields, D.R., Soumerai, S.S., and Avorn, J. Resident Behavior and Staff Distress in the Nursing Home. *Journal of the American Geriatrics Society* 39:792–798, 1991.

Fagin, C.M., Marek, K.D., Krejci, J.W., and Amor, G.E. The Nursing Home Reform Act: Progress and Outcomes. Final Report. Grant identification no. 19584. Philadelphia: University of Pennsylvania School of Nursing, 1995.

Feder, J., and Scanlon, W. Case-Mix Payment for Nursing Home Care: Lessons from Maryland. *Journal of Health Politics, Policy and Law* 14(3):523–547, 1989.

Feldstein, A., Valanis, B., Vollmer, W., et al. The Back Injury Prevention Project Pilot Study: Assessing the Effectiveness of "Back Attack," an Injury Prevention Program Among Nurses, Aides, and Orderlies. *Journal of Occupational Medicine* 35(2):114–120, 1993.

Fielding, J., and Weaver, S.M. A Comparison of Hospital- And Community-Based Mental Health Nurses: Perceptions of their Work Environment and Psychological Health. *Journal of Advanced Nursing* 19(6):1196–1204, 1994.

Folkemer, D. *State Use of Home and Community-Based Services for the Aged Under Medicaid: Waiver Programs, Personal Care, Frail Elderly Services and Home Health Services.* Washington, D.C.: Intergovernmental Health Policy Project, 1994.

Foner, N. Nursing Home Aides: Saints or Monsters? *The Gerontologist* 34:245–250, 1994.

Fottler, M.D., Smith, H.L., and James, W.L. Profits and Patient Care Quality in Nursing Homes: Are they Compatible? *The Gerontologist* 21:532–538, 1981.

Foxall, M.J., Zimmerman, L., Standley, R., and Bene, B. A Comparison of Frequency and Sources of Nursing Job Stress Perceived by Intensive Care, Hospice and Medical-Surgical Nurses. *Journal of Advanced Nursing* 15(5):577–584, 1990.

Friedman, B. Economic Aspects of the Rationing of Nursing Home Beds. *Journal of Human Resources* 17:59–71, 1982.

Fries, B.E., and Cooney, L. Resources Utilization Groups: A Patient Classification System for Long-term Care. *Health Care Financing Review* 23(2):110–122, 1985.

Fries, B.E., Schneider, D., Foley, W., and Dowling, M. Case-Mix Classification of Medicare Residents in Skilled Nursing Facilities. *Medical Care* 9:843–858, 1989.

Fries, B.E., Schneider, D., Foley, W., et al. Refining a Case-mix Measure for Nursing Homes: Resources Utilization Groups (RUGS-III). *Medical Care* 32:668–685, 1994.

Ganroth, L. Long-term Care Resource Requirements Before and After the Prospective Payment System. *Image: Journal of Nursing Scholarship* 20(1):7–11, 1988.

GAO (General Accounting Office). *Medicaid: Methods for Setting Nursing Home Rates Should Be Improved.* Report to the Secretary of HHS. Pub. no. HRD-86-26. Washington, D.C.: U.S. GAO, 1986.

GAO. *Medicare and Medicaid: Stronger Enforcement of Nursing Home Requirements Needed.* Report to the Ranking Minority Member, Special Committee on Aging, U.S. Senate. Pub. no. HRD-87-113. Washington, D.C.: U.S. GAO, July 1987.

GAO. *Long-term Care for the Elderly: Issues of Need, Access, and Cost.* Report to the Chairman, Subcommittee on Health and Long-term Care, Select Committee on Aging, U.S. House of Representatives. Pub. no. HRD-89-4. Washington, D.C.: U.S. GAO, November 1988a.

GAO. *Medicare: Improved Patient Outcome Analyses Could Enhance Quality Assessment.* Report to the Ranking Minority Member, Special Committee on Aging, U.S. Senate. Pub. no. PEMD-88-23. Washington, D.C.: U.S. GAO, June 1988b.

Garg, A., Owen, B.D., and Carlson, B. An Ergonomic Evaluation of Nursing Assistants' Job in a Nursing Home. *Ergonomics* 35(9):979–995, 1992.

Garrett, B., Singiser, D., and Banks, S.M. Back Injuries Among Nursing Personnel: The Relationship of Personal Characteristics, Risk Factors, and Nursing Practices. *AAOHN (American Association of Occupational Health Nursing) Journal* 40(11):510–516, 1992.

Geberding, J.L., Bryant-LeBlanc, C.E., Nelson, K., et al. Risk of Transmitting the Human Immunodeficiency Virus, Cytomegalovirus, and Hepatitis B Virus to Health-Care Workers Exposed to Patients with AIDS and AIDS-related Conditions. *Journal of Infectious Diseases* 156:1–8, 1987.

Geron, S.M. Regulating the Behavior of Nursing Homes Through Positive Incentives: An Analysis of Illinois' Quality Incentive Program (QUIP). *The Gerontologist* 31:292–301, 1991.

Gertler, P.J. Subsidies, Quality, and The Regulation of Nursing Homes. *Journal of Public Economics* 38:33–52, 1989.

GHAA (Group Health Association of America). *Patterns in HMO Enrollment.* Washington, D.C.: GHAA, 1995.

Girard, N. The Case Management Model of Patient Care Delivery. *AORN (Association of Operating Room Nurses) Journal* 60(3):403–405, 408–412, 415, 1994.

Goetz, R.R., Bloom, J.D., Chenell, S.L., and Moorhead, J.C. Weapons Possession by Patients in a University Emergency Department. *Annals of Emergency Medicine* 20(1):8–10, 1991.

Gold, D.R., Rogacz, S., Bock, N., et al. Rotating Shift Work, Sleep, and Accidents Related to Sleepiness in Hospital Nurses. *American Journal of Public Health* 82(7):1011–1013, 1992.

Gold, M.F. Bridging the Salary Gap in Long Term Care. *Provider: The Magazine for Long Term Care Professionals* 21(4)42–46, 48, 1995.

Goldin, G.J. The Influence of Self-Image upon the Performance of Nursing Home Staff. *Nursing Homes* 34:33–38, 1985.

Goodman, R.A., Jenkins, E.L., and Mercy, J.A. Workplace-Related Homicide Among Health Care Workers in the United States, 1980 through 1990. *Journal of the American Medical Association* 272:1686–1688, 1994.

Graber, D.R., and Sloane, P.D. Nursing Home Survey Deficiencies for Physical Restraint Use. *Medical Care* 33:1051–1063, 1995.

Grady, G.F., Lee, V.A., Prince, A.M., et al. Hepatitis B Immune Globulin for Accidental Exposures Among Medical Personnel. Final Report of a Multicenter Controlled Trial. *Journal of Infectious Diseases* 138:625–638, 1978.

Greene, V.L., and Monahan, D.J. Structure and Operational Factors Affecting Quality of Patient Care in Nursing Homes. *Public Policy* 29:399–415, 1981.

Greenfield, S., Nelson, E.C., Zubkoff, M., et al. Variations in Resource Utilization Among Medical Specialties and Systems of Care: Results from the Medical Outcomes Study. *Journal of the American Medical Association* 267:1624–1630, 1992.

Greenwood, J.G. Back Injuries Can be Reduced with Worker Training, Reinforcement. *Occupational Health and Safety* 55(5):26–29, 1986.

Griffin, K.M., Leftwich, R.A., and Smith, M.S. Current Forces Shaping Long-term Care in the 1990s. *The Journal of Long Term Care Administration* 17(3):8–11, 1989.

Gurny, P., Hirsch, M.B., and Gondek, K.E. Chapter 11: A Description of Medicaid-Covered Services. *Health Care Financing Review* Annl. Suppl.:227–234, 1992.

Gustafson, D.H., Sainfor, F.C., Van Konigsveld, R., and Zimmerman, D.R. The Quality Assessment Index (QAI) for Measuring Nursing Home Quality. *HSR (Health Services Research)* 25:97–127, 1990.

Guterman, S., Eggers, P., Riley, G., et al. The First 3 Years of Medicare Prospective Payment: An Overview. *Health Care Financing Review* 9(3):67–77, 1988.

Harber, P., Billet, E., Gutowski, M., et al. Occupational Low Back Pain in Hospital Nurses. *Journal of Occupational Medicine* 27(7):518–524, 1985.

Hare, J., and Pratt, C. Burnout: Differences Between Professional and Paraprofessional Nursing Staff in Acute and Long-term Care Health Facilities. *Journal of Applied Gerontology* 7(1):60–71, 1988.

Harrington, C., and Estes, C.L. Trends in Nursing Homes in the Post Medicare Prospective Payment Period. San Francisco: Institute for Health and Aging, 1989.

Harrington, C., Preston S., Grant, L.A., and Swan, J.H. Revised Trends in States' Nursing Home Capacity. *Health Affairs* 11(2):170–180, 1992a.

Harrington, C., Tompkins, C., Curtis, M., and Grant, L. Psychotropic Drug Use in Long Term Care Facilities: A Review of the Literature. *The Gerontologist* 32:822–833, 1992b.

Harrington, C., Curtis, M., and DuNah, R., Jr. Trends in State Regulation of the Supply of Long Term Care Services. Paper prepared for the U.S. Department of Housing and Urban Development and the Health Care Financing Administration. San Francisco: University of California, 1994a.

Harrington, C., DuNah, R., Jr., and Bedney, B. The Supply of Community-Based Long Term Care Services in 1992. Paper prepared for the Department of Housing and Urban Development and the Health Care Financing Administration. San Francisco: University of California, 1994b.

Harrington, C., DuNah, R., Jr., and Curtis, M. State Variations and Trends in Preadmission Screening. Paper prepared for the U.S. Department of Housing and Urban Development and the Health Care Financing Administration. San Francisco: University of California, 1994c.

Harrington, C., Thollaug, S.C., and Summers, P.R. Nursing Facilities, Staffing, Residents and Facility Deficiencies, 1991–93. Paper prepared for the Health Care Financing Administration. San Francisco: University of California, 1995.

Harrington et al. 1993 State Data Book on Long-term Care Programs and Market Characteristics. Baltimore, Md.: Health Care Financing Administration, in press.

Hartz, A., Krakauer, H., Kuhn, E., et al. Hospital Characteristics and Mortality Rates. New England Journal of Medicine 321:1720–1725, 1989.

Hawes, C., and Phillips, C.D. The Changing Structure of the Nursing Home Industry and the Impact of Ownership on Quality, Cost, and Access. Pp. 492–538 in: Institute of Medicine. For-Profit Enterprise in Health Care. B.H. Gray, ed. Washington, D.C.: National Academy Press, 1986.

Hawkins, A.M., Burgio, L.D., Langford, A., and Engel, B.T. The Effects of Verbal and Written Supervisory Feedback on Staff Compliance with Assigned Prompted Voiding in a Nursing Home. Journal of Organizational Behavior Management 13:137–150, 1992.

Hawley, M.P. Sources of Stress for Emergency Nurses in Four Urban Canadian Emergency Departments. Journal of Emergency Nursing 18(3):211–216, 1992.

Hay, D.G. Health Care Services in 100 Superior Nursing Homes. Long-term Care and Health Services Administration Quarterly 1: 300–313, 1977.

HCFA (Health Care Financing Administration). State Medicaid Manual. Part 2, State Organization and General Administration. Transmittal no. 79. Pub. no. 45-2. Washington, D.C.: HCFA, U.S. Department of Health and Human Services, 1992a.

HCFA. Medicaid spDATA System. Characteristics of Medicaid State Programs. Volume 1. National Comparisons. Pub. no. 02178. Washington, D.C.: Medicaid Bureau, HCFA, U.S. Department of Health and Human Services, 1992b.

HCFA. Medicare and Medicaid Programs: Survey, Certification, and Enforcement of Skilled Nursing Facilities and Nursing Facilities. Final Rule. 42 CFR Part 401. Federal Register 59(217): 56116–56252, 1994a.

HCFA. Report to Congress on Nursing Facility Staffing Requirements. Washington, D.C.: Medicaid Bureau, HCFA, U.S. Department of Health and Human Services, 1994b.

HCIA and Arthur Andersen. The Guide to the Nursing Home Industry. Baltimore, Md.: HCIA, Inc., and Arthur Andersen and Company, 1994.

Hegyvary, S.T. Issues in Outcomes Research. Journal of Nursing Quality Assurance 5(2):1–6, 1991.

Heine, C.A. Burnout Among Nursing Home Personnel. Journal of Gerontological Nursing 12(3): 14–18, 1986.

Henderson, D.K., Fahey, B.J., Willy, M., et al. Risk for Occupational Transmission of Human Immunodeficiency Virus Type 1 (HIV-1) Associated with Clinical Exposures: A Prospective Evaluation. Annals of Internal Medicine 113(10):740–746, 1990.

Hing, E. Effects of the Prospective Payment System on Nursing Homes. PHS-89-1759. Hyattsville, Md.: National Center for Health Statistics, 1989.

Hiscott, R.D., and Connop, P.J. The Health and Well-Being of Mental Health Professionals. Canadian Journal of Public Health 81(6):422–426, 1990.

Holahan, J. *Nursing Home Care Under Alternative Patient-Related Reimbursement Systems.* Washington, D.C.: The Urban Institute, 1984.

Holahan, J., and Cohen, J. Nursing Home Reimbursement: Implications for Cost Containment, Access, and Quality. *Milbank Quarterly* 65(1):112–147, 1987.

Holahan, J., and Sulvetta, M.B. Assessing Medicare Reimbursement Options for Skilled Nursing Facility Care. *Health Care Financing Review* 10(3):13–27, 1989.

Holahan, J., Rowland, D., Feder, J., and Heslam, D. Explaining the Recent Growth in Medicaid Spending. *Health Affairs* 12(3):177–193, 1993.

Hospital and Healthcare Compensation Service. *The 1994–1995 Home Care Salary and Benefits Report.* Oakland, N.J.: Hospital and Healthcare Compensation Service, 1994.

HRSA (Health Resources and Services Administration, Public Health Service). *Health Personnel in the United States: Eighth Report to Congress.* Washington, D.C.: Bureau of Health Professions, HRSA, Public Health Service, U.S. Department of Health and Human Services, 1992.

HRSA. *Trends in Hospital Personnel: 1983–1990.* Pub. no. HRSA-P-OD-93-1. Washington, D.C.: HRSA, Public Health Service, U.S. Department of Health and Human Services, September, 1993.

HRSA. 1991 National Employment Estimates of Selected Health Care Personnel in Home Health Care Agencies, Hospices, Nursing Homes, and Board and Care (Residential) Homes. Data from the 1991 National Health Provider Inventory. Unpublished report. Washington, D.C.: Division of Nursing, Bureau of Health Professions, HRSA, Public Health Service, U.S. Department of Health and Human Services, 1994.

Hu, T., Huang, L., and Cartwright, W.S. Differences Among Black, Hispanic, and White People in Knowledge about Long Term Care Services. *Health Care Financing Review* 2:51–67, 1986.

Husted, G.L., Miller, M.C., and Wilczynski, E.M. Retention Is the Goal: Extinguish Burnout with Self-Esteem Enhancement. *Journal of Continuing Education in Nursing* 20(6):244–248, 1989.

ICONS (Interagency Conference on Nursing Statistics). *Research on Nursing Resources: Definitions and Calculations.* Photocopied document, June, 1993.

Iezzoni, L.I., Foley, S.M., Heeren, T., et al. A Method for Screening the Quality of Hospital Care Using Administrative Data: Preliminary Validation Results. *QRB (Quality Review Bulletin)* 18:361–371, 1992.

Iezzoni, L.I., Daley, J., Heeren, T., et al. Using Administrative Data to Screen Hospitals for High Complication Rates. *Inquiry* 31:40–55, 1994.

Immigration Nursing Relief Advisory Committee. *Report to the Secretary of Labor on the Immigration Nursing Relief Act of 1989.* Washington, D.C.: Office of the Assistant Secretary for Policy, Department of Labor, 1995.

IOM (Institute of Medicine). *For-Profit Enterprise in Health Care.* B.H. Gray, ed. Washington, D.C.: National Academy Press, 1986a.

IOM. *Improving the Quality of Care in Nursing Homes.* Washington, D.C.: National Academy Press, 1986b.

IOM. *Allied Health Services: Avoiding Crises.* Washington, D.C.: National Academy Press, 1989.

IOM. *Medicare: A Strategy for Quality Assurance,* volumes I and II. K.N. Lohr, ed. Washington, D.C.: National Academy Press, 1990.

IOM. *Real People, Real Problems: An Evaluation of the Long-term Care Ombudsman Programs of the Older Americans Act.* J. Harris-Wehling, J.C. Feasley, and C.L. Estes, eds. Washington, D.C.: National Academy Press, 1995.

IOM. *Best at Home: Assuring Quality of Long-term Care in Home- and Community-based Settings.* J.C. Feasley, ed. Washington, D.C.: National Academy Press, 1996.

Jagger, J. Preventing HIV Transmission in Health Care Workers with Safer Needle Devices. In Proceedings and Abstracts of the Sixth International Conference on AIDS, San Francisco, June 20–24, 1990, p. 99. University of California at San Francisco, 1990.

JCAHO. *1995 Comprehensive Accreditation Manual for Hospitals: Standards, Scoring Guidelines, Aggregation Rules, Decision Rules.* Oakbrook Terrace, Ill.: JCAHO, 1994.

Jensen, R.C. Back Injuries Among Nursing Personnel: Research Needs and Justifications. *Research in Nursing and Health* 10:29–38, 1987.

Johnson, C. Coping with Compassion Fatigue. *Nursing* 22(4):116–119, 1992.

Johnson-Pawlson, J. The Relationship Between Nursing Staff Variables and Quality of Care in Nursing Homes. UMI Dissertation Services. O.N. 9316112, 1993.

Johnson-Pawlson, J. Study of Surveyor Performance. Final Report Prepared for the American Health Care Association, December, 1994.

Jorgensen, S., Hein, H.O., and Gyntelberg, F. Heavy Lifting at Work and Risk of Genital Prolapse and Herniated Lumbar Disc in Assistant Nurses. *Occupational Medicine* 44(1):47–49, 1994.

Justice, D. State Long Term Care Reform: Development of Community Care Systems in Six States. Washington, D.C.: National Governors' Association, April, 1988.

Kahn, K.L., Keeler, E.B., Sherwood, M.J., et al. Comparing Outcomes of Care Before and After Implementation of the DRG-Based Prospective Payment System. *Journal of the American Medical Association* 264:1984–1988, 1990a.

Kahn, K.L., Rogers, W.H., Rubenstein, L.V., et al. Measuring Quality of Care with Explicit Process Criteria Before and After Implementation of the DRG-Based Prospective Payment System. *Journal of the American Medical Association* 264:1969–1973, 1990b.

Kahn, K.L., Rubenstein, L.V., Draper, D., et al. The Effects of the DRG-Based Prospective Payment System on Quality of Care for Hospitalized Medicare Patients. An Introduction to the Series. *Journal of the American Medical Association* 264:1953–1955, 1990c.

Kanda, K., and Mezey, M. Registered Nurse Staffing in Pennsylvania Nursing Homes: Comparison Before and After Implementation of Medicare's Prospective Payment System. *The Gerontologist* 31:318–324, 1991.

Kandolin, I. Burnout of Female and Male Nurses in Shiftwork. *Ergonomics* 36(1–3):141–147, 1993.

Kane, R.A. Assessing Quality in Nursing Homes. *Clinics in Geriatric Medicine* 4:655–666, 1988.

Kane, R.A. Expanding the Home Care Concept: Blurring Distinctions Among Home Care, Institutional Care, and Other Long-Term-Care Services. *Milbank Quarterly* 73(2):161–186, 1995.

Kane, R.L. Improving the Quality of Long-term Care. *Journal of the American Medical Association* 273:1376–1380, 1995.

Kane, R.A., and Kane, R.L. Long-term Care: Variations on a Quality Assurance Theme. *Inquiry* 25:132–146, 1988.

Kane, R.A., Kane R.L., Arnold, S., et al. Geriatric Nurse Practitioners as Nursing Home Employees: Implementing the Role. *The Gerontologist* 28:469–477, 1988.

Kane, R.L., Jorgenson, L.A., Teteberg, B., and Kuwahara, J. Is Good Nursing Home Care Feasible? *Journal of the American Medical Association* 235:516–519, 1976.

Kane, R.L., Bell, R., Riegler, S., et al. Assessing the Outcomes of Nursing Home Patients. *Journal of Gerontology* 38(4):385–393, 1983.

Kayser-Jones, J. The Use of Nasogastric Feeding Tubes in Nursing Homes: Patient, Family and Health Care Provider Perspectives. *The Gerontologist* 30:469–479, 1990.

Kayser-Jones, J.S., Wiener, C.L., and Barbaccia, J.C. Factors Contributing to the Hospitalization of Nursing Home Residents. *The Gerontologist* 29:502–510, 1989.

Keeler, E.B., Kahn, K.L., Draper, D., et al. Changes in Sickness at Admission Following the Introduction of the Prospective Payment System. *Journal of the American Medical Association* 264:1962–1968, 1990.

Keeler, E.B., Rubenstein, L.V., Kahn, K.L., et al. Hospital Characteristics and Quality of Care. *Journal of the American Medical Association* 268:1709–1714, 1992.

Kemper, P., and Murtaugh, C.M. Lifetime Use of Nursing Home Care. *New England Journal of Medicine* 324:595–600, 1991.

Kennedy, L., Neidlinger, S., and Scroggins, K. Effective Comprehensive Discharge Planning for Hospitalized Elderly. *The Gerontologist* 27(5):577–580, 1987.

Kichen, S. Annual Report on American Industry. *Forbes* 155(1):122–125, January 2, 1995.

Knaus, W.A., Draper, E.A., Wagner, D.P., and Zimmerman, J.E. An Evaluation of Outcome from Intensive Care in Major Medical Centers. *Annals of Internal Medicine* 104(3):410–418, 1986.

Koerner, J. Differentiated Practice: The Evolution of Professional Nursing. *Journal of Professional Nursing* 8:335–341, 1992.

Koetting, M. *Nursing Home Organization and Efficiency.* Lexington, Mass.: Lexington Books, 1980.

Kosciesza, I. What's Ahead in the Post-Health Planning Era? *Health Policy Week Special Report* (June 1):1–5, 1987.

Kosecoff, J., Kahn, K.L., Rogers, W.H., et al. Prospective Payment System and Impairment at Discharge: The Quicker-and-Sicker Story Revisited. *Journal of the American Medical Association* 264:1980–1983, 1990.

Kramer, M., and Schmalenberg, C. Magnet Hospitals: Part I: Institutions of Excellence. *Journal of Nursing Administration* 18(1):13–24, 1988a.

Kramer, M., and Schmalenberg, C. Magnet Hospitals: Part II: Institutions of Excellence. *Journal of Nursing Administration* 18(2):11–19, 1988b.

Krapohl, G., and Larson, E. Utilization of Unlicensed Assistive Personnel in Nursing Care Delivery: Examination, Evaluation and Recommendations for the Future. Submitted for publication, 1995.

Kravitz, R.L., Greenfield, S., Rogers, W., et al. Differences in the Mix of Patients Among Medical Specialties and Systems of Care: Results from the Medical Outcomes Study. *Journal of the American Medical Association* 267:1617–1623, 1992.

Kruzich, J.M., Clinton, J.F., and Kelber, S.T. Personal and Environmental Influences on Nursing Home Satisfaction. *The Gerontologist* 32:342–350, 1992.

Lachs, M.S., and Pillemer, K. Abuse and Neglect of Elderly Persons. *New England Journal of Medicine* 332:437–443, 1995.

Lanza, M.L. The Reactions of Nursing Staff to Physical Assault by a Patient. *Hospital and Community Psychiatry* 34(1):44–47, 1983.

Larese, F., and Fiorito, A. Musculoskeletal Disorders in Hospital Nurses: A Comparison Between Two Hospitals. *Ergonomics* 37(7):1205–1211, 1994.

LaRocco, J.M., House, J.S., and French, J.R.P., Jr. Social Support, Occupational Stress, and Health. *Journal of Health and Social Behavior* 21:202–218, 1980.

Larson, P.F., Osterweis, M., and Rubin, E.R., eds. *Health Workforce Issues for the 21st Century.* Washington, D.C.: Association of Academic Health Centers, 1994.

Lathrop, J.P. The Patient-focused Hospital. *Healthcare Forum Journal* 35(3):76–78, 1992.

Latta, V.B., and Keene, R.E. Use and Cost of Skilled Nursing Facility Services Under Medicare, 1987. *Health Care Financing Review* 11(1):105–116, 1989.

Lavoie, F., Carter, G.L., Danzl, D.F., and Berg, R.L. Emergency Department Violence in United States Teaching Hospitals. *Annals of Emergency Medicine* 17(11):1227–1233, 1988.

Letsch, S.W., Lazenby, H.C., Levit, L.R., and Cowan, C.A. National Health Expenditures, 1991. *Health Care Financing Review* 14(2):1–30, 1992.

Levit, K.R., Sensenig, A.L., Cowan, C.A., et al. National Health Expenditures, 1993. *Health Care Financing Review* 16(1):247–294, 1994.

Lewin/ICF. *Synthesis of Medicaid Reimbursement Options for Nursing Home Care.* Submitted to the Health Care Financing Administration. Washington, D.C.: Lewin/ICF, 1991.

Lewin-VHI. Nursing Care Report Card for Acute Care. Report prepared for the American Nurses Association. Washington, D.C.: American Nurses Publishing, 1995.

Lewis, M., Kane, R., Cretin, S., and Clark, V. The Immediate and Subsequent Outcomes of Nursing Home Care. *American Journal of Public Health* 75(7):758–762, 1985.

Libow, L.S., and Starer, P. Care of the Nursing Home Patient. *New England Journal of Medicine* 321:93–96, 1989.

Linn, M.W., Gurel, L., and Linn, B.S. Patient Outcome as a Measure of Quality of Nursing Home Care. *American Journal of Public Health* 67:337–344, 1977.

Lipscomb, J.A., and Love, C.C. Violence Toward Health Care Workers: An Emerging Occupational Hazard. *AAOHN (American Association of Occupational Health Nursing) Journal* 40(5):219–227, 1992.

Lipson, L., and Laudicina, S. *State Home and Community-Based Services for the Aged Under Medicaid: Waiver Programs, Optional Services Under the Medicaid State Plan, and OBRA 1990 Provisions for a New Optional Benefit.* Washington, D.C.: American Association of Retired Persons, 1991.

Lucas, M.D., Atwood, J.R., and Hagaman, R. Replication and Validation of Anticipated Turnover Model for Urban Registered Nurses. *Nursing Research* 42(1):29–35, 1993.

Lurie, N., Moscovice, I.S., Finch, M., et al. Does Capitation Affect the Health of the Chronically Mentally Ill? *Journal of the American Medical Association* 267:3300–3304, 1992.

Lusk, S.L. Violence Experienced by Nurses' Aides in Nursing Homes: An Exploratory Study. *AAOHN (American Association of Occupational Health Nursing) Journal* 40(5):237–242, 1992.

Lutz, S. Let's Make a Deal: Healthcare Mergers, Acquisitions Take Place at Dizzying Pace. *Modern Healthcare* 24(51):47–52, 1994.

Lyles, Y. Impact of Medicare DRGs on Nursing Homes in the Portland Oregon Metropolitan Area. *Journal of the American Geriatrics Society* 34(8):573–578, 1986.

Lyman, K.A. *Work-Related Stress for Staff in an Alzheimer's Day Care Center: The Effects of Physical Environments.* Paper presented at the 40th annual meeting of The Gerontological Society of America, Washington, D.C., 1987.

Maas, M., Buckwalter, K., Kelley, L., and Stolley, J. Family Members' Perceptions: How They View Care of Alzheimer's Patients in a Nursing Home. *Journal of Long Term Care Administration* 19(1):21–25, 1991.

Maas, M., Buckwalter, K., Swanson, E., et al. The Caring Partnership: Staff and Families of Persons Institutionalized with Alzheimer's Disease. *Journal of Alzheimer's Disease and Related Disorders* 9(6):21–30, 1994.

MacNeil, J.M., and Weisz, G.M. Critical Care Nursing Stress: Another Look. *Heart and Lung: The Journal of Critical Care* 16(3):274–277, 1987.

Manthey, M. Primary Practice Partners: A Nurse Extender System. *Nursing Management* 19(3):58–59, 1988.

Manthey, M. Practice Partners: Humanizing Healthcare. *Nursing Management* 23(5):18–19, 1992.

Manton, K.G., Corder, L.S., and Stallard, E. Estimates of Change in Chronic Disability and Institutional Incidence and Prevalence Rates in the U.S. Elderly Population from the 1982, 1984, and 1989 National Long Term Care Survey. *Journal of Gerontology* 48(4):S153–S165, 1993.

Maraldo, P.J. Quality in Long-term Care. Pp. 1–11 in: *Mechanisms of Quality in Long-term Care: Service and Clinical Outcomes.* Pub. no. 41–2382. New York: National League for Nursing Press, 1991.

Marchette, L., and Marchette, B. Back Injury: A Preventable Occupational Hazard. *Orthopaedic Nursing* 4(6):25–29, 1985.

Marcus, R. CDC Cooperative Needlestick Study Group: Surveillance of Health-care Workers Exposed to Blood from Patients Infected with the Human Immunodeficiency Virus. *New England Journal of Medicine* 319:1118–1123, 1988.

Marcus, R.A., Tokars, J.I., Culver, P.S., and McKibben, D.M. Zidovudine Use After Occupational Exposure to HIV-infected Blood. Abstract no. 979. Presented by R.A. Marcus at the 1991 31st Interscience Conference on Antimicrobial Agents and Chemotherapy (ICAAC), Chicago, 1991.

Masterson-Allen, S., Mor, V., and Laliberte, L. Turnover in National Hospice Study Sites: A Reflection of Organizational Growth. *Hospital Journal* 3(2–3):147–164, 1987.

McAbee, R. Nursing and Back Injuries. *AAOHN (American Association of Occupational Health Nursing Journal)* 36:200–209, 1988.

McCorkle, R., Benoliel, J.Q., Donaldson, G., et al. A Randomized Clinical Trial of Home Nursing Care for Lung Cancer Patients. *Cancer* 64:1375–1382, 1989.

McCulloch, L.E., McNeil, D.E., Binder, R.L., and Hatcher, C. Effects of a Weapon Screening Procedure in a Psychiatric Emergency Room. *Hospital and Community Psychiatry* 37:837–838, 1986.

McDonald, C.A. Recruitment, Retention, and Recognition of Frontline Workers in Long Term Care. *Generations* XVIII(3):41–49, 1994.

McEvoy, M., Porter, K., Mortimer, P., et al. Prospective Study of Clinical, Laboratory, and Ancillary Staff with Accidental Exposures to Blood or Body Fluids from Patients Infected with HIV. *British Medical Journal* 294:1595–1598, 1987.

Meddaugh, D.I. Staff Abuse by the Nursing Home Patient. *The Clinical Gerontologist* 6:45–47, 1987.

Meiners, M., Thornburn, P., Roddy, P., and Jones, B. *Nursing Home Admissions: The Results of an Incentive Reimbursement Experiment.* Long Term Care Studies Program Research Report. PHS 86–3397. Rockville, Md.: National Center for Health Services Research and Health Care Technology Assessment, 1985.

Mendelson, D.N., and Arnold, J. Certificate of Need Revisited. *Spectrum* (Winter):36–44, 1993.

Mezey, M.D. Institutional Care: Caregivers and Quality. Pp. 155–166 in: *Indices of Quality in Long Term Care: Research and Practice.* Pub. no. 20–2292. New York: National League for Nursing Press, 1989.

Mezey, M.D. Presentation at a special invitational session on Quality and Staffing in Nursing Homes sponsored by the National Institute for Nursing Research on behalf of the IOM study, and held in conjunction with the 1994 annual meeting of the Gerontology Society of America in Atlanta, November 1994.

Mezey, M.D., and Lynaugh, J.E. The Teaching Nursing Home Program: Outcomes of Care. *Nursing Clinics of North America* 24(3):769–780, 1989.

Mezey, M.D., and Lynaugh, J.E. Teaching Nursing Home Program: A Lesson in Quality. *Geriatric Nursing* (March/April):76–77, 1991.

Mezey, M.D., and Scanlon, W. *Registered Nurses in Nursing Homes: Secretary's Commission of Nursing.* Washington, D.C.: U.S. Department of Health and Human Services, 1988.

Miller, N.A. Medicaid 2176 Home and Community-Based Care Waivers: The First Ten Years. *Health Affairs* 11(4):162–171, 1992.

Miller, R.H., and Luft, H.S. Managed Care Plan Performance since 1980: A Literature Analysis. *Journal of the American Medical Association* 271:1512–1519, 1994.

Mitchell, P.H., Armstrong, S., Simpson, T.F., and Lentz, M. American Association of Critical-Care Nurses Demonstration Project: Profile of Excellence in Critical Care Nursing. *Heart and Lung: The Journal of Critical Care* 18:219–237, 1989.

Mobily, P.R., Maas, M.L., Buckwalter, K.C., and Kelley, L.S. Taking Care of the Caregivers: Staff Stress and Burnout on a Special Alzheimer's Unit. *Journal of Psychosocial Nursing* 30(9):25–31, 1992.

Mohler, M. Combined Federal and State Nursing Services Staffing Standards. Washington, D.C.: National Committee to Preserve Social Security and Medicare, 1993.

Mor, V. Invest in your frontline worker: Commentary. *The Brown University Long-term Care Quality Letter* 7(1):4–5, 1995.

Moritz, P. Outcomes Research: Examining Clinical Effectiveness. *Communicating Nursing Research* 28 (3):113–137, 1995.

Morris, J.N., Hawes, C., Fries, B.E., et al. Designing the National Resident Assessment Instrument for Nursing Homes. *The Gerontologist* 30:293–307, 1990.

Morrisey, M.A., Sloan, F.A., and Valvona, J. Medicare Prospective Payment and Posthospital Transfers to Subacute Care. *Medical Care* 26:685–698, 1988.

Moses, E.B. *The Registered Nurse Population. Findings from the National Sample Survey of Registered Nurses, March 1988.* Washington, D.C.: Division of Nursing, Bureau of Health Professions, Health Resources and Services Administration, Public Health Service, U.S. Department of Health and Human Services, 1990.

Moses, E.B. *The Registered Nurse Population. Findings from the National Sample Survey of Registered Nurses, March 1992.* Washington, D.C.: Division of Nursing, Bureau of Health Professions, Health Resources and Services Administration, Public Health Service, U.S. Department of Health and Human Services, 1994.

Munroe, D.J. The Influence of Registered Nursing Staffing on the Quality of Nursing Home Care. *Research in Nursing and Health* 13(4):263–270, 1990.

Murtaugh, C.M., Kemper, P., and Spillman, B.C. The Risk of Nursing Home Use in Later Life. *Medical Care* 28:952–962, 1990.

NAHC (National Association for Home Care). *Basic Statistics About Home Care, 1992.* Washington, D.C.: NAHC, 1993.

Naylor, M.D. Comprehensive Discharge Planning for Hospitalized Elderly: A Pilot Study. *Nursing Research* 39(3):156–161, 1990.

Naylor, M., Brooten, D., Jones, R., et al. Comprehensive Discharge Planning for the Hospitalized Elderly: A Randomized Clinical Trial. *Annals of Internal Medicine* 120:999–1006, 1994.

NCCNHR (National Citizens Coalition for Nursing Home Reform). *Consumer Statement of Principles for the Nursing Home Regulatory System—State Licensure and Federal Certification Programs.* Washington, D.C.: NCCNHR, 1983.

NCHS (National Center for Health Statistics). Nursing Home Characteristics: Preliminary Data From the 1985 National Nursing Home Survey. Prepared by G. Strahan. *Advance Data from Vital and Health Statistics,* no. 131. Hyattsville, Md.: NCHS, U.S. Department of Health and Human Services, 1987.

NCHS. Characteristics of Registered Nurses in Nursing Homes: Preliminary Data from the 1985 National Nursing Home Survey. *Advanced Data from Vital and Health Statistics,* no. 152. Prepared by G. Strahan. Hyattsville, Md.: NCHS, U.S. Department of Health and Human Services, 1988.

NCHS. An Overview of Home Health and Hospice Care Patients: Preliminary Data from the 1993 Home Health and Hospice Care Survey. Prepared by G. Strahan. *Advance Data from Vital and Health Statistics,* no. 256. Hyattsville, Md.: NCHS, U.S. Department of Health and Human Services, 1993a.

NCHS. *Vital Statistics of the United States, 1989.* Vol. II, Mortality, part A. Hyattsville, Md.: NCHS, U.S. Department of Health and Human Services, 1993b.

NCHS. Nursing Homes and Board and Care Homes: Data From the 1991 National Health Provider Inventory. *Advance Data from Vital and Health Statistics,* no. 244. Prepared by A. Sirrocco. Hyattsville, Md.: NCHS, U.S. Department of Health and Human Services, 1994.

Neidlinger, S.H., Scroggins, K., and Kennedy, L.M. Cost Evaluation of Discharge Planning for Hospitalized Elderly. *Nursing Economic$* 5(7):225–230, 1987.

Neu, C.R., and Harrison, S.C. *Posthospital Care Before and After the Medicare Prospective Payment System.* Santa Monica, Calif.: Rand Corporation, 1988.

Neuberger, J.S., Kammerdiener, A.M., and Wood, C. Traumatic Injuries Among Medical Center Employees. *American Association of Occupational Health Nursing Journal* 36(8):318–325, 1988.

NLN (National League for Nursing) Division of Research. *Nursing Datasource 1994: Volume I, Trends in Contemporary Nursing Education.* Pub. no. 19-2642. New York: NLN Press, 1994a.

NLN Division of Research. *Nursing Datasource 1994: Volume III, Focus on Practical/Vocational Nursing.* Pub. no. 19–2644. New York: NLN Press, 1994b.

NLN Division of Research. *Profiles of the Newly Licensed Nurse: Historical Trends and Future Implications,* second ed. Prepared by P. Rosenfeld. Pub. no. 19–2530. New York: NLN Press, 1994c.

NLN Division of Research. *Nursing Datasource 1995: Volume I, Trends in Contemporary Nursing Education.* Pub. no. 19–6649. New York: NLN Press, 1995.

Norton, E.C. Incentive Regulation of Nursing Homes. *Journal of Health Economics* 11:105–128, 1992.

Nyman, J.A. Prospective and "Cost-Plus" Medicaid Reimbursement, Excess Medicaid Demand, and the Quality of Nursing Home Care. *Journal of Health Economics* 4:237–259, 1985.

Nyman, J.A. The Effect of Competition on Nursing Home Expenditures Under Prospective Reimbursement. *HSR (Health Services Research)* 23:555, 1988a.

Nyman, J.A. Improving the Quality of Nursing Home Outcomes: Are Adequacy- or Incentive-Oriented Policies More Effective. *Medical Care* 26(12):1158–1171, 1988b.

Nyman, J.A. Analysis of Nursing Home Use and Bed Supply, Wisconsin, 1983. *HSR (Health Services Research)* 24:511–538, 1989a.

Nyman, J.A. Excess Demand, Consumer Rationality, and the Quality of Care in Regulated Nursing Homes. *HSR (Health Services Research)* 24:105–127, 1989b.

Nyman, J.A., Breaker, D.L., and Link, D. Technical Efficiency in Nursing Home. *Medical Care* 28:541–551, 1990.

OASH (Office of the Assistant Secretary of Health). *Registered Nurse Chart Book.* Washington, D.C.: OASH, U.S. Department of Health and Human Services, 1994.

Oehler, J.M., Davidson, M.G., Starr, L.E., and Lee, D.A. Burnout, Job Stress, Anxiety, and Perceived Social Support in Neonatal Nurses. *Heart and Lung* 20(5):500–505, 1991.

Oermann, M. Professional Nursing Education in the Future: Changes and Challenges. *JOGNN (Journal of Obstetric, Gynecologic, and Neonatal Nursing)* 23:153–159, 1994a.

Oermann, M. Reforming Nursing Education for Future Practice. *Journal of Nursing Education* 33:215–219, 1994b.

OIG (Office of the Inspector General). *State Progress in Carrying Out the Nursing Home Survey Reforms.* OEI–01–91–01580. Washington, D.C.: OIG, U.S. Department of Health and Human Services, 1993.

O'Brien, J., Saxberg, B.O., and Smith, H.L. For Profit or Not-For-Profit Nursing Homes: Does It Matter? *The Gerontologist* 23:341–348, 1983.

OTA (Office of Technology Assessment). *Biological Rhythms: Implications for the Worker.* Pub. no. OTA–BA–463. Washington, D.C.: OTA, U.S. Congress, September 1991.

Ouslander, J., and Kane, R. The Costs of Urinary Incontinence in Nursing Homes. *Medical Care* 22:69–79, 1984.

Ouslander, J.G, Kane, R.L., and Abrass, I.B. Urinary Incontinence in Elderly Nursing Home Patients. *Journal of the American Medical Association* 248:1194–1198, 1982.

Owen, B.D. The Lifting Process and Back Injury in Hospital Nursing Personnel. *Western Journal of Nursing Research* 7(4):445–459, 1985.

Owen, B.D. Low Back Problems in Nursing. *Western Journal of Nursing Research* April, 1989.

Patchner, M.A and Patchner, L.S. Essential Staffing for Improved Nursing Home Care: The Permanent Assignment Model. *Nursing Homes and Senior Citizen Care* 42(4):37–39, 1993.

Pearson, L.J. Annual Update of How Each State Stands on Legislative Issues Affecting Advanced Nursing Practice. *Nurse Practitioner* 20(1):13–14, 16–18, 21–22, 1995.

Penner, L.A., Luderria, K., and Mead, G. Staff Attitudes: Image or Reality. *Journal of Gerontological Nursing* 10:110–117, 1984.

Peppard, N. Alzheimer's Special Care Nursing Home Units. *Nursing Homes* 34(5):25–28, 1984.

Phillips, C.D., Hawes, C., and Fries, B.E. Reducing the Use of Physical Restraints in Nursing Homes: Will it Increase Costs? *American Journal of Public Health* 83(3):342–348, 1993.

Phillips, C.D., Mor, V., Hawes, C. et al. Development of Resident Assessment System and Data Base for Nursing Home Residents. Executive Summary of Implementation Report submitted to the Health Standards and Quality Bureau, Health Care Financing Administration, under contract no. 500–88–0055, January, 1994.

Phillips, J.A., and Brown, K.C. Industrial Workers on a Rotating Shift Pattern: Adaptation and Injury Status. *AAOHN (American Association of Occupational Health Nursing) Journal* 40(10): 468–476, 1992.

Pillemer, K. Maltreatment of Patients in Nursing Homes: Overview and Research Agenda. *Journal of Health and Social Behavior* 29:227–238, 1988.

Pillemer, K., and Hudson, B. A Model Abuse Prevention Program for Nursing Assistants. *The Gerontologist* 33(1):128–131, 1993.

Pines, A., and Maslach, C. Characteristics of Staff Burnout in Mental Health Settings. *Hospital and Community Psychiatry* 29:233–237, 1978.

Poster, E.C., and Ryan, J.A. Nurses Attitudes Toward Physical Assaults by Patients. *Archives of Psychiatric Nursing* 3(6):315–322, 1989.

Prescott, P.A. Nursing: An Important Component of Hospital Survival under a Reformed Health Care System. *Nursing Economic$* 11(4):192–199, 1993.

ProPAC (Prospective Payment Assessment Commission). *Medicare and the American Health Care System: Report to Congress.* Washington, D.C.: ProPAC, 1994.

ProPAC. *Report and Recommendations to the Congress, March 1, 1995.* Washington, D.C.: ProPAC, 1995.

Ray, G.L., and Hardin, S. Advanced Practice Nursing: Playing a Vital Role. *Nursing Management* 26(2):45–47, 1995.

Reagan, J. Management of Nurse's Aides in Long Term Care Settings. *Journal of Long Term Care Administration* 14:9–14, 1986.

Rees, D., and Cooper, C.L. Occupational Stress in Health Service Workers in the UK. *Stress Medicine* 8(2):79–90, 1992.

Ribeiro, B.J., and Smith, S.R. Evaluation of Urinary Catheterization and Urinary Incontinence in a General Nursing Home Population. *Journal of the American Geriatrics Society* 33(7):479–482, 1985.

Robertson, J.F., Herth, K.A., and Cummings, C.C. Long-term Care: Retention of Nurses. *Journal of Gerontological Nursing* 20(11):4–10, 1994.

Rodgers, S. Back Pain Four: Positive Lifting. *Nursing Times* 81:43–45, 1985.

Rogers, W.H., Draper, D., Kahn, K.L., et al. Quality of Care Before and After Implementation of the DRG-Based Prospective Payment System: A Summary of Effects. *Journal of the American Medical Association* 264:1989–1994, 1990.

Rohrer, J.E., Buckwalter, K.C., and Russell, D.W. The Effects of Mental Dysfunction on Nursing Home Care. *Social Science and Medicine* 28(4):399–403, 1989.

Rubenstein, L.V., Kahn, K.L., Reinisch, E.J., et al. Changes in Quality of Care for Five Diseases Measured by Implicit Review, 1981 to 1986. *Journal of the American Medical Association* 264:1974–1979, 1990.

Rubin, H.R., Gandek, B., Rogers, W.H., et al. Patients' Ratings of Outpatient Visits in Different Practice Settings: Results from the Medical Outcomes Study. *Journal of the American Medical Association* 270:835–840, 1993.

Rudder, C. *New York State's Nursing Home Industry: Profit, Losses, Expenditures and Quality.* New York: Nursing Home Community Coalition of New York State, 1994.

Rudman, D., Alverno, L., and Mattson, D.E. A Comparison of Physically Aggressive Behavior in Two VA Nursing Homes. *Hospital and Community Psychiatry* 44(6):571–575, 1993.

Russell, L.C. Cost containment of modified radical mastectomy: The impact of the clinical nurse specialist. *ETHICON* 26(3):18–19, 1989.

Ryden, M.B., Bossenmaier, M., and McLachlan, C. Aggressive Behavior in Cognitively Impaired Nursing Home Residents. *Research in Nursing and Health* 14(2):87–95, 1991.

Safran, D.G., Tarlov, A.R., and Rogers, W.H. Primary Care Performance in Fee-for-Service and Prepaid Health Care Systems: Results from the Medical Outcomes Study. *Journal of the American Medical Association* 271:1579–1586, 1994.

Satinsky, M.A. *An Executive Guide to Case Management Strategies.* Chicago: American Hospital Association Publishing, 1995.

Schieber, G., Wiener, J., Liu, K., and Doty, P. Prospective Payment for Medicare Skilled Nursing Facilities: Background and Issues. *Health Care Financing Review* 8(1):79–85, 1986.

Schlenker, R.E. Comparison of Medicaid Nursing Home Payment Systems. *Health Care Financing Review* 13(1):93–109, 1991a.

Schlenker, R.E. Nursing Home Costs, Medicaid Rates, and Profits Under Alternative Medicaid Payment Systems. *HSR (Health Services Research)* 26:623–649, 1991b.

Schlenker, R.E., Shaughnessy, P.W., and Yslas, I. Estimating Patient-Level Nursing Home Costs. *HSR (Health Services Research)* 20:103–128, 1985.

Schneider, E.L., and Guralnik, J.M. The Aging of America. Impact on Health Care Costs. *Journal of the American Medical Association* 263(17):2354–2355, 1990.

Schneider, D.P., Fries, B.E., Foley, W.J., et al. Case Mix for Nursing Home Payment: Resource Utilization Groups, Version II. *Health Care Financing Review* Annl. Suppl.:39–52, 1988.

Schnelle, J. Treatment of Urinary Incontinence in Nursing Home Patients by Prompted Voiding. *Journal of the American Geriatrics Society* 38:256–360, 1990.

Schnelle, J. Presentation at a special invitational session on Quality and Staffing in Nursing Homes sponsored by the National Institute for Nursing Research on behalf of the IOM study, and held in conjunction with the 1994 annual meeting of the Gerontology Society of America in Atlanta, November 1994.

Schnelle, J.F., Newman, D.R., and Fogarty, T. Management of Patient Continence in Long Term Care Nursing Facilities. *The Gerontologist* 30:373–376, 1990.

Schultz, B.M., Ward, D., and Knickman, J.R. RUG-II Impacts on Long-term Care Facilities in New York. *Health Care Financing Review* 16(2):85–99, 1994.

Scott, W., and Shortell, S. Organizational Performance: Managing for Efficiency and Effectiveness. In: S. Shortell, and A. Kaluzny, eds. *Health Care Management: A Text in Organizational Theory and Behavior.* New York: John Wiley & Sons, 1983.

Seeff, L.B., Wright, E.C., Zimmerman, H.J., et al. Type B Hepatitis After Needlestick Exposure: Prevention with Hepatitis B Immunoglobulin. Final Report of the Veterans Administration Cooperative Study. *Annals of Internal Medicine* 88:285–293, 1978.

SEIU (Service Employees International Union). *Back Injuries Among Nursing Home Workers in Pennsylvania: A Crippling Epidemic.* Washington, D.C.: SEIU, AFL-CIO, CLC, 1991.

SEIU. *The National Nurse Survey: 10,000 Dedicated Healthcare Professionals Report on Staffing, Stress and Patient Care in U.S. Hospitals and Nursing Homes.* Washington, D.C.: SEIU, AFL-CIO, CLC, 1993.

SEIU. *Caring Til it Hurts: How Nursing Home Work Is Becoming the Most Dangerous Job in America.* Washington, D.C.: SEIU, AFL-CIO, CLC, 1994.

SEIU. *Falling Short: The Staffing Crisis in Beverly Enterprises' Texas Nursing Homes and the Need for a Minimum Standard.* Washington, D.C.: SEIU, AFL-CIO, CLC, 1995a.

SEIU. *System Breakdown: How Quality Assurance Failed at Beverly Enterprises, the Nation's Largest Nursing Home Operator.* Washington, D.C.: SEIU, AFL-CIO, CLC, 1995b.

Shaughnessy, P., and Kramer, A. The Increased Needs of Patients in Nursing Homes and Patients Receiving Home Health Care. *New England Journal of Medicine* 322:21–27, 1990.

Shaughnessy, P.W., Schlenker, R.E., and Kramer, A.M. Quality of Long-term Care in Nursing Homes and Swing-Bed Hospitals. *HSR (Health Services Research)* 25:65–96, 1990.

Shelley, G.A., and Howard, R.J. A National Survey of Surgeons' Attitudes About Patients with Human Immunodeficiency Virus Infections and Acquired Immunodeficiency Syndrome. *Archives of Surgery* 127(2):206–211, 1992.

Sheridan, J., Hogstel, M., and Fairchild, T.J. Organization Climate in Nursing Homes: Its Impact on Nursing Leadership and Patient Care. Pp. 90–94 in: L.R. Jouch and J.L. Wall, eds. *Best Papers Proceedings 1990.* San Francisco: Academy of Management, 1990.

Shortell, S.M., and Hughes, E.F.X. The Effects of Regulation, Competition, and Ownership on Mortality Rates Among Hospital Inpatients. *New England Journal of Medicine* 318:1100–1107, 1988.

Shortell, S.M., and Hull, K.E. Chapter 1: New Organization of Health Care—Managed Care/Integrated Health Care Systems. In: S.H. Altman and U.E. Reinhardt. *Baxter 2: Health Policy Book. Strategic Choices for a Changing Health Care System.* Ann Arbor, Mich.: Health Administration Press, in press.

Shortell, S.M., Zimmerman, J.E., Rousseau, D.M., et al. The Performance of Intensive Care Units: Does Good Management Make a Difference? *Medical Care* 32:508–525, 1994.

Shortell, S.M., Gillies, R.R., and Devers, K.J. Reinventing the American Hospital. *The Milbank Quarterly* 73(2):131–160, 1995.

Silber, J.H., Rosenbaum, P.R., Schwartz, J.S., et al. Evaluation of the Complication Rate as a Measure of Quality of Care in Coronary Artery Bypass Graft Surgery. *Journal of the American Medical Association* 274:317–323, 1995.

Soldo, B.J., and Agree, E.M. *America's Elderly. Population Bulletin,* vol. 43, no. 3. Washington, D.C.: Population Reference Bureau, 1988.

Sovie, M.D. Tailoring Hospitals for Managed Care and Integrated Health Systems. *Nursing Economic$* 13:72–83, March-April 1995.

Spector, W.D., and Takada, H.A. Characteristics of Nursing Homes that Affect Resident Outcomes. *Journal of Aging and Health* 3(4):427–454, 1991.

Spence, D.A., and Wiener, J.M. Nursing Home Length of Stay Patterns: Results from the 1985 National Nursing Home Survey. *Gerontologist* 30(1):16–20, 1990.

Spillman, B.C., and Kemper, P. Lifetime Patterns of Payment for Nursing Home Care. *Medical Care* 33:280–296, 1995.

Stahl, D.A. 1995 Leadership Challenges for SNFs. *Nursing Management* 26(3):16–17, 19, 1995a.

Stahl, D.A. Maximizing Reimbursement for Subacute Care. *Nursing Management* 26(4):16–7, 19, 1995b.

Stewart, A.L., Greenfield, S., Hays, R.D., et al. Functional Status and Well-Being of Patients with Chronic Conditions. *Journal of the American Medical Association* 262:907–913, 1989.

Stolley, J.M., Buckwalter, K.C., and Shannon, M.D. Caring for Patients with Alzheimer's Disease: Recommendations for Nursing Education. *Journal of Gerontological Nursing* 17(6):34–38, 1991.

Straus, M.A. Domestic Violence and Homicide Antecedents. *Bulletin of the New York Academy of Medicine* 62:446–465, 1986.

Strumpf, N. Presentation at a special invitational session on Quality and Staffing in Nursing Homes sponsored by the National Institute for Nursing Research on behalf of the IOM study, and held in conjunction with the 1994 annual meeting of the Gerontology Society of America in Atlanta, November 1994.

Strumpf, N.E., and Knibbe, K.K. Long Term Care: Fulfilling Promises to the Old Among Us. Pp. 217–225 in: J. McCloskey and H. Grace, eds. *Current Issues in Nursing.* St. Louis, Mo.: C.V. Mosby, 1990.

Suzman, R.M., Willis, D.P., and Manton, K.G., eds. *The Oldest Old.* New York: Oxford University Press, 1992.

Swan, J.H., and Harrington, C. Estimating Undersupply of Nursing Home Beds in States. *HSR (Health Services Research)* 21:57–83, 1986.

Swan, J.H., and Harrington, C. Certificate of Need and Nursing Home Bed Capacity in States. *Journal of Health and Social Policy* 2(2):87–105, 1990.

Swan, J., Torre, A., and Steinhart, R. Ripple Effects of PPS on Nursing Homes: Swimming or Drowning in the Funding Stream? *The Gerontologist* 30:323–331, 1990.

Swan, J.H., Harrington, C., DuNah, R. et al. Estimating Adequacy of Nursing Home Bed Supply in the States. Paper prepared for the U.S. Department of Housing and Urban Development and the Health Care Financing Administration. Wichita, Kans.: Wichita State University, 1993a.

Swan, J.H., Harrington, C., and Grant, L.A. State Medicaid Reimbursement for Nursing Homes, 1978–88. *Health Care Financing Review* 14(4):111–131, 1993b.

Swan, J.H., Dewit, S., and Harrington, C. State Medicaid Reimbursement Methods and Rates for Nursing Homes, 1993. Paper prepared for the Department of Housing and Urban Development and the Health Care Financing Administration. Wichita, Kans.: Wichita State University, 1994.

Tan, C.C. Occupational Health Problems Among Nurses. *Scandinavian Journal of Work Environment Health* 17:221–230, 1991.

Tarlov, A.R., Ware, J.E., Greenfield, S., et al. The Medical Outcomes Study: An Application of Methods for Monitoring the Results of Medical Care. *Journal of the American Medical Association* 262:925–930, 1989.

Teresi, J., Holmes, D., Benenson, E., et al. A Primary Care Nursing Model in Long Term Care Facilities: Evaluation of Impact on Affect, Behavior, and Socialization. *The Gerontologist* 33:667–674, 1993.

Thomas, J.W., Holloway, J.J., and Guire, K.E. Validating Risk-Adjusted Mortality as an Indicator for Quality of Care. *Inquiry* 30:6–22, 1993.

Treas, J. *Older Americans in the 1990s and Beyond. Population Bulletin,* vol. 50, no. 2. Washington, D.C.: Population Reference Bureau, 1995a.

Treas, J. U.S. Aging: "Golden Oldies" Remain Variable. *Population Today: News, Numbers, and Analysis* 23(5):1–2, 1995b.

U.S. Department of Justice. *Crime in the United States.* Washington, D.C.: U.S. Government Printing Office, 1985.

U.S. DHHS (U.S. Department of Health and Human Services). *Federal Register: 42 CFR Part 401.* November 10, 1994.

U.S. House of Representatives, Committee on Ways and Means. *Overview of Entitlement Programs, 1990 Green Book.* Washington, D.C.: U.S. Government Printing Office, p. 147–149, 1990.

U.S. Senate, Special Committee on Aging. *Nursing Home Care: The Unfinished Agenda.* 1 (Special Hearing and Report, May 21, 1986). Washington, D.C.: U.S. Government Printing Office, 1986.

U.S. Senate, Special Committee on Aging. Reducing the Use of Chemical Restraints in Nursing Homes. Workshop Before the Special Committee. Pub. no. SN 102-6. Washington, D.C.: U.S. Government Printing Office, 1991.

VHA. The Impact of Organizational Redesign on Nurse Executive Leadership: A VHA, Inc., Survey of 423 Nurse Executives with Analysis by the Hay Group. Irving, Tex.: VHA, 1995.

Wagnild, G. A Descriptive Study of Nurse's Aide Turnover in Long Term Care Facilities. *Journal of Long-term Care Administration* 16(Spring):19–23, 1988.

Wagnild, G., and Manning, R. The High Runover Profile: Screening and Selecting Applicants for Nurse's Aides. *Journal of Long-term Care Administration* 14(Summer):2–4, 1986.

Wallace, C. Chains Plan Growth in Response to Rising Demand for Services. *Modern Healthcare* (June 6):116–126, 1986.

Wanich, C.K., Sullivan-Marx, E.M., Gottlieb, G.L., and Johnson, J.C. Functional Status Outcomes of a Nursing Intervention in Hospitalized Elderly. *Image: The Journal of Nursing Scholarship* 24(3):201–207, 1992.

Weiler, K., Buckwalter, K.C., and Curry, J. Nurses, Work-Related Stress, and Ethical Dilemmas. In: D.M. Corr and C.A. Corr, eds. *Nursing Care in an Aging Society.* New York, N.Y.: Springer, 1990.

Weissert, W.G., and Cready, C.M. Determinants of Hospital-to-Nursing Home Placement Delays: A Pilot Study. *HSR (Health Services Research)* 23:619–646, 1988.

Weissert, W.G., and Musliner, M.C. *Access, Quality, and Cost Consequences of Case-Mix Adjusted Reimbursement for Nursing Homes.* Pub. no. 9109. Washington, D.C.: American Association of Retired Persons, 1992a.

Weissert, W.G., and Musliner, M.C. Case Mix Adjusted Nursing-Home Reimbursement: A Critical Review of the Evidence. *The Milbank Quarterly* 70(3):455–490, 1992b.

Weissert, W.G., Scanlon, W.J., Wan, T.T.H., and Skinner, D.E. Care for the Chronically Ill: Nursing Home Incentive Payment Experiment. *Health Care Financing Review* 5:41–49, 1983.

Wells, K.B., Hays, R.D., Burnam, A., et al. Detection of Depressive Disorder for Patients Receiving Prepaid or Fee-for-Service Care: Results from the Medical Outcomes Study. *Journal of the American Medical Association* 262:3298–3302, 1989a.

Wells, K.B., Steward, A., Hays, R.D., et al. The Functioning and Well-Being of Depressed Patients: Results from the Medical Outcomes Study. *Journal of the American Medical Association* 262:914–919, 1989b.

White, C.M. The Nurse-Patient Encounter: Attitudes and Behavior in Action. *Journal of Gerontological Nursing* 3:16–20, 1977.

Whitley, M.P., and Putzier, D.J. Measuring Nurses' Satisfaction with the Quality of their Work and Work Environment. *Journal of Nursing Care Quality* 8(3):43–51, 1994.

Wilging, P.R. OBRA as a Measure of Quality. Pp. 21–25 in: E.L. Mitty, ed. *Quality Imperatives in Long-term Care: The Elusive Agenda.* New York, N.Y.: National League for Nursing Press, 1992a.

Wilging, P.R. A Strategy for Quality Assurance in Long-term Care. Pp. 13–19 in: E.L. Mitty, ed. *Quality Imperatives in Long-term Care: The Elusive Agenda.* New York, N.Y.: National League for Nursing Press, 1992b.

Wilkinson, W. Occupational Injury at a Midwestern Health Science Center and Teaching Hospital. *AAOHN (American Association of Occupational Health Nursing) Journal* 35(8):367–376, 1987.

Willcocks, D., Peace, S., and Kellaher, L. *Private Lives in Public Places.* London: Tavistock, 1987.

Willemain, T.R. A Comparison of Patient-Centered and Case Mix Reimbursement for Nursing Home Care. *HSR (Health Services Research)* 15:365–377, 1980.

Winger, J. Schirm, V., and Steward, P. Aggressive Behavior in Long-term Care. *Journal of Psychosocial Nursing and Mental Health Services* 25:28–33, 1987.

Witt Associates. Today's Nurse Executive: Data Analysis, 1990 Survey. Survey cosponsored by the American Organization of Nurse Executives. Oak Brook Terrace, Ill.: Witt/Kieffer, Ford, Hadelman and Lloyd, 1990.

Wright, L.K. A Reconceptualization of the "Negative Staff and Poor Care in Nursing Homes" Assumption. *The Gerontologist* 28:813–820, 1988.

Yordy, K.D. Implications of the Changing Market on the Nursing Workforce: Integrated Systems and Changing Sites of Service. In: C.L. Hopper, H.R. Manasse, C.J. McLaughlin, and M. Osterweis. *The Health Workforce: Power, Politics, and Policy.* Washington, D.C.: Association of Academic Health Centers, in press.

Yu, L.C., Mansfield, P.K., Packard, J.S., et al. Occupational Stress Among Nurses in Hospital Settings. *AAOHN (American Association of Occupational Health Nursing) Journal* 37(4):121–128, 1989.

Zimmer, J.G. Quality of Care Assessment in Long-term Care Facilities. *Evaluation and the Health Professions* 6:339–344, 1983.

Zimmer, J.G. Quality Assurance. In: P.R. Katz and E. Calkins, eds. *Principles and Practice of Nursing Home Care.* New York: Springer, 1989.

Zimmer, J.G., Watson, N., and Treat, A. Behavioral Problems Among Patients in SNFs. *American Journal of Public Health* 74(10):1118–1121, 1984.

Zimmer, J.G., Bentley, D.W., Valenti, W.M., and Watson, N.M. Systemic Antibiotic Use in Nursing Homes: A Quality Assessment. *Journal of American Geriatrics Society* 34:703–710, 1986.

Zimmerman, D.R. Impact of New Regulations and Data Sources on Nursing Home Quality of Care. Madison, Wisc.: Center for Health Systems Research and Analysis, 1990.

Zimmerman, D.R., Egan, J.R., Gustafson, D., et al. Evaluation of the State Demonstrations in Nursing Home Quality Assurance Processes. Final Report to the Health Care Financing Administration. Madison, Wisc.: Mathematica Policy Research, 1985.

Zimmerman, D.R., Karon, S.L., Arling, G., et al. Development and Testing of Nursing Home Quality Indicators. *Health Care Financing Review* 16(4):107–127, 1995.

Zimmerman, J.E., Shortell, S.M., Rousseau, D.M, et al. Improving Intensive Care: Observations Based on Organizational Case Studies in Nine Intensive Care Units: A Prospective, Multicenter Study. *Critical Care Medicine* 21(10):1443–1451, 1993.

Zinn, J.S. Inter-SMSA Variation on Nursing Home Staffing and Management Practices. *Journal of Applied Gerontology* 12(2):206–224, 1993a.

Zinn, J.S. The Influence of Nurse Wage Differentials on Nursing Home Staffing and Resident Care Decisions. *The Gerontologist* 33:721–729, 1993b.

Zinn, J.S., Aaronson, W.E., and Rosko, M.D. The Use of Standardized Indicators as Quality Improvement Tools: An Application in Pennsylvania Nursing Homes. *American Journal of Medical Quality* 8:456–465, 1993a.

Zinn, J.S., Aaronson, W.E., and Rosko, M.D. Variations in Outcomes of Care Provided in Pennsylvania Nursing Homes: Facility and Environmental Correlates. *Medical Care* 31:475–487, 1993b.

Biographical Sketches of
Committee Members

CAROLYNE K. DAVIS *(Chair)*, R.N., Ph.D., is a national and international health care adviser to Ernst & Young. She received her B.S. in nursing from the Johns Hopkins University, and the M.S. in nursing and the Ph.D. in higher education administration from Syracuse University. She has been chair of the baccalaureate nursing program at Syracuse University and held many positions at the University of Michigan, Ann Arbor, including dean of the school of nursing, professor of both nursing and education, and associate vice president for academic affairs. Following this, she became the fourth administrator of the Health Care Financing Administration and held that position from 1981 to 1985. As administrator, Dr. Davis oversaw the functions of the Medicare and Medicaid programs, which finance health care services for 54 million poor, elderly, and disabled Americans. She is a member of the editorial board of the journal *Nursing Economics* and has more than 100 publications on a wide variety of issues concerning the health care system. Dr. Davis has received many honorary degrees and alumni awards, is on the board of directors or is a member of the board of several corporations, and is a member of the Institute of Medicine.

FRANK A. SLOAN *(Cochair)*, Ph.D., is the Alexander McMahon professor of health policy and management and professor of economics at Duke University. He did his undergraduate work at Oberlin College and received his Ph.D. in economics from Harvard University. Before joining the faculty at Duke last summer, he was a research economist at the RAND Corporation and was on the faculties of the University of Florida and Vanderbilt University. His current research interests include long-term care and medical malpractice. Dr. Sloan also has a long-standing interest in the costs and financing of medical education. He has served on several national advisory groups, is a member of the Institute of Medicine (IOM) and until recently was a member of the IOM's Council.

DYANNE D. AFFONSO, Ph.D., is dean and professor at the Nell Hodgson Woodruff School of Nursing, Emory University, and associate professor in the Women's and Children's Division of the School of Public Health. Previously, she was a faculty member at the School of Nursing of the University of California at San Francisco and the College of Nursing, University of Arizona. Beginning in the late 1970s, Dr. Affonso conducted research exploring women's experiences with cesarean childbirth. Her publications of these important findings resulted in national recognition of her contribution to perinatal health care, including her appointment as the first nurse to serve on the Advisory Council of the National Institute of Child Health and Human Development (NICHD) at the National Institutes of Health (NIH). In this capacity, she was an active participant in the 1980 Consensus Conference on Vaginal Birth After Cesarean, which led to a major change in obstetrical philosophy and practice regarding methods of childbirth. She continues to be a productive leader in a variety of maternal–child health topics, and plays an active role in recruitment and mentoring of minority women in biomedical careers. In addition to her work on the NICHD Advisory Council, Dr. Affonso was a member of the Task Force on Recruitment, Retention, Re-entry, and Advancement of Women in Biomedical Careers for the Office of Research on Women's Health; and the Panel on Women's Health of the American Academy of Nursing. She cochaired the Priority Expert Panel on Prevention and Care of Low Birth Weight Infants for the National Center for Nursing Research, NIH, and participated in a workshop on mental disorders in pregnancy and postpartum for the National Institute of Mental Health. She is the first non-Nordic citizen to be appointed to the Scientific Council of Sweden's Nordic School of Public Health and has been elected to the Institute of Medicine and the American Academy of Nursing. Her other honors include March of Dimes National Nurse of the Year and American Nurses Association Maternal–Child Nurse of the Year. She is a member of the International Council of Psychology, the Society of Behavioral Medicine, and the Nursing Association of the American College of Obstetrics and Gynecology. Dr. Affonso is a frequent invited speaker at international, national, and regional conferences. She has served as a reviewer for leading journals on women's health issues and is the author of numerous publications, including *Childbearing: A Nursing Perspective*, which won an *American Journal of Nursing* Book of the Year Award. Recent publications focus on health issues for women from ethnically diverse and rural backgrounds, with an emphasis on Asian Pacific Islanders.

JAMES F. BLUMSTEIN, LL.B., holds a B.A. in economics from Yale College, an M.A. in economics from Yale University, and an LL.B. from Yale Law School. He is currently a professor of law at Vanderbilt Law School, a senior fellow at the Vanderbilt Institute for Public Policy Studies, and an adjunct professor of health law at Dartmouth Medical School. He was the John M. Olin Visiting Professor of Law at the University of Pennsylvania Law School in the spring of 1989, and a visiting associate professor of law and policy sciences at Duke Law School during 1974–1975. He is a recipient of the Earl Sutherland Prize for Research at Vanderbilt University and the Paul Hartman Award for Teaching at the Vanderbilt Law School. Professor Blumstein is an elected member of the Institute of Medicine and is a contributor to professional journals on health policy issues.

DONALD L. CHENSVOLD, R.N., is president of Healthcare of Iowa, Inc., a nursing facility management corporation based in Cedar Rapids, Iowa. The company operates 19 for-profit and not-for-profit facilities in the State of Iowa. Mr. Chensvold is licensed as a nursing home administrator in Iowa, Wisconsin, and Nebraska; as a licensed practical nurse; and as a registered nurse. He is chairman of the Iowa Health Care Association Facility Standards Committee, which deals with regulatory issues related to long-term care, and is vice president of the Iowa Health Care Association. Mr. Chensvold is a regional representative to the American Health Care Association (AHCA) Facility Standards Committee and served as a member of the AHCA Clinical Practice Guideline Subcommittee for Nutrition Care and Services for Long-Term Care Residents. He has also served on numerous state and national committees dealing with long-term care issues, and chaired a Model Standards Committee for the development of clinical practice guidelines on the use of physical and chemical restraints in long-term care facilities. Mr. Chensvold has served in the capacity of orderly, licensed practical nurse, registered nurse, director of nursing, or administrator in numerous nursing facilities in Iowa, Wisconsin, and Nebraska. He attended Upper Iowa University in Fayette, Iowa.

LINDA HAWES CLEVER, M.D., founding chairman of the Department of Occupational Health at California Pacific Medical Center and editor of the *Western Journal of Medicine,* received undergraduate and medical degrees from Stanford University. After interning at Stanford, she had several years of medical residency and fellowships at Stanford and the University of California, San Francisco. Dr. Clever is board certified in internal medicine and occupational medicine. In 1970, Dr. Clever became the first medical director of the teaching clinic at St. Mary's Hospital in San Francisco, where she started a nurse practitioner training and research program. In 1977, she became the founding chairman of the Department of Occupational Health at the Pacific Medical Center and began her activities in the American College of Physicians in which she now serves on the Board of Regents. She is a member of the Institute of Medicine and the Western

Association of Physicians, and is a clinical professor of medicine at the University of California, San Francisco. Her areas of special interest include the health of health care workers, AIDS, leadership, managed care, ethics, medical journalology, care of elders (her father is a resident of a convalescent center), and numerous organizations including Stanford University, the radio station KQED, and White House Fellows. Dr. Clever chaired the development committee for senior services at California Pacific Medical Center and serves on the Lucile Packard Children's Hospital Board of Directors.

JOYCE C. CLIFFORD, R.N., M.S.N., F.A.A.N., is vice president for nursing and nurse-in-chief at Beth Israel Hospital in Boston and holds a visiting scholar appointment at Boston College School of Nursing. She is an established author and consultant on the subject of organizational restructuring and the development of a professional practice model and has spoken both nationally and internationally. Her past nursing experiences include multiple nursing positions and both active and reserve duty in the U.S. Air Force Nurse Corps. She has also served on the faculty of several nursing schools, has been recognized with numerous awards and honorary doctorates, and serves on the editorial advisory boards of several nursing journals. Among many other affiliations and honors, she is a fellow of the American Academy of Nurses, former president of the American Organization of Nurse Executives, and a former trustee of the American Hospital Association. She is a graduate of St. Anselm College, received the masters' in nursing from the University of Alabama, and is currently a Ph.D. candidate in the field of health planning and policy analysis at the Heller School of Brandeis University.

EDWARD J. CONNORS is president emeritus of Mercy Health Services (MHS) and former chair of the American Hospital Association (AHA) Board of Trustees. Mr. Connors served as president and chief executive officer of MHS from 1976 to 1993. Mercy Health Services is a Farmington Hills, Michigan, based nonprofit health care system sponsored by the Sisters of Mercy Regional Community of Detroit. Mr. Connors has more than 35 years of experience in the health care field. He has held academic and management leadership positions at the University of Michigan and the University of Wisconsin Hospitals. Mr. Connors is a member of the Joint Commission on Accreditation of Healthcare Organizations Board of Commissioners and serves on the boards of AHA's Hospital Research and Educational Trust; Eastern Mercy Health System in Radnor, Pennsylvania; and Sisters of Providence Health System in Springfield, Massachusetts. He is also the former chair of the American Healthcare Systems Board of Governors. In 1988, Mr. Connors completed a 1-year appointment to the Secretary's Commission on Nursing, U.S. Department of Health and Human Services. He is an International King's Fund Fellow and a member of the Institute of Medicine, and has lectured and published extensively on the topic of health care. Mr. Connors holds a master's degree in hospital administration from the University of Minnesota and currently provides consultation services to health care organizations through the Connors/Roberts and Associates firm.

ARTHUR COOPER, M.D., is associate professor of clinical surgery at the College of Physicians and Surgeons of Columbia University and chief of pediatric surgical critical care at the Harlem Hospital Center, as well as attending surgeon at the Babies' and Children's Hospital of New York of the Columbia-Presbyterian Medical Center. He obtained his baccalaureate at Harvard College and his doctorate at the University of Pennsylvania School of Medicine, where he also undertook training in general surgery, pediatric surgery, and surgical critical care; he is certified by the American Board of Surgery in all three specialties. Dr. Cooper also holds a master's degree in human nutrition from Columbia University, is a member of numerous professional and scientific societies, has written more than 100 articles and textbook chapters, serves on a variety of national and regional expert committees, and is a recognized authority in the fields of pediatric surgical nutrition, critical care, trauma, and emergency medical services—particularly pediatric prehospital emergency care—as well as physical child abuse and the surgical care of children with human immunodeficiency virus infection.

ALLYSON ROSS DAVIES, Ph.D., M.P.H., is an independent health care consultant. Until March 1994, she was the senior program advisor to the Measurement & Monitoring Initiative at the New England Medical Center. In that role, Dr. Davies facilitated hospital-wide efforts to build into ongoing quality assurance and improvement activities the collection, interpretation, and use of patient-based assessments of their health status and consumers' assessments of the quality of care and services. From 1988 through 1992, she was the first director of the New England Medical Center's Department of Quality Assessment. From 1975 to 1988, she was a health policy analyst at the RAND Corporation. Dr. Davies received her M.P.H. and Ph.D. from the University of California at Los Angeles. Dr. Davies has published and lectured widely on the development of patient-based assessments of health status and quality of care and their use in outcomes assessment and quality improvement, and her consulting practice focuses on these topics.

ERIKA SIVARAJAN FROELICHER, R.N., Ph.D., is a professor of Nursing and Epidemiology at the University of California, San Francisco. She is a graduate of the University of Washington, Seattle, School of Nursing where she earned a B.S. and an M.A. in nursing (Minoring in business administration). Her masters' degree in public health, doctorate in public health-epidemiology, and Minor in biostatistics were earned at the University of California, Los Angeles, School of Public Health. She has more than 20 years' experience in clinical practice, teaching, and research in cardiovascular disease prevention and rehabilitation. Dr. Froelicher is a Fellow of the American Academy of Nursing, the American

Heart Association Council of Cardiovascular Nursing, and the American Association of Cardiovascular and Pulmonary Rehabilitation. She is one of 12 founding editorial board members of the *Journal of Cardiac Rehabilitation.* She serves on the editorial boards of *Health and Lung, American Journal of Critical Care,* and *Progress in Cardiovascular Nursing.* She is a member of the American Heart Association Committee on Exercise and Rehabilitation and has served on the American College of Cardiology Prevention Committee. She has served as a peer reviewer for the Health Failure and Unstable Angina Clinical Practice Guidelines and has participated in numerous Agency for Health Care Policy and Research meetings to identify priorities for guideline development. Dr. Froelicher's program of research has focused on studying the efficacy of activity and exercise prescription, education, and counseling in patients with heart disease, as well as risk factor reduction using education-counseling and behavioral interventions to reduce risk, improve adherence, and enhance quality of life. Dr. Froelicher has published extensively: textbook, chapters, and scientific and professional articles on exercise testing, patient and family education, counseling, and behavioral interventions.

CHARLENE A. HARRINGTON, Ph.D., R.N., F.A.A.N., professor and chair of the Department of Social and Behavioral Sciences, School of Nursing, University of California, San Francisco. She is a nurse and sociologist who is a fellow in the American Academy of Nursing and a member of the American Nurses Association Task Force on Reimbursement. She has been the principal investigator for several large national research studies on state policies in long-term care and their effects on utilization and expenditures, funded by the Health Care Financing Administration (HCFA). After conducting the National Evaluation of the Social/Health Maintenance Organization (SHMO) Demonstration Projects with her colleagues for 7 years, she and her colleagues are providing technical assistance to the new second generation of SHMOs for the HCFA. In 1994, she coedited a book entitled *Health Policy and Nursing* and she teaches courses on health care economics and health policy.

MARK C. HORNBROOK, Ph.D., is a health economist and a senior investigator and director of the research program in health services, social, and economic studies at the Kaiser Permanente Center for Health Research (CHR). His current research focuses on payment systems for health maintenance organizations (HMO) under private and public health insurance programs. With support from the Health Care Financing Administration, he is developing morbidity-based risk models to adjust payments to health plans to counter selection bias. In collaboration with the Washington State Health Care Authority and the University of Washington, he is working to develop morbidity and demographic prediction models to adjust payments to health plans participating in the Washington public employee health benefits program. In a third project, he is collaborating with the

Pacific Business Group on Health and the University of California, San Francisco, to create social survey risk models to assist employers in evaluating health plan premiums. The Robert Wood Johnson Foundation supports these latter two projects. Dr. Hornbrook's other research activities have included a demonstration of an HMO-based geriatric assessment and care coordination model for primary care; a randomized trial of a physical fitness program to reduce the incidence and severity of fall-related injuries among older persons; a randomized trial of outreach and treatment of depressed adolescents in an HMO; and cost–benefit and cost-effectiveness analyses of several innovative health promotion and health care delivery programs related to smoking cessation, cancer screening, mental illness, and childhood asthma. Dr. Hornbrook received a master's degree in economics from the University of Denver in 1969 and a Ph.D. in medical care organization, with emphasis in health economics, from the University of Michigan in 1975. As a program director at the CHR, he directs a team of 12 other senior and junior investigators along with their scientific support staff. He also holds a part-time academic appointment as professor in the Community Health Care Systems Department of the School of Nursing, Oregon Health Sciences University. Currently, Dr. Hornbrook also serves on the Scientific Review and Evaluation Board of the Health Services Research and Development Service, Department of Veterans Affairs.

RONALD E. KUTSCHER is associate commissioner, Office of Employment Projections, Bureau of Labor Statistics. He is responsible for the program in the Bureau of Labor Statistics that (1) develops 5- to 10-year projections of the U.S. economy, covering the gross national product, industry output, productivity, and employment by industry and occupation; and (2) prepares the *Occupational Outlook Handbook* and other career guidance and training materials. Mr. Kutscher has held many positions within the Bureau of Labor Statistics, including economist, assistant chief for research, and assistant commissioner for economic growth. His expertise in the areas of the labor market, employment forecasting, technical aspects of converting statistical programs, and secondary education has resulted in invitations to act in various capacities, including consultant, lecturer, and member of two U.S. delegations in the former republics of the Soviet Union, Hungary, South Korea, Indonesia, and France. He received the B.A. from Doane College, Nebraska, with a major in economics and pursued graduate work in economics at the University of Illinois and Washington, D.C., area universities.

SUE LONGHENRY, M.S., R.N., is a certified gerontological nurse practitioner. She started her career in long-term care more than 12 years ago when she was a clinical instructor for practical nurse students. She has been a care plan coordinator, assistant director of nursing, and for the past 8 years, director of nursing in a 260 skilled-bed facility in Columbus, Ohio. This facility has been delivering subacute care for more than 10 years and has a 30-bed adult ventilator unit, a 20-bed pediatric ventilator unit, a hospice unit, a short-term orthopedic rehabilitation unit, and a 16-bed medical-complex unit. Ms. Longhenry now works part-time for the Joint Commission on the Accreditation of Healthcare Organizations as a field surveyor for long-term care and subacute facilities, and also consults with facilities needing help in developing subacute units. She is a past president of the National Association of Directors of Nursing Administration/Long Term Care.

ELLIOTT C. ROBERTS, SR., M.A., is a professor in the Department of Health Systems Research and Public Health at the Louisiana State University Medical School. He is also an adjunct professor and preceptor in the Department of Health Systems Management at Tulane University School of Public Health and Tropical Medicine. In his previous position as chief executive officer of the Medical Center of Louisiana (formerly Charity Hospital at New Orleans), he assisted in the implementation of the reorganization of the Louisiana State Department of Health and Human Resources, which ultimately became the Louisiana Health Care Authority. Mr. Robert's prior positions include chief executive officer of Cook County Hospital in Chicago, vice president and associate project director for Hyatt Medical Management Services, and commissioner of hospitals and executive director of Detroit General Hospital. He also served as executive director at Harlem Hospital Center and Mercy Douglass Hospital in Philadelphia. An active member of the American Hospital Association, Mr. Roberts served on its board of trustees for 5 years as well as on the nominating committee, in the House of Delegates, and in other capacities. He is a past chairman of the Metropolitan Hospital Constituency Section of the AHA. Mr. Roberts has held similar positions of responsibility at the National Association of Public Hospitals and the Association of American Medical Colleges' Council on Teaching Hospitals. He is also a diplomate of the American College of Healthcare Executives. In addition to many other appointments, Mr. Roberts served on the Secretary's Commission on Nursing, Department of Health and Human Services. He received a B.A. from Morgan State College and an M.A. in business administration-hospital administration from the George Washington University.

Part II

RESOURCES FOR THE STUDY

OVERVIEW

In the course of its deliberations the Institute of Medicine (IOM) Committee on the Adequacy of Nurse Staffing in Hospitals and Nursing Homes relied on a variety of sources of information. Part II of this report is designed to make some of these resources available to the reader, specifically, a discussion of the study activities; statistical resources used by the committee members; and the background papers commissioned by the committee.

The study activities are described in that section of the report, which immediately follows this introduction, as well as in the introduction to Part I (Chapter 1). The statistical resources are data from the American Hospital Association's annual hospital surveys and its National Hospital Panel Surveys, and data from the Bureau of Labor Statistics, the Public Health Service, and other sources; these were used to better understand trends in the delivery of, and market for, acute care. Several chapters in the report benefited from these data. The commissioned papers provided scholarly background information on a range of issues for the committee's benefit.

1

Study Activities

Two major information-gathering activities were conducted by the Institute of Medicine (IOM) in the course of its congressionally mandated study of the adequacy of nurse staffing in hospitals and nursing facilities. The first activity was the committee's wide-ranging request for written and oral testimony, and the second was a series of four site visits by small subgroups of the committee.

WRITTEN AND ORAL TESTIMONY
SUBMITTED TO THE COMMITTEE

Many IOM studies use requests for testimony to elicit a broader expression of views on the main topics of the project than would otherwise be available from committee members, published literature, and site visits. Providing testimony is an opportunity for interested parties to express their views and for committee members to obtain, firsthand, an extensive range of opinion on matters under consideration. Written testimony is solicited from a wide group of respondents and, based in part on the testimony received, selected groups and individuals may then be invited to present their testimony before the committee at a public hearing.

Because of the high level of interest among many organizations and individuals, the IOM committee requested testimony in the early stages of its study to help identify issues and resources. Following general guidance received from the committee and other IOM staff, the study staff developed a mailing list of organizations and individuals from whom written testimony related to the committee's mandate could be requested. In addition, some of the study's liaison panel members, nursing and nursing home associations, labor unions, other interest groups, and study sponsors provided names or sent their mailing lists for the committee's use. Selections were made from these and other lists, with the goal of representing all points of view.

A general announcement, containing the committee's mandate, its purpose in requesting testimony, a guide to assist in preparing written statements, and "key questions" around which the testimony could be organized, was then developed. (See Exhibit 1.1, at the back of this appendix, for a facsimile of the announcement/request for testimony.) In all, 511 announcements were mailed during July 1994; responses were requested by September 26, 1994. Some organizations and individuals who received the announcements also distributed them further to their memberships and acquaintances. By May 1995, staff had received and reviewed 108 testimonies. (See Table 1.1 for an alphabetical listing of the organizations and individuals that responded; for those that presented oral testimony, the site of the hearing is indicated.)

In addition to the request for written testimony, the mailed announcements also included information about 2 half-day public hearings at which the committee would hear oral testimony from a smaller group of individuals. The announcement specifically stated that if testimony were received by the September 1994 deadline, the organization or individual would be considered for one of the two hearings. After that deadline, potential testifiers for the two hearings were contacted.

Because travel costs could limit the ability of some groups and individuals to testify, the committee deliberately held one public hearing on each coast. This strategy also made it easier to distinguish broad, region-based differences across the country. The first public hearing was held in Washington, D.C., on October 19, 1994, in conjunction with committee's second meeting; 23 witnesses appeared before the committee. The second public hearing was held in Irvine, California, on January 22, 1995, in conjunction with the third committee meeting; 21 witnesses presented testimony. To the extent feasible, the preferences for dates and location of those invited to testify were honored.

Those presenting oral testimony were grouped into panels, asked to confine their remarks to 5 minutes, and requested to be prepared to respond to committee members' questions. In addition to those invited and scheduled to testify, at both public hearings the meetings were opened to general comments at the end of the day and were not adjourned until all those who wished to speak had done so.

Written and oral testimony received equal weight in the committee's deliberations. The written testimony ensured input from all interested parties, and the information, references, referrals, and suggestions provided in the statements were of considerable benefit to the study. The public hearings were convened to give committee members an opportunity to engage in discussion with—or to observe discussions among—an extensive range of health care providers, consumers and consumer advocates, professional organizations, and others. Both

TABLE 1.1 Organizations Submitting Written Statements

Name of Organization	Presented Testimony at Public Hearing
Academy of Medical-Surgical Nurses	
Affiliated Organization of Nurse Managers	
Aging Services for the Upper Cumberlands, Inc.	
Alcanter, B.J.	
American Association of Colleges of Nursing	DC
American Association of Homes and Services for the Aging	DC
American Association of Occupational Health Nurses	
American Federation of State, County and Municipal Employees	DC
American Health Care Association	DC
American Nephrology Nurses' Association	
American Nurses Association	DC
American Organization of Nurse Executives	DC
American Psychiatric Nurses Association	DC
American Public Health Association	
American Radiological Nurses Association	
American Society for Parenteral and Enteral Nutrition	
Association of Child and Adolescent Psychiatric Nurses, Inc.	
Association of Operating Room Nurses	CA
Association of Rehabilitation Nurses	
Baptist Hospital of East Tennessee	
Belew, John	
Bureau of Aging and In-Home Services	
California Advocates for Nursing Home Reform	CA
California Association of Hospitals and Health Systems	CA
California Nurses Association	CA
Career Nurse Assistants' Programs	DC
Catlett, Carter Williams	
Commonwealth of Pennsylvania, Department of Aging	
Connecticut Nurses Association	
Danbury Hospital Professional Nurses Association	
Davenport, Jennie	
Davis, Feather Ann	CA
East Tennessee Human Resource Agency	
Emergency Nurses Association	DC
Federation for Accessible Nursing Education and Licensure	CA
Federation of Nurses and Health Professionals	DC
Florida Nurses Association	DC
Gerontological Nursing Consulting Services	CA
Graves, Ruby	
Hannigan, Hank	CA
Harvard Medical School, Center for National Health Program Studies	DC
Harvard School of Public Health	
HBO & Company	DC
Healthcare Association of New York State	

continued on next page

TABLE 1.1 Continued

Name of Organization	Presented Testimony at Public Hearing
Illinois Nurses Association	
Intravenous Nurses Society	
Kaiser Permanente Medical Care Program	CA
Kansans for Improvement of Nursing Homes, Inc.	
Kentucky Nurses Association	
Kroposki, Margaret	
Legal Services of South Central Tennessee, Inc.	
Lewis, Nancy	
Marshall, Sarah	
Massachusetts Hospital Association	DC
Massachusetts Nurses Association	DC
Miller, Maura Farrell	
Minnesota Alliance for Health Care Consumers	
Minnesota Nurses Association	CA
Montana Coalition for Nursing Home Reform	CA
Mount St. Vincent	CA
Nagy, Mary	
National Association for Practical Nurse Education and Service, Inc.	
National Association of Hispanic Nurses	CA
National Association of Neonatal Nurses	
National Citizens' Coalition for Nursing Home Reform	DC
National Committee to Preserve Social Security and Medicare	DC
National Council of State Boards of Nursing, Inc.	DC
National League for Nursing	DC
New York City Substate Long Term Care Ombudsman Program	
New York State Nurses Association	
Nurses Organization of Veterans Affairs	
Nursing Home Advisory and Research Council, Inc.	
Nursing Home Community Coalition of New York State	
Ohio Board of Nursing	
Ohio Nurses Association	
Oliver, Pauline	
Oregon Federation of Nurses and Health Professionals	CA
Oregon Nurses Association	CA
Organization of Nurse Executives-California Organization for Nurse Leaders	CA
Parma School of Practical Nursing	
Peer Review Systems	CA
Pennsylvania Nurses Association	
Rehabilitation Care Consultants, Inc.	
Revolution	
Service Employees International Union	DC
Smith, Judy	
Stanford University Hospital	
Streeter, Janyce	
Tennessee Hospital Association	

TABLE 1.1 Continued

Name of Organization	Presented Testimony at Public Hearing
Tennessee LTC Ombudsman Program	
Texas Nurses Association	
The Children's Hospital, Denver, Colorado	
The University of Tennessee Medical Center at Knoxville	DC
Town of Amherst LTC Ombudsman Program	
Turner Healthcare Associates, Inc.	CA
Unicare Health Facilities	DC
University of California, Irvine, California Strategic Planning Committee for Nursing	CA
University of Missouri-Columbia	
Vermont Ombudsman Project	
Villa, Marina	CA
Walsh, James F. (Ombudsman, Indiana Area II)	DC
Wilder Foundation Residence West	CA

forms of public participation in the study were vital parts of the committee's fact-finding efforts.

The following section presents an overview of the concerns and issues raised in the testimony submitted to the committee. The testimony is divided into four categories: hospitals, nursing homes, nursing education, and individual comments (e.g., from academics, self-employed geriatric nurse practitioners, a nursing journal). The testimony is usually grouped by the affiliation, membership, or area of concern of the testifying organization (e.g., professional nursing organizations, hospital industry, resident advocacy groups). The concerns of the relatively few individuals and organizations that testified about both settings are included in both categories.

Hospital-Related Testimony

Nursing Personnel

Testimony presented by nursing personnel, including unions, state nurse associations, and nursing organizations formed around clinical specialties, careers, or ethnic groups, is discussed below. The following section addresses testimony from institutional providers of health care such as hospitals and hospital associations.

Unions and Union Members　With the exception of one association, all of whose members are registered nurses (RNs), the unions that testified have memberships that include RNs, licensed practical and licensed vocational nurses (LPN),[1] and nurse assistants (NA). All unions providing statements for this study noted that in their opinion, patient acuity levels are increasing and managed care is delaying hospital admissions and shortening hospital lengths of stay. In general, the unions do not take issue with the cost containment goals of restructuring hospital care, but they are concerned that these changes are being poorly implemented. Many anecdotes were provided describing the perceived negative effects of understaffing on the quality of patient care and on nurses' stress and health.

Other reports involved changes such as the sudden elimination of all positions at a certain level (e.g., all LPNs). The staff currently in those positions are told they no longer have a job, but they may apply for newly created positions at an hourly wage several dollars lower than their current wage and essentially provide the same care. Several examples of such practices were supplied in the testimony and in the committee's site visits (see later discussion).

The unions reported that, in a time of greater patient needs and shorter hospital stays, a variety of changes in staffing patterns have made it more difficult for licensed nurses to provide direct patient care. Many hospitals have established higher ratios of patients to licensed staff; others have reduced the number of supporting ancillary nursing personnel (ANP) or have replaced more highly skilled ANP with those having less training. At other locations, according to testimony, specialized nursing is being replaced with "generic" nursing: intravenous care teams are disbanded, scrub nurses in operating rooms are replaced with cursorily trained technicians, and nurses are sent to provide care on short-staffed, specialized units (e.g., pediatrics) without training or experience in that area.

In addition to concerns about the quality and safety of patient care, the unions expressed concern about the safety and quality of the workplace. Many nursing personnel stated that their work environment is unsafe for employees as well as for patients. Hospital nurses, in particular, report that rates of injuries (e.g., needlesticks, back strains) and illness (e.g., hypertension) have increased due to overwork, stress, and the need to work even if sick. These nurses also had strong feelings that hospital management is not responding to the increases in injury, illness, and stress.

Some testimony did provide examples of successful cooperation between unions and hospitals in addressing concerns. The testimony from a nurses' union and from the administration of one hospital was presented jointly. After significant difficulties over a restructuring initiative, the union and the administration used federal "mutual gains bargaining" to resolve some of their differences, with the result that they are now more able to focus, together, on patient care.

---

[1]As noted in Part I of the report, for simplicity's sake both licensed practical nurses and licensed vocational nurses will be referred to as LPNs.

State Nurse Associations State nurse associations are membership organizations of RNs; many of them also act as collective bargaining units or unions for their members. The testimony in this category was almost completely about acute care and, because of the membership composition, consisted of RN-specific experiences, perceptions, and concerns.

The widespread restructuring and downsizing within hospitals, as well as some implementations of patient-focused models of acute care delivery, are not well regarded by some RNs. Experience with these models has led them to question the value of such changes because the restructuring does not seem to benefit patients or improve the delivery of care. In the testimony, RNs' primary concerns, like those of the unionized health professionals, were about their job performance and security and their patients' safety and quality of care. Many reported being at "the end of their rope," either because they are trying to maintain the quality of care at enormous personal cost or because they are trying very hard simply to maintain a uniform level of safety. They argued that restructuring efforts are often poorly planned and implemented, and are seldom evaluated for the quality of nursing care; furthermore, there is sometimes no consultation with nurses about these changes.

Registered nurses are also unhappy with having less patient contact and more delegating and supervisory responsibilities. Several witnesses noted that the educational preparation for such managerial responsibilities is inadequate. Others pointed out that opportunities for learning on the job are now greatly reduced because many hospitals have fired their clinical nurse specialists, given their charge nurses patient care loads (sometimes full loads), and eliminated or reduced orientation programs for new nurses.

One general perception was that changes are cost driven and poorly and hastily planned; another was that no data support such changes, whereas data suggesting that higher levels of RNs improve the quality of care are felt to exist. The growth of for-profit institutions; the trend toward business, rather than medical and nursing, leadership in hospitals; and the profitability of the hospital industry were also matters for comment. Registered nurses believe they are bearing the brunt of financially motivated cost-saving efforts.

Concern was also expressed about "a loss of understanding that nursing is not a series of tasks, but an integrated process which may include a series of tasks to achieve a [patient] assessment and a [care] plan." Some witnesses worried that inflexible, task-oriented, top-down systems were being imposed on care givers who are educated to make judgments and who are ultimately responsible for care. Acuity systems for determining staffing levels, for instance, were seen as valuable tools but not more valuable than RNs' clinical judgment. Some testifiers also expressed concern that hospitals are altering the threshold on their acuity systems as a means of justifying lower staffing levels.

Both the state nurse organizations and the unions were concerned about licensed nurses' professional, legal, and ethical responsibility—and liability—for providing safe and adequate care. Under the nursing practice acts of each state, nurses are responsible for all care delivered under their supervision; furthermore, they are liable for patient abandonment if they do not accept reasonable assignments, but they must not accept unreasonable work assignments. Many state nursing organizations and unions have responded by encouraging their members to use "assignment despite protest" forms to document their concerns; this is not, however, considered a solution to the concerns about patient safety and quality of patient care. Furthermore, according to one union, some hospitals are pushing for "reinterpretation or revisions in state nurse practice acts so as to allow unlicensed personnel to perform significant nursing duties, while leaving ultimate responsibility and legal liability in nurse hands."

Most of the testimony noted the current challenges of delivering nursing care: higher levels of patient acuity; an aging population; shorter lengths of stay in which to deliver care and teach patients self-care; the use of ANP in place of RNs; and sometimes the loss of support services. Many RNs expressed concern that ANP are replacing RNs rather than supporting them, and a few mentioned that at their institution new and less knowledgeable ancillary personnel were replacing those with greater skills and better training. Others spoke of a general "de-skilling" of nursing practice.

Specific concerns about the quality of patient care included less preventive care; more "near misses," considered by many RN organizations to be a critical "invisible" indicator; inappropriate transfers to other units or to the home; and more unsafe patient loads. Another perception was reduced continuity of care, especially with the growth of cross-training, and increased reliance on floating and per diem nurses. Cross-training and floating,[2] it should be noted, are regarded as appropriate solutions for both hospitals and nurses if implemented properly, but many testifiers believe that these tactics are often poorly implemented and, as a consequence, the risks to quality of care are high.

Specific problems involving injuries, illness, and stress were also mentioned. Violence, back injuries, and the risk of infectious diseases are all serious occupational hazards. One example raised was that equipment that could prevent or minimize injuries is not being used because of cost considerations. In addition, strains on family life and personal time, job security worries and layoffs, and either mandatory overtime or days without work are significant sources of stress. Some complaints about increased stress and risks to their health came from experienced nurses who have been providing care for decades.

By and large, most representatives of the state associations expressed con-

---

[2]*Cross-training* is on-the-job training of nursing personnel to deliver specialized clinical care in an area outside their primary expertise and experience. *Floating* is the temporary assignment of nursing personnel to a clinical unit other than the one to which they are usually assigned.

cern about the deteriorating quality of patient care, job safety and security for their members, and nurses' abilities to meet their professional, legal, and ethical responsibilities in their current situations.

Nursing Organizations Formed Around Clinical Specialties, Careers, or Ethnic Groups Although most of these organizations are national in scope and organized around areas of RN clinical specialization, they form a somewhat varied group and their testimony reflected this variety. As an example, two organizations affiliated with state-level hospital associations represent the interests of nurse executives and managers. Understandably, the positions taken by these associations differ somewhat from those of the nurses in clinical specialty organizations. The testimony of the former, for instance, exhibit greater awareness of the cost pressures on hospitals and the tensions between clinical and administrative responsibilities that can be felt by nurse managers. The American Organization of Nurse Executives, which represents nurse executives and managers at the national level, made three points: (1) the "[a]dequacy of nurse staffing in hospitals and nursing homes needs to be determined in the context of the future, restructured health care delivery system—not in the context of today's needs"; (2) "[n]urse and other staffing needs are and will continue to be unique to each health care delivery organization and the community it serves. No single approach fits the needs of each situation in determining appropriate staffing levels"; and (3) "[c]urrent data on the number of nurses in institutional settings and on nursing's impact on the quality of patient care is limited."

Of the 17 organizations testifying in this group, the majority represent nurses who have a specific clinical specialization. Some organizations expressed concerns similar to those noted previously; for instance, reductions in staffing are seen as hazardous to patients and, over the long term, debilitating to nurses' abilities and health. Clinical specialty organizations tended, however, to add a broader perspective to the discussion of concerns and issues, often paying more attention to the movement of patients across sites of care delivery and the need to track patients after discharge. The need for continuity of care was a strong theme in some of the testimony and several organizations expressed confidence that cost-effectiveness considerations would demonstrate the value of nursing once factors such as rehospitalization and increased morbidity after discharge are taken into account. Some also expressed greater approval of the concept of team nursing—perhaps because nurses with clinical specialties are more likely to function as part of an established nursing team and thus to have had positive experiences with team nursing.

Finally, several of the organizations in this subgroup, such as the National Association of Neonatal Nurses and the National Association of Hispanic Nurses, noted the need for more minority RNs and higher-level nurses. This was seen as particularly important because of demographic predictions that cultural diversity and patient acuity will continue to increase nationally.

Institutional Providers of Acute Care

Organizations representing providers of acute care included two hospitals; the national association representing hospitals; three state-level chapters of the same; one health maintenance organization (HMO); and one organization with both hospital and nursing facility membership that was reporting on behalf of its hospital members.

The hospital associations, HMO, and dual membership organization provided analyses of recent changes in the delivery of acute care. This testimony was generally in agreement on two issues. First, that there have been significant changes in hospital utilization. This is a time of retrenchment, when the movement of inpatient care into outpatient settings is resulting in lowered census and fewer beds. In many states, the growth in managed care has been dramatic and some acute care hospitals have either closed or merged. Second, hospital associations were able to provide some data suggesting that despite declines in hospital utilization and the high costs of nursing labor to hospitals, RN utilization in hospitals—that is, the total number of RNs employed—has either remained constant or increased.

In general, hospital associations did not see notable changes in the levels stress felt by nursing personnel, patient satisfaction, or mortality rates. Most organizations in this category noted the lack of data on the number of nurses in institutional settings and the effect of nursing on quality of patient care. This information is not uniformly collected or linked, and often is not collected at all. Several of these organizations urged that valid and reliable patient care outcome data, particularly outcome data associated with nursing care, be collected.

Nursing Homes-Related Testimony

Resident Advocacy Groups and Long-term-Care Ombudsmen

Testimony from nursing home resident advocacy groups, family members, and long-term-care (LTC) ombudsmen exhibited great concern about poor-quality care and inadequate staffing.[3] This testimony is useful because these insights are often not available directly from residents.

Mandated tasks in a nursing home include, at a minimum, turning bed-bound residents every 2 hours and keeping them clean; getting wheelchair residents up

---

[3]Long-term care ombudsman "advocate to protect the health, safety, welfare, and rights of the institutionalized elderly" (IOM, 1995, p. 1). For more information on long-term care ombudsmen see the IOM report from which this quotation was taken: IOM. *Real People, Real Problems: An Evaluation of the Long-term Care Ombudsman Programs of the Older Americans Act.* J. Harris-Wehling, J.C. Feasley, and C.L. Estes, eds. Washington, D.C.: National Academy Press, 1995.

to exercise; giving residents adequate food and water; and assisting them in toileting. Often, however, NAs do not have time to get all of this done: "There are times I have been there when there has been only one aide on the floor with the charge nurse and the med nurse. . . . One aide isn't enough for, roughly, I would say sixty-two beds." The equipment for delivering care may also be inadequate.

Basic care is sometimes not given frequently or quickly enough—patients are often left in dirty diapers or on the toilet for extended periods of time, baths may be given infrequently, and basic dental care is sometimes forgotten. Neglect is sometimes so extreme as to become abuse. Other concerns are the lack of dignity accorded to residents in terms of not leaving them naked or exposed in public areas or respecting their wishes about daily activities such as eating and dressing. Even such simple things as providing sufficient water are often neglected. Water pitchers may be missing or out of reach. Many residents need to have water handed to them or must be reminded to drink.

Residents' family members expressed high levels of concern about neglect, unnecessary pain, endangerment, loss of health or life, and abuse. Testimony from family members sometimes mentioned unreported falls; errors such as a nondiabetic resident being given an insulin shot; and the widespread loss of bladder and bowel control by residents because aides do not have the time to toilet them.

Although much of the testimony from resident advocacy groups and LTC ombudsmen concerned examples of poor quality of care and poor quality of life for residents, overall points specific to nurse staffing levels were also made. Most of the problems with the delivery of long-term care were felt to be tied, in some way, to inadequate staffing or to inadequately trained staff.

One national organization estimated that almost half of all hospitalizations of nursing home residents could be eliminated with adequate staffing, which would save more than $942 million per year. This same organization calculated, in addition to less morbidity and pain, substantial savings of both money and time from improved levels of care and staffing. Citing annual national costs from more than $3 billion for the care of urinary incontinence to between $1.2 billion and $12 billion for preventable pressure sores, this organization argued that many of these expenses are preventable and that higher-quality care would be more cost-effective than the current approach to long-term care.

Nursing Personnel

Unions and Union Members Union concerns about nursing homes are somewhat different from those about hospitals. Structural changes and managed care do not pose immediate issues in nursing facilities; consequently, union testimony tended to focus more on concerns in acute care than in long-term care. Nevertheless, in the words of one union, "Nurses and nurse aides in nursing homes, already laboring under chronic understaffing, inadequate training, and other adversities, face growing numbers of persons discharged from hospitals, with new and more intensive needs."

Some individual union members provided examples of their concerns. One noted that at her institution an NA is typically responsible for 10 residents during the day shift. The evening shift has one NA for 13 to 18 residents, and on the overnight shift the ratio is usually one NA for 22 residents. She described how impossible it is to provide for the needs of all residents—even in such basics as turning them to prevent bed sores and providing hot food on time—with staff-to-patient ratios that low. Nevertheless, she noted, these ratios are deemed sufficient under the state's minimum required staffing levels for nursing facilities. Some of those presenting testimony attributed injuries such as back strain to inadequate staffing levels, because when facilities are understaffed nursing personnel often attempt difficult physical tasks (e.g., lifting and turning patients) with insufficient help.

Compensation levels for RNs and NAs in long-term care are low compared to those in acute care. Certified nurse assistants, in particular, are paid low wages for arduous work; consequently, turnover is high. This contributes to poor continuity of care, working short staffed, and high injury rates compared to most other occupations. To summarize, the unions appear to believe that "[w]hile adequate staffing levels in themselves do not guarantee good care, consistently good care is not possible in their absence."

Professional Nursing Organizations Formed Around Clinical Specialties or Careers   Although there were 17 testifiers from professional nursing organizations for the hospital testimony, only 1 such organization focused on nursing home care. The Career Nurse Assistants' Programs "promotes recognition, education and peer support development for experienced nurse assistants in long term care settings."

The Career Nurse Assistants' Programs (CNAP) made three points in its testimony. First, being realistic about the number of tasks any NA can perform, and therefore the number of bodies needed to provide care. The organization believes that guidelines must be developed for assigning NAs on the basis of acuity level and complexity of care, and that no NA should be required to perform more than 40 to 50 different tasks, each requiring 5 minutes or more, within a 4-hour period. The second recommendation related to NA supervision. NAs want daily direct access to a clinical supervisor who has the responsibility and time to help prompt, shape, coach, and adapt care for patients. The third recommendation concerned the issue of responsibility and authority, particularly as it relates to the new NA. Career NAs want to complement the role of trainer, not usurp it. Their tasks associated with training new nurse assistants must be clearly defined, properly assigned, and supervised.

In summary, CNAP noted, the quality-of-life experience of the resident is largely determined by the person who provides the hands-on, daily care. If the issue of quality is to be addressed, the experienced career nurse assistant should be recognized as a valuable resource and provided with a supportive work environment and the supplies necessary to the provision of care.

Providers of Care in Nursing Facilities

Three associations representing nursing facilities (two are national and one is on the state level), are discussed first. The testimony of a national chain of nursing facilities and of two individual nursing facilities is discussed later.

The three nursing facility associations agreed on several points, specifically on the challenges faced by nursing facilities and their strong opposition to mandatory minimum staffing ratios. On the first topic, the associations noted the numerous regulations and expectations confronting nursing facilities and the low reimbursement rates that make meeting those tasks so difficult. They also noted the increase in resident acuity levels, the challenges of providing subacute care, and how the levels of nursing skills and the documentation required have grown with the increase in acuity and regulation.

On the second topic, the associations articulated several arguments against minimum required staffing ratios. Both national organizations expressed the view that the use of mandatory staffing ratios would be, essentially, a step backwards: "the shift from process to outcomes embodied in OBRA [the Omnibus Budget Reconciliation Act of] 1987 was supported by both consumers and providers. Establishing required staffing ratios would reverse this and shift the emphasis back to processes." These associations expressed their general belief that there is no proven correlation between higher staffing levels and positive care outcomes. The American Health Care Association (AHCA), for instance, noted that available data suggest that staffing levels explain only a very small portion of the variation in number of "outcome-related" deficiencies issued to facilities. The following were additional arguments against minimum staffing levels:

- The leadership and management of a facility are more important to the delivery of quality care than having a specific minimum number of staff.
- It is difficult to determine what particular measure could be used to assess nurse staffing levels and skill mix in all facilities because of myriad differences in areas such as structure, patient mix, acuity levels, and state requirements.
- The health care environment continues to change every day, making it likely that any preordained staffing levels would poorly address the needs and care environments of the future.

In addition to the areas in which all three nursing home associations agreed, each individually made points that were useful to the committee's work. California has more than 400 surveyors who conduct 200 to 300 hours of inspections, annually, in each nursing facility. Despite this, the California Association of Health Facilities (CAHF) reported that reliable data about quality of care are difficult to find, especially since there is no general agreement on a definition of quality of care. Furthermore, surveys performed by state and federal surveyors provide only partially reliable information because no two surveyors perform their function in the exact same way. The California Association of Health Facilities urged that any changes to the workforce in nursing facilities take into consideration growth projections, educational opportunities, and actual workplace dynamics.

Testimony from the American Health Care Association stated that the number of nursing staff in nursing homes is adequate. Rather, turnover among NAs is the real problem. It does not believe such expenditures should be recommended by the IOM committee without supporting information that shows a correlation between greater numbers of nursing staff and higher levels of quality of care.

The American Association of Homes and Services for the Aging (AAHSA) asserted that a mission, philosophy, and principles must be established within nursing facilities; also, that care should be delivered through a team approach that relies on education, training, coaching, checking, and correction and clearly communicates the expectations of staff members. AAHSA believes that the goal of high-quality, individualized long-term care can be achieved only through "(1) continued movement toward quality of care assessment based on resident outcomes rather than process; (2) ongoing efforts to define positive outcomes within the context of [resident] populations; (3) maintenance of facilities' ability to achieve these outcomes while determining staffing needs and targeting resources based on the populations they serve; (4) the development of valid, reliable quality monitoring systems that incorporate not only clinical indicators, but also resident perceptions and satisfaction; (5) the assurance of adequate reimbursement rates by State Medicaid programs and an increase in Medicare cost limits, specifically for nurse staffing; and (6) by increasing academic awareness and opportunities for nursing experience in these long term care settings."

Unicare Health Facilities (UHF) currently operates 160 health facilities in 14 states. Their services include skilled nursing care, therapeutic and rehabilitative care, dementia units, and subacute care, as well as services in assisted living and retirement settings. Their testimony identified three challenges: (1) the need to increase staffing in skilled nursing facilities, in terms of both numbers and skill mix, as patient acuity levels continue to rise, and (2) the difficulty of considering quality-of-care outcomes across the clinical settings of hospitals and nursing homes. Computerization of the minimum data set, as mandated by the Health Care Financing Administration, should provide an opportunity to analyze a variety of factors in relation to quality outcome indicators. UHF also recommended that new studies be conducted to provide data to help design staffing models (e.g., time-motion studies based on resident acuity within the long-term-care setting).

(3) current reimbursement systems have lagged behind the delivery of care, and this has had a prohibitive effect on facilities' use of higher staff-to-residents ratios.

The testimony from UHF also reported that the organization has not seen a significant correlation between current staffing levels and either quality of care or work-related injuries and stress, probably because its facilities responded to the needs of higher-acuity residents with higher staffing ratios. UHF believes that a great deal of additional research and analysis of existing data are needed.

Two different examples of restructured nursing facilities, both of which reported that these changes were essentially cost-neutral, were provided in testimony to the committee. The first was from Robert Ogden, representing the Mt. St. Vincent Nursing Home; the second was from Jan Olson, speaking on behalf of Wilder Residence West.

Robert Ogden described how a 200-bed nursing facility at the Mt. St. Vincent Nursing Home was restructured both physically and programatically to shift the emphasis toward "resident-directed" services. He believes that long-term-care services should meet the needs and wants of residents, not of regulations, facility management, or physicians. He noted that this may not sound radical but that it is, in fact, a major change for staff to truly internalize and act on this new perspective.

Ogden believes that the use of nurse assistants or aides is a critical aspect of long-term care and stressed that nurse aides are the key to both quality of life and quality of care. He believes that the ratios of NAs need to be changed, and he also strongly urged that their title in nursing facilities be changed from nurse aides, or nursing assistants, to resident assistants. Along with such a change, he recommends training. At his facility, NAs are required to have 12 hours of continuing education each year. To make this possible, the facility brings in replacement staff. Ogden concluded by noting that at present, when acuity cannot really be used to set staffing levels, he and his facility feel the need for regulations that require some kind of minimum staffing levels of resident assistants or nurse assistants.

Jan Olson described a new model of care delivery that was implemented on the 50-bed Wilder Residence West unit. It changed nursing care from a task-oriented system to a resident-oriented system by assigning primary nurses and their associates ongoing responsibility to care for a designated group of residents. The number of hours of care did not increase, but the skill mix did; the percentage of licensed staff coverage over a 24-hour period increased from 24 to 38 percent at the time of implementation and to 45 percent when the testimony was submitted. Olson noted that the increase of licensed staff is perceived as having improved quality of care and of life for residents and quality of work for staff, while remaining cost-effective. Ongoing data collection supports this assertion, documenting notable reductions in the use of restraints and antipsychotic drugs; a dramatic decrease in hospitalization rates; high resident satisfaction rates, along with reduced staff turnover rates; and high levels of success with various forms of rehabilitation despite a continuously rising acuity level and an average resident age of 91 years.

Education-related Testimony

Most education-related testimony either was site neutral or focused on the hospital setting. In general, if organizations discussed hospital restructuring, cost containment efforts, and the use of ANP, they agreed with the concerns raised in testimony from other hospital-focused nursing groups. Unlike the prior grouping of testimony, however, the seven organizations in this category have fairly varied perspectives on nursing education and practice. None of these education-focused groups addressed the training needs of NAs and ANP, probably because these health care workers are not among their membership. Testimony provided by the Career Nurse Assistants Program did provide the committee with general comments on the educational and training needs of NAs and LPNs and suggestions on how to organize and provide continuing education to NAs.

The American Association of Colleges of Nursing (AACN) represents nursing education programs at universities and 4-year colleges, so its concerns are baccalaureate and graduate education, nursing research, and the development of academic leaders. In its testimony, AACN explicitly considered the bachelor's degree in nursing "the critical first step to a professional nursing career" and supported it as "the minimum educational requirement for professional nursing practice." The AACN also offered an agenda for nursing education in the twenty-first century, noting that schools of nursing must redefine the role and rewards of nursing scholarship to include nursing practice in an expanding array of settings, as well as nursing theory. The movement from delivering services in acute care settings to delivering them in outpatient and home-based settings also implies a need to retrain and redeploy health care professionals in the future.

The Federation for Accessible Nursing Education and Licensure (FANEL) represents the educational interests of "nurses" defined more broadly to include LPNs and RNs with associate degrees or diplomas. In contrast to the AACN, FANEL advocates recognition of the value of different, coexisting levels of education: "There is a wide spectrum of health care needs which can be met more cost efficiently if there is a choice of educational programs to enable anyone, regardless of economic or social condition, to enter the program that best fits that person's situation. Then, upon entering the workforce they can render valuable services and through articulation can go on into advanced nursing, *if they so choose* [emphasis in original]." Expressing concern that funds for diploma and associate degree programs for educating nurses might be diverted into baccalaureate programs, FANEL noted that this would be "highly unjustified" and provided information to demonstrate that nurses without RN baccalaureate degrees, as well as those with them, can provide critical types of care and meet high levels of competency and responsibility.

Testimony from the Parma School for Practical Nursing seconded FANEL's point, adding that practical nursing programs also provide "experienced, pre-screened" individuals a way to finance their RN education. The National Association for Practical Nurse Education and Service (NAPNES), an organization with the mission of promoting the standards of practical nursing education and practice, also noted that "[m]ultiplicity of choice in nursing programs will continue to attract citizens from all backgrounds and educational preparation. This diversity will reflect the broad spectrum of patients and nursing needs."

The National Council of State Boards of Nursing (NCSBN) and the Ohio Board of Nursing (OBN) are organizations charged with the regulation of nursing practice. State boards of nursing are created by statute to administer the licenses of RNs and LPNs in accordance with a state's nurse practice act, and complaints against licensed nursing personnel would be filed with state boards. The NCSBN testimony emphasized the value of licensing as "a mechanism to assure the public of the competence of the licensee to practice safely and effectively." The testimony from OBN agreed with this and also noted that the concept of delegation is becoming critical. According to OBN, boards of nursing "must define and regulate delegation by rule language and enforce disciplinary action when there is non-compliance."

The National League for Nursing (NLN) considered nursing practice from a policy and research perspective rather than a regulatory one. Expressing concern about the effects on nursing practice of staffing models that are task oriented and prescribed, NLN urged the articulation of a "clear and universal definition of nursing practice" and the development and use of outcome measures of nursing practice, rather than of nursing tasks or process. The design of staffing models should recognize the "central role and accountability of the clinical nurse in achieving optimal outcomes for patients and families."

A few unions raised the issue of education; they expressed concern that the swift national movement from inpatient to outpatient care leaves many nursing personnel unprepared to provide care in the settings where it will have to be provided. Reeducation and retraining in primary and preventive care, and advanced education at the clinical specialist or nurse practitioner levels, were seen as solutions. Other issues were a lack of qualified faculty in some regions and salary levels for faculty that are lower than hospital salaries. As far as continuing their education, some instances were cited in which staff RNs have been unable to attend mandatory in-service programs because of low staffing levels and were (understandably) very unhappy later to be rebuked in performance reviews for those absences.

Testimony from Observers

Other observers include individual testifiers and a nursing journal; academics and representatives of universities; self-employed nurses, such as gerontological nurse practitioners; and consulting groups. Individual testifiers—for the most part either nursing personnel or people whose relatives were in nursing homes—expressed some of the same concerns as the state nurse associations, unions, resident advocates, and consulting groups. The nursing journal testimony provided a critique of the current changes in nurse staffing, including mandatory floating, mandatory overtime, unsafe nurse-to-patient ratios, retaliation against nurses who object to changes, and increased use of unlicensed assistive personnel.

The testimony from four academics or university representatives made several different points. One presented information on a state-level strategic plan for summarizing data about the current nurse supply and predicting the future need for RNs in California. Another argued strongly that current staffing levels for direct care are insufficient while staffing levels for administrative tasks are excessive. Testimony from another academic presented information on the implementation, at a large nursing facility, of a professional practice and participatory management model for nursing. This model resulted in reduced mortality, despite increases in resident acuity, as well as high levels of job satisfaction for staff nurses and nurse managers. The final academic testimony emphasized the effects on decisions about nurse staffing of the changing economic incentives experienced by hospitals.

Testimony from consulting groups addressed several broad areas. Two consulting firms were data-focused organizations whose primary clients were acute care institutions. One of these firms emphasized the value of data analysis, while the other discussed the opportunities provided by sophisticated information and documentation systems. This second firm argued that in addition to the goal of cutting costs, a true restructuring of hospital care requires a deep commitment to reinventing delivery processes and to removing inefficiencies and redundancies so as to improve patient care.

The remaining three consulting groups are nurse consultant organizations concerned with long-term care. One articulated the need for skilled management, upgrading of employee education and supervision, and role modeling. The second argued that nurses are complaining without data to back them up and that there are no data or correlations between staffing ratios and any of the following concerns: poor patient outcomes, decreased quality of care, or decreased well-being of nurses. Rather, this testimony strongly stated, an evolving health care environment is requiring nurses to take responsibility for decisions about, and the implementation of, change. The final testimony from a consulting group offered the committee a research-based staffing methodology and urged the use of case-mix classifications systems to determine the nursing needs of specific nursing facility residents. This testimony also argued for reimbursement based on resident classification systems that (1) are evaluated systematically for the adequacy of nursing time and (2) require facilities to use funds allocated on the basis of high acuity to increase staffing.

Concluding Remarks on Testimony

The IOM committee did not look to the testimony for quantitative data. Indeed, many of those affected by proposed or implemented staffing changes—hospital patients, nurse assistants, hospital and nursing home administrators, managed care organizations, licensed practical nurses, and others—were not necessarily represented through the submitted testimony in numbers commensurate with their potential interests. Rather, as noted above, the testimony provided the study with a rich set of materials representing a broad range of opinions, expertise, and experience in the matters under consideration. The hearings additionally represented an opportunity for interested parties to express their views directly to committee members, respond to committee members' requests for clarification or additional information, and reply to other panelists with different positions on some of the issues.

The submitted documents and statements enriched and broadened the study by greatly informing the committee's deliberations, helping committee members to understand better the concerns of specific groups, and alerting them to additional issues. The committee is grateful for the insights provided, and it acknowledges the generosity of time and effort of those who prepared and contributed to the testimony.

SITE VISITS CONDUCTED BY THE COMMITTEE

This section describes site visits conducted by the IOM committee. Because members bring diverse backgrounds and experience to the committee, site visits are often used to educate them, give them common reference points, and help them develop some collective understanding on a variety of issues. Site visits also provide vivid circumstances and specific instances that can be extremely useful during committee discussions. During the fall and winter of 1994–1995, therefore, site visits were a central activity of the IOM committee.

A principal objective of these visits was to increase the committee's understanding of the issues of nurse staffing levels and skill mixes, quality of patient care, and nurses' work-related stress and injuries. The visits were an opportunity for committee members to benefit from the experiences and opinions of those directly involved in the questions posed by the study's mandate. Because individual locales (as well as organizations and individuals) were chosen for the insights they could provide, the site visits were not intended to result in a broad, quantitative analysis of national nurse staffing patterns. Rather, the visits sensitized committee members to a broad range of issues and informed them, in rich detail, about myriad points of view.

Approach

The committee conducted intensive site visits in Mississippi, Missouri, New York, and Oregon between November 1994 and March 1995. Site visit teams were usually composed of four committee members and one staff member, and the visits usually consisted of 2 full days of meetings with host facilities, agencies, and individuals in specific regions. The states to be visited were chosen by committee members at the first committee meeting. The specific organizations and individuals with which the site visit teams met were chosen on the basis of suggestions from members of the committee, various interest groups, and the liaison panel, and on the basis of staff research. An effort was made to achieve representation of

- geographic areas of the country (e.g., urban, suburban, and rural areas and the four census regions);
- a range of health care delivery environments in hospitals and nursing facilities (e.g., from areas with high rates of managed care to those in which managed care is minimally present);
- a variety of facilities and institutions in terms of size, ownership and governance, organization of health care delivery, and other characteristics; and
- a wide sampling of local professional groups, associations, and individuals concerned about the issues in the committee's mandate.

Overall, the committee heard a broad range of perspectives, including (but not limited to) staff and management at hospitals and nursing homes; representatives and members of labor unions, professional organizations, and the business community; state-level hospital and nursing home associations; federal and state government officials; nursing home residents, their family members, and resident advocacy groups; and nurse educators in a range of educational institutions.

A "typical" site visit would include (1) 2 ½-hour visits to 2 hospitals and 2 nursing homes and (2) shorter appointments with others such as health care professionals, state regulators, patients, and educators.[4] The committee members held a total of 41 meetings and spoke with approximately 350 people in a variety of settings. During site visits the committee members referred to an interview guide developed by staff but were also led by their own interests and those of the groups being visited.

---

[4]The specific facilities, organizations, and individuals visited by the site visit team were promised confidentiality. For this reason, descriptive information rather than names and locations is used here.

General Issues in Health Care Delivery

Information derived from site visits documented several broad issues: increasing patient acuity-of-care needs; an aging population; the movement from inpatient to outpatient delivery of care; and cost containment approaches to the delivery of care, which ranged from managed care to low Medicaid reimbursement rates to the "restructuring" being undertaken in many hospitals.

Both acute care and long-term-care settings reported increased acuity levels and the need for higher intensities of services in the past few years. This change in the needs of the patient populations was attributed to several factors, including the aging of the U.S. population. For acute care settings, a primary reason cited in the facilities visited was the change in lengths of stay and the incentives to delay admissions. A significant change in the kinds of illness presented has also altered hospital acuity levels. In some regions, many cases of AIDS and drug-resistant tuberculosis and an increase in the numbers of trauma patients have compounded the general increases in acuity levels.

Similar issues—changes in the kinds of residents, their acuity of illness, and age and comorbidities—were also described in nursing facilities. The staff at some facilities pointed out, first, that many or most of their residents have been in the facility for a while and are "aging in place," and, second, that they are getting more short-term rehabilitative patients discharged from the hospital and more patients classified as "subacute." This means that nursing homes are now receiving people with such care needs as in-house kidney dialysis, tracheotomy care, and intravenous pain management; 10 or 15 years ago, these patients would have remained in an acute care setting.

Alternative models for delivering long-term care, such as increased placement of the elderly in community-based care settings, are extensively used in some areas. This also increases the acuity level in nursing homes because the existence of alternate forms of long-term-care services essentially results in the selection of relatively healthier persons for placement elsewhere. Consequently, higher concentrations of severely ill or debilitated individuals can be found in nursing facilities.

In some urban areas, the age groups served appear to be expanding. Urban facilities are providing chronic, but intense, care to younger populations, in part because of AIDS and violent trauma. Another specific reason for the increased acuity is the closing of mental hospitals. Whatever the various causes, however, the concentration of high-acuity residents—those who need extensive help with eating and elimination and are less mobile; those who have greater psycho-behavioral problems; and those with intravenous pumps, oxygen concentrators, and other such devices—is straining the staff and, at times, the physical plant of nursing facilities.

Managed care and other cost containment efforts are also greatly affecting the environment in which health care is delivered. Hospitals are currently feeling the immediate effects of these pressures, but managed care for Medicaid patients is starting to affect nursing home residents. Committee members heard some concern that managed care for Medicaid patients may mean, for long-term care, more focus on cost, a lower priority for quality, and, therefore, the possibility of further reductions in staffing levels.

Staffing Issues

The ability of institutions to recruit and retain nursing staff has changed in recent years. In both acute care and nursing facilities, positions for RNs and, to some extent, LPNs are generally filled without much problem. Retention rates for nurse assistants, however, particularly in nursing facilities, are often poor. The sections below draw a picture of recruiting and retention issues in hospitals and nursing homes.

Staffing Issues in Hospitals

Hospital staffing ratios are usually determined by the administrative staff of an individual facility or of the health care system with which the hospital is affiliated. Consequently, in acute care, many approaches are used in determining the levels of staff needed and scheduled. These approaches can be broadly divided into census-based systems and acuity-based systems, although most staffing systems combine aspects of both. A true census-based system for determining staffing is one in which the number of patients determines staffing levels. An acuity-based system is one in which the patient's health status and needs are rated to help determine staffing levels.

In general, most of those with whom the committee met were not in favor of across-the-board mandated minimum staffing ratios (i.e., ratios based only on census levels) not only because individual patients' health status and needs can differ broadly, but also because each hospital differs in terms of the population served and organizational variables. The number of nursing staff required, for example, will be affected by available support systems as well as by patient acuity levels and medical practices. These systems include such components as medication administration technology, transportation and messenger services, and computerized information systems. During site visits the development and use of patient classification systems based on acuity levels were frequently mentioned as the most desirable approach to determining staffing levels. Site visit teams also heard concerns from several different groups of hospital nursing staff about the fact that some hospitals have "backtracked" from an acuity-based system to a census-based system for determining staffing levels.

In urban areas, RN positions are infrequently vacant because of a number of changes in recent years, not the least of which are various cost containment and efficiency models that have resulted in the downsizing and restructuring of hospitals and comparatively high RN salaries in acute care settings. Those salaries have led the administrative levels of hospitals to put pressure on nursing management to find and use care providers, such as NAs, who are cheaper than RNs. Several hospitals reported experiencing high turnover rates among NAs.

Committee members saw a variety of alternative models for delivering care and reengineering the delivery of nursing services. These included cuts in staff positions (either direct cuts or through attrition), implementation of team nursing, movement of some RNs into float pools, and use of "flexing"—(e.g., sending nurses home or calling them in partway through a shift). Until recently, facilities in some areas relied heavily on recruiting foreign-trained RNs. With one notable exception among the group of hospitals visited, these facilities are no longer actively recruiting from other countries to fill their positions and are not experiencing great difficulties in recruiting and retaining RNs. In fact, the overall supply of LPNs and RNs in hospitals appears sufficient, and new RN graduates are having difficulty finding jobs because facilities prefer to hire experienced RNs.

RNs and LPNs reacted to the changes in the way acute care is delivered—the restructuring and new models of patient care delivery—with strong concern about the quality and safety of future care. For some of those interviewed, this concern extended to the belief that current levels of care are a threat to the quality of patient care. Others believed that the overall quality of patient care is being maintained, but at a high personal and professional cost to nursing staff that cannot be sustained indefinitely.

Staffing Issues in Nursing Facilities

Three staffing issues for nursing facilities are notable: turnover and retention rates for NAs; adequacy of staffing levels, particularly in light of increasing patient acuity; and reimbursement levels for care. These issues did not differ dramatically from site to site because federal regulations have a significant and fairly uniform effect on both staffing and reimbursement levels. Nevertheless, labor markets, regulatory environments, and state reimbursement policies did differ by site; consequently, recruitment and retention also vary somewhat.

Almost all nursing facilities visited reported high turnover rates among NAs. As mandated by federal regulations, states and facilities provide training and certification for nursing-home-based NAs. Once trained and certified, however, these NAs often chose to leave long-term-care for positions in hospitals, which can afford to pay a little more per hour. Still other NAs leave the health care industry entirely when other jobs become available. Committee members heard reports of NAs leaving health care for retail jobs when a K-Mart opened or to waitress or clean in locations where the tourist industry was growing. In some areas the redesign of hospital staffing is causing NAs to move into acute care at a greater rate, which is increasing the demand for NAs in long-term care.

The need for more staff, particularly NAs, was expressed almost universally.

Many NAs try to provide good care but there are not enough of them, particularly on weekends when staffing ratios are lower and getting people out of bed, giving baths, and other care tasks may be omitted. The same kinds of problems noted in the written and oral testimony were reported during some of the site visits: patients not being turned as required to prevent bed sores, being left on the toilet for prolonged periods, or not having their physiological needs attended to on time. Furthermore, the staffing levels mandated in some states were reported to have little relevance to the level of patient needs and work at most of the facilities visited.

In economically depressed areas, many of the NAs in nursing facilities hold permanent second jobs, either as NAs in other facilities or in retail settings. Their incomes as NAs are sometimes less than those they could receive as welfare recipients. Frequently, NAs must worry about child care. At one site, NAs could not afford health insurance coverage offered by the facility because it would cost approximately 75 percent of their salary; they were better off if they and their children were eligible to receive Medicaid.

Working as an NA is physically and emotionally grueling; it is hard physical labor for comparatively low compensation. Not surprisingly, NA turnover is one of the most pressing issues facing those who deliver long-term care. Even at facilities where NAs were fairly satisfied with working conditions, turnover rates were still 50 to 70 percent. Nationally, some facilities have annual turnover rates as high as 200 percent, and at most facilities a cycle of recruiting, hiring, and providing the mandated training to new NAs never ends. Consequently, facilities are not always very selective and do not always perform such quality control measures as criminal record checks on applicants.

In general, what site visit teams seemed to hear was that delivering care was much more difficult because of the increase in patient acuity and other factors, including the higher concentrations of extremely ill residents in nursing homes resulting from new care options such as board and care, home health, and hospital subacute units. Nevertheless, many NAs were doing what they could to deliver, despite static staffing levels and rising needs, at least a basic level of care.

Site visit teams heard reasons NAs continue to work at a facility. By and large, retention of NAs occurs despite low salary levels and little opportunity for advancement. Of those who stay, a personal commitment to the residents is often one of the primary reasons for doing so. Leaving is not, however, only a response to salary levels or to physical and emotional demands—"life events," such as the NA moving or seeking further education, are also factors. Nevertheless, it seemed as though those who stay have found sources of satisfaction and pride: one woman who had been an NA at a single facility for more than 20 years said "to me, a CNA [certified nurse assistant] is a high ranking people in a nursing home," while another noted that although she is injured and will never be able to do the full range of work she used to, she has an important educational role: "the younger ones come to me for help."

Different facilities have taken innovative approaches to recruiting and retaining NAs. One facility tries to assign NAs to residents on a permanent basis. Another has an NA leadership position that allows for recognition of the knowledge and achievements of senior NAs. Other approaches include tracking NA job satisfaction, offering health benefits to part-time employees, and providing financial assistance in becoming a licensed nurse. In contrast, most of the nursing facilities visited experienced relatively few problems with turnover of RNs and LPNs.

Quality of Patient Care and Quality of Life

Site visit teams heard many anecdotes about how inadequate staffing levels and mixes have threatened or diminished the quality of patient care. Many specific factors considered either to increase or to dilute the quality of care were mentioned and are discussed below. One issue applicable in all settings, however, is the need to meet the cultural and language needs of patients and residents.

Quality of Patient Care and Patient Life in Hospitals

Acute care institutions had quite varied responses to what sounded to the committee like fairly similar concerns about the quality of patient care and the costs of delivering care. The following example provides specific details of how one hospital changed the delivery of nursing services in order to improve the quality of patient care.

One of the committee's teams visited an acute care hospital that had recently restructured the delivery of nursing care. This facility operates in an area with high levels of managed care and has 5-year goals of maintaining and improving quality, decreasing costs, and shifting from inpatient to outpatient programs.

When committee members visited this hospital system, they saw the first test unit in which a new model for patient care had been implemented. Before implementation, 18 months were spent in planning. Job classifications were reduced from 80 or 90 to approximately 8, and service associate (SA) positions were developed. Three-person teams composed of an SA, an RN, and either a CNA or an LPN were formed to deliver care on the test unit. These changes were staff- and budget-neutral; the purpose was to make better use of nursing personnel.

High levels of staff participation and representation were reported in planning for use of the new patient care delivery model. Each test unit had its own implementation team, and techniques such as surveys, shadowing, and focus groups were used for planning purposes. A notable amount of time and money was also budgeted to train the teams. Registered nurses, for example, reported initially needing considerable coaching in delegation and supervision, and SAs needed to learn hospital policies and procedures, as well as ergonomic principles.

All participants in the 4-week competency-based training module received large amounts of training in team building skills, including conflict resolution.

Some RNs had negative responses to the proposed changes before the new patient care model was implemented. Registered nurse tenures at the 2 campuses in this facility were 7 and 10 years, respectively, and some RNs did resign before implementation of the model. The RNs, LPNs, CNAs, and SAs with whom committee members spoke, however—whether already delivering care in teams or anticipating this change—appeared genuinely enthusiastic about the new model. The consensus, among both nursing and administrative staff, was that the new approach, along with many specific organizational or structural changes, allowed nursing staff to concentrate on patients and provide better-quality care.

Each team with an LPN was typically assigned 7 or 8 patients, while a team with a CNA would be assigned 6 patients; on a 12-hour shift, the total number of patients would go no higher than 10. Members of the care teams almost always work together and plan their shifts together, deciding among themselves whether to work four 12-hour shifts or five 8-hour shifts. They report knowing each others' capabilities well, trusting in and relying on each other, and cooperating to accomplish tasks. The satisfaction and enthusiasm of team members were most impressive, as was their acknowledgment of each individual's part in providing care.

The administrative staff with whom committee members met were cautiously optimistic, while the nursing personnel were extremely enthusiastic. Morale was high, and there appeared to be a pervasive conviction that the quality of patient care had improved. Even though the plan was staff-neutral, nursing staff spoke of feeling as though there were more staff than before implementation of the new model. All levels of team members reported feeling less stress and being more confident about the care delivered, because of the trust and communication among the three members of the team. More patient teaching was reported, and RNs reported feeling secure that in a time of crisis with a patient, other patients would be taken care of and they would be notified if an additional patient needed their attention. In terms of patients' responses to the change, staff related anecdotes of patients returned to the hospital demanding "their" care team and of positive comments from patients who had been on the unit prior to implementation of the new approach and could therefore compare the two models of care delivery. Administrative staff confirmed that patient responses were positive.

In conclusion, this new patient care model was instigated by the top levels of the health care system to improve the quality of care delivered. The leadership appears to have successfully created a system and environment in which a reorganization of patient services could take place that improved both the quality of patient care and the morale. Key factors identified by participants in this process were keeping staff aware of planned changes, involving them in decision making aspects of the new model, empowering the care giving staff, and leadership from top levels. The patient care model is still being improved; anxiety about the new model no doubt remains for some personnel, as do the stresses of transition. Additional facets of the plan have to be improved or clarified, such as ways of increasing communication along some lines (e.g., among teams or between teams and charge nurses). Nevertheless, care giver satisfaction with, and commitment to, the new patient care delivery model appear extremely high, and preliminary indications are that patient satisfaction has also noticeably improved. At the time of the site visit, the entire hospital system was expected to have converted to the new care model by 1 to 2 years after the first unit-level test of the new model began. Pre-implementation evaluations and two evaluations conducted during the implementation process should eventually provide data upon which to base an assessment of the model's success.

The level of involvement of nursing personnel in the shaping and implementation of change seems to account for some of the critical differences in the success of institutional restructuring. Based on insights provided by the site visits, hospitals appear more likely to be successful in restructuring when all or most of the following is true:

- the top management levels of the institutions provide a strong vision, clear goals, and steady commitment to the reorganization;
- nursing staff have the time and the opportunity to discuss with management both the goals of restructuring care and the ways in which these might be met;
- nursing staff have autonomy and accountability in the delivery of care;
- top management is open to discussion and suggestions and negotiates in good faith; and
- reorganizations focus on improving the quality of patient care rather than on cost-cutting measures (e.g., are budget- and staff-neutral).

Collaborative change, where successful, resulted in visible confidence among the nursing staff in their ability to deliver quality care, unusually high levels of trust and teamwork, and clearer responsibility for the quality of patient care. In situations where relations between administration and health professionals appeared particularly bad, top-level administrators may have given insufficient value to nursing and not included nursing staff in the strategic plan processes at a decision making level.

Quality of Patient Care and Patient Life in Nursing Facilities

One factor that can positively affect the quality of patient care in long-term care is RN clinical leadership. Physicians have a minimal presence in most nursing homes, and the number of RNs in a facility is extremely low compared to other nursing staff; despite the high levels of acuity in most nursing homes, nationally RNs comprise less than 10 percent of the total nursing staff in long-term-care facilities. Some site visit hosts believed that RNs' administrative and documentation responsibilities reduce the quality of patient care because RNs spend the majority of their time on paperwork rather than with residents. Combined, these factors lead to a deficiency of clinical expertise, minimal direct resident care by RNs or physicians, and lack of RN supervision and clinical leadership for LPNs and NAs. One facility seen by a site visit team used clinical nurse specialists to address these concerns and to implement programs such as a restraint reduction effort.

The extremely high turnover of NAs also exacerbates quality-of-care problems. NAs are the residents' primary care givers. According to some NAs with whom committee members met, LPNs provide little supervision and are unable to deliver adequate clinical support and care. Despite the fact that NAs spend the most time with residents and know them best, they have little or no input into residents' care plans.

Resident comfort is also an element of high-quality care. When one group of residents was asked what they valued, they cited security, medical care and the availability of physicians, and private rooms. (Residents may share a room with as many as three other people.) Other residents wanted more staff and more experienced staff on the night shift. At most of the sites visited by committee members, residents with whom the site visit teams met reported the care to be either good or adequate.

Yet another issue in the areas of quality of care and quality of life involves the assumptions and expectations of family members. Some care givers pointed out with frustration that a demanding individual or active family member can result in fairly elaborate attention being devoted to one resident, while someone who cannot speak up or has no family nearby—but who requires more care—may be shortchanged on basic care. On the other hand, site visit teams were sometimes informed that scheduled visits by inspectors or family members typically present a reassuring picture but that unannounced visits can be a different matter. If visitors are not expected, care may be limited or inadequate. Yet residents and family members are often afraid to complain for fear—whether realistic or not—of retaliation from care givers. At a meeting with LTC ombudsmen, site visit team members heard some grim stories of neglect, intimidation, abuse, and theft. The stories pointed out the many ways in which both the quality and the quantity of staff in nursing facilities can directly affect the quality of care and quality of life for residents.

Another quality-of-care point that was raised frequently in nursing home visits is that the current survey process and standards can override the clinical judgment of care givers and negatively affect the quality of patient care and quality of life. In at least one example recounted to the site visit team, the problem seems to have been rote enforcement of the OBRA guidelines without permitting the facility to explain the rationale for the restraint or discuss the resident's care plan and without consultation with the resident's family members.

Finally, a few of the larger, more diversified long-term-care facilities are starting to use outcome measures of quality of care that will be meaningful to managed care entities; these include admissions to the hospital or emergency room, length of stay, and resident and family satisfaction.

Injuries and Stress

In general, discussions during site visits were more about stress than injuries. Information on injuries is equivocal. Some hospitals and nursing homes are maintaining or reducing rates of problems such as back injuries, needlestick incidents, and nosocomial infections. Other facilities expressed concern that injury rates have been reduced through education and training but will soon rise again because of the physical demands of nursing the current resident populations.

Nursing personnel are more subject to injuries than other workers; this is particularly true of NAs who work in nursing homes where many residents must be turned, lifted, or assisted in their toileting. Nevertheless, a noticeable number of facilities and nursing personnel did not seem to be concerned about traditional work-related injuries, probably because they are taking steps to reduce these. Such steps include the use of back supports when lifting, as well as educational programs, and the results seem to indicate that such efforts are often effective in reducing back injury rates.

A possible solution to the physical demands of providing long-term care is the provision of equipment and the use of technology. When NAs at one site were asked to list the equipment they would like to have, their wishes appeared surprisingly modest: hospital beds, bathtubs, shower chairs, bedside commodes, bed linen with rubber backing, and adult diapers were all mentioned as equipment that staff needed but often did not have. At first glance, these technologies might seem relatively unlikely to affect injury rates but the NAs explained that many of them do reduce the physical strain of caring for and lifting residents. Aides were open to the possibility of more technologically sophisticated equipment but were more aware of the basic tools they lacked.

Stress appears to affect nursing staff in a variety of ways. In acute care settings at least, anger, frustration, and confusion about restructuring and cost-cutting measures were often evident. It appeared to committee members that lack of empowerment or participation in the planning and implementation of restructuring, combined with uncertainty about their jobs or new responsibilities, clearly increased the stress level among nurses.

Many licensed nurses in acute care were concerned about the use of ANP, particularly since they are held responsible for the care provided by these unlicensed staff whether or not they are the ANP's supervisors. Committee members also heard reports of mandatory overtime and double shifts being common on weekends. "Floating" from one unit to another and reduced staffing levels because some staff are out on sick leave were frequently mentioned sources of stress, even at institutions with fairly satisfactory staffing levels. Even under good conditions and with sufficient training to establish the familiarity and competence of floating nurses, nursing personnel usually hate floating, often because of strong concerns about the quality of patient care that they can deliver when they are shifted from one location and one type of care to another.

Many of the complaints to LTC ombudsmen about care delivered in nursing facilities concern the inadequacy of staff, particularly at night and on weekends. Other complaints involve patient abuse. Many of those interviewed believed that abuse is most likely when nursing personnel are understaffed or are taking care of unfamiliar residents. Complaints to ombudsmen often result in formal surveys by the state units that handle licensure and certification; the survey process is a mechanism for identifying inadequate care that can result in the issuance of statements of deficiencies against facilities.

More generally, patient acuity levels are up in long-term-care facilities, and staffing levels are insufficient; this situation is compounded by turnover rates that leave staff habitually working shorthanded. Not surprisingly, overall staff stress is high. Specific sources of stress for NAs are lack of time, constant turnover of staff, inadequate time to orient and help new staff, and the addition of unpredictable, poorly prioritized tasks to their responsibilities.

As noted earlier, many facilities and staff in highly urban areas are concerned about the vulnerability of nursing staff to increased stress and injury inflicted by patients. The increase in patient violence toward nurses seems to be more prevalent in settings where a general societal increase in violence and other social ills is evident (e.g., emergency rooms, municipal hospitals, psychiatric units, and nursing home dementia units). The increased violence appears most likely to occur when care is being provided to prisoners, drug abusers, the homeless, and the mentally ill. The level of experience and training of the care provider becomes an issue in these situations. Sometimes the danger is augmented because a less prepared provider is unable to control a situation or does not have the assessment skills to identify such a situation far enough in advance to avoid conflict. A few facilities reported that nonviolent crisis intervention is taught to all emergency room staff.

Reimbursement Issues

Most reimbursement issues raised to committee members were concerned with long-term care. Medicare and Medicaid reimbursement rates are seldom sufficient to cover the actual costs of providing care and can easily be half the average costs. For this reason, private-pay residents are preferred. The rates charged private-pay residents differ widely by facility, region, and resident, but they ranged in just one facility from $27,600 to $59,000 per year. Inadequate reimbursement from Medicaid also makes it difficult for administrators to get physicians into the facilities for routine, required visits to Medicaid patients.

The response of one facility to financial concerns was to set a goal of converting the entire facility into a subacute unit, which yields better (Medicare) reimbursement rates that the current (Medicaid) payments for long-term-care residents. Two facilities, in contrast, were very diversified; they offered many services such as a profitable home health agency or assisted living facility; educational programs, consultations, and workshops; on-site, ongoing NA training; and a day care center. Such facilities may also be seeking more managed care contracts, which some facility administrators consider critical for future financial stability.

Some hosts argued that the current system for reimbursement needs to be improved because it offers no motivation or reward for providing restorative or preventive nursing care. They recommended that the base reimbursement rate be tied to acuity (e.g., activity-of-daily-living factors) and that incentive payments be given for achieving positive outcomes. These outcomes should not necessarily be limited to improvements in health; the avoidance of poor outcomes (e.g., low decubitus, incontinence, or hospitalization rates) should also be considered.

Education

Throughout the site visits, the topic of education—whether initial, continuing, clinical, academic, or managerial—was frequently raised. The majority of those interviewed on site visits felt that the educational preparation of new RNs is insufficient. Assessment skills may be adequate but judgment, experience, knowledge of medications, and leadership and delegation skills are lacking. The need for baccalaureate-prepared RNs was noted by both educators and nursing leaders. Some spoke of the need for nurses in intensive care units to be trained with 6-month internships after graduation. Many mentioned that new graduates need more rehabilitation and geriatrics in their educational program, and some expressed the opinion that 2-year associate degree programs are inadequate to prepare nurses for their roles in the current evolving health care system. Adequate preparation is especially necessary when nurses have to plan the care for patients who require exceptional assessment.

According to some staff nurses in hospitals, one difficulty facing new RN graduates is that they simply have not been prepared for the work. Their schooling is mostly theoretical, and these staff nurses felt that neither associate degree nor bachelor's degree RNs have received the necessary preparation and orientation. Educators, in contrast, point out that changes in the delivery of acute care have exacerbated the difficulty of the transition from school to work because facilities no longer have time to teach new staff, and often those who used to teach them (e.g., staffing coordinators, clinical nurse specialists) have heavy patient loads or have been dismissed.

The need for clinical leadership for nursing personnel and for educational preparation and training was a topic that recurred several times and across settings. Registered nurses' difficulties in delegation and the importance of being good nurse managers were noted. Some nurses spoke of the role of the RN "becoming expensive" and the need to maximize these nurses by delegating functions to others such as LPNs and NAs whom RNs would then supervise. It was suggested at more than one site visit that RNs need to be explicitly instructed in delegation, management, and supervision and that these subjects ought to be in the curriculum of the educational program.

On the topic of NA training, several CNAs who had worked as uncertified NAs while attending certification classes believed that this combination of learning and experience prepared them better than only attending classes would have. They also pointed out that it might be an efficient way to "weed out" those student NAs who would not continue working in long-term care once they experienced the day-to-day work. The disadvantage is that this double load of work and learning can be tiring. They also identified a need for additional training and, most particularly, additional supervision of newly certified NAs after they have started working; this is the time when new CNAs need explicit guidance and reinforcement in translating their training into clinical care.

Concluding Remarks About Site Visits

The site visits were a vital part of the IOM committee's information gathering efforts. They provided committee members with opportunities to learn about a variety of staffing issues in acute and long-term care and to ground their discussions and deliberations in an appreciation of the complex ways such issues play out in the actual delivery of bedside care. Furthermore, the site visit teams benefited from the opinions, expertise, and experiences of a number of individuals and organizations in the areas of health care delivery and policy; nursing care and nursing administration; hospital and nursing home administration; labor relations; state-level regulation and oversight of nursing facilities; nursing education; resident advocacy; business concerns; and health care policy.

Despite the fact that committee members often had quite different experiences on site visits, analysis of all this information enabled them to reach several overarching conclusions:

• Issues such as increased patient acuity, difficulties in recruiting and retaining NAs, and the effects of reimbursement systems and rates on the ways in which care is delivered are increasingly crucial factors influencing the quality of care and the safety of the workplace.

• Hospitals are restructuring the delivery of health care in many diverse ways, and gathering and using data on these changes are difficult challenges for hospitals, nursing personnel, consumers, payers, and other concerned groups.

- The links between reimbursement and patient acuity levels or case-mix could be strengthened.
- In both nursing homes and hospitals, flexibility in staffing arrangements and in nursing personnel's approaches to work can result in improved morale and quality of care.
- High-level leadership and direction within a facility are critical for maintaining and improving the quality of patient care.

The committee is grateful to the individuals and organizations that hosted its visits. In addition to the information conveyed in person, many sites and individuals provided information before and after the visits. It is impossible to document the myriad forms of assistance that were provided, but the committee wishes to express here its recognition of the expenditure of time and energy on the part of all those who helped committee members.

EXHIBIT 1.1   Request by the Committee on the Adequacy of Nurse Staffing for written testimony.

INSTITUTE OF MEDICINE
2101 Constitution Avenue, Washington, D.C. 20418

Division of Health Care Services   TEL (202) 334-1321
Committee on the Adequacy of Nurse Staffing   FAX (202) 334-2031

The Adequacy of Nurse Staffing:
Stress, Injury, and Quality of Care

REQUEST FOR TESTIMONY

The following is an open invitation to prepare written testimony for submission to the Institute of Medicine (IOM) Committee on the Adequacy of Nurse Staffing, with the opportunity for oral presentation before the committee at a later date. Any organization or individual may submit testimony to the committee, but written statements are to be received no later than September 26, 1994. Please read further for more details.

Background

The Congress of the United States, following 1993 hearings on the current state of staffing of nursing personnel in hospitals and nursing homes, directed the Secretary of the Department of Health and Human Services to request a study from the Institute of Medicine, National Academy of Sciences, to determine whether and to what extent there is a need for an increase in the number of nurses in hospitals and nursing homes in order to promote the quality of patient care and reduce the incidence among nurses of work-related injuries and stress. For the purposes of this legislative mandate "nurses" includes registered nurses, licensed practical and vocational nurses, and nursing assistants and aides. The Congress has requested a formal report at the conclusion of this study.

Providing Testimony

To respond to this request, the IOM has established a committee of 15 experts representing a wide range of expertise (the committee roster is attached). As part of the committee's activities, written testimony is being solicited from organizations and groups representing all points of view on the subject, with the opportunity for oral presentation before the committee and to respond to the committee's questions. Two invitational sessions, each one-half-day long, will be convened — one in Washington, D.C., and the other in Irvine, California. The committee will make every effort to accommodate as many oral presentations as possible within the very limited time available for each session. Those organizations and individuals asked to present oral statements will be grouped in panels, asked to confine their remarks to about 5-7 minutes summarizing their written testimonies, and requested to be prepared to respond to committee members' questions. These sessions will be open to the public for observation. **Reporters interested in attending the oral presentation sessions should contact the Office of News and Public Information at 202-334-2138, or through Internet at NEWS@NAS.EDU.**

These hearings are an opportunity for the committee members to obtain firsthand an extensive range of opinion on the matters under consideration. Written and oral statements will be summarized by staff for the committee after they are completed. The topics to be addressed in the written testimony are provided in the following *Guide to Preparing Testimony.*

Guide to Preparing Testimony

First, as background, briefly describe your organization and its activities; existing brochures or publications are acceptable. Then, to the extent possible, please address at least the topics listed below. Your written statement may be as long as you choose and you may confine your remarks to only hospitals or only nursing homes, if you prefer. Please note that, in accordance with the legislative mandate for this study, the term "nurses" is used to cover registered nurses, licensed practical and vocational nurses, and nursing assistants and aides. All testimony should include a one-page executive summary and a cover letter identifying the name, affiliation, address, and telephone number of the contact person.

1. Your experiences with and conclusions about the current status of nurse staffing and its adequacy (both for numbers and skill mix), effects on the quality of patient care, and effects on nurses' work-related well-being.

2. The gaps in knowledge and documented evidence in the areas that the committee is studying, and priority areas and concerns.

3. The measures that are or should be used to assess the impact of nurse staffing levels and skill mix on the quality of nursing care and patient well-being.

4. The measures that are or should be used to assess the impact of nurse staffing levels and skill mix on nurses' work-related well-being (including stress and injuries).

5.   Beyond anecdotes, what data are available to support the committee's analysis? What resources and mechanisms exist to confirm and strengthen anecdotal information? Can you provide any of these resources or data?

6.   The appropriateness and adequacy of current nursing undergraduate, graduate, and in-service education and training in addressing the changing delivery and organization of health care.

7.   What data or information are available relating to the institutional cost benefits, quality of patient care, and nurses' work-related well-being associated with restructuring of the delivery of nursing care utilizing different skill mixes? What information is available about patients' satisfaction with different skill mixes in nursing care?

8.   Keeping in mind the current national environment for cost containment, please note any suggestions you have for the committee.

Please note that all written statements are to be received no later than September 26, 1994. Feel free to distribute this announcement to others who may wish to submit written testimony. Questions regarding the written statements may be directed to Gooloo S. Wunderlich, Ph.D., Study Director, at Institute of Medicine, 2101 Constitution Avenue, NW, Washington, DC 20418.

2

Statistical Resources

CONTENTS

TABLE 2.1 Utilization of Community Hospitals by Geographic Division for Selected Years, United States, 1983–1993

TABLE 2.2 Use of Inpatient Services in Community Hospitals by Persons 65 Years of Age and Over (Medicare population) by Geographic Division for Selected Years, United States, 1983–1993

TABLE 2.3 Number of Inpatient Beds in Community Hospitals by Geographic Division for Selected Years, United States, 1983–1993

TABLE 2.4 Number of Acute Care Beds and Intensive Care Unit Beds as a Percent of Total Beds by Geographic Division for Selected Years, United States, 1983–1993

TABLE 2.5 Number of Community Hospitals Offering Selected Services by Geographic Division for Selected Years, United States, 1983–1993

TABLE 2.6 Number of Community Hospitals Contracting with HMOs and PPOs by Geographic Division for Selected Years, United States, 1983–1993

TABLE 2.7 Percent Change in Selected Hospital Performance Indicators, United States, 1993–1995

TABLE 2.8 Number of Registered Nurses as a Percent of Total Nursing Personnel by Geographic Division for Selected Years, United States, 1983–1993

TABLE 2.9 Number of Full-Time Equivalent (FTE) Personnel in Community Hospitals by Geographic Division for Selected Years, United States, 1983–1993

TABLE 2.10 Number of Registered Nurses per 1,000 Admissions by Geographic Division for Selected Years, United States, 1983–1993

TABLE 2.11 Number of Registered Nurse Full-Time Equivalents (FTE) per 100 Adjusted Average Daily Census by Geographic Division for Selected Years, United States, 1983–1993

TABLE 2.12 Number of Registered Nurse (RN) Basic Education Programs, Enrollments, and Graduations and Percent Change, United States, 1983–1993

TABLE 2.13 Percent Distribution of Registered Nurse (RN) Basic Education Programs, Enrollments, and Graduations, United States, 1983–1993

TABLE 2.14 Number of Licensed Practical Nurse (LPN) Education Programs, Enrollments, and Graduations and Percent Change, United States, 1983–1993

TABLE 2.15 Employment in Selected Health Occupations, United States, 1983–1993

TABLE 2.1 Utilization of Community Hospitals by Geographic Division for Selected Years, United States, 1983–1993

	Year							Average Annual Percent Change					
	1983	1984	1987	1990	1991	1992	1993	1983–1984	1984–1987	1987–1990	1992–1993	1990–1993	1983–1993
Total hospitals													
U.S. total	5,783	5,759	5,611	5,384	5,342	5,292	5,261	−0.4	−0.9	−1.4	−0.6	−0.8	−0.9
Metropolitan	3,070	3,063	3,012	2,924	2,921	3,007	3,012	−0.2	−0.6	−1.0	0.2	1.0	−0.2
Nonmetropolitan	2,713	2,696	2,599	2,460	2,421	2,285	2,249	−0.6	−1.2	−1.8	−1.6	−2.9	−1.7
Geographic divisions													
New England	251	249	243	229	228	230	227	−0.8	−0.8	−2.0	−1.3	−0.3	−1.0
Middle Atlantic	608	603	586	568	563	560	561	−0.8	−0.9	−1.0	0.2	−0.4	−0.8
South Atlantic	820	823	827	803	801	790	790	0.4	0.2	−1.0	0.0	−0.5	−0.4
E. North Central	900	888	852	818	819	813	809	−1.3	−1.4	−1.3	−0.5	−0.4	−1.0
E. South Central	488	491	481	464	461	454	449	0.6	−0.7	−1.2	−1.1	−1.1	−0.8
W. North Central	796	792	767	742	726	722	714	−0.5	−1.1	−1.1	−1.1	−1.3	−1.0
W. South Central	845	842	810	765	758	746	743	−0.4	−1.3	−1.9	−0.4	−1.0	−1.0
Mountain	371	371	373	355	353	352	350	0.0	0.2	−1.6	−0.6	−1.0	−1.2
Pacific	704	700	672	640	633	625	618	−0.6	−1.4	−1.6	−1.1	−0.5	−0.6
Total admissions													
U.S. total	36.152	35.155	31.601	31.181	31.064	31.034	30.748	−2.8	−3.5	−0.4	−0.9	−0.5	−1.5
Metropolitan	28.284	27.706	25.601	25.490	25.508	25.885	25.751	−2.0	−2.6	−0.1	−0.5	0.3	−0.9
Nonmetropolitan	7.868	7.449	6.000	5.691	5.556	5.149	4.997	−5.3	−7.0	−1.7	−3.0	−4.1	−3.6

Number

Number (in millions)

continued on next page

TABLE 2.1 Continued

	Year							Average Annual Percent Change					
	1983	1984	1987	1990	1991	1992	1993	1983–1984	1984–1987	1987–1990	1992–1993	1990–1993	1983–1993
	Number (in millions)												
Geographic divisions													
New England	1.793	1.772	1.615	1.621	1.625	1.638	1.603	-1.2	-3.0	0.1	-2.1	-0.4	-1.1
Middle Atlantic	5.728	5.710	5.363	5.249	5.282	5.316	5.294	-0.3	-2.1	-0.7	-0.4	0.3	-0.8
South Atlantic	6.042	5.919	5.456	5.512	5.452	5.489	5.503	-2.0	-2.7	0.3	0.3	-0.0	-0.9
E. North Central	6.695	6.450	5.640	5.404	5.363	5.295	5.222	-3.7	-4.4	-1.4	-1.4	-1.1	-2.2
E. South Central	2.852	2.738	2.377	2.323	2.286	2.272	2.256	-4.0	-4.6	-0.8	-0.7	-1.0	-2.1
W. North Central	3.006	2.808	2.398	2.335	2.309	2.268	2.200	-6.6	-5.1	-0.9	-3.0	-1.9	-2.7
W. South Central	4.247	4.088	3.382	3.322	3.299	3.298	3.267	-3.7	-6.1	-0.6	-0.9	-0.6	-2.3
Mountain	1.604	1.546	1.434	1.426	1.451	1.444	1.431	-3.6	-2.5	-0.2	-0.9	0.1	-1.1
Pacific	4.184	4.125	3.935	3.990	3.998	4.014	3.974	-1.4	-1.6	0.5	-1.0	-0.1	-0.5
	Number of days (in millions)												
Total inpatient days													
U.S. total	273.2	256.6	227.0	226.0	222.9	221.0	215.9	-6.1	-4.0	-0.1	-2.3	-1.5	-2.1
Metropolitan	216.6	205.0	183.3	182.6	180.0	180.7	176.5	-5.4	-3.7	-0.1	-2.3	-1.1	-1.9
Nonmetropolitan	56.6	51.6	43.7	43.4	42.9	40.3	39.3	-8.8	-5.4	-0.2	-2.5	-3.1	-3.1
Geographic divisions													
New England	14.6	14.1	12.2	12.0	11.7	11.5	11.2	-3.4	-4.7	-0.5	-2.6	-2.2	-2.3
Middle Atlantic	50.9	49.9	44.5	45.8	45.5	46.4	46.3	-2.0	-3.7	1.0	-0.2	0.4	-0.9
South Atlantic	45.1	42.0	38.6	38.8	38.6	38.5	37.7	-6.9	-2.8	0.2	-2.1	-0.9	-1.6
E. North Central	52.7	48.3	40.2	38.6	37.7	36.5	35.3	-8.3	-5.9	-1.3	-3.3	-2.8	-3.3
E. South Central	20.3	18.6	16.2	16.2	15.9	15.9	15.5	-8.4	-4.5	0.0	-2.5	-1.4	-2.4
W. North Central	24.8	22.5	20.0	19.6	19.3	19.0	18.2	-9.3	-3.9	-0.7	-4.2	-2.4	-2.7

Number of days

W. South Central	27.7	25.6	21.4	21.5	21.1	20.9	20.4	-7.6	-5.8	0.2	-2.4	-1.7	-2.6
Mountain	10.7	10.0	9.2	9.3	9.2	9.0	8.9	-6.5	-2.7	0.4	-1.1	-1.4	-1.7
Pacific	26.5	25.6	24.8	24.2	23.8	23.4	22.5	-3.4	-1.1	-0.8	-3.8	-2.3	-1.5
Average length of stay													
U.S. total	7.55	7.29	7.18	7.24	7.17	7.13	7.03	-3.4	-0.5	0.3	-1.4	-1.0	-0.7
Metropolitan	7.65	7.40	7.16	7.16	7.06	6.98	6.84	-3.3	-1.1	0.0	-1.9	-1.5	-1.1
Nonmetropolitan	7.16	6.97	7.28	7.61	7.66	7.90	7.86	-2.7	1.5	1.5	-0.5	1.1	1.0
Geographic divisions													
New England	8.11	7.83	7.63	7.50	7.31	7.19	7.00	-3.4	-0.9	-0.5	-2.6	-2.2	-1.4
Middle Atlantic	8.93	8.75	8.24	8.81	8.58	8.75	8.74	-2.0	-2.0	2.2	-0.2	-0.3	-0.2
South Atlantic	7.52	7.12	7.02	7.05	7.02	7.00	6.85	-5.3	-0.5	0.2	-2.1	-0.9	-0.9
E. North Central	7.87	7.55	7.18	7.15	6.98	6.89	6.79	-4.1	-1.7	-0.1	-1.4	-1.7	-1.4
E. South Central	7.00	6.89	6.75	7.04	6.91	6.91	6.74	-1.6	-0.7	1.4	-2.5	-1.4	-0.4
W. North Central	8.27	8.04	8.33	8.52	8.39	8.26	8.27	-2.8	1.2	0.7	0.1	-1.0	0.0
W. South Central	6.60	6.24	6.29	6.52	6.39	6.33	6.18	-5.3	0.3	1.2	-2.4	-1.7	-0.6
Mountain	6.69	6.67	6.57	6.64	6.13	6.43	6.36	-0.3	-0.5	0.4	-1.1	-1.4	-0.5
Pacific	6.31	6.24	6.36	6.05	5.95	5.85	5.63	-1.0	0.6	-1.6	-3.8	-2.3	-1.1

SOURCE: American Hospital Association, Annual Surveys, 1983–1993, special tabulations.

TABLE 2.2 Use of Inpatient Services in Community Hospitals by Persons 65 Years of Age and Over (Medicare Population) by Geographic Division for Selected Years, United States, 1983–1993

	Year							Average Annual Percent Change					
	1983	1984	1987	1990	1991	1992	1993	1983–1984	1984–1987	1987–1990	1992–1993	1990–1993	1983–1993
Discharges	Number (in millions)												
U.S. total	11.562	11.462	10.295	10.693	10.776	11.127	11.354	-0.9	-3.5	1.3	2.0	2.1	-0.2
Metropolitan	8.673	8.680	8.022	8.382	8.505	8.931	9.152	0.0	-2.6	1.5	2.5	3.1	0.6
Nonmetropolitan	2.889	2.782	2.273	2.311	2.271	2.196	2.202	-3.7	-6.5	0.6	0.3	-1.6	-2.4
Geographic divisions													
New England	0.613	0.625	0.544	0.568	0.598	0.616	0.634	2.0	-4.5	1.4	2.9	3.9	0.3
Middle Atlantic	1.811	1.855	1.777	1.819	1.852	1.905	1.950	2.4	-1.4	0.8	2.4	2.4	0.8
South Atlantic	2.008	1.975	1.800	1.879	1.899	2.011	2.083	-1.6	-3.0	1.4	3.6	3.6	0.4
E. North Central	2.056	2.059	1.831	1.873	1.908	1.950	1.984	0.1	-3.8	0.8	1.7	2.0	-0.4
E. South Central	0.940	0.908	0.827	0.859	0.850	0.861	0.882	-3.4	-3.1	1.3	2.4	0.9	-0.6
W. North Central	1.070	1.015	0.837	0.880	0.897	0.913	0.906	-5.1	-6.2	1.7	-0.8	1.0	-1.5
W. South Central	1.288	1.247	1.043	1.134	1.114	1.161	1.178	-3.2	-5.8	2.8	1.5	1.3	-0.9
Mountain	0.465	0.462	0.428	0.458	0.449	0.463	0.476	-0.6	-2.5	2.3	2.8	1.3	0.2
Pacific	1.312	1.314	1.206	1.225	1.209	1.247	1.261	0.2	-2.8	0.5	1.1	1.0	-0.4
Inpatient Days	Number of days (in millions)												
U.S. total	115.1	106.7	92.1	97.2	96.7	97.1	95.7	-7.3	-4.8	1.8	-1.4	-0.5	-1.7
Metropolitan	90.2	84.7	74.8	79.1	79.0	80.2	79.3	-6.1	-4.1	1.9	-1.1	0.0	-1.2
Nonmetropolitan	24.9	22.0	17.3	18.1	17.7	16.9	16.4	-11.6	-7.7	1.5	-3.0	-3.1	-3.4

Geographic divisions

New England	6.7	6.6	5.6	5.8	5.7	5.8	5.6	-1.5	-5.3	1.2	-3.4	-1.1	-1.6
Middle Atlantic	22.2	21.9	19.4	20.7	20.5	20.9	21.1	-1.4	-4.0	2.2	1.0	0.6	-0.5
South Atlantic	19.3	17.6	16.0	17.0	16.9	17.3	17.0	-8.8	-3.1	2.0	-1.7	0.0	-1.2
E. North Central	21.7	19.8	16.3	16.7	16.5	16.4	16.1	-8.8	-6.3	0.8	-1.8	-1.2	-2.6
E. South Central	8.6	7.8	6.8	7.3	7.3	7.3	7.2	-9.3	-4.5	2.4	-1.4	-0.5	-1.6
W. North Central	10.4	8.9	7.2	7.7	7.6	7.7	7.4	-14.4	-6.8	2.3	-3.9	-1.3	-2.9
W. South Central	11.1	10.1	8.4	9.4	9.4	9.5	9.4	-9.0	-6.0	3.8	-1.1	0.0	-1.5
Mountain	4.0	3.7	3.2	3.4	3.4	3.3	3.3	-7.5	-4.7	2.0	0.0	-1.0	-1.8
Pacific	11.1	10.3	9.3	9.2	9.1	9.0	8.6	-7.2	-3.3	-0.4	-4.4	-2.2	-2.3

Average length of stay

Number of days

U.S. total	10.0	9.3	8.9	9.1	9.0	8.7	8.4	-6.5	-1.3	0.5	-3.4	-2.4	-1.5
Metropolitan	10.4	9.8	9.3	9.4	9.3	9.0	8.7	-6.2	-1.5	0.4	-3.5	-2.7	-1.7
Nonmetropolitan	8.6	7.9	7.6	7.8	7.8	7.7	7.4	-8.2	-1.3	1.0	-3.2	-1.6	-1.4

Geographic divisions

New England	10.9	10.6	10.3	10.2	9.5	9.4	8.8	-3.4	-0.8	-0.3	-6.2	-4.5	-1.9
Middle Atlantic	12.3	11.8	10.9	11.4	11.1	11.0	10.8	-3.7	-2.6	1.4	-1.4	-1.6	-1.2
South Atlantic	9.6	8.9	8.9	9.0	8.9	8.6	8.2	-7.3	-0.0	0.6	-5.1	-3.3	-1.5
E. North Central	10.6	9.6	8.9	8.9	8.6	8.4	8.1	-8.9	-2.5	0.0	-3.5	-3.0	-2.3
E. South Central	9.1	8.6	8.2	8.5	8.6	8.5	8.2	-6.1	-1.4	1.1	-3.7	-1.3	-1.1
W. North Central	9.7	8.8	8.6	8.8	8.5	8.4	8.2	-9.8	-0.6	0.6	-3.2	-2.2	-1.6
W. South Central	8.6	8.1	8.1	8.3	8.4	8.2	8.0	-6.0	-0.2	1.0	-2.5	-1.2	-0.7
Mountain	8.6	8.0	7.5	7.4	7.6	7.1	6.9	-6.9	-2.3	-0.2	-2.7	-2.2	-1.9
Pacific	8.5	7.8	7.7	7.5	7.5	7.2	6.8	-7.3	-0.5	-0.9	-5.5	-3.1	-1.4

SOURCE: American Hospital Association, Annual Surveys, 1983–1993, special tabulations.

TABLE 2.3 Number of Inpatient Beds in Community Hospitals by Geographic Divisions for Selected Years, United States, 1983–1993

	Year							Average Annual Percent Change					
	1983	1984	1987	1990	1991	1992	1993	1983–1984	1984–1987	1987–1990	1992–1993	1990–1993	1983–1993
Total beds													
U.S. total	1,020,378	1,012,611	954,977	928,055	923,861	921,294	916,227	-0.8	-1.9	-0.9	-0.5	-0.4	-1.0
Metropolitan	785,066	781,024	738,552	721,743	719,284	728,809	726,704	-0.5	-1.8	-0.8	-0.3	0.2	-0.7
Nonmetropolitan	235,312	231,587	216,425	206,312	204,577	192,485	189,523	-1.6	-2.2	-1.6	-1.5	-2.7	-1.9
Geographic divisions													
New England	50,794	50,894	46,262	44,214	44,023	43,691	43,053	0.2	-3.1	-1.5	-1.5	-0.9	-1.5
Middle Atlantic	167,614	167,985	156,580	156,218	156,087	159,556	161,790	0.2	-2.3	-0.1	1.4	1.2	-0.3
South Atlantic	165,966	165,374	158,885	158,207	158,744	158,938	159,083	-0.4	-1.3	-0.1	0.1	0.2	-0.4
E. North Central	196,612	191,647	174,812	163,178	160,914	158,588	155,083	-2.5	-3.0	-2.3	-2.2	-1.7	-2.1
E. South Central	75,475	75,053	73,123	71,036	71,140	70,291	69,776	-0.6	-0.9	-1.0	-0.7	-0.6	-0.8
W. North Central	100,267	96,289	90,632	86,810	85,936	85,364	83,671	-4.0	-2.0	-1.4	-2.0	-1.2	-1.7
W. South Central	111,264	112,185	104,719	101,550	101,352	100,406	100,277	0.8	-2.3	-1.0	-0.1	-0.4	-1.0
Mountain	43,587	43,986	42,856	42,254	41,883	41,487	42,130	0.9	-0.9	-0.5	1.5	-0.1	-0.3
Pacific	108,799	109,198	107,108	104,588	103,782	102,973	101,364	0.4	-0.6	-0.8	-1.6	-1.0	-0.7

SOURCE: American Hospital Association, Annual Surveys 1983–1993, special tabulations.

TABLE 2.4 Number of Acute Care Beds and Intensive Care Unit Beds as a Percent of Total Beds by Geographic Division for Selected Years, United States, 1983–1993

Hospital Beds	Year						
	1983	1984	1987	1990	1991	1992	1993
				Number			
Total hospital beds	1,020,378	1,012,611	954,977	928,055	923,861	921,294	916,227
				Percent of Total Beds			
Acute care beds							
U.S. total	81.6	80.4	78.7	69.2	67.4	66.3	64.3
Metropolitan	82.9	81.5	79.9	69.7	67.8	66.8	64.7
Nonmetropolitan	77.2	76.8	74.6	67.6	66.1	64.6	62.5
Geographic divisions							
New England	87.6	87.1	87.0	78.6	75.4	74.1	72.6
Middle Atlantic	82.7	81.2	81.6	72.5	71.4	70.0	66.4
South Atlantic	81.6	81.9	79.0	72.6	70.5	68.6	68.8
E. North Central	84.6	83.4	81.1	69.0	67.3	66.4	64.8
E. South Central	82.4	82.4	82.0	69.8	68.7	66.4	62.8
W. North Central	75.5	74.3	73.1	61.8	59.8	59.9	57.7
W. South Central	81.6	79.7	78.8	71.1	69.9	69.2	67.5
Mountain	89.5	74.4	73.2	63.5	59.5	59.6	55.5
Pacific	78.7	75.3	71.1	62.0	59.5	59.0	56.5

continued on next page

TABLE 2.4 Continued

Hospital Beds	Year						
	1983	1984	1987	1990	1991	1992	1993
				Percent of Total Beds			
Intensive care beds							
U.S. total	7.5	7.8	9.0	9.9	10.3	10.7	10.8
Metropolitan	8.2	8.6	10.0	11.0	11.5	11.9	12.0
Nonmetropolitan	5.0	5.2	5.7	6.1	6.1	6.1	6.0
Geographic divisions							
New England	7.1	7.2	7.9	8.8	8.7	9.1	9.3
Middle Atlantic	6.8	7.0	7.7	8.2	8.5	8.7	8.7
South Atlantic	7.8	8.3	9.7	11.1	11.7	12.2	12.5
E. North Central	7.0	7.4	8.8	9.8	10.3	10.8	11.0
E. South Central	7.1	7.7	8.8	9.3	9.9	10.1	9.9
W. North Central	6.9	7.2	8.2	8.8	9.0	9.4	9.2
W. South Central	7.2	7.9	9.4	10.7	10.9	11.5	11.9
Mountain	8.1	8.5	9.7	10.7	10.8	11.1	11.1
Pacific	10.0	9.9	10.6	11.6	12.6	12.6	12.4

SOURCE: American Hospital Association, Annual Surveys, 1983–1993, special tabulations.

TABLE 2.5 Number of Community Hospitals Offering Selected Services by Geographic Division for Selected Years, United States, 1983–1993

Service	Year							Average Annual Percent Change					
	1983	1984	1987	1990	1991	1992	1993	1983–1984	1984–1987	1987–1990	1992–1993	1990–1993	1983–1993
	Number												
Home health care													
U.S. total	795	1,167	1,843	1,801	1,798	1,873	2,047	46.8	16.5	-0.8	9.3	4.6	15.7
Metropolitan	501	703	989	943	934	997	1,092	40.3	12.1	-1.6	9.5	5.3	11.8
Nonmetropolitan	294	464	854	858	864	876	955	57.8	22.5	0.2	9.0	3.8	22.5
Geographic divisions													
New England	51	55	58	40	38	37	45	7.8	1.8	-11.6	21.6	4.2	-1.2
Middle Atlantic	110	124	183	174	173	173	184	12.7	13.9	-1.7	6.4	1.9	6.7
South Atlantic	58	92	199	207	215	225	258	58.6	29.3	1.3	14.7	8.2	34.5
E. North Central	136	198	298	292	292	297	310	45.6	14.6	-0.7	4.4	2.1	12.8
E. South Central	55	80	124	118	119	130	146	45.5	15.7	-1.6	12.3	7.9	16.5
W. North Central	121	214	353	321	316	338	356	76.9	18.2	-3.1	5.3	3.6	19.4
W. South Central	84	164	291	281	289	315	362	95.2	21.1	-1.2	14.9	9.6	33.1
Mountain	53	87	132	147	144	155	176	64.2	14.9	3.7	13.5	6.6	23.2
Pacific	127	153	205	221	212	203	210	20.5	10.2	2.5	3.4	-1.7	6.5
Skilled nursing units													
U.S. total	752	829	861	1,073	1,158	1,269	1,354	10.2	1.3	7.6	6.7	8.7	8.0
Metropolitan	266	271	345	514	559	660	721	1.9	8.4	14.2	9.2	13.4	17.1
Nonmetropolitan	486	558	516	559	599	609	633	14.8	-2.6	2.7	3.9	4.4	3.0

continued on next page

TABLE 2.5 Continued

Service	Year 1983	1984	1987	1990	1991	1992	1993	1983–1984	1984–1987	1987–1990	1992–1993	1990–1993	1983–1993
				Number				Average Annual Percent Change					
Geographic divisions													
New England	25	26	13	17	18	21	25	4.0	-20.6	9.4	19.0	15.7	0.0
Middle Atlantic	98	97	87	115	113	124	125	-1.0	-3.6	9.7	0.8	2.9	2.8
South Atlantic	82	78	88	126	142	164	175	-4.9	4.1	12.7	6.7	13.0	11.3
E. North Central	106	113	145	173	184	209	219	6.6	8.7	6.1	4.8	8.9	10.7
E. South Central	55	50	58	69	77	93	96	-9.1	5.1	6.0	3.2	13.0	7.5
W. North Central	185	247	196	201	205	222	229	33.5	-7.4	0.8	3.2	4.6	2.4
W. South Central	32	42	84	142	176	177	202	31.3	26.0	19.1	14.1	14.1	53.1
Mountain	91	97	84	96	100	104	109	6.6	-4.7	4.6	4.8	4.5	2.0
Pacific	78	79	106	134	143	155	174	1.3	10.3	8.1	12.3	10.0	12.3
Hospice													
U.S. total	513	578	764	817	825	874	964	12.7	9.7	2.3	10.3	6.0	8.8
Metropolitan	367	406	499	523	527	552	576	10.6	7.1	1.6	4.3	3.4	5.7
Nonmetropolitan	146	172	265	294	298	322	388	17.8	15.5	3.5	20.5	10.7	16.6
Geographic divisions													
New England	35	40	39	33	28	31	38	14.3	-0.8	-5.4	22.6	5.1	0.9
Middle Atlantic	98	109	120	113	112	111	123	11.2	3.3	-2.0	10.8	2.9	2.6
South Atlantic	47	56	82	103	98	103	114	19.1	13.6	7.9	10.7	3.6	14.3

E. North Central	116	126	141	141	149	154	175	8.6	3.8	0.0	13.6	8.0	5.1
E. South Central	23	24	35	41	41	45	52	4.3	13.4	5.4	15.6	8.9	12.6
W. North Central	78	89	138	165	178	202	212	14.1	15.7	6.1	5.0	9.5	17.2
W. South Central	17	23	44	57	62	72	75	35.3	24.1	9.0	4.2	10.5	34.1
Mountain	27	28	46	54	48	53	65	3.7	18.0	5.5	22.6	6.8	14.1
Pacific	72	83	119	110	109	103	110	15.3	12.8	-2.6	6.8	0.0	5.3
Outpatient visits													
U.S. total	210.0	212.0	245.5	301.3	322.0	348.5	366.9	1.0	5.0	7.1	5.3	7.3	7.5
Metropolitan	171.9	173.1	198.5	242.1	259.3	283.8	298.2	0.7	4.7	6.8	5.1	7.7	7.3
Nonmetropolitan	38.1	38.9	47.0	59.2	62.7	64.7	68.7	2.1	6.5	8.0	6.2	5.3	8.0
Geographic divisions													
New England	15.6	16.1	16.7	19.5	20.8	23.3	23.4	3.2	1.2	5.3	0.4	6.7	5.0
Middle Atlantic	44.8	44.2	48.0	60.2	61.8	65.6	69.5	-1.3	2.8	7.8	5.9	5.1	5.5
South Atlantic	28.2	30.1	35.3	43.5	45.4	48.5	52.7	6.7	5.5	7.2	8.7	7.0	8.7
E. North Central	44.6	44.0	52.0	63.4	66.4	71.3	73.8	-1.3	5.7	6.8	3.5	5.5	6.5
E. South Central	9.7	9.7	12.9	16.4	17.6	19.6	21.4	0.0	10.0	8.3	9.2	10.2	12.1
W. North Central	13.9	13.6	17.1	20.6	22.3	23.9	26.1	-2.2	7.9	6.4	9.2	8.9	8.8
W. South Central	15.8	15.3	18.4	23.4	25.0	28.6	30.8	-3.2	6.3	8.3	7.7	10.5	9.5
Mountain	9.5	9.6	12.4	13.9	15.9	17.5	18.3	1.1	8.9	3.9	4.6	10.6	9.3
Pacific	27.9	29.4	32.7	40.2	46.9	50.4	50.9	5.4	3.6	7.1	1.0	8.9	8.2

Number (in millions)

SOURCE: American Hospital Association, Annual Surveys, 1983–1993, special tabulations.

TABLE 2.6 Number of Community Hospitals Contracting with Health Maintenance Organizations (HMO) and Prospective Payment Organizations (PPO) by Geographic Divisions for Selected Years, United States, 1983–1993

Hospital Contract	Year							Average Annual Percent Change					
	1983	1984	1987	1990	1991	1992	1993	1983–1984	1984–1987	1987–1990	1992–1993	1990–1993	1983–1993
HMO													
U.S. total	1,103	1,378	2,488	2,433	2,502	2,558	2,649	24.9	21.8	-0.7	3.6	3.0	14.0
Metropolitan	967	1,222	1,939	1,941	1,987	2,058	2,089	26.4	16.6	0.0	1.5	2.5	11.6
Nonmetropolitan	136	156	549	492	515	500	560	14.7	52.1	-3.6	12.0	4.6	31.2
Geographic divisions													
New England	96	114	153	156	156	157	165	18.8	10.3	0.6	5.1	1.9	7.2
Middle Atlantic	163	184	299	312	321	345	368	12.9	17.6	1.4	6.7	6.0	12.6
South Atlantic	102	163	335	320	335	338	366	59.8	27.1	-1.5	8.3	4.8	25.9
E. North Central	256	322	558	538	538	542	549	25.8	20.1	-1.2	1.3	0.7	11.4
E. South Central	32	40	139	130	150	155	156	25.0	51.5	-2.2	0.6	6.7	38.8
W. North Central	104	142	295	266	260	261	265	36.5	27.6	-3.4	1.5	-0.1	15.5
W. South Central	52	78	220	218	237	248	274	50.0	41.3	-0.3	10.5	8.6	42.7
Mountain	57	72	134	131	134	145	145	26.3	23.0	-0.8	0.0	3.6	15.4
Pacific	241	263	355	362	371	367	361	9.1	10.5	0.7	-1.6	-0.0	5.0

PPO											
U.S. total	a	807	2,290	2,674	2,802	2,980	3195	a	41.6	5.3	7.2	6.5	32.9
Metropolitan		719	1,713	1,929	1,973	2,122	2189		33.6	4.0	3.2	4.5	22.7
Nonmetropolitan		88	577	745	829	858	1006		87.2	8.9	17.2	11.7	115.9
Geographic divisions	a							a					
New England		26	80	103	117	125	137		45.4	8.8	9.6	11.0	47.4
Middle Atlantic		20	154	204	220	260	298		97.5	9.8	14.6	15.4	154.4
South Atlantic		113	370	432	461	485	540		48.5	5.3	11.3	8.3	42.0
E. North Central		155	505	570	578	601	611		48.2	4.1	1.7	2.4	32.7
E. South Central		58	240	247	260	263	262		60.5	1.0	-0.4	2.0	39.1
W. North Central		64	173	244	265	308	351		39.3	12.1	14.0	14.6	49.8
W. South Central		49	217	321	347	379	455		64.2	13.9	20.1	13.9	92.1
Mountain		67	140	149	146	162	164		27.8	2.1	1.2	3.4	16.1
Pacific		155	411	404	408	397	377		38.4	-0.6	-5.0	-2.2	15.9

[a]This item was not collected on the 1983 survey.

SOURCE: American Hospital Association, Annual Surveys, 1983–1993, special tabulations.

TABLE 2.7 Percent Change in Selected Hospital Performance Indicators, United States, 1993–1995

Indicator	Quarter Ending March		Year-to-Date March		Year Ending March	
	1993–1994	1994–1995	1993–1994	1994–1995	1993–1994	1994–1995
Utilization						
Staffed beds	−1.2	−1.5	−1.2	−1.5	−0.8	−1.6
Admissions	0.2	3.2	0.2	3.2	0.8	1.6
Inpatient days	−2.9	−2.6	−2.9	−2.6	−2.4	−2.9
Average length of stay	−3.1	−5.6	−3.1	−5.6	−3.2	−4.4
Outpatient visits	3.9	13.0	3.9	13.0	5.9	9.3
Surgical operations	0.3	6.4	0.3	6.4	1.0	4.1
Births	−2.3	−1.0	−2.3	−1.0	−1.9	−1.5
65-and-over admissions	2.3	5.2	2.3	5.2	3.0	2.8
65-and-over inpatient days	−1.1	−3.0	−1.1	−3.0	−1.9	−2.8
65-and-over length of stay	−3.4	−7.8	−3.4	−7.8	−4.8	−5.3
Under-65 admissions	−1.1	1.9	−1.1	1.9	−0.5	0.9
Under-65 inpatient days	−4.6	−2.1	−4.6	−2.1	−2.8	−3.0
Under-65 length of stay	−3.5	−4.0	−3.5	−4.0	−2.3	−3.9

SOURCE: American Hospital Association, *Economic Trends*, 1995.

TABLE 2.8 Number of Registered Nurses as a Percent of Total Nursing Personnel by Geographic Division for Selected Years, United States 1983–1993

	Year							Average Annual Percent Change					
	1983	1984	1987	1990	1991	1992	1993	1983–1984	1984–1987	1987–1990	1992–1993	1990–1993	1983–1993
U.S. total	57.0	59.9	64.8	64.7	65.2	66.3	67.1	5.1	2.6	-0.0	1.2	1.2	1.8
Metropolitan	59.5	62.2	67.1	66.8	67.1	68.1	68.8	4.5	2.6	-0.2	1.1	1.0	1.6
Nonmetropolitan	45.8	49.4	54.7	54.6	55.5	56.9	57.9	7.9	3.5	-0.0	1.9	2.0	2.7
Geographic divisions													
New England	66.9	66.9	70.4	70.9	72.5	73.1	73.1	3.3	1.7	0.2	-0.6	1.0	0.9
Middle Atlantic	62.5	62.5	66.2	65.8	66.5	68.1	68.1	2.9	1.9	-0.2	1.5	1.2	0.9
South Atlantic	57.7	57.7	63.4	62.7	63.3	64.3	64.3	6.2	3.2	-0.4	1.7	0.8	1.1
E. North Central	60.5	60.5	66.6	67.1	67.7	69.4	69.4	5.6	3.3	0.2	0.3	1.1	1.5
E. South Central	50.2	50.2	57.3	58.0	57.6	59.2	59.2	10.0	4.5	0.4	1.8	0.7	1.8
W. North Central	60.5	60.5	67.0	65.7	66.0	67.7	67.7	6.0	3.5	-0.7	0.7	1.0	1.2
W. South Central	50.6	50.6	55.3	54.1	54.8	56.2	56.2	8.1	3.0	-0.8	3.7	1.3	1.1
Mountain	65.3	65.3	70.2	70.0	69.1	69.0	69.0	4.1	2.4	-0.0	1.7	-0.5	0.6
Pacific	66.6	66.6	70.1	71.1	71.6	71.6	71.6	2.1	1.7	0.5	0.2	0.2	0.8

SOURCE: American Hospital Association, Annual Surveys, 1983–1993, special tabulations.

TABLE 2.9 Number of Full-Time Equivalent (FTE) Personnel in Community Hospitals by Geographic Division for Selected Years, United States, 1983–1993

Region	Year			
	1983	1984	1987	1990
U.S. Total				
FTE personnel	3,095,638	3,016,850	3,113,608	3,419,519
Nursing personnel	1,225,200	1,164,791	1,171,474	1,251,568
RNs	698,162	697,814	758,973	809,927
LPNs	229,751	204,578	174,027	167,933
Ancillary nursing personnel	294,181	259,220	234,162	268,113
New England				
FTE personnel	189,759	188,900	190,693	197,689
Nursing personnel	68,105	66,033	63,286	65,400
RNs	44,121	44,195	44,578	46,372
LPNs	11,090	9,997	7,716	6,966
Ancillary nursing personnel	12,508	11,441	10,587	11,630
Middle Atlantic				
FTE personnel	550,698	552,467	574,012	628,648
Nursing personnel	211,808	208,783	207,484	220,700
RNs	128,750	130,539	137,273	145,252
LPNs	33,771	31,267	25,965	25,529
Ancillary nursing personnel	48,762	46,334	43,507	48,234
South Atlantic				
FTE personnel	492,137	481,070	509,370	578,299
Nursing personnel	205,380	192,443	203,392	226,259
RNs	111,553	110,975	129,044	141,841
LPNs	39,697	35,229	31,168	30,999
Ancillary nursing personnel	53,554	45,564	42,390	52,365
E. North Central				
FTE personnel	614,812	589,151	588,045	627,134
Nursing personnel	238,361	223,350	213,763	221,337
RNs	136,581	135,180	142,460	148,600
LPNs	41,600	35,764	26,387	24,478
Ancillary nursing personnel	59,362	51,676	43,824	47,330
E. South Central				
FTE personnel	200,846	193,586	197,870	223,715
Nursing personnel	86,693	81,627	80,545	87,954
RNs	39,576	40,989	46,129	51,010
LPNs	20,664	18,482	15,811	16,742
Ancillary nursing personnel	26,405	22,087	18,501	20,067

			Average Annual Percent Change					
1991	1992	1993	1983–1984	1984–1987	1987–1990	1992–1993	1990–1993	1983–1993
3,535,294	3,619,849	3,676,642	−2.5	1.1	3.2	1.6	2.5	1.9
1,289,465	1,295,271	1,302,840	−4.9	0.2	2.2	0.6	1.4	0.6
840,509	858,909	874,127	0.0	2.8	2.2	1.8	2.6	2.5
165,858	157,220	148,855	−11.0	−5.2	−1.2	−5.3	−3.8	−3.5
278,125	274,015	274,195	−11.9	−3.3	4.6	0.0	0.8	−0.7
200,614	204,786	206,533	−0.5	0.3	1.2	0.9	1.5	0.9
65,168	64,355	64,489	−3.0	−1.4	1.1	0.2	−0.5	−0.5
47,267	47,052	46,855	0.2	0.3	1.3	−0.4	0.3	0.6
6,232	5,786	5,314	−9.9	−8.3	−3.4	−8.2	−7.9	−5.2
11,174	11,049	11,786	−8.5	−2.6	3.2	6.7	0.4	−0.6
641,669	659,512	680,003	0.3	1.3	3.1	3.1	2.7	2.3
224,900	226,717	230,694	−1.4	−0.2	2.1	1.8	1.5	0.9
149,511	154,413	159,494	1.4	1.7	1.9	3.3	3.3	2.4
25,048	23,452	22,303	−7.4	−6.0	−0.6	−4.9	−4.2	−3.4
49,375	47,757	47,582	−5.0	−2.1	3.5	−0.4	−0.5	−0.2
601,829	615,982	632,779	−2.2	1.9	4.3	2.7	3.1	2.9
232,352	235,593	235,683	−6.3	1.9	3.6	0.0	1.4	1.5
146,992	151,369	153,969	−0.5	5.2	3.2	1.7	2.9	3.8
31,055	29,310	27,704	−11.3	−4.0	−0.2	−5.5	−3.5	−3.0
53,303	53,895	53,059	−14.9	−2.4	7.3	−1.6	0.4	−0.0
646,070	652,507	653,314	−4.2	−0.0	2.2	0.1	1.4	0.6
228,302	225,975	225,234	−6.3	−1.5	1.2	−0.3	0.6	−0.6
154,520	156,805	156,767	−1.0	1.8	1.4	−0.0	1.8	1.5
23,960	21,954	20,198	−14.0	−9.6	−2.5	−8.0	−5.8	−5.1
48,978	46,475	47,528	−12.9	−5.3	2.6	2.3	0.1	−2.0
235,286	246,627	248,865	−3.6	0.7	4.2	0.9	3.7	2.4
92,411	94,328	96,357	−5.8	−0.4	3.0	2.2	3.2	1.1
53,200	55,833	58,086	3.6	4.0	3.4	4.0	4.6	4.7
17,413	17,120	16,541	−10.6	−5.1	1.9	−3.4	−0.4	−2.0
21,686	21,233	21,547	−16.4	−5.7	2.7	1.5	2.5	−1.8

TABLE 2.9 Continued

Region	Year			
	1983	1984	1987	1990
W. North Central				
FTE personnel	254,313	236,836	246,427	268,978
Nursing personnel	98,918	89,005	90,605	98,024
RNs	56,457	53,870	60,738	64,419
LPNs	18,555	15,950	12,651	12,511
Ancillary nursing personnel	23,736	19,039	16,881	20,886
W. South Central				
FTE personnel	309,830	296,416	299,223	341,100
Nursing personnel	128,414	121,404	120,232	134,828
RNs	60,066	61,403	66,492	72,898
LPNs	32,821	29,561	26,979	29,099
Ancillary nursing personnel	35,398	30,371	26,558	32,494
Mountain				
FTE personnel	126,349	122,243	133,244	145,195
Nursing personnel	49,095	47,064	49,330	52,584
RNs	30,790	30,733	34,611	36,790
LPNs	8,460	7,390	5,974	5,875
Ancillary nursing personnel	9,609	8,750	8,526	9,679
Pacific				
FTE personnel	356,894	356,181	374,724	408,761
Nursing personnel	138,420	135,084	139,239	144,481
RNs	90,268	89,930	97,648	102,745
LPNs	23,093	20,938	17,776	15,734
Ancillary nursing personnel	24,846	23,960	23,389	25,427

NOTE: LPN = licensed practical nurse; RN = registered nurse.
SOURCE: American Hospital Association, Annual Surveys, 1983–1993, special tabulations.

1991	1992	1993	Average Annual Percent Change					
			1983–1984	1984–1987	1987–1990	1992–1993	1990–1993	1983–1993
279,526	283,347	280,527	−6.9	1.3	3.0	−1.0	1.4	1.0
99,989	99,393	97,003	−10.0	0.6	2.7	−2.4	−0.3	−0.2
66,007	67,278	66,144	−4.6	4.1	2.0	−1.7	0.9	1.7
12,128	11,360	10,673	−14.0	−7.4	−0.4	−6.0	−4.9	−4.2
21,612	20,476	19,924	−19.8	−3.9	7.4	−2.7	−1.5	−1.6
355,751	370,412	383,415	−4.3	0.3	4.5	3.5	4.1	2.4
139,926	144,688	147,419	−5.5	−0.3	3.9	1.9	3.1	1.5
76,663	81,377	85,990	2.2	2.7	3.1	5.7	6.0	4.3
29,030	28,089	27,037	−9.9	−3.0	2.6	−3.7	−2.4	−1.8
33,790	34,750	33,814	−14.2	−4.4	7.0	−2.7	1.4	−0.4
151,922	158,281	166,062	−3.2	2.9	2.9	4.9	4.8	3.1
57,133	56,412	58,368	−4.1	1.6	2.2	3.5	3.7	1.9
39,492	38,918	40,941	−0.2	4.0	2.1	5.2	3.8	3.3
5,851	5,586	5,301	−12.6	−6.8	−0.6	−5.1	−3.3	−3.7
11,503	11,599	11,815	−8.9	−0.9	4.3	1.9	7.4	2.3
422,627	428,395	425,144	−0.2	1.7	2.9	−0.8	1.3	1.9
149,284	147,811	147,593	−2.4	1.0	1.2	−0.1	0.7	0.7
106,857	105,864	105,881	−0.4	2.8	1.7	0.0	1.0	1.7
15,141	14,563	13,784	−9.3	−5.3	−4.0	−5.3	−4.1	−4.0
26,704	26,781	27,139	−3.6	−0.8	2.8	1.3	2.2	0.9

TABLE 2.10 Number of Registered Nurses per 1,000 Admissions by Geographic Division for Selected Years, United States, 1983–1993

	Year							Average Annual Percent Change					
	1983	1984	1987	1990	1991	1992	1993	1983–1984	1984–1987	1987–1990	1992–1993	1990–1993	1983–1993
U.S. total	19.3	19.8	24.0	26.0	27.0	27.7	28.5	2.8	6.6	2.6	2.8	3.2	4.8
Metropolitan	21.0	21.5	25.4	27.2	28.3	28.7	29.2	2.3	5.7	2.3	2.0	2.5	3.9
Nonmetropolitan	13.0	13.7	18.1	20.2	21.4	22.8	23.9	5.4	9.5	3.8	4.9	6.1	8.3
Geographic divisions													
New England	24.5	24.6	27.9	29.0	29.5	29.4	29.3	1.4	3.4	1.2	1.9	0.3	1.9
Middle Atlantic	22.6	22.9	25.4	27.9	28.2	29.1	30.1	1.8	3.9	2.8	3.8	2.6	3.3
South Atlantic	18.6	18.8	23.5	25.8	26.7	27.5	28.0	1.6	8.1	2.9	1.4	2.9	5.1
E. North Central	20.4	21.1	25.4	27.5	28.6	29.6	30.1	2.7	6.5	2.8	1.4	3.2	4.8
E. South Central	13.6	15.2	19.2	22.2	23.1	24.3	25.3	7.9	9.1	4.2	4.8	4.6	8.5
W. North Central	18.8	19.2	25.3	28.0	28.7	29.3	30.1	2.1	9.8	2.8	1.3	2.4	6.0
W. South Central	14.3	15.0	19.6	22.1	23.2	24.7	26.1	6.1	9.5	3.8	6.8	6.0	8.2
Mountain	19.2	20.5	24.7	26.3	26.3	27.8	29.2	3.4	6.7	2.3	6.1	3.8	5.2
Pacific	21.5	21.9	25.0	25.7	26.7	26.5	26.5	1.1	4.5	1.3	1.2	1.0	2.3

SOURCE: American Hospital Association, Annual Surveys, 1983–1993, special tabulations.

TABLE 2.11 Number of Registered Nurse Full-Time-Equivalents (FTE) per 100 Adjusted Average Daily Census by Geographic Division for Selected Years, United States 1983–1993

	Year							Average Annual Percent Change					
	1983	1984	1987	1990	1991	1992	1993	1983–1984	1984–1987	1987–1990	1992–1993	1990–1993	1983–1993
U.S. Total	80.82	85.06	97.82	99.65	102.48	103.81	105.55	5.2	4.8	0.6	1.7	1.9	2.6
Metropolitan	86.95	91.16	105.05	107.72	111.09	112.25	114.34	4.8	4.8	0.8	1.9	2.0	2.9
Nonmetropolitan	57.44	61.08	69.21	68.64	69.90	70.14	71.05	6.3	4.3	-0.3	1.3	1.2	2.2
Geographic divisions													
New England	90.04	92.27	101.08	102.14	104.80	104.79	105.29	2.5	3.1	0.3	0.5	1.0	1.6
Middle Atlantic	78.51	80.68	89.78	89.22	91.11	91.91	93.93	2.8	3.6	-0.2	2.2	1.7	1.9
South Atlantic	79.12	83.57	99.57	103.61	105.30	107.05	108.35	5.6	6.0	1.3	1.2	1.5	3.3
E. North Central	81.83	87.27	102.27	104.06	107.75	110.27	111.02	6.6	5.4	0.6	0.7	2.2	3.2
E. South Central	64.14	71.29	86.06	89.81	92.52	95.28	97.95	11.1	6.5	1.4	2.8	2.9	4.5
W. North Central	73.42	76.20	89.06	90.10	90.92	91.53	91.23	3.8	5.3	0.4	-0.3	0.4	2.3
W. South Central	70.58	76.95	93.00	96.43	100.21	105.68	110.39	9.0	6.5	1.2	4.4	4.6	4.7
Mountain	90.56	95.44	108.84	107.89	113.81	113.13	116.31	5.4	4.5	-0.3	2.8	2.6	2.6
Pacific	105.82	108.61	115.02	118.51	123.39	120.99	123.55	2.6	1.9	1.0	2.1	1.4	1.6

SOURCE: American Hospital Association, Annual Surveys, 1983–1993, special tabulations.

TABLE 2.12 Number of Registered Nurse (RN) Basic Education Programs, Enrollments, and Graduations and Percent Change, United States, 1983–1993

Academic Year	Total RN Programs Number	Percent Change	Baccalaureate Programs Number	Percent Change	Associate Degree Programs Number	Percent Change	Diploma Programs Number	Percent Change
Programs								
1983	1,466	—	421	—	764	—	281	—
1984	1,477	0.8	427	1.4	777	1.7	273	-2.8
1985	1,473	-0.2	441	3.3	776	-0.1	256	-6.2
1986	1,469	-0.3	455	3.2	776	0.0	238	-7.0
1987	1,465	-0.3	467	2.6	789	1.7	209	-12.2
1988	1,442	-1.6	479	2.6	792	0.3	171	-18.7
1989	1,457	1.0	488	1.9	812	2.5	157	-8.2
1990	1,470	0.9	489	0.2	829	2.1	152	-3.2
1991	1,484	1.0	501	2.4	838	1.1	145	-4.6
1992	1,484	0.0	501	0	848	1.2	135	-6.9
1993	1,493	0.6	507	1.2	857	1.1	129	-4.4

Enrollments

Year								
1982–83	250,553	—	98,941	—	109,605	—	42,007	—
1983–84	237,232	-5.3	95,008	-4.0	104,968	-4.2	37,256	-11.3
1984–85	217,955	-8.1	91,020	-4.2	96,756	-7.8	30,179	-19.0
1985–86	193,712	-11.1	81,602	-10.3	89,469	-7.5	22,641	-25.0
1986–87	182,947	-5.6	73,621	-9.8	90,399	1.0	18,927	-16.4
1987–88	184,924	1.1	70,078	-4.8	95,986	6.2	18,860	-0.4
1988–89	201,458	8.9	74,865	6.8	106,175	10.6	20,418	8.3
1989–90	221,170	9.8	81,788	9.2	117,413	10.6	21,969	7.6
1990–91	237,598	7.4	90,877	11.1	123,816	5.4	22,905	4.3
1991–92	257,983	8.6	102,128	12.4	132,603	7.1	23,252	1.5
1992–93	270,228	4.7	110,693	8.4	137,300	3.5	22,235	-4.4

Graduations

Year								
1982–83	77,408	—	23,855	—	41,849	—	11,704	—
1983–84	80,312	3.8	23,718	-0.6	44,394	6.1	12,200	4.2
1984–85	82,075	2.2	24,975	5.3	45,208	1.8	11,892	-2.5
1985–86	77,027	-6.2	25,170	0.8	41,333	-8.6	10,524	-11.5
1986–87	70,561	-8.4	23,761	-5.6	38,528	-6.8	8,272	-21.4
1987–88	64,839	-8.0	21,504	-9.5	37,397	-2.9	5,938	-28.2
1988–89	61,660	-4.9	18,997	-11.6	37,837	1.2	4,826	-18.7
1989–90	66,088	7.2	18,571	-2.2	42,318	11.8	5,199	7.7
1990–91	72,230	9.3	19,264	3.7	46,794	10.6	6,172	18.7
1991–92	80,839	11.9	21,415	11.2	52,896	13.0	6,528	5.8
1992–93	88,149	9.0	24,442	14.1	56,770	7.3	6,937	6.3

SOURCE: NLN Division of Research, 1994a, Tables 1, 17, and 26 in Section 3.

TABLE 2.13 Percent Distribution of Registered Nurse (RN) Basic Education Programs, Enrollments, and Graduations, United States, 1983–1993

Academic Year	Total RN Programs	Baccalaureate Programs (%)	Associate Degree Programs (%)	Diploma Programs (%)
Programs				
1983	1,466	28.72	52.11	19.17
1984	1,477	28.91	52.61	18.48
1985	1,473	29.94	52.68	17.38
1986	1,469	30.97	52.83	16.20
1987	1,465	31.88	53.86	14.27
1988	1,442	33.22	54.92	11.86
1989	1,457	33.49	55.73	10.78
1990	1,470	33.27	56.39	10.34
1991	1,484	33.76	56.47	9.77
1992	1,484	33.76	57.14	9.10
1993	1,493	33.96	57.40	8.64
Enrollments				
1982–1983	250,553	39.49	43.75	16.77
1983–1984	237,232	40.05	44.25	15.70
1984–1985	217,955	41.76	44.39	13.85
1985–1986	193,712	42.13	46.19	11.69
1986–1987	182,947	40.24	49.41	10.35
1987–1988	184,924	37.90	51.91	10.20
1988–1989	201,458	37.16	52.70	10.14
1989–1990	221,170	36.98	53.09	9.93
1990–1991	237,598	38.25	52.11	9.64
1991–1992	257,983	39.59	51.40	9.01
1992–1993	270,228	40.96	50.81	8.23
Graduations				
1982–1983	77,408	30.82	54.06	15.12
1983–1984	80,312	29.53	55.28	15.19
1984–1985	82,075	30.43	55.08	14.49
1985–1986	77,027	32.68	53.66	13.66
1986–1987	70,561	33.67	54.60	11.72
1987–1988	64,839	33.17	57.68	9.16
1988–1989	61,660	30.81	61.36	7.83
1989–1990	66,088	28.10	64.03	7.87
1990–1991	72,230	26.67	64.78	8.54
1991–1992	80,839	26.49	65.43	8.08
1992–1993	88,149	27.73	64.40	7.87

SOURCE: NLN Division of Research, 1994a, tables 1, 17, and 26 in Section 3.

TABLE 2.14 Number of Licensed Practical Nurse (LPN) Education Programs, Enrollments, and Graduations and Percent Change, United States, 1983–1993

	Total LPN Programs	
Academic Year	Number	Percent Change
Programs		
1983	1,297	—
1984	1,254	−3.3
1985	1,165	−7.1
1986	1,087	−6.7
1987	1,068	−1.7
1988	1,095	0.4
1989	1,171	6.9
1990	1,154	−1.4
1991	1,125	−2.5
1992	1,154	2.6
1993	1,159	0.4
Enrollments		
1982–1983	55,446	—
1983–1984	48,840	−11.9
1984–1985	39,345	−19.4
1985–1986	38,510	−2.1
1986–1987	40,035	4.0
1987–1988	42,808	6.9
1988–1989	46,720	9.1
1989–1990	52,749	12.9
1990–1991	56,762	7.1
1991–1992	59,095	4.1
1992–1993	61,007	3.2
Graduations		
1982–1983	45,174	—
1983–1984	44,654	−2.5
1984–1985	36,955	−17.2
1985–1986	29,599	−19.9
1986–1987	27,285	−7.8
1987–1988	26,912	−1.4
1988–1989	30,368	12.8
1989–1990	35,417	16.6
1990–1991	38,100	7.0
1991–1992	41,951	10.1
1992–1993	44,822	6.8

SOURCE: NLN Division of Research, 1994b, tables 1, 13, and 17 in Section 3.

TABLE 2.15 Employment in Selected Health Occupations, United States, 1983–1

Occupation	Year				
	1983	1984	1985	1986	1987
	Number (in thousands)				
Total, all occupations	92,586	96,748	99,651	101,552	104,184
Health occupations	4,711	4,798	4,920	5,069	5,186
Nursing occupations					
Registered nurses	1,287	1,309	1,341	1,381	1,489
Licensed practical nurses	576	587	602	620	587
Nurse aides, orderlies, attendants	1,116	1,136	1,164	1,199	1,110
Dental occupations					
Dental assistants	145	147	150	155	158
Dental hygienists	81	82	84	86	87
Dieticians	35	36	37	38	36
Therapists					
Physical therapists	49	50	51	53	58
Recreational therapists	26	26	27	28	24
Respiratory therapists	53	53	54	56	53
Health technologists and technicians					
Clinical laboratory technologists	227	231	236	243	237
Emergency medical technicians	61	62	64	66	73
Nuclear medicine technologists	9	9	9	10	10
Radiologic technologists	107	109	111	114	126

NOTE: Wage and salary workers only.

[a]Home health aides are classified as personal service rather than health workers. If they were included, the change would be 45.2 percent.

SOURCE: Bureau of Labor Statistics, Industry-Occupation Matrix.

1988	1989	1990	1991	1992	1993	Percent Change 1983–1993
107,389	110,059	111,510	110,340	110,746	112,312	21.3
5,394	5,708	5,927	6,202	6,654	6,654	41.2[a]
1,551	1,635	1,700	1,756	1,820	1,887	46.6
613	610	635	629	654	679	17.8
1,151	1,194	1,234	1,227	1,279	1,324	18.6
165	168	174	175	182	188	29.7
90	92	96	104	108	112	38.3
38	40	42	44	46	47	34.3
61	69	72	75	78	81	65.3
25	27	28	25	26	27	3.8
56	57	60	70	73	75	41.5
246	244	254	257	267	276	21.6
76	86	89	111	114	117	91.8
10	10	10	12	12	13	44.4
131	141	147	155	161	167	56.1

3

Commissioned Papers

Institute of Medicine (IOM) committees frequently commission papers on specific topics related to the committee's charge. The authors usually have expertise in the area and have published already in subject areas related to the committee's charge. At times, the work commissioned by the IOM is a reconfiguration of work already familiar to the author; at other times, a paper involves quantitative analysis of unpublished data available only on public use tapes. Generally, however, these background papers contribute to the committee members' knowledge of selected aspects of the study topic, and information from such papers is frequently incorporated into the text of the committee's report.

When the IOM commissions a paper, no promises are made as to whether the paper will be published by National Academy Press. That decision is made after the committee has reviewed the final paper and is based on a variety of factors, including the quality of the paper and the need for such a document in the relevant field of investigation.

The papers that follow are

- "Quality of Care, Organizational Variables, and Nurse Staffing," by Joyce A. Verran
- "Professional Nursing Education—Today and Tomorrow," by Angela Barron McBride
- "Nursing Staff and Quality of Care in Nursing Homes," by Meridean Maas, Kathleen Buckwalter, and Janet Specht
- "Quality of Care and Nursing Staff in Nursing Homes," by Jean Johnson, C. McKeen Cowles, and Samuel J. Simmens

- "Nursing Facility Quality, Staffing, and Economic Issues," by Charlene A. Harrington
- "Nursing Injury, Stress, and Nursing Care," by Bonnie Rogers

These papers were reviewed by committee members in the course of the study, but the views and conclusions reached in each paper are those of the individual author(s) and in no way reflect the views or conclusions of the IOM, the National Research Council, the study committee, or the funders of the study.

Quality of Care, Organizational Variables, and Nurse Staffing

Joyce A. Verran, Ph.D., R.N., F.A.A.N.

INTRODUCTION: THE STATE OF THE SCIENCE

Nurses in acute health care settings are convinced that there is a link between organization variables, including the numbers and types of nursing staff available to provide care, and the quality of nursing care that patients receive. It is plausible to assume that nursing organizational variables interact with clinical treatments to influence patient care outcomes. However, the data to support such an assumption are generally unavailable.

Most health outcomes research to date has focused on treatment effects during a single episode of care and the specific individual patient outcomes that can be related directly to that treatment. An examination of the effect of organizational variables on outcomes requires a different kind of outcome measure that can be attributed to all patients without regard to medical diagnosis. Research that includes these broad measures of outcome (e.g., mortality) invariably focuses on broad structural and organizational variables such as ownership and reimbursement type. Only tangentially have most studies included nursing organizational variables (e.g., number of nursing staff, number of registered nurses, nursing practice pattern). Research that does include nursing level organizational variables most likely have insufficient sample sizes to have adequate statistical power to detect difference, or use inappropriate level of analysis.

Even though empirical data to support the link among nursing organizational

Dr. Verran is a professor in the College of Nursing, University of Arizona, Tucson.

variables and patient outcomes are limited, such links continue to be assumed in the profession and its literature. The American Nurses Association (ANA, 1995) nursing care report card for the acute care setting proposes six broad areas of outcomes to be examined. These areas are mortality rate, length of stay, adverse incidents, complications, patient and family satisfaction with nursing care, and patient adherence to discharge plan. The ANA also attests to the lack of conclusive research supporting the inclusion of these outcomes that are reflective of quality nursing care.

The purpose of this manuscript is to summarize the state of the science on the relationship among nursing organizational variables and patient outcomes. Because a number of recent research projects have included broad patient outcomes as part of their projects, several approaches to the examination of the science are used. First, information is presented from a special conference convened by the American Academy of Nursing. Participants at this conference included researchers with current projects that include elements of nursing care and patient outcomes. Much of the information from these studies is yet to be published. Second, published research related to selected quality-of-care variables is reviewed. In addition, methodological issues related to the research in this area is discussed and gaps in the research base are identified.

AMERICAN ACADEMY OF NURSING INVITATIONAL CONFERENCE

In October of 1994, the American Academy of Nursing convened a special conference for researchers who were involved with projects examining the relationship among organizational variables and quality of care. The purposes for this conference were to (1) define linkages between organizational variables, staffing variables, and patient care outcomes; and (2) discuss the current state of knowledge, identify promising trends in preliminary analysis of ongoing projects, and define the problematic issues in this type of research.

Those individuals invited to participate in the conference represented six recently completed or ongoing studies examining patient outcomes, experts in the area of research methodology, and representatives of funding agencies and national foundations or organizations interested in quality-of-care measurement. A more detailed review of the six studies presented in this conference follows.

Current and Recently Completed Research Projects

Six research projects were represented at the special conference. Three of these projects were combined demonstration and research studies, while three were descriptive research that examined existing nursing care delivery and the impact of this delivery on a variety of outcomes.

Demonstration Research

The three demonstration projects began in 1988–1989 as a response to the nursing shortage. The purpose of all three projects was to create and evaluate the effect of innovative nursing practice models in hospitals with the intention of improving retention. All three studies, which were unit-based models, also examined the costs of care delivery and the effect of the delivery systems on a variety of client outcomes.

Study 1: Baltimore   The first project took place at Johns Hopkins Hospital in Baltimore (Gordon et al., 1989). Twenty-four nursing units eventually would implement the "Professional Practice Model," which is a unit-level self-management model including participant decision making, use of primary nursing, peer review, and a salaried status for registered nurse (RN) staff. For the purpose of the research component of the project, eight practice model units and eight comparison units were included in the analysis, which examined three sets of outcomes. Nursing outcomes included work satisfaction and retention; cost outcomes included personnel expenditures, recruitment costs, and orientation costs; patient outcomes included satisfaction, health status, and perceived functional status at discharge and two weeks after discharge. In addition, information was gathered on unanticipated health plan usage. Results of this study have been reported in two articles (Weisman et al., 1993; Wong et al., 1993) and two others are in press and expected to be published in 1995. A full description of the practice model has also been published (Rose and DiPasquale, 1990).

Study 2: Rochester   The second project took place at the University of Rochester (Ingersoll et al., 1988). In this project, an "Enhanced Professional Practice Model" consisting of five interdependent conceptual elements was introduced and tested in five experimental units and contrasted with five comparable units. Urban, community, and rural settings were observed. Model components included: control over practice; continuing education responsive to staff nurse need; continuity of care delivery; collaborative practice; and professional compensation reflective of education and experience. The goal of the Rochester project was to invest nurse managers and staff with increased control over practice and decision making authority to produce higher levels of work satisfaction, decreased staff nurse turnover, improved patient outcomes, and increased cost effectiveness of care delivery.   Specific nurse outcomes measured were job satisfaction, unscheduled absences, peer group relationships, professional identity, intent to leave, autonomy, leadership responsiveness, perceived RN workload, and advancement opportunity. Cost data included both direct and indirect nursing costs. Patient outcome information included satisfaction, morbidity, mortality, length of stay, untoward hospital incidents, and infections. Three papers discussing the practice model for this research and methodological problems have been published (Ingersoll et al., 1990, 1991, 1993).

Study 3: Arizona   The third demonstration project was located at the University of Arizona (Verran et al., 1988). The practice model for this research was entitled the "Differentiated Group Professional Practice" (DGPP) Model, which was implemented in 4 demonstration hospitals for a total of 10 nursing units. In September 1991, one rural hospital dropped from the project leaving a total of nine units (three intensive care units, two telemetry units, and four general medical-surgical units) in one rural, one community, and one tertiary hospital. For the first 2 years of the project 10 units in 3 other hospitals were included for comparison purposes. The initial plan for the project included the elimination of comparison hospital data collection after 2 years. Since three of these units were in the same hospital as three demonstration units, it was believed that diffusion of innovation could only be controlled for this 2-year period. The original data analysis plan included procedures to project comparison unit data to the last two data collection times. Components of the DGPP Model include group governance (participative unit management, shared decision making by staff bylaws, peer review and professional salary structure), differentiated care delivery (differentiated RN practice, use of nurse extenders, primary case management), and shared values in a culture of excellence (quality of care, support for intrapreneurship, internal and external recognition). The research goals of the Arizona project were to test the effectiveness of the unit-based DGPP Model on (1) professional practice as measured by group cohesion, control over practice, autonomy, and organization commitment, (2) nurse satisfaction as measured by job satisfaction subscales of professional status, task requirements, organizational policies, pay, interaction with nurses, interaction with physicians, and autonomy, (3) nurse resources as measured by rates of turnover, vacancy, stability, activity, positive activity, and negative activity, (4) quality outcomes as measured by rates of intravenous fluid errors, skin injury, patient falls, nosocomial infections, nursing documentation, and (5) fiscal outcomes as measured by operating costs, personnel costs, RN costs, RN agency costs, RN overtime costs, and RN absence costs. An article describing the innovative practice model on this project has been published (Milton et al., 1992) and other methodological and measurement papers are also in print (Milton et al., 1990, 1995; Verran et al., 1995). In addition, a partial report of data for one hospital has been published (Verran et al., 1994).

Descriptive Research

The three descriptive studies vary considerably from each other in their initial impetus and their approach. The first of these examines the environment in which nurses practice in the critical care setting and is like the previous intervention studies, in that it was an attempt to examine factors that would influence nurse retention. The second study also has an organizational base but is attempting to identify factors associated with patient-centered care. The third study is not nursing-unit-based and is directed at the quality of care delivered by nurses to patients with the specific condition of acquired immunodeficiency syndrome (AIDS).

Study 4: Seattle   The first descriptive study took place around Seattle in 17 hospitals and involved 25 critical care units. The research, entitled "Critical Care Nursing Systems, Retention and Patient Outcomes" (Mitchell et al., 1991), was a correlational study to examine the predictors of patient care outcomes related to the organization vectors in critical care nursing. The study was built on a demonstration project from the American Association of Critical Care Nurses (Mitchell et al., 1989). The underlying framework of the current research is taken from industrial organizations and proposes that high outcomes will result when there is a match between the pattern of structures and processes and the work being done. For nursing, technology includes elements of a professional practice model as described in some of the previous intervention research projects. The model for critical care indicates that the more the actual practice environment approaches the ideal, then the greater will be the organizational and patient care outcomes. Specific hypotheses indicated that the closer a unit was to the idealized score on variables such as expertise, discretion, and standardization, the higher would be the organizational variables such as job satisfaction, propensity to stay on the job, retention of nursing expertise, and documented quality of care, and the lower would be the severity-adjusted mortality rate and length of stay.

Study 5: New York   The second descriptive study took place in 17 hospitals in New York with 116 to 119 adult, nonpsychiatric, nonobstetric nursing units. The project, entitled "Improving Patient Centered Care Through Initiatives in Nursing" (Minnick, 1991) examined the variables that contribute to reports of patient-centered care in nursing. A set of hypotheses were developed that examined (1) the effect of labor and capital on outcomes; (2) whether satisfied (contented) employees provide patient-centered care; and, (3) the impact of patient characteristics on patient-centered care. Data have been analyzed from this research and articles are in review for publication. Findings were not shared at the invitational conference, however methodological issues from the study are included. Three articles from this study have been accepted for publication with anticipated publication dates in 1995–1996 (Minnick et al., in press[a,b,c]).

Study 6: San Francisco   The final research study presented at the conference was a prospective research project entitled "Quality of Nursing Care for People with AIDS" (Holzemer and Henry, 1989). This descriptive study is examining the quality of care for clients with AIDS across the trajectory of health care from the inpatient hospital setting, home care, and skilled nursing facilities. Data are collected from nurses about specific patient problems in nursing care activities and from the patients about their perceptions of their problems. Extensive audits of care plans, progress records, and shift reports are also conducted. Unlike the other studies presented at the conference, this research proceeds from a microlevel to examine the relationship between patient problems, nursing care activities, and outcomes. Structural or organizational characteristics are not included. Currently data have been entered on approximately 300 subjects representing over 15,000 patient problems. A number of microlevel findings related to patient problems and nursing interventions are available from this research. In addition, methodological issues related to care planning and measurement have been identified. Published articles from the research include Janson-Bjerklie and colleagues (1992), Holzemer and colleagues (1993), and Henry and coworkers (1994a,b).

Variables Addressed in Current Research

This section will summarize the independent variables and the outcome variables examined in the current research projects. Outcome variables may be organized under three classifications: staff outcomes, organizational outcomes, and client outcomes. None of the studies described included a direct measurement of staffing mix and staff numbers as one of the independent or outcome variables.

Independent Variables

The independent variables for the three demonstration projects and two of the descriptive studies involved the environment of the hospital unit within which nurses practice. The intent of demonstration models was to increase the degree of control over nursing practice through a variety of mechanisms and to establish professional practices consistent with previous research.

Although the models differed on specific components, most included some form of self-governance to increase control and could be said to be based upon the characteristics associated with magnet hospitals (McClure et al., 1983; Kramer and Schmalenberg, 1988a,b; Kramer, 1990). This environment includes the following characteristics: (1) high status of nurses within the organization; (2) autonomy in the area of clinical decisions related to nursing practice; (3) decentralized decision making at the unit level; (4) assignment patterns that allow continuity and accountability; and (5) an organizational culture that values excellence and provides rewards commensurate with excellent practice. For the purposes of this paper, the environment just described has been labeled a professional practice environment.

In two descriptive studies, the existing environment of the nursing unit was examined as the independent variable. Specific aspects of the environment studied included some of the variables associated with professional practice. Individual patient problems were the independent variables identified in the final descriptive study. These problems were identified by nurses and patients and have been categorized with a variety of classification schemes, primarily nursing diagnosis as developed by the North American Nursing Diagnosis Association. One finding of particular interest from this last study is the lack of agreement on the identified problems that was found between patients and nurses. This suggests that patients' perceptions of their problems need to be captured to enhance care and provide data for the analysis of outcomes. The study also confirmed the impression that the chart does not capture well the data required to measure the quality of nursing care.

Staff Outcomes

Staff outcomes were viewed in most of the studies as intervening variables influenced by the independent variable and influencing other outcomes. The primary staff variable included in four of the studies was job satisfaction. In addition, some measure of autonomy was also included. In two of these studies this concept was divided into a measure of control over practice and control over job. Various other measures that represent some aspect of a professional practice environment were also included in one or more of the studies. These variables included organizational commitment, work group cohesion, and work group culture.

In the microlevel research project with patients with AIDS, the staff outcome was nursing care activities. These activities were thought to be influenced by the independent variable, patient problems, and to influence client outcomes.

Organizational Outcomes

Two types of organizational outcomes were included in the macrolevel research projects. The first included various retention measures of actual turnover rates or intent-to-leave measures. The second type of organizational variable involved costs of delivering care on a nursing unit. Cost measures were primarily related to various aspects of personnel costs. In none of the studies were charges to the patient or third-party payer included as variables. All costs were those associated with the organization. In the San Francisco microlevel study, work is currently in progress to link quality and cost data across the continuum of care.

Organizational variables were considered to be both intervening and final outcome variables in the studies and were influenced by the practice environment of the nursing unit. Retention outcomes were primarily considered to be intervening variables affecting both quality and cost of service. Organizational costs were considered final outcomes.

Client Outcomes

For all the studies described, client outcomes as indicators of quality were the final variable examined. These outcomes were thought to be influenced by a combination of the independent variable, staff outcomes, and organizational outcomes related to retention.

Two of the research projects, the Rochester demonstration study and the Seattle critical care study, included severity-adjusted mortality rates as an outcome. The San Francisco microlevel study also includes the measurement of mortality, although results on this variable are not available for report.

Other common client outcome measures included some form of client satisfaction for two of the demonstration and one of the descriptive studies. Two of the intervention studies used negative indicators of client outcomes in the form of untoward hospital incidents and nosocomial infection.

A variety of other client outcome measures were used for individual studies, including unanticipated health care service utilization, length of stay, health status and functional status. In the San Francisco study, the investigators developed a 10-item, 3 factor (self-care, ambulation, and psychological distress) instrument that evidences excellent psychometric properties including predictive validity of mortality at 3 and 6 months (Holzemer et al., 1993).

Findings Related to the Independent Variable

Studies that implemented models that were designed to create a professional practice environment on nursing units had variable success with that implementation. These projects cited the need for strong administrative support and a committed cohort of staff in order for full implementation to take place. Variable levels of implementation led to a methodological recommendation that will not be detailed further in this paper. That recommendation involved the need for the systematic evaluation of the level of professional practice model implementation on the nursing unit in order to assess strength of the intervention. Both the Rochester and Arizona studies developed scales to assess the level of model implementation.

Findings Related to Staff and Organizational Outcomes

For the studies examining the effect of a professional practice environment, findings consistently confirm an increase in job satisfaction when this environment is in place to a high degree. In addition, measures such as autonomy or control over practice tend to increase. One of the projects (Rochester) found limited differences between their comparison units and demonstration units in terms of job satisfaction, however the evidence from this research, in general, tends to support previous studies' findings that a professional practice environment will increase job satisfaction. In terms of the autonomy variable, for those studies that included both a measure of control over practice and a measure of control over job, control over practice had a greater predictive value on job satisfaction than did control over aspects of the job.

The staff variable for the microlevel study in San Francisco involved the identification of nursing care activities. Over 80 percent of the activities identified could be classified into the 2 categories of monitoring the patient's condition and medication administration. The nursing intervention classification system from the University of Iowa has been adopted for activity classification. For some identified patient problems, no nursing care activities were identified. In general, nurses also did not document individualized problems or interventions for their patients. Standardized care plans and nursing activity lists are usually organized by body systems. Twenty-two percent of patients studied had no care plan under any system (manually generated, computer supported, or standardized). There were no differences on selected outcome variables for patients with or without a care plan.

The results from the macrolevel research also support the belief that professional practice environments will increase retention of nurses on the unit and in the hospital. All of the studies that examined the cost of care delivery found that the professional practice models were cost neutral. In other words, there were no significant increases or decreases in costs under these practice frameworks.

Findings Related to Client Outcomes

In general, there were no relationships among any of the independent variables, staff or organizational outcomes, and the client outcomes examined in the studies reported at the invitational conference. In neither of the research projects that examined mortality were any differences noted. In none of the demonstration or descriptive macrolevel studies were there positive differences in other quality indicators across time or comparison units. The microlevel San Francisco study did not report the examination of nursing care on client outcomes.

Discussion of Findings

The findings of the current macrolevel research projects are consistent with the literature in terms of staff outcomes and organizational outcomes, and support the contention that a professional practice environment will improve these variables. However, there were no significant findings associated with quality measures. There are a variety of methodological issues that help to explain these results, that will be addressed at the end of this paper.

PUBLISHED RESEARCH

A review of published studies in the area of client outcomes and organizational variables will be presented next. Only research published in the last 10 years was examined. Earlier research tended to examine, primarily, the effect of new nursing care delivery models such as primary vs. team care. In the majority of these studies staff outcomes, including the process of care, were considered to be of primary significance and client outcomes were seldom addressed. More recent studies, like those at the invitational conference, were conducted due to the nursing shortage and attempted to increase retention of nurses. Relatively few national studies with large samples have been reported.

As with treatment effectiveness research, there exists a body of literature related to specific nursing interventions and the effect of these interventions on individual client outcomes. Most of these studies are directed at patients with specific diagnoses and will not be reviewed in this paper. However, five meta-analyses of many of these studies have been conducted and may be of interest (Mumford et al., 1982; Devine and Cook, 1983; Smith and Naftel, 1984; Hathaway, 1986; Heater et al., 1988).

The following sections report on the results of published research that is related to more generalized client outcomes. The primary outcomes that have been examined in the literature are mortality, nosocomial complications, adverse incidents, service utilization, and patient satisfaction. Although there is a beginning attempt to examine health status on discharge and postdischarge, this research is not summarized in this paper for several reasons. First, there are few studies that include nursing variables as predictors to changes in health status. Second, health status is conceptualized in a variety of different ways, from the very abstract to very specific measures related to specific diagnoses. Third, even when the same variable is conceptualized (e.g., functional status) it is measured in such a variety of ways that comparisons are difficult.

Mortality

The literature on the variables influencing severity-adjusted mortality rates is extensive. When considering qualities of nursing services that influence this variable, two areas are pertinent. Studies have consistently found that the proportion of RNs on the nursing staff or the total number of RNs will have a positive influence on mortality rates. Prescott (1993) has done a complete review of this research base and it will not be detailed further.

More pertinent to the research reported at the invitational conference is the second aspect of nursing that has been shown to have some effect on mortality. These studies have taken place in the critical care setting and indicate that the level of interdisciplinary collaboration has a positive influence on mortality. This finding was originally reported by Knaus and colleagues (1986) and was supported by the original Critical Care Nurses Association Demonstration Project (Mitchell et al., 1989). More recent findings by the same team as the original research (Zimmerman et al., 1993, 1994) failed to support the original result. The Seattle critical care study described at the invitational conference also failed to find a relationship between units that were closer to the ideal level of practice and adjusted mortality rates.

In an extensive investigation, Aiken and colleagues (1994) reported a strong relationship between the nursing organization found in magnet hospitals and lower adjusted Medicare mortality rates. The hypothesis was also tested that decreased mortality rates were a result of staffing mix, which is traditionally richer in magnet hospitals. No evidence was found to support the contention that skill mix or the proportion of RNs was the key variable in affecting mortality. Instead the authors conclude that the mortality decrease (5 deaths per 1,000 Medicare discharges) stems from ". . . the greater status, autonomy and control afforded nurses in the magnet hospitals, and their resulting impact on nurses' behaviors on behalf of patients.—i.e., this is not simply an issue of the number of nurses, or their mix of credentials." (Aiken et al., 1994, p. 783). This finding was not supported in the studies that examined mortality and were reported at the invitational conference. In these cases, there were no difference in mortality rates on the high professional practice units and nonprofessional practice units.

Complications

Flood and Diers (1988) examined two general medical units with differing staffing levels to determine the effect of staffing on patient complications. The most frequently occurring complications were infections, heart conditions, and gastrointestinal disorders. They found that the mean number of complications per patient was higher on the "short-staffed" unit than on the unit with adequate staffing. Both generalized infections and urinary tract infections evidenced the greatest difference between units, with rates being almost double those of other complications. For this research, staffing was determined by an index of required staff hours (based on patient acuity) to actual staff hours. Data confirmed that one unit in the study was consistently below the staffing level required while the other was at or above that level. No data were found that indicated that patients were different in terms of age, gender, and diagnosis-related group (DRG) between the two units, although some evidence was found that acuity on the short-staffed unit was slightly higher. This higher rate could have been due to either the increased level of complications or simply the type of patient.

More recently, Taunton and colleagues (1994) reported on research that examined the effect of three organizational variables (absenteeism, unit separation, and work load) on nosocomial infections. This study took place in 4 large Midwestern acute care urban hospitals for a total of 65 patient care units in the sample. Specific units within the sample included 15 critical care units, 5 telemetry units, 22 medical-surgical units, 6 pediatric units, 6 obstetric-gynecological units, 4 long-term care/rehabilitation units, and 7 other (type not specified) units. Findings supported a relationship between patient infections and staff RN absenteeism. No other organizational variable evidenced a significant relationship with the outcome variable.

Both of these studies indicate that nurse staffing has some effect on the incidence of nosocomial infection rates. These increased rates were also associated with increased length of hospital stay in the Flood and Diers (1988) research. Disruption in the continuity of care due to absences and inadequate staffing were cited as reasons for the increased incidents of infections.

Other research has examined the effect of practice models on complications. Mitchell and colleagues (1989) found that complications related to infections, immobility, and fluid balance represented nonresolution of problems on admission to the intensive care unit rather than new problems. Brett and Tonges (1990) in a one-unit pilot evaluation of the ProACT™ Model at the Robert Wood Johnson University Hospital found no increase in nosocomial infections despite the planned decrease in the number of RNs.

Two of the intervention studies reported at the invitational conference also included nosocomial infections as part of their research. Neither study found a significant relationship between infection rates and any other included study variable.

Adverse Incidents

Adverse incidents that occur during hospitalization include errors in medication delivery (wrong patient, wrong drug, wrong dose, wrong route, wrong time), patient falls, treatment errors, and skin injury or breakdown. Again, two of the demonstration projects included these items in their research model with no significant findings. The study by Taunton and colleagues (1994) cited earlier also examined the effect of organizational variables on patient falls and medication errors. No significant associations were discovered.

A comprehensive investigation by Wan and Shukla (1987) examined the relationship of contextual and organizational variables with the quality of nursing care. Contextual variables were considered to be attributes of the hospital and region that are beyond control of the hospital. Organizational variables include structural and design variables. Only the design variables are amenable to change. These variables include the nursing care delivery model, staff skill mix, and staffing levels. The patient incidents included in the study were rates of medication errors, patient falls, patient injuries, and testing or treatment errors. Forty-five community acute care hospitals were included in the study. Results indicate that the independent variables did not account for a large portion of the variation in incident rates. Nursing skill mix, nursing model, and nursing resource consumption were not significantly related to any of the dependent variables. The authors suggest these findings support an earlier study that found that the most significant nursing variable affecting the quality of nursing care was nursing competence. This research[1] was unavailable for review. A further explanation may involve the interrelatedness of patient factors, hospital support systems, and nursing variables. Even though a support system index was included in this research, the interaction effect with nursing variables was not examined. Of significance, however, is the fact that patient age had the greatest impact on falls and that age, along with acuity, were the two significant variables in the regression of patient injury on contextual and organizational variables. This suggests that patient characteristics are the most influencing factor for the occurrence of adverse incidents and any research examining these factors should control for the risk of injury.

Currently, there is no evidence to support the belief that nursing variables are directly associated with adverse hospital incidents. There is some suggestion that nursing competence has an effect on quality.

Service Utilization

Primarily, the research on the relationship of nursing to service utilization has concentrated on types of care delivery systems rather than staffing variables. An exception to this is the article by Flood and Diers (1988) that found that although total length of stay adjusted by DRG was similar between the two study units, two specific DRGs showed differences in length of stay. Patients within these DRGs (GI hemorrhage [174] and CVA [14]) had longer length of stays on the short-staffed unit and, in addition, developed more complications during their hospital stay.

Brooten and colleagues (1986) designed a clinical trial to examine the effect of nurse specialist care on early discharge of low-birthweight infants on selected patient outcomes. The experimental intervention included early discharge of low-birthweight infants meeting specific criteria, to be followed by master's prepared nurse specialists for 18 months after hospitalization. Random assignment resulted in 39 infants in the experimental group and 40 infants in the control group. Groups were equivalent on a number of demographic family variables and infant treatment variables. Findings showed that the experimental group was discharged a mean of 11.2 days earlier that the controls and that there were no differences in rehospitalizations, acute-care visits, failure to thrive, child abuse, foster placement, or developmental quotient of infants. There were also no differences in outcomes for the mothers.

---

[1]Shukla, R.K. *Structure vs People and Nursing Performance: An Evaluation Study.* Report no. PB86-150588/AS. Washington, D.C.: National Center for Health Services Research, U.S. Department of Health and Human Services, 1986.

Research on the case management system at Carondolet St. Mary's Medical Center also has found that the content of nursing care has an impact on length of stay. The nursing delivery system at this facility involves a network of home care, hospice, community wellness centers, and hospital nursing with a nurse case manager bridging community and in-hospital care. Case managers, prepared at least at the bachelor's level, are the hub of the health care delivery system. Ethridge and Lamb (1989) report on the effects of the nursing case management intervention with patients who received total hip replacements and those with respiratory disease. For the first group, length of stay was reduced by 2.1 days while it was reduced by 3.5 days for the second group. The authors hypothesize that the reduction for acute illness (hip replacement) occurs at the end of hospitalization and that case management allowed earlier discharge of these patients. For the chronically ill (respiratory disease), length of stay appeared to be reduced at the beginning of the hospitalization. Those patients who were case-managed prior to hospitalization entered the hospital at lower acuity levels and shortened their length of stay by seeking care before illness severity reached a level that would require longer hospitalization.

A further report by Ethridge (1991) examines more than 700 case-managed patients enrolled in a health maintenance organization's senior plan. The data for the case managed clients were compared with national and state statistics for Medicare patients and health maintenance organization service use statistics. Results indicate that the case-managed patients had 53 fewer annualized hospital admissions, 895 fewer bed-days, and an average length of stay 1.73 days lower than other Medicare patients in the state.

Two reports by Naylor and colleagues (Naylor, 1990; Naylor et al., 1994) examine the effects of gerontological nurse specialist care. This care primarily involved a discharge planning protocol for hospitalized elders that was implemented by clinical nurse specialists while the client was hospitalized and 2 weeks after discharge. The earlier manuscript reports on the pilot study for the full project and included 40 hospitalized patients, age 70 and older, who were randomly assigned to the discharge planning or control group. No statistical differences were found in initial hospital length of stay or posthospital infection rate. However, there were significant differences in the number of rehospitalizations during the 12 weeks after discharge. In the larger, second study, 276 patients were included. Findings indicated that patients in the medical intervention group had fewer readmissions and fewer total days rehospitalized than the control group. No differences were found between the surgical intervention group and the control. Again, there were no differences in initial hospital length of stay.

Studies such as those described above indicate that nursing care does have an impact on the utilization variables of length of hospital stay and readmission rates. However, the research has more to do with the practice pattern of nurses than with the mix of staff or staffing ratios. These studies also indicate the advantages of nurses in specialized advanced practice. Unfortunately, no research has been reported that describes such practice patterns with less well educated staff to determine whether results would be similar.

Methodological Note

Research on the utilization of health care services has included primarily the variables of readmission and length of hospital stay. Continued use of these variables, particularly hospital length of stay, is problematic due to increased implementation of critical paths and prospective payment that essentially predetermines length of hospitalization. What appears to be of greater significance in the future is a measure of episode of illness that would include both length of stay and readmission.

Patient Satisfaction

Many studies that examine models of nursing practice also investigate the effect of these models on patient and family satisfaction. Both Burnes-Bolton and colleagues (1990) and Brett and Tonges (1990) report the results from one nursing unit. The first report notes increases in satisfaction, while the second indicates that two measures of satisfaction remained stable. This latter finding has some significance since the practice model implemented included a decrease in the number of RNs and an increase in unlicensed personnel. However, the data presented from both studies are considered pilot work from only one involved nursing unit.

Lamb and Huggins (1990) in another report of the Carondolet nurse case management system also reported increase in patient satisfaction over time. The study by Mitchell and colleagues (1989) previously mentioned under the heading of "Mortality" also noted higher levels of patient satisfaction in the ideal critical care environment.

In a 1985 publication, Koerner and colleagues (1985) report the results of the implementation of a system of professional nursing practice through collaboration with physicians. The system contained the five interrelated parts as specified by the National Joint Practice Commission in 1977: a joint practice committee of physicians and nurses; primary nursing; nursing clinical decision making within the scope of nursing practice as defined by the joint practice committee; integrated patient records; and joint practice review. Again this study contained only one demonstration unit and one control unit. The sample included 280 patients (100 from the control unit and 180 from the demonstration unit). The researchers evaluated patient satisfaction with a self-developed instrument designed to measure patient-provider interaction, quality of care, health education, knowledge of practitioners, and environment of the unit. Patients from the collaborative practice unit reported significantly greater patient-provider interaction, provider knowledge, health education, and respectful treatment. No differences were noted in patient satisfaction with the physical environment or expectations of care. The authors note a limitation to the study in that the satisfaction instrument was designed with an emphasis on items pertinent to a collaborative practice environment and results may be biased toward the positive evaluation of the experimental treatment.

These research studies tend to indicate an increase in patient satisfaction with the implementation of a more professional model of practice, which is consistent with that previously described as part of the magnet hospital studies. However, there is also some indication that satisfaction remains stable even when the mix of nursing staff is altered to fewer professional nurses and more unlicensed personnel.

Methodological Note

The popularity of patient satisfaction as an outcome measure is reflected in the number of instruments that have been developed for evaluation and research purposes (McDaniel and Nash, 1990). While there are many ways to measure patient satisfaction, not all are accurate or reliable. Specifically, the construct validity of many instruments designed for individual studies is questionable. Often, it appears that patients are being asked to evaluate quality of care rather than their satisfaction with that care. A further limitation of patient satisfaction with nursing care as an outcome measure is that patients traditionally report high levels of satisfaction, thus decreasing the variability of responses that are needed for analysis (LaMonica et al., 1986). Measures of satisfaction that are clinically feasible for use because of their parsimony often lack the sensitivity required to tap fine differences in patient perception.

Relationship of Staff Satisfaction to Client Outcomes

Much of the research investigating factors to increase staff nurse satisfaction makes the assumption that increased levels of satisfied staff will directly lead to increased quality of care. Two projects have examined this relationship as their primary hypothesis and will be described here, even though one of the studies occurred prior to the 1985 review date.

Holland and associates (1981) examined resident mental health patients and staff from 22 units in 3 psychiatric hospitals. Of the eligible staff, 98 percent (N = 297) were included in the analysis. However, exact titles and preparation were not delineated in the report. Sixty-eight percent (N = 249) of the total patients were selected with stratified random sampling to be included in the study. The focal unit for this research was the nursing unit and when individual data were aggregated to that level an analysis sample of 22 resulted. The outcome examined was potential posthospital adjustment as measured at discharge by a standardized scale. Improvement in resident functioning was moderately associated with staff satisfaction. Greater staff participation in resident treatment affected the outcome only indirectly through staff satisfaction. The total effect of staff satisfaction, using path analysis, was .55 (.38 direct and .17 indirect).

A 1985 publication by Weisman and Nathanson (1985) reported on a study of teenage clients who attended 1 of 77 family planning clinics. Although this research does not involve the acute care setting, findings may still be pertinent. The 77 clinics involved in the research represented data from 344 nurses and 2,900 clients. Outcomes investigated were client satisfaction and rate of compliance with contraceptive prescriptions. Using path analysis, a significant direct effect (.32) of job satisfaction on client satisfaction was discovered. There was no direct effect of this variable on compliance rates. However, there was a significant indirect effect (.08) of job satisfaction on compliance through client satisfaction. Hays and White (1987) reanalyzed the Weisman and Nathanson (1985) data using structural equation modeling with LISREL. They supported the model proposed in the original study and proposed an alternative model that also fits the data. Both models supported the significant relationship between job satisfaction and client outcomes.

Of the four studies at the invitational conference that were also looking at the relationship between staff satisfaction and outcomes, none reported significant direct or indirect relationships. However, final data analyses were not completed for all of the studies.

SUMMARY: LINKAGES AND GAPS

Although some of the findings from investigations are limited by the number of studies supporting the relationship, small sample sizes, or both, some tentative conclusions can be drawn from the research presented. Research, either previously published or reported through the invitational conference, has supported the following linkages:

(1)   There is a relationship between a professional practice environment and perceptions of control over practice and autonomy.

(2)   There is a relationship between a professional practice environment and job satisfaction.

(3)   A professional practice environment and job satisfaction improve retention of staff.

(4)   The implementation of a professional practice model is cost neutral.

(5)   The proportion of RNs on a nursing staff has positive influence on severity-adjusted Medicare mortality rates.

(6)   A professional practice environment has a positive influence on severity-adjusted Medicare mortality rates, over and above the influence of staffing mix.

(7)   There is inconsistent evidence of the effect of nursing-staff-related

variables on the development of nosocomial infection rates. It is likely, however, that when continuity of care is assured through various staffing mechanisms infection rates are lower.

(8)   Despite the existence of some research, there is currently no evidence that nurse staffing variables have an effect on adverse patient incidents. There is some indication, however, that nurse competence may have a positive effect on these rates.

(9)   There is sufficient evidence to suggest that innovative nursing delivery patterns (e.g., case management; transitional models of hospital to home care) will reduce utilization of health care services through either decreased length of hospital stay or reduced readmissions.

(10) Findings on the effect of nursing on patient satisfaction are inconsistent. Published studies indicate that satisfaction is stable or increased with professional practice environments even when staffing levels are reduced; current unpublished research as presented at the invitational conference does not support this conclusion.

(11) In outpatient and inpatient psychiatric settings there is a relationship between job satisfaction and client satisfaction; this result has not been supported for acute care hospitals and does not hold for outcomes other than client satisfaction.

In addition to needing more research to further support or clarify some of the tentative findings indicated above, research is needed to fill the gaps in the state of the science. Some of the gaps in our current empirical knowledge include:

(1)   Whether satisfied staff in acute care give better care, resulting in improved client outcomes.

(2)   Whether there is a link between professional practice and staffing needs.

(3)   Whether there is a relationship between professional practice environments and patient outcomes other than mortality.

(4)   Whether there is a connection between staffing mix and client outcomes of health status.

(5)   What the interaction is between productivity and quality care and the main effect and interactive effect of these variables on client outcomes.

(6)   What the influence of leadership is on the productivity and quality of nursing care.

METHODOLOGICAL ISSUES

A number of methodological problems and issues in research involving the investigation of nursing's effect on client outcomes were identified at the invitational conference. Only those that directly relate to the impact of nursing on client outcomes and the measurement of those outcomes are addressed in this paper. These issues tend to categorize into three areas: sampling, sensitivity of measures, and consistency of measures.

Sampling

The first issue under the area of sampling involves the sample size of research projects that examine nursing interventions that are unit based. These interventions include practice patterns, staffing mix, collaboration, and a number of other aspects of the work environment. Since the environment in which nurses deliver care is often determined by the unit or the hospital in which they practice, the unit of analysis for most of these studies is not at the individual level. In general, the cost to implement a practice model requires a smaller sample size than would normally be desired when the sampling unit is the work group. A further cost factor has to do with the expense of collecting data in a number of sites or on a number of units. Since some data must be collected at the individual level and aggregated to the unit (e.g., staff satisfaction) researchers generally expend scarce resources to collect the individual staff data and identify already existing measures of outcomes that can be considered unit or hospital based. Such information is normally collected and reported by hospitals. This approach results in outcome measures with a high degree of variability that are unit based from a limited number of units and a subsequent reduction in power. Under such conditions, it is extremely difficult to find statistical significance. It is quite likely that this effect explains the inconsistent findings in the research on nursing's impact on mortality rates. Those studies with larger sample sizes yield significant findings; those with smaller ($N \leq 30$–40) sample sizes have no significant results. The same may be true for other measures of client outcomes such as untoward hospital incidents and nosocomial infections. The good news about these measures is they are rare events; the bad news is that nursing's effect cannot be shown unless, like mortality data, the information is included in large databases to which researchers have access.

A further result of small sample sizes is the resultant inability to use sophisticated statistical procedures that consider the multivariate nature of nursing practice and the complexity of factors that lead to positive client outcomes. In the Arizona study we were limited, primarily, to the most basic inferential statistics. When we were able to use individual data and, thus, increased our sample size, we found highly significant results. Also, when we examined patterns of response we had important findings—they may not be statistically significant but they are clear patterns that result from the use of more complex statistical techniques.

A second issue with sampling has to do with the number of patients who are ineligible to participate in the research for a variety of reasons. This problem is exemplified in the descriptive New York study (Study 5). For this project, individual patients were interviewed. The potential sample was approximately 4,600. Of these, 956 subjects refused to be part of the study and 577 were ineligible. These may be the patients who are most sensitive to quantity and quality of nursing care. However, when individual patient responses are required, these data are never collected (e.g., patient satisfaction). In addition, patients are lost to studies for a variety of reasons and those reasons may, again, be critical in determining outcomes.

Measurement Sensitivity

The need to identify nurse-sensitive patient outcomes has been discussed in a number of settings with both clinicians, managers, and researchers. Although this need is critical, there remains a concurrent need to continue to use more traditional outcome measures (e.g., mortality, morbidity, length of stay). These client outcomes are recognized by consumers and other providers as being important in examining patient welfare. It must be recognized, however, that large sample sizes will be needed to increase the sensitivity of these measures and the measures must be readily available in large data sets to which researchers have access.

When nurse-sensitive outcome measures are discussed, usually they are considered to be those that relate to specific patient problems or conditions. For macrolevel research as described above, other outcomes must be identified. These outcomes need to be applicable across settings and conditions, and they must be reflective of the pattern of nursing care delivered. In order to be useful such outcomes must also be easy to measure on large numbers of patients, and when aggregated to the unit or hospital level they must have validity and reliability at that level. The issue of aggregation has been examined recently and criteria for examining reliability and validity have been described (Verran et al., 1992, 1995). Existing and ongoing work, such as that by the researchers in the San Francisco study, may provide a model for the development of such outcome measures. Their 10-item instrument is clinically feasible, reliable, and valid with predictive power. We need more of these measures that are applicable to a wide variety of clients, including the family of a client, and that can be used across units, hospitals, and settings. Such measures could eventually be included in databases and if used in a number of research projects will allow comparability. Currently, an expert panel of the American Academy of Nursing is beginning work on the identification of a set of these outcomes. What may be needed is to expand this work into a nationally supported nursing Patient Outcomes Research Team similar to those established for specific patient conditions through the Agency for Health Care Policy and Research.

A further issue in the area of sensitivity has to do with the timing of outcome measurement. Research that examines outcomes at one point in time, such as discharge, will probably not see significant results. In today's health care environment, positive outcomes usually occur in the community a significant period of time after the client leaves the hospital. In order to show the effect of nursing on outcomes, longitudinal studies need to be conducted. Hospital effects probably don't occur while the client is in the hospital. It is after they are home for a while that they realize they don't know how to care for themselves or that they know a variety of techniques to relieve pain or discomfort. In association with this timing issue is the need to examine timing expectancies. There is an ideal outcome level to be achieved and there are benchmarks along the trajectory toward that achievement that need to be identified.

Consistency of Measures

The third area of concern with researching the relationship of nursing to patient outcomes has to do with the consistency of outcomes measurement. Definitions of terms need to be very specific in order to compare findings across studies. With the complexity of nursing processes and small sample sizes, the only way firm conclusions can be drawn is by synthesizing the results from several research projects. One way to establish this specificity is to establish standardized nursing vocabularies for outcomes. These are not medical vocabularies—they are nursing oriented. We have some consistent work on a vocabulary for nursing problems and one for nursing interventions. A group of researchers at the University of Iowa is also working on a taxonomy for outcomes.

These taxonomies or categorization schemes are less meaningful, however, if the variables are not included in national databases. Nursing information on practice, staffing patterns, problems, interventions, and outcomes need to be incorporated into health care systems information. A national effort needs to be mounted to establish standardized vocabularies, incorporate them into databases, and encourage research using such systems.

SUMMARY

This paper has been presented in four sections. The first reported on six current research projects examining the interrelationship of staff, organizational, and client outcome variables. Second, a review of literature from 1985 to 1995 on the effect of nursing care on general client outcomes was presented. From these two approaches, the linkages and gaps in our current knowledge about the effects of nursing care on client outcomes on a macrolevel were identified. Finally, methodological issues with research in this field were discussed. These issues were organized into the three categories of sampling, sensitivity of measures, and consistency of measures.

REFERENCES

Aiken, L.H., Smith, H.L., and Lake, E.T. Lower Medicare Mortality Among a Set of Hospitals Known for Good Nursing Care. *Medical Care* 32:771–787, 1994.

ANA (American Nurses Association). *Nursing Care Report Card for Acute Care.* Washington, D.C.: American Nurses Publishing, 1995.

Brett, J.L.L., and Tonges, M.C. Restructured Patient Care Delivery: Evaluation of the ProACT™ Model. *Nursing Economic$* 8:36–44, 1990.

Brooten, D., Kuman, S., Brown, L.P., et al. A Randomized Clinical Trial of Early Hospital Discharge and Home Follow-up of Very Low Birthweight Infants. *New England Journal of Medicine* 315:934–939, 1986.

Burnes-Bolton, L., Daviver, M.A., Voxburgh, M.M., et al. A Cost Containment Model of Primary Nursing at Cedars-Sinai Medical Center. Pp. 129–149 in: G.G. Mayer, M.J. Madden, and E. Lawrenz, eds. *Patient Care Delivery Models.* Rockville, Md.: Aspen, 1990.

Devine, E.C., and Cook, T.D. A Meta-Analytic Analysis of Psychoeducational Interventions on Length of Postsurgical Hospital Stay. *Nursing Research* 32:267–274, 1983.

Ethridge, P. A Nursing HMO: Carondelet St. Mary's Experience. *Nursing Management* 22:22–27, 1991.

Ethridge, P., and Lamb, G.S. Professional Nursing Case Management Improves Quality, Access and Costs. *Nursing Management* 20:30–35, 1989.

Flood, S.D., and Diers, D. Nurse Staffing, Patient Outcome And Cost. *Nursing Management* 19:34–43, 1988.

Gordon, D., Weisman, C., Bergner, M., and Wong, R. *A Model for Reorganizing Nursing Resources.* Funded by the National Institute of Nursing Research, National Institutes of Health (NR02091), 1989.

Hathaway, D. Effect of Preoperative Instruction on Postoperative Outcomes: A Meta-Analysis. *Nursing Research* 35:269–275, 1986.

Hays, R.D., and White, K. Professional Satisfaction and Client Outcomes. *Medical Care* 25:259–262, 1987.

Heater, B.S., Becker, A.M., and Olson, R.K. Nursing Interventions and Patient Outcomes: A Meta-Analysis of Studies. *Nursing Research* 37:303–307, 1988.

Henry, S.B., Holzemer, W.L., and Reilly, C.A. The Relationship Between Type of Care Planning System and Patient Outcomes in Hospitalized AIDS Patients. *Journal of Advanced Nursing* 19:691–698, 1994a.

Henry, S.B., Holzemer, W.L., Reilly, C.A., and Campbell, K.E. Terms Used By Nurses To Describe Patient Problems: Can SNOMED III Represent Nursing Concepts in the Patient Record? *Journal of the American Medical Informatics Association* 1:61–74, 1994b.

Holland, T.P., Konick, A., Buffum, W., et al. Institutional Structure and Resident Outcomes. *Journal of Health and Social Behavior* 22:433–444, 1981.

Holzemer, W.L., and Henry, S.B. "Quality of Nursing Care for People with AIDS." Funded by the National Institute of Nursing Research, National Institutes of Health (R01 NR02215), 1989.

Holzemer, W.L., Henry, S.B., Stewart, A., and Janson-Bjerklie, S. The HIV Quality Audit Marker (HIV-QAM): An Outcome Measure for Hospitalized AIDS Patients. *Quality of Life Research* 3:99–107, 1993.

Ingersoll, G.M., Schultz, A.W., Ryan, S.A., et al. "The Enhanced Professional Practice Model." Cooperative agreement award jointly funded by the National Institute of Nursing Research, National Institutes of Health and the Division of Nursing, Public Health Service (U01 NR02156), 1988.

Ingersoll, G.M., Ryan, S.A., and Schultz, A.W. Enhanced Professional Practice Model for Nursing. *Research Review: Studies for Nursing Practice* 7:3, 1990.

Ingersoll, G.M., Ryan, S.A., and Schultz, A.W. Evaluating the Impact of Enhanced Professional

Practice on Patient Outcome. Pp. 301–313 in: I.E. Goertzer, ed. *Differentiating Nursing Practice into the Twenty-First Century.* Kansas City, Mo.: American Academy of Nursing, 1991.

Ingersoll, G.M., Bazar, M., and Zentner, J. Use of a Process Evaluation Map to Measure Program Implementation Progress. *Nursing Economic$* 11:137–142, 1993.

Janson-Bjerklie, S., Holzemer, W.L., and Henry, S.B. Patients' Perceptions of Pulmonary Problems and Nursing Interventions During Hospitalization for *Pneumocystis carinii* Pneumonia. *American Journal of Critical Care* 1:114–121, 1992.

Knaus, W.A., Draper, E.A., Wagner, D.P., and Zimmerman, J.E. An Evaluation of Outcome from Intensive Care in Major Medical Centers. *Annals of Internal Medicine* 104:410–418, 1986.

Koerner, B.L., Cohen, J.R., and Armstrong, D.M. Collaborative Practice and Patient Satisfaction. *Evaluation and the Health Professions* 8:299–321, 1985.

Kramer, M. The Magnet Hospitals: Excellence Revisited. *Journal of Nursing Administration* 18:20–25, 1990.

Kramer, M., and Schmalenberg, C. Magnet Hospitals: Institutions of Excellence, Part I. *Journal of Nursing Administration* 18(1):13–24, 1988a.

Kramer, M., and Schmalenberg, C. Magnet Hospitals: Institutions of Excellence, Part II. *Journal of Nursing Administration* 18(2):11–19, 1988b.

Lamb, G.S., and Huggins, D. The Professional Nursing Network. Pp. 169–184 in: G.G. Mayer, M.J. Madden, and E. Lawrenz, eds. *Patient Care Delivery Models.* Rockville, Md.: Aspen, 1990.

LaMonica, E.L., Oberst, M.T., Madea, A.R., and Wolf, R.M. Development of a Patient Satisfaction Scale. *Research in Nursing and Health* 9:43–50, 1986.

McClure, M., Poulin, M., Sovie, M.D. et al. *Magnet Hospitals: Attraction and Retention of Professional Nurses.* Kansas City, Mo.: American Academy of Nursing, 1983.

McDaniel, C., and Nash, J.G. Compendium of Instruments Measuring Patient Satisfaction with Nursing Care. *QRB (Quality Review Bulletin)* 16:182–188, 1990.

Milton, D., Verran, J.A., Murdaugh, C., and Gerber, R. Implementing Differentiated Practice as Part of a Professional Practice Model. Pp. 279–285 in: I.E. Goertzer, ed. *Differentiating Nursing Practice into the Twenty-First Century.* Kansas City, Mo.: American Academy of Nursing, 1990.

Milton, D., Verran, J.A., Murdaugh, C., and Gerber, R. Differentiated Group Professional Practice in Nursing: A Demonstration Model. *Nursing Clinics of North America* 27:23–30, 1992.

Milton, D.A., Verran, J.A., Gerber, R.M., and Fleury, J. Tools To Evaluate Reengineering Progress. Pp. 195–202 in: S.S. Blancett and D.L. Flarey, eds. *Reengineering Nursing and Health Care.* Gaithersburg, Md.: Aspen, 1995.

Minnick, A. Improving Patient Centered Care Through Initiatives in Nursing. Funded by the Picker/Commonwealth Fund, 1991.

Minnick, A. Kleinpell, R., Micek, W., and Dudley, D. The Management of a Multi-Site Study. *Journal of Professional Nursing,* in press(a).

Minnick, A., Roberts, M.J., Young, W., et al. Telephone Survey Response Rates and the Measurement of Patient Centered Care. *Nursing Research,* in press(b).

Minnick, A., Young, W., and Roberts, M.J. Reports of Service, Ratings of Quality and Intent to Recommend: 2000 Patients Relate Their Hospital Experiences. *Nursing Management,* in press(c).

Mitchell, P.H., Armstrong, S., Simpson, T.F., and Lentz, M. American Association of Critical-Care Nurses Demonstration Project: Profile of Excellence in Critical Care Nursing. *Heart and Lung* 18:219–237, 1989.

Mitchell, P., Hegevary, S., and Secrest, K. "Critical Care Nursing Systems, Retention and Patient Outcomes." Funded by the National Institute of Nursing Research, National Institutes of Health (R01 NR02343), 1991.

Mumford, E., Schlesinger, H.J., and Glass, G.V. The Effects of Psychoeducational Intervention on Recovery from Surgery and Heart Attacks: An Analysis of the Literature. *American Journal of Public Health* 72:141–151, 1982.

Naylor, M.D. Comprehensive Discharge Planning for Hospitalized Elderly: A Pilot Study. *Nursing Research* 39:156–161, 1990.

Naylor, M., Brooten, D., Jones, R., et al. Comprehensive Discharge Planning for the Hospitalized Elderly. *Annals of Internal Medicine* 120:999–1006, 1994.

Prescott, P.A. Nursing: An Important Component of Hospital Survival Under a Reformed Health Care System. *Nursing Economic$* 11:192–199, 1993.

Rose, M., and DiPasquale, B. The Johns Hopkins Professional Practice Model. Pp. 85–97 in: G.G Mayer, M.J. Madden, and E. Lawrenz, eds. *Patient Care Delivery Models.* Rockville, Md.: Aspen, 1990.

Smith, M.C., and Naftel, D.C. Meta-Analysis: A Perspective for Research Synthesis. *Image: The Journal of Nursing Scholarship* 16:9–13, 1984.

Taunton, R.L., Kleinbeck, S.V.M., Stafford, R., et al. Patient Outcomes. Are They Linked to Registered Nursing Absenteeism, Separation or Work Load? *Journal of Nursing Administration* 24:48–55, 1994.

Verran, J.A., Murdaugh, C., Gerber, R., and Milton, D. Differentiated Group Professional Practice in Nursing. Cooperative agreement award jointly funded by the National Institute of Nursing Research, National Institutes of Health, and the Division of Nursing, Public Health Service (U01 NR02153), 1988.

Verran, J.A., Mark, B.A., and Lamb, G. Psychometric Examination of Instruments Using Aggregated Data. *Research in Nursing and Health* 15:237–240, 1992.

Verran, J.A., Gerber, R., Milton, D., and Murdaugh, C. Differentiated Group Professional Practice in Nursing Project: Pathfinding for Patient Care Restructuring. Pp. 26–42 in: M.L. Parsons and C.L. Murdaugh, eds. *Patient-Centered Care: A Model for Restructuring.* Gaithersburg, Md.: Aspen, 1994.

Verran, J.A., Gerber, R., and Milton, D. Data Aggregation: Criteria for Psychometric Evaluation. *Research in Nursing and Health* 18:77–80, 1995.

Wan, T.T., and Shukla, R.K. Contextual and Organizational Correlates of the Quality of Hospital Nursing Care. *QRB (Quality Review Bulletin)* 13:61–65, 1987.

Weisman, C.S., and Nathanson, C.A. Professional Satisfaction and Client Outcomes. A Comparative Organizational Analysis. *Medical Care* 23:1179–1192, 1985.

Weisman, C.S., Gordon, D.L., Cassard, S.D., et al. The Effects of Unit Self-Management on Hospital Nurses' Work Process, Work Satisfaction, and Retention. *Medical Care* 31:381–393, 1993.

Wong, R., Gordon, D.L., Cassard, S.D., et al. A Cost Analysis of a Professional Practice Model for Nursing. *Nursing Economic$* 11:292–297, 323, 1993.

Zimmerman, J.E., Shortell, S.M., Rousseau, D.M., et al. Improving Intensive Care: Observations Based on Organizational Case Studies in Nine Intensive Care Units: A Prospective, Multicenter Study. *Critical Care Medicine* 21:1443–1451, 1993.

Zimmerman, J.E., Rousseau, D.M., Duffy, J., et al. Intensive Care at Two Teaching Hospitals: An Organizational Case Study. *American Journal of Critical Care* 3(2):129–138, 1994.

APPENDIX

Attendees at the Invitational Workshop "Quality of Care:
Examining the Influences of Nursing Resources"
October 23–24, 1994
Phoenix, Arizona

The workshop was sponsored and organized by the American Academy of Nursing.

Chairperson: Margaret Sovie

Researchers: Dorothy Gordon
                    Gail Ingersoll
                    Joyce Verran
                    Rose Gerber
                    Doris Milton
                    Ann Minich
                    Pam Mitchell
                    William Holzemer
                    Sue Henry

Methodologists: Sandra Ferketich
                    Lee Secrest
                    Ada Sue Hinshaw

Organizations: Jan Heinrich, American Academy of Nursing
                    Pat Moritz, National Institute of Nursing Research
                    Gooloo Wunderlich, Institute of Medicine
                    Angela McBride, American Academy of Nursing
                    Barbara Donohoe, American Academy of Nursing and
                      the Robert Wood Johnson and Pew Foundations
                    Marjorie Beyers, American Organization of
                      Nurse Executives
                    Deborah Nansom, Joint Commission on Accreditation
                      of Healthcare Organizations
                    Marilyn Chow, American Nurses Association

Professional Nursing Education—
Today and Tomorrow

Angela Barron McBride, Ph.D., R.N., F.A.A.N.

So there is recognition of the fact that not one but several types of nurses are needed in the life of the country. . . . The gist of the matter is that (1) intelligent nurses are better than unintelligent; (2) physicians and hospitals demand much more of their nurses than formerly; (3) preparation for bedside nursing needs good basic teaching; preparation for public health nursing, which is largely instructing, needs further teaching; while those who are to teach other nurses, hold executive positions, and become leaders must not only be of a higher grade mentally but have had a more extended formal schooling (pp. 276–277).

Minnie Goodnow, R.N.
Outlines of Nursing History, fifth ed., 1937

Nurse Goodnow's words serve well as an introduction to a consideration of professional nursing education today and tomorrow, with their emphasis on the country's long-standing need for different kinds of nurses and on the importance to differentiated practice of different levels of formal education. This paper will summarize within a historical context how the existing programs of study, from associate degree through postdoctoral training, singly and collectively strive to meet the demand for professional nursing within the United States. Because nursing as a practice profession exists at the interface between the service sector

---

Dr. McBride is distinguished professor and dean, Indiana University School of Nursing, Indianapolis.

and academia, the current state of affairs will then be analyzed in terms of the forces shaping both health care delivery and higher education. Existing at the interface between these two major social institutions affords nursing both advantages and disadvantages, which will be articulated. The major challenges ahead for professional nursing education will then be summarized with an emphasis at the end on the importance of addressing fundamentals. Although the opinions expressed are those of the author, a number of nurses responded with helpful comments to a very detailed outline of the paper. They included the leadership of six major nursing organizations—the American Academy of Nursing, the American Association of Colleges of Nursing (AACN), the American Nurses Association, the American Organization of Nurse Executives (AONE), the National League for Nursing, and Sigma Theta Tau International (nursing's honor society). See the "Author's Note" section at the end for a full listing of respondents.

A BRIEF HISTORY OF NURSING EDUCATION

To understand the present, one must always have some sense of the past. The first "modern" school of nursing was founded in 1860 by Florence Nightingale at St. Thomas Hospital in London. A little more than a decade later, the first schools in the United States to build on her curriculum and philosophy (i.e., put patients in the best situation for nature to heal) came into existence; they were associated with Bellevue Hospital in New York City, New England Hospital for Women and Children (which became Massachusetts General), and New Haven Hospital in Connecticut. Hospital diploma schools were a boon to their institutions, since student nurses provided most of needed patient care as inexpensive apprentices. By 1900, an infrastructure for nursing education was taking shape; the American Society of Superintendents of Training Schools (which became the National League for Nursing), the Nurses Associated Alumnae of United States and Canada (which became the American Nurses Association), and the *American Journal of Nursing* had all been founded.

The demanding working conditions soon contributed to a shortage of student applicants. In an attempt to de-emphasize apprenticeship training, nursing schools began to be affiliated with academic institutions. The earliest university-based nursing education took place at Howard University, Teachers College of Columbia University, Johns Hopkins University, what is now known as the University of Texas at Galveston, Rush Medical College in Chicago, and the University of Minnesota, which in 1909 became the first university to have an official school of nursing. By 1920, 180 nursing schools reported having college affiliations (Goodnow, 1937).

In 1922, Sigma Theta Tau, nursing's honor society, was founded at Indiana University with the expectation that the baccalaureate degree was to be required for entry into professional practice; this has yet, however, to become the agreed-upon norm for the field. The 1920s saw the formation of two committees—the

TABLE 1   Entry Into Practice: Nursing Programs, 1950–1990

	1950	1961	1970	1973	1978	1990
Program						
Diploma	1129	875	636	494	367	152
ADN	3	84	437	574	656	829
BSN	61	176	267	305	349	489

SOURCE: DeBack (1994) and Murphy (1979).

Committee on the Study of Nursing Education (1923) and the Committee on the Grading of Nursing Schools (1928)—that issued reports on themes that would concern nursing for the remainder of the twentieth century: the standardization of nursing education, restriction of the supply to ensure adequately paid work, and distribution and specialization of the aggregate work force. The 1930s were a period when hospitals expanded and private duty nursing declined, as the sick were unable to pay for home care because of the economic depression.

Two reports in the 1940s were to sound once again the theme of the need for standardized nursing education. The Brown Report (1948), considered to be "the nursing equivalent of the 1910 Flexner Report in medicine" (Friss, 1994, p. 604), urged that only college graduates be regarded as truly professional. That same year, the Committee on the Function of Nursing (1948) recommended upgrading standards for both the licensed practical nurse (LPN) and the registered nurse (RN), the former with an associate degree and the latter with a bachelor's of science in nursing (BSN) degree. In 1951, Montag elaborated on the growing distinction between technical training, which was to be established under the ægis of the community college, and professional education, which belonged at the bachelor's level (Montag, 1951). The first associate degree in nursing (ADN) program was started in 1952 at Fairleigh Dickinson University.

Programs offering ADNs have largely replaced diploma programs in the last four decades (see Table 1), but they became another means of acquiring the RN rather than the LPN (Deloughery, 1977; Murphy, 1979; Fondiller, 1983). Entry into professional nursing practice has been further complicated by the development of generic master's and doctoral programs on the grounds that undergraduate education is foundational to truly professional practice, just as it is for dentistry, law, and medicine (Dolan et al., 1983). For example, the first generic nursing doctorate (ND) was started at Case Western Reserve University in 1979, and there are now three such programs (Watson and Phillips, 1992).

Graduate education for nurses, however, first took the form of additional preparation in the functional areas of education and administration as nurse leaders prepared for academic or supervisory roles. The first master's degree was awarded by Teachers College of Columbia University in the 1920s, and that institution also took the lead in doctoral education a decade later. The establishment of programs to develop advanced clinical skills occurred later. By 1949, Yale University Graduate School offered a master's of science in mental health (this program moved to the School of Nursing in 1958). In 1954, Hildegard Peplau founded at Rutgers one of the first master's programs to prepare clinical nurse specialists. The first nurse practitioner program was started a decade later by Loretta Ford at the University of Colorado.

Three phases of doctoral education have been distinguished (Grace, 1978; Murphy, 1985; Hart, 1989). Before 1960, the emphasis was on functional role preparation, because nurses largely needed the EdD degree to develop the baccalaureate and higher education programs that began to be established during those years. In the 1960s, the importance of the PhD for research training gained favor as nurses sought degrees in other disciplines so as to apply that learning in developing the scientific base of their profession. Since the 1970s, the emphasis has largely been on research training within nursing. The clinical research orientation that began to take hold in the 1960s (Wald and Leonard, 1964) reached fruition in 1986 with the establishment of the National Center for Nursing Research, now the National Institute of Nursing Research (NINR), within the National Institutes of Health (McBride, 1987). That agency is organized to promote study of three general areas: (1) fostering health and preventing disease, (2) facilitating care of persons who are acutely or chronically ill, and (3) improving the delivery of nursing services (Merritt, 1986).

UNCONTROLLED DIVERSITY VERSUS INNOVATIVE CAREER LADDER

Nursing in 1995 is a heterogeneous field; it covers the full spectrum of academic degrees from the associate degree through postdoctoral training. (See Table 2 for an overview of graduations from nursing programs in the last academic year for which full data exist, 1991–1992.) Seventy-one percent of the undergraduate degrees awarded that year were at the ADN level; if anything, "the proportion of new entrants into nursing that come from baccalaureate programs has declined" in recent years (Friss, 1994, p. 615). Of the 1,853,024 employed nurses in March 1992 (out of about 2.2 million altogether), 31 percent had baccalaureate degrees in nursing or a related field, 31 percent had associate degrees in nursing, and 30 percent were graduates of diploma programs; only 8 percent had graduate degrees in nursing or a related field (Moses, 1994).

The traditional academic ladder for nurses begins with basic preparation at the undergraduate level—with a distinction between more technical preparation with the 2-year ADN and more professional preparation with the 4-year BSN—then presupposes advanced preparation in a specialty area at the master's level. At the doctoral level, the emphasis is on in-depth study of some specific problems within the specialty area for the purpose of expanding the field's knowledge base.

TABLE 2 Graduations from Nursing Programs, 1991–1992

Degree	Number of Programs	Graduations
Associate	848	52,896
Baccalaureate	501	21,415
Master's	243	7,345
Doctorate	54	391

SOURCE: NLN (1994).

The purpose of postdoctoral training is to enable new doctorally prepared nurses to set in motion a program of research. (See Figure 1 for an overview of nursing education pathways.) Existing programs have encouraged entry into the profession at various points, transitions from one academic level to the next, acceleration when career goals are clear, the acquisition of dual degrees as appropriate, and considerable experimentation.

Professional nursing can be both criticized for its seemingly uncontrolled diversity and lauded for its innovative career ladder. Traditionally, such diversity has been regarded as antithetical to being a profession, since one of the characteristics of a profession was thought to be *one* entry point. There is a growing opinion, however, that such diversity can be an asset if the practice at each level is differentiated in terms of education, experience, and demonstrated competence (Pew Health Professions Commission, 1991; Conway-Welch, 1994). That is a very big IF.

Historically, many employers have not encouraged differentiated practice according to type of education, ostensibly because both ADN and BSN graduates, as well as generic master's and doctoral students, sit for the same licensure exam to become an RN. What is more, ADN graduates tend to score somewhat higher on the examination largely for two reasons: basic knowledge is being tested, and that is the strength of the ADN program; and the BSN graduate, who has a longer program of study, is disadvantaged by taking the examination longer after having learned the material. The lack of differentiation in the examination has emboldened employers to compress salaries accordingly. Economic returns for BSN education "are modest at best, and well below the national averages for other professions" (Lowry, 1992, p. 52). Efforts are under way by the National Council of State Boards of Nursing to create a second level of licensure that would evaluate the complex decision making, community health, and management skills of BSN graduates, but widespread implementation has not yet occurred.

Nurses themselves have contributed to the lack of differentiated practice. Faculty in the ADN and BSN programs do not always have different expectations

Licensed practical nurse (LPN) to associate degree nurse (ADN)
LPN to baccalaureate in nursing (BSN)
LPN to master's of science in nursing (MSN)
Diploma
ADN
Generic baccalaureate (BSN)
Registered nurse (RN) to BSN
Accelerated RN to BSN
Accelerated BSN for nonnursing college graduates
RN to BSN (external degree baccalaureate)
MSN
Accelerated BSN to MSN
RN to MSN
MSN for nonnursing college graduates
Accelerated MSN for nonnursing college graduates
MSN for *nurses* with nonnursing college degrees
MSN/master's in business administration
MSN/master's of public health
MSN/master's of hospital administration
MSN/master's of public administration
Generic nursing doctorate (ND)
Doctorate (DNS, DNSc, DSN/PhD)
Postdoctorate

FIGURE 1   Nursing education pathways.

PROGRAM DEFINITIONS FOR FIGURE 1

Licensed practical nurse (LPN) to associate degree nurse (ADN); LPN to baccalaureate in nursing (BSN); LPN to master's of science in nursing (MSN)—Programs that admit licensed practical nurses and award an associate, baccalaureate, or master's degree in nursing.

Generic baccalaureate (BSN)—A program of instruction that admits students with no previous nursing education and requires at least four but not more than five academic years of full-time-equivalent college academic work, the completion of which results in a bachelor of science in nursing.

Registered nurse (RN) to BSN—A program that admits registered nurses with associate degrees or diplomas in nursing and awards a baccalaureate degree in nursing.

"Accelerated" option or pathway—Programs that accomplish the programmatic objectives in a shorter time frame than the traditional program, usually through a combination of "bridge" or transition courses and core courses.

BSN for nonnursing college graduates—A program that admits students with baccalaureate degrees and with no previous nursing education and, at completion, awards a baccalaureate degree in nursing.

RN to BSN (external degree baccalaureate)—A degree awarded by transcript evaluation, academically acceptable cognitive and performance examinations, or both, without residency and classroom attendance requirements.

Master of Science in Nursing (MSN)—A program of instruction that admits students with baccalaureate degrees in nursing and, at completion, awards a master of science in nursing.

RN to MSN—A program that admits registered nurses without a baccalaureate degree in nursing and awards a master's degree in nursing.

MSN for nonnursing college graduates—A program that admits students with baccalaureate degrees and with no previous nursing education and, at completion, awards a master's degree in nursing.

MSN for *nurses* with nonnursing college degrees—A program that admits registered nurses with nonnursing baccalaureate degrees and, at completion, awards a master's degree in nursing.

MSN/master's in business administration; MSN/master's of public health; MSN/master's of hospital administration; MSN/master's of public administration—Dual degree programs that admit registered nurses with a baccalaureate degree in nursing and award a master's degree in nursing in combination with a master's degree in business administration, public health, hospital administration, or public administration.

Generic Nursing Doctorate (ND)—A generic doctoral program with a clinical focus primarily designed for baccalaureate-prepared college graduates with no nursing experience.

Doctorate—A program of instruction requiring at least three academic years of full-time-equivalent academic work beyond the baccalaureate in nursing, the completion of which results in a doctoral degree that is either a doctorate of nursing science (DNS, DNSc, or DSN) or the doctor of philosophy degree (PhD).

Postdoctorate—A program environment for multidisciplinary research training involving more than one unit of a university and a recruitment plan that will attract the most highly qualified candidates (individuals must have received a doctoral degree) from throughout the nation. In such a program environment the nursing unit has the ability to demonstrate that graduates of the program remain active in research.

NOTE: These program definitions are based on the typology used by the American Association of Colleges of Nursing in their annual institutional data survey.

regarding the competencies to be developed (Conway, 1983). Graduates of ADN programs, who are on average more mature and experienced at graduation (the mean age was 35.7 years in 1992), have resisted the notion that they were less professional than their younger BSN colleagues (29.2 years old on average). This tension between undergraduate programs is further exacerbated by all of the tensions between community colleges and universities. To the extent that different kinds of RNs are educated in different educational systems, there is little opportunity for learning how to work together.

Matters have been further complicated by the fact that ADN graduates are regarded by the public at large, and especially by many a state legislature, as the success story of community colleges because of their speedy access to a relatively well-paid field. Graduates of BSN programs, in contrast, are regarded as requiring an expensive undergraduate education by universities, which tend to equate professional education with graduate education. Legislators would resist efforts to limit the production of ADN graduates, while some universities may countenance the elimination of BSN programs (as has happened, for example, in the University of California system). The more that RN production is relegated to ADN programs, the more nursing is seen solely in vocational terms by the public, including career counselors, rather than as a career choice for the best and brightest. Nursing is so equated in the public mind with doing procedures and giving medications that nurses who manage complex systems and conduct research are viewed by many as not being "real" nurses.

What has frequently been confused in ADN versus BSN discussions is the question of whether one is working at the bottom or the top of one's scope of practice. While the ADN and the BSN recipient may look relatively comparable technically and interpersonally at graduation, their progress from novice to competent practitioner, and on to expert, will not be comparable (Conway, 1983). The liberal education that is considered foundational to the development of critical thinking, decision making, and independent judgment in the BSN graduate is likely to facilitate the acquisition of the imaginal and systems skills required of advanced practice (Koerner, 1993). Considerable efforts are under way to articulate a model for differentiated nursing practice; Table 3 provides a schematic synthesis of current thinking based on the recent AACN-AONE Task Force on Differentiated Nursing Practice (1995) and the work of Davis and Burnard (1992) as well as that of Koerner (1992). It should be noted that a characteristic of recent consensus development in this area has been giving up the technical versus professional distinctions of previous ADN-BSN debates, because of the pejorative implications in characterizing ADN graduates as *not* professional, in favor of distinguishing between practice in structured and unstructured environments.

Celebrating 40 years of ADN education, Simmons (1993) noted that that degree is no longer considered to be "terminal" in nature, but a pathway for career and educational mobility. Nursing education must move to an interconnected system of distinct educational levels with differentiated outcomes (Fagin

TABLE 3 Toward Differentiated Practice

	Associate Degree	Bachelor's Degree	Master's Degree	Doctoral Degree
Characteristic(s) of knowledge	Broad	Broad and deep, with integration across subjects	Specific and deep	Very specific; expected to extend or generate new knowledge
Relationship between teacher and student	Contact high; courses structured	Contact high; courses structured with opportunities for independent study	Partnership, but within relatively structured curriculum	Emphasis on expert guided study
Practice	Provides care in structured settings where policies and procedures are established	Provides and coordinates care, health promotion, and illness prevention in structured and unstructured environments	Applies specialized knowledge and skills within a broad range of practice settings; develops policies and procedures for routine care; solves complex care problems	Extends the knowledge base for policymaking and resolving care problems

and Lynaugh, 1992; Hanner et al., 1993), but do so with pride in the articulations across pathways that are already in place and that build on experience and demonstrated competence (Shalala, 1992). The need to address these issues is crucial, because too many ADN graduates and too few BSN and higher degree nurses are being produced relative to future needs (Aiken and Salmon, 1994). As health care delivery systems become increasingly primary care oriented and boundary spanning, the roles in which nurses will be needed will require more professional judgment and clinical autonomy (Clifford, 1990).

Expectations regarding educational level and competencies for advanced practice nursing roles are also in need of some clarification. The American Association of Colleges of Nursing (1994) has taken the position that all advanced practice nurses (APN) should hold a graduate degree in nursing and be certified, and that the American Board of Nursing Specialties should serve as the umbrella board to assist member-certifying bodies adopt professional and educational standards for the evaluation and certification of APNs. The effectiveness of this level of nurse has been documented (Office of Technology Assessment, 1986; Safriet, 1992); APNs provide needed services with consumer satisfaction, demonstrable effectiveness, and significant cost savings (Brooten et al., 1986; Pew Health Professions Commission, 1994a,b). The term APN is used, however, to refer to a number of roles—clinical nurse specialists, nurse practitioners, certified nurse midwives, and nurse anesthetists. Nurse practitioners have a history of providing primary health care services, while clinical nurse specialists have traditionally worked with less educated nurses to solve complex care problems, although psychiatric clinical nurse specialists and those majoring in community health or gerontology have also provided considerable first contact care. There is substantial debate as to whether the clinical nurse specialist role, with its systems orientation, should merge with the nurse practitioner role, with its emphasis on delivering primary care, so that the public will be less confused by different titles (Fenton and Brykczynski, 1993; Page and Arena, 1994).

At the doctoral level, the debate centers on whether the research focus of PhD programs should supplant the clinical focus of professional-degree programs (e.g., a doctorate of nursing science (DNS) program) (Flaherty, 1989; Martin, 1989). Most of the original DNS programs were as research minded as any PhD program; the decision to establish a DNS program rather than a PhD program was often a political decision rather than an academic decision (Downs, 1989). Professional-degree programs were more numerous when graduate schools were not very welcoming and took the attitude that a doctorally prepared nurse was an oxymoron. As the quality of nursing research became established, so, too, did PhD programs in nursing. There is, however, some renewed interest in professional-degree programs as a means of preparing clinical leaders capable of the evaluation research that is needed for a quickly changing health care delivery system (Starck et al., 1993).

All of the emphasis within nursing education on the spectrum of academic degrees has had the unintended consequence that continuing education (CE) has received comparatively short shrift. Many states do not have mandatory CE requirements for maintaining RN licensure. This state of affairs is particularly problematic because of the knowledge explosion and the many forces dramatically reshaping health care delivery. As with other professions, learning in nursing must be a lifelong enterprise that cannot stop with the awarding of a degree (IOM, 1995).

FORCES SHAPING HEALTH CARE DELIVERY

Health care delivery is changing dramatically, with the drive toward cost effectiveness leading to: shorter hospital stays; the downsizing of acute care hospitals and corresponding increase in acuity levels within those institutions; more judicious use of high-priced technology; the advance of capitated payment and growth of health maintenance organizations (HMO); expansion of home health care and corresponding increase in acuity levels within the community; encouragement of health promotion and informed consumers; downward substitution of personnel (from LPN to aide, from RN to LPN, from physician to APN); and less emphasis on specialization but more on primary care delivery and cross training. These trends and their work force implications have been chronicled in a number of publications and reports (Pew Health Professions Commission, 1991, 1993; de Tornyay, 1992; Bureau of Health Professions, 1993; AAMC, 1994; Fineberg et al., 1994; Iliffe and Zwi, 1994; IOM, 1994; Larson et al., 1994).

Professional nursing is, therefore, experiencing paradigm shifts. (See Table 4 for an overview of some major changes as care moves away from traditional conceptualizations to expanded ones.) Most nurses are still hospital based, but a shift is taking place away from nursing at the bedside to nursing at the patient's side wherever (s)he may be. In the future, nurses must be able to span boundaries in providing continuity of care, particularly as case managers. Heretofore nursing, like medicine, has been organized to manage diseases and illness episodes, but henceforth emphasis will be placed on disease prevention and health promotion as cost containment measures. This means a renewed interest in compressing morbidity and facilitating quality of life, as opposed to focusing largely on limiting mortality. Instead of the military metaphor of health, with its view of the patient's body as a battlefield and the physician as captain of the ship, the ecologic metaphor offers the promise of "halfway technology," more concern about wastefulness, and a community orientation (Annas, 1995). It should be noted, however, that the market metaphor with its language of "covered lives," market share, vertical integration, and customer satisfaction may be an intermediary step in reframing the debate.

Traditionally, nurses have been expected to meet as many of a patient's needs as possible. Those unbounded expectations are being superseded by the

TABLE 4 Some of the Paradigm Shifts that Professional Nurses Are Experiencing

Traditional	Expanded
Nursing at bedside (hospital)	Nursing at patient's side (spanning boundaries)
Disease management	Disease prevention and health promotion
Limit mortality	Limit mortality, compress morbidity, and facilitate quality of life
Organized by illness episodes	Organized to provide continuity of care
Shaped by the military metaphor	Shaped by the ecologic metaphor
Unbounded expectations for meeting a patient's needs	Expectations bound by resources, hierarchy of needs
Nursing seen as providing care	Nursing seen as providing care, directing care provided by others, developing population-based programs, and managing systems
All-RN staff models of care	Partner models of care with RN mix
Process oriented	Outcomes oriented
Oblivious to costs	Mindful of costs
Nurses support the primary care provider (dependent)	Nurses provide primary care (independent/interdependent)
Nurses have responsibility	Nurses have responsibility *and* corresponding authority
Discipline-specific education and practice	Interdisciplinary education and practice
Diversity seen as antithetical to being professional	Differentiated practice emphasized
Job security	Career development

notion that needs should be triaged in terms of available resources, and that there should be fewer nursing imperatives—e.g., everyone should be bathed every day. Nursing has been equated with providing care, but care as a one-to-one relationship will not be as large a component of professional nursing in the future because the RN is increasingly expected to direct the care provided by others (Hines et al., 1994), develop programs for vulnerable populations, and manage complicated, boundary-spanning systems. These changes are prompted, in part, because all-RN staff models of care are giving way to so-called partner models of care, with the RN skill mix dropping from 76 to 100 percent to 52 to 79 percent in some settings (Smeltzer et al., 1993). The in-process component of nursing will be less emphasized than what is actually achieved by way of outcomes, particularly cost-effective outcomes. Where the nurse has traditionally supported the physician as the primary care provider, there will be increasing emphasis on the nurse, particularly the APN, as a primary care provider, which means that responsibility must be balanced with corresponding authority (e.g., prescriptive authority).

Up until now, the emphasis has been on discipline-specific education and practice, but this is shifting to become more interdisciplinary as cost-effective care requires all health care providers to avoid duplication of efforts and make full use of the best, least expensive care giver according to need. Such differentiated practice will replace the notion that the physician is *the* health care provider of choice for all situations. Collectively, these shifts make it impossible to promise job security to any nurse, because of the extent to which institutions and systems are being reconfigured. In place of job security, nurses need to take comfort from the career opportunities that will continue to hold for individuals who are skilled, as they are, in health promotion, boundary spanning, and clinical decision making.

Nurses will continue to be in demand with the graying of America and the move toward community-centered practice, with its emphasis on a broad range of practice sites—schools, day care and senior centers, outpatient clinics, shelters, workplaces, homes, shopping malls, and church basements. Computer literacy will become more important as technologies are developed to connect care givers in remote sites to information and assessment systems. The outcomes orientation of health care will also increase the demand for competencies like those of nurses who collect and analyze data to evaluate their own effectiveness and that of their institutions (Oermann, 1994b). A return to community-centered care also requires that health care professionals "look like" the communities served; this means taking steps to recruit minority faculty and students in numbers proportionate to their representation in the area (Morris and Wykle, 1994), and to expand the number of men in the profession.

A TIME OF REDIRECTION ON CAMPUS

Higher education is changing almost as fundamentally as health care delivery systems and in the same general direction toward greater accountability at a time of restricted taxpayer support. In the name of cost effectiveness, there have been a number of changes: the adoption of responsibility-centered budgeting; increased emphasis on teaching and credit hour production; increased use of part-time faculty with corresponding decreases in full-time and tenure track faculty; examination of faculty entitlements and productivity; increases in class size and setting minimum expectations for class size; some experimentation with capitated payment; examination of administrative bloat; and stemming the proliferation of programs through greater clarity about mission. These shifts have been chronicled in a number of publications (Lynton and Elman, 1987; Shulman, 1987; Rice, 1991; El-Khawas, 1994; Brand, 1995; Magrath, 1995).

The traditional university activities of teaching, research, and service are being rethought. (See Table 5 for an overview of some major changes as these activities are reconceptualized.) The emphasis has shifted away from teaching to learning, with a concomitant new regard for the teacher as "guide by side" rather than "sage on stage." Instead of stressing the accumulation of facts, the thrust is on the application of knowledge to real problems, many of which may demand an

TABLE 5 Some of the Paradigm Shifts That Academia Is Experiencing

	Traditional	Expanded
Teaching	• Emphasis on teaching • "Sage on stage" • Obtain and retain facts • Obtain degree • Process oriented • Discipline based • Place bound	• Emphasis on learning • "Guide by side" • Apply knowledge to real problems • Develop portfolio of competencies • Outcomes oriented • Interdisciplinary • "Virtual university"
Research	• Scholarship narrowly defined • Congruent with personal interests • Emphasis on refereed publications • Supported largely by federal government	• Scholarship broadly defined • Congruent with institutional mission • Emphasis on dissemination to professionals and public alike • Supported increasingly by private sector
Service	• Undervalued and discouraged • Confused with volunteer community activities • Seen as quasi-charity • Emphasis on university and disciplinary service	• Valued and encouraged • Based on professional expertise • Seen as a profit center for university • Emphasis on public service

interdisciplinary perspective. This moves the educational goal away from degree acquisition toward the development of a portfolio of competencies that can be described to prospective employers. Outcomes have replaced the curriculum as the preoccupation of pedagogical attention. Furthermore, all of these activities are less and less place bound as the advent of new technologies and distance learning techniques make the "virtual university" possible.

Thanks to Boyer's landmark work (1990), scholarship is no longer narrowly defined to include only the scholarship of discovery (i.e., traditional basic research), but also includes the scholarship of integration, utilization, and teaching or pedagogy. Where once the emphasis was solely on the investigator's interests, the expectation increasingly is that faculty research should be congruent with the campus mission. The product of that research should not only be scholarly publications but also contributions to the public good, which means that the private sector may be more interested in supporting some efforts with entrepreneurial possibilities.

Where service was once undervalued and discouraged, the opposite is increasingly the case. Indeed, there has been renewed interest in the concept of service learning. When the emphasis is on applying professional expertise for the public's well-being, these activities can even be conceptualized as a possible profit center for the university. Most professional schools are beginning to explore practice plans, contracts with local agencies, and continuing education for professionals and the public alike as possible new revenue streams.

Like the health care delivery system, higher education is increasingly sensitive to community need, focused on performance-based outcome measures, and concerned about differentiated faculty roles with a concomitant reliance on some mix in expertise. Data management systems assume a new importance in an environment concerned about policy-making to achieve efficiency and effectiveness. New initiatives are increasingly being funded by redirecting existing resources rather than acquiring new ones from traditional public sources. The lifting of mandatory retirement requirements has created an additional concern about whether the faculty in place have the skills and knowledge base needed for the future.

HEALTH CARE AND ACADEMIA: NURSING'S ADVANTAGES AND DISADVANTAGES

With the two social institutions of health care delivery and higher education undergoing such fundamental change, nursing will have distinct advantages and disadvantages. In the reconfigured health care delivery system, nursing has much to offer: a comfortableness about operating within systems; conceptual models capable of analyzing the person-environment fit; a family-centered care focus; a history of interdisciplinary collaboration; community assessment skills; experience with health promotion and consumer education; the ability to span boundaries; a nonreductionist philosophy of care; relationship-centered care (Tresolini and the Pew-Fetzer Task Force, 1994); established links with community agencies and long-term care facilities; long-standing encouragement of functional ability and quality of life; expertise in behavioral outcomes research; and several hundred community-based nursing centers attached to schools of nursing. In a reconfigured health care delivery system, a major advantage is that the cost of educating an APN may be as little as one-third of the cost of physician training, and that nurse practitioner can provide about 80 percent of primary care services at an equivalent level of positive outcomes and patient satisfaction (Pew Health Professions Commission, 1994a,b).

Nursing also is disadvantaged in the reconfigured health care delivery system. The downsizing of hospitals is displacing RNs more than any other worker, and those in place may be more prone to burnout because of increased workload (McClure, 1991; Gordon, 1995). Many of the changes that are taking place are not based on tried-and-true principles, but on a frustration with current realities. The downsizing of nursing within hospitals is also taking place at the same time that nurses are being expected to supervise the work of more unlicensed assistive personnel, which is itself a time-consuming task (ANA, 1992). Joel (1994) has noted that coordination of care is further complicated when these assistive personnel are assigned directly to patients as if they operated on their own authority, rather than being assigned to nurses for delegation purposes.

High-level strategic planning for fundamental institutional change frequently does not include RNs, yet they are regularly expected to work out the operational details of restructuring, mergers, and consolidations. There is a move in many hospitals to incorporate nursing with other patient care services under a single vice president for patient care services. This has diminished the importance of the nursing director in the senior hierarchy, who was previously comparable to the medical director. Although nurses are best suited to take these new positions, the emphasis has shifted in many institutions away from the patient-care focus of nursing to "patient-focused care" which is sometimes used as a rallying cry for providing services at the lowest cost. These trends are disturbing because lower mortality has been associated with a higher ratio of RNs to patients (Hartz et al., 1989; Prescott, 1993) and with nurses having control over their practice (Aiken et al., 1994).

Advanced practice nurses are typically hired by physicians or administrators to staff a particular service and have no formal ties to nursing service delivery in other parts of the institution, so their connection to their profession can easily weaken over time, particularly if they are utilized only as physician substitutes rather than for their nursing expertise. The danger is that the growing use of APNs may replicate what happened to psychiatric clinical nurse specialists in the 1960s with the development of community mental health centers, when they were used as interchangeable members of the mental health team and consequently forsook nursing's traditional focus on maximizing functional ability in favor of "doing therapy" in 50-minute hours. As managed care systems grow in size across state boundaries, they have begun to push for institutional licensure to promote uniform practice, but such a move could further remove individuals from control over their profession's practice. Considerable legal and institutional barriers do exist to prevent reimbursement for nurse-provided primary care, for example, Medicare policies (Inglis and Kjervik, 1993).

Nursing may be in a more advantageous position in the universities of tomorrow for a number of reasons. The emphasis on service learning has made the activities of nursing students and faculty much more valued, particularly in those instances in which course requirements or contracted faculty time have benefited participating clinical or community agencies. The areas of scholarship that are being regarded with renewed appreciation—the scholarship of integration, utilization, and teaching—have been areas where nursing faculty have traditionally excelled. Nursing's accrediting body, the National League for Nursing, shifted to an outcomes orientation well ahead of other professional associations.

Nursing has a long history of being interdisciplinary; for example, the doctoral preparation of nurses has actively made use of the models of various disciplines such as ethics, education, anthropology, psychology, sociology, public health, and physiology. Nursing has never emphasized just regurgitating facts, but weaving those facts into clinical decision making (Tanner, 1987, 1993). Nontraditional educational methods are not new to nursing (Lenburg, 1986). Distance learning has become a staple in many nursing schools with outreach commitments (Billings et al., 1994). The problem-solving orientation, consensus-building techniques, and interpersonal skills of nurses enable them to demonstrate competencies in great demand across settings.

On the other hand, nursing is likely to be disadvantaged in the universities of tomorrow. Because it is a field that has come later to research (i.e., the scholarship of discovery), an infrastructure to support that mission within schools of nursing is not fully in place. The current devaluation of research in support of teaching is likely to have more negative consequences for a field that has long valued teaching but only recently made research a priority, for it will be more difficult to get the resources for research in a climate less supportive of that activity.

Clinical teaching is labor intensive, particularly when students are spread throughout the community rather than concentrated in a single hospital (Rothert et al., 1994), so universities will be increasingly critical of such costs, particularly in the face of dropping enrollments occasioned by a tight job market. This problem is also likely to be an issue in the merger or consolidation of university hospitals with other kinds of hospitals that are less inclined to believe they should subsidize clinical teaching even indirectly. The demand for master's and doctorally prepared faculty is outstripping supply (Mullinix, 1990; Rosenfeld, 1992); indeed, today's "nursing shortage" is at those levels of preparation. What is more, the nature of practice is changing faster than the curriculum of most schools of nursing and the knowledge base of existing nursing faculty (VanOrt et al., 1989; Oermann, 1994a).

MAJOR CHALLENGES AHEAD

The major challenges ahead for professional nursing education reflect the key themes of this paper.

Differentiating Practice

Both nurse educators and employers must be encouraged to differentiate nursing practice by education, experience, and demonstrated competence. This movement can be facilitated by deliberately encouraging different levels of nurses to work together as part of their educational preparation, standardizing the second level of licensure for BSN graduates, and requiring advanced practice nurses to have a graduate degree and certification from a professional association approved by the American Board of Nursing Specialties. It should be recognized that one of the difficulties that is likely to complicate differentiated practice between ADN and BSN nurses is the extent to which there also needs to be differentiated practice between the RN and the LPN or unlicensed aide; the American Association of Critical Care Nurses (1990) has recommended five criteria to facilitate these distinctions.

Levels of nursing must be particularly differentiated with regard to the needs of an aging society because society still has the mistaken notion that the least well prepared are best suited to provide gerontological care when the converse is true (Aiken, 1990; McBride and Burgener, 1994). State strategies for health care work force reform must be encouraged (Pew Health Professions Commission, 1994c), particularly the establishment of a methodology for modeling work force needs by competency sets across the educational continuum.

Creating a More Educated RN Work Force

The aggregate supply of nurses is impressive, but there are too many ADN graduates and too few baccalaureate and higher degree nurses (Moccia, 1990; Aiken and Salmon, 1994). The Pew Health Professions Commission (1994a) has estimated, for example, that the number of graduates from nurse practitioner programs needs to double by the year 2000. Something must be done to provide incentives to community colleges to limit their number of graduates. Depictions of nursing must portray the career opportunities that are only available to baccalaureate and higher degree nurses, so the public is less likely to think that "a nurse is a nurse is a nurse." Recruitment efforts must communicate in a visionary way the extent to which the professional nurse of the future is not like the traditional nurse of the past, so applicants can make informed career choices.

New kinds of articulation agreements (e.g., RN-BSN, RN-MSN) between community colleges and universities must be forged to facilitate mobility across programs and educational systems. This is of pressing concern because articulation strategies exist (Mathews and Travis, 1994), but the percentage of RN-BSN graduates has remained flat over the last decade (about 10 percent) despite the large number of ADN graduates and the many mobility programs (Salmon, 1995). Federal policies that deliberately encourage diploma nursing and ADN education are outmoded and must be reformulated to encourage baccalaureate and higher degree nurses who are in limited supply. For example, Medicare currently supports diploma nursing education, which is hospital owned; the Department of Education supports only ADN programs through the Perkins Act; and graduate education in nursing has none of the supports that are available to medicine through graduate medical education (GME) funds.

Reconfiguring RN Work Force Demographics

The nursing work force is aging more rapidly than the overall population. More traditional college-aged students must be recruited to the field since the proportion of RNs under age 30 declined from 25 to 11 percent between 1980 and

1992; "by 2000, two thirds of all RNs are expected to be over age 40" (Aiken et al., 1995, p. 4). If the average ADN graduate is over 35 and the overwhelming majority of new RNs are ADN graduates, then the aging of the RN work force is easy to understand. The BSN is the most cost-effective route for the individual to the RN (Lowry, 1992), and the one with the highest percentage of minority graduates (Aiken and Salmon, 1994). It is also the program most likely to supply applicants to APN and doctoral programs. Expectations must change to encourage RNs to obtain graduate education and research training at an earlier age, so that the expertise obtained can be utilized over a longer period of time. This approach is not intended to deny opportunities because of age, but to limit practices that discourage and disadvantage younger students.

It is also vitally important that recruitment and retention policies encourage underrepresented populations to enter the profession. About 23 percent of the U.S. population consists of racial and ethnic minorities, but only 9 percent of nurses are from these groups. What is more, these groups are further underrepresented in APN, doctoral and postdoctoral programs, and in management roles. The accelerated growth of specific populations, for example Hispanics, has consequences for the language skills to be expected of nurses. The diversification of the citizenry in general also requires all health care professionals to be able to deliver culturally competent care (Andrews, 1992). Only 4 percent of all nurses are male, although they are better educated than their female counterparts and more prominent among nurse managers (Salmon, 1995).

Supporting Creative Pedagogy and Community-Centered Care

Nursing education must test the validity of its most cherished practices, such as reliance on person-to-person transmission of information or the practice of keeping education separate from the "business" side of health care (Hegyvary, 1991, 1992). Creative pedagogy must become the order of the day, particularly with respect to clinical teaching in community settings (Aiken, 1990; Alexander, 1991; Barger and Kline, 1993; Benner, 1993; Baird et al., 1994; de Tornyay, 1994; Knuteson and Wielichowski, 1994). The majority of existing faculty are not prepared to advance models that collapse boundaries between education and practice (Andreoli and Musser, 1986; Chickadonz, 1987). Developmental supports must be provided for faculty renewal and experimentation in light of the needs created by quickly changing practice conditions, including the need for nurses to be preventionists and not just interventionists; the need to bridge experiences to help new graduates handle the escalating acuity level of hospitals; and the use of nurses as house staff (Mallison, 1993); the reorganization of master's education programs to emphasize core competencies across specialty areas; the role of nursing in health maintenance organizations and reconfigured academic health centers (Moore et al., 1994; Valberg et al., 1994); and the development of greater competencies in community assessment and in teaching clinical skills to family members.

Encouraging Interdisciplinary Collaboration

With the blurring of disciplinary lines, the education and practice of health care professionals must become more interdisciplinary. This will necessitate the development of new models of collaboration that are not rigidly hierarchical, but that provide for differentiated practice by education, experience, and demonstrated competence (Fagin, 1992; Pike et al., 1993). Studies of such collaboration have demonstrated improvements in care (Knaus et al., 1986; Garcia et al., 1993). Perhaps no phrase is more bandied about, despite any agreement about its meaning, than "interdisciplinary collaboration." Indeed, some physicians think it refers to cooperation across medical specialties (e.g., pediatricians and psychiatrists working respectfully together) rather than to practice involving different kinds of providers working collegially together (e.g., a mental health strategy involving psychiatrists, psychologists, psychiatric nurses, and psychiatric social workers).

Supporting Informatics and Health Systems Delivery Research

Computers and telecommunications are likely to become more important in the education and practice of RNs as nurses organize patients into electronic self-help groups and customize health promotion (Rheingold, 1993). Technology will be increasingly regarded as an aid to clinical decision making, particularly in ensuring that guidelines and standards are implemented appropriately (Donaldson and Sox, 1992). Electronic links offer the promise of consultation across vast distances, easy access to the latest information, and the possibility of lifelong learning opportunities across state lines. For this promise to be realized, informatics must be mainstreamed into the curriculum.

Nurses must become adept at evaluation research and develop the corresponding technologic and data management skills to achieve that objective (Fagin and Jacobsen, 1985). The large data bases that will be developed to monitor quality and cost effectiveness must include variables of concern to nursing, and nurses must be prepared to make use of these data sets in shaping their practice and policies (NLN, 1993). There is no obvious home for such research, however, since the Agency for Health Care Policy Research is biased toward *medical* outcomes and work force issues and NINR is geared toward clinical interventions and biomedical research rather than health systems delivery research. Efficacy (what works under relatively ideal conditions) and effectiveness (what works under ordinary conditions) must be monitored not only in terms of patient outcomes, but in terms of what happens to vulnerable populations as a group. There is an important role for the nurse researcher to play in clinical and community settings (Chaska, 1992; Kirchhoff, 1993), and both doctoral and postdoctoral research training should develop those competencies.

Removing Practice Barriers

An extremely broad scope of practice is accorded physicians in some states, which makes it possible for the medical profession to occupy the entire health care field (Safriet, 1992). Barriers to practice (e.g., lack of prescriptive authority) and to reimbursement of APNs must be systematically removed. "In view of the serious access problems among poor and minority Medicare beneficiaries in urban areas, the continued systematic exclusion of nurse practitioners from Medicare is striking" (Aiken and Salmon, 1994, p. 323). Medicaid and Medicare laws should be revised to cover those services provided by APNs within their scope of practice.

Renewing Displaced Nurses

Programs must be provided to renew displaced nurses. Such programs will, for example, develop severance packages that support additional education, enable nurses who have previously been hospital-based to learn how to work effectively in community settings, and help MSN graduates who are not certified as nurse practitioners to move quickly in that direction. Mandatory CE should be required and supported in all states, given the knowledge explosion and the quickening pace of changes in practice. Related to this is the obligation of universities and professional associations to provide CE programs on career assessment and the transformational leadership skills necessary in times of rapid change (Wolf et al., 1994a,b; Feldman, 1995). Relationships between employee and employer are much more explicit with regard to task outcomes and development expectations than they once were (Noer, 1993), and it is incumbent on nursing education both to prepare a work force capable of revitalizing itself in a time of fundamental organizational change and to act accordingly as it, too, becomes reconfigured.

ADDRESSING FUNDAMENTALS

In an article humorously entitled "Nursing Studies Laid End to End Form a Circle," Friss (1994) acknowledged that nurses have been one of the most studied groups in history, but that fundamental problems remain: no single route to entry into professional practice; lack of differentiated practice and corresponding salary compression; an impressive aggregate supply of nurses but the wrong educational mix; a scope of practice too often shaped by what others permit nurses to do rather than by what they can do; and periodic nurse shortages that lead to the attraction of casual workers rather than to a stable dedicated core. Her conclusion is that nursing alone cannot address these fundamental issues, but must press physicians and administrators to change those practices of theirs that promote inefficient and ineffective use of nurses. It should be noted that the time is ripe for such fundamental change because nursing's work force has itself undergone a major shift in the last quarter century—away from a situation in which the personal flexibility of nursing was valued as the overarching consideration, to one of being largely peopled by individuals with a full-time work commitment. Workers with a career orientation are more likely to be prepared to change the conditions of practice.

Now that the health care delivery system is downsizing acute care hospitals in favor of community-centered care, the need for nursing in unstructured environments will become more visible and with it the need for a more educated nursing work force. (Recall Nurse Goodnow's words at the beginning of this paper that public health nursing requires more educated nurses.) Drucker (1994) identifies the fastest growing work force group as being knowledge workers who take responsibility for making themselves understood by people who do not have the desired knowledge base. That actually is a very accurate depiction of nursing—using knowledge to help people do for themselves what they would do unaided if they knew what to do. Alas, the popular conception of nursing still emphasizes carrying out discrete tasks more than the weaving together of various knowledge bases into a coherent plan of care. But such situation-specific integration of diverse knowledge from the behavioral and biological sciences is the promise of professional nursing in the twenty-first century.

AUTHOR'S NOTE

The author wishes to acknowledge the many nurses who were asked to review an outline of this paper and who made very helpful suggestions:

Dyanne Affonso
Carole Anderson
Margaret Applegate
Joan Austin
Geraldine "Polly" Bednash
Ginna Betts
Marge Beyers
Diane Billings
Donna Boland
Rachel Booth
Faye Bower
Judy Campbell
Sara Campbell
Janie Canty

Penny Cass
Bianca Chambers
Luther Chrisman
Dawn Daniels
Donna Diers
Jerry Durham
Geraldene Felton
Linda Finke
Joyce Fitzpatrick
Juanita Fleming
Janet Gerkensmeyer
Nancy Dickenson Hazard
Jan Heinrich
Thomas Hicks

Bill Holzemer	Jane Norbeck
Gail Ingersoll	Nancy Opie
Norma Lang	Marla Salmon
Carol Lindeman	Catherine Scott
Brenda Lyon	Mary Lou de Leon Siantz
Barbara Manz	Phyllis Stern
Geraldine Marillo	Diana Weaver
Patricia Moccia	Judy Williams
Sue Morrissey	May Wykle

REFERENCES

AACN (American Association of Colleges of Nursing). *Certification and Regulation of Advanced Practice Nurses.* Washington, D.C.: AACN, 1994.

AACN-AONE (American Association of Colleges of Nursing and American Organization of Nurse Executives) Task Force on Differentiated Nursing Practice. *A Model for Differentiated Nursing Practice.* Washington, D.C.: AACN, 1995.

AAMC (Association of American Medical Colleges). *Academic Medicine and Health Care Reform. Roles for Medical Education in Health Care Reform.* Washington, D.C.: AAMC, 1994.

Aiken, L.H. *Educational Innovations in Gerontology: Teaching Nursing Homes and Gerontological Nurse Practitioners.* Washington, D.C.: Association for Gerontology in Higher Education, 1990.

Aiken, L.H., and Salmon, M.E. Health Care Workforce Priorities: What Nursing Should Do Now. *Inquiry* 31:318–329, 1994.

Aiken, L.H., Smith, H.L., and Lake, E.T. Lower Medicare Mortality Among a Set of Hospitals Known for Good Nursing Care. *Medical Care* 32:771–787, 1994.

Aiken, L.H., Gwyther, M.E., and Friese, C.R. The Registered Nurse Workforce: Infrastructure for Health Care Reform. *Statistical Bulletin* 76(1):2–9, 1995.

Alexander, B.W. Team Learning. *Geriatric Nursing* 12:248, 1991.

American Association of Critical Care Nurses. *Delegation of Nursing and Non-Nursing Activities in Critical Care: A Framework for Decision Making.* Newport Beach, Calif.: The Association, 1990.

ANA (American Nurses Association). *Progress Report on Unlicensed Assistive Personnel: Informational Report.* Report no. CNP-CNE-B. Washington, D.C.: ANA, 1992.

Andreoli, K.G., and Musser, L.A. Faculty Productivity. Pp. 177–193 in: H.H. Werley, J.J. Fitzpatrick, and R.L. Taunton, eds. *Annual Review of Nursing Research* (vol. 4). New York: Springer, 1986.

Andrews, M.M. Cultural Perspectives on Nursing in the 21st Century. *Journal of Professional Nursing* 8:7–15, 1992.

Annas, G.J. Reframing the Debate on Health Care Reform by Replacing Our Metaphors. *New England Journal of Medicine* 332:744–747, 1995.

Baird, S.C., Bopp, A., Schofer, K.K.K. et al. An Innovative Model for Clinical Teaching. *Nurse Educator* 19(3):23–25, 1994.

Barger, S.E., and Kline, P.M. Community Health Service Programs in Academe. *Nurse Educator* 18(6):22–26, 1993.

Benner, P. Transforming RN Education: Clinical Learning and Clinical Knowledge Development. Pp. 3–14 in: N.L. Diekelmann and M.L. Rather, eds. *Transforming RN Education: Dialogue and Debate.* New York: National League for Nursing Press, 1993.

Billings, D., Durham, J., Finke, L., et al. Faculty Perceptions of Teaching on Television: One School's Experience. *Journal of Professional Nursing* 10:307–312, 1994.

Boyer, E.L. *Scholarship Reconsidered: Priorities of the Professoriate.* Princeton, N.J.: Carnegie Foundation, 1990.

Brand, M. Higher Education and Obligations to the Future. *The IU Newspaper* 19(2):9–12, January 1995.

Brooten, D., Jumar, S., Brown, L., et al. A Randomized Clinical Treatment of Early Hospital Discharge and Home Followup of Very Low Birth Weight Infants. *New England Journal of Medicine* 315:934–939, 1986.

Brown, E.L. *Nursing for the Future: A Report Prepared for the National Nursing Council.* New York: Russell Sage Foundation, 1948.

Bureau of Health Professions. *An Agenda for Health Professions Reform.* Washington, D.C.: U.S. Government Printing Office, 1994.

Chaska, N.L. The Staff Nurse Role. Pp. 185–203 in: J.J. Fitzpatrick, R.L. Taunton, and A.K. Jacox, eds. *Annual Review of Nursing Research* (vol. 10). New York: Springer, 1992.

Chickadonz, G.H. Faculty Practice. Pp. 137–151 in: J.J. Fitzpatrick and R.L. Taunton, eds. *Annual Review of Nursing Research* (vol. 5). New York: Springer, 1987.

Clifford, J.C. The Future of Nursing Practice. Pp. 617–623 in: N. Chaska, ed. *The Nursing Profession—Turning Points.* St. Louis, Mo.: Mosby, 1990.

Committee on the Function of Nursing. *A Program for the Nursing Profession.* New York: Macmillan, 1948.

Committee on the Grading of Nursing Schools. *Nurses, Patients, and Pocketbooks.* New York: The Committee, 1928.

Committee on the Study of Nursing Education. *Nursing and Nursing Education in the United States.* New York: MacMillan, 1923.

Conway, M. E. Socialization and Roles in Nursing. Pp. 183–208 in: H.H. Werley and J.J. Fitzpatrick, eds. *Annual Review of Nursing Research* (vol. 1). New York: Springer, 1983.

Conway-Welch, C. National Initiatives for Change. Pp. 196–201 in: J.C. McClosky and H.K. Grace, eds. *Current Issues in Nursing* (4th ed.). St. Louis, Mo.: Mosby Year Book, 1994.

Davis, B.D., and Burnard, P. Academic Levels in Nursing. *Journal of Advanced Nursing* 17:1395–1400, 1992.

DeBack, V. Debate: Diversity in Nursing Education. Does it Help or Hinder the Profession? Pp. 153–157 in: J.C. McCloskey and H.K. Grace, eds. *Current Issues in Nursing* (4th ed.). St. Louis, Mo.: Mosby Year Book, 1994.

Deloughery, G.L. *History and Trends of Professional Nursing.* St. Louis, Mo.: C.V. Mosby, 1977.

de Tornyay, R. Reconsidering Nursing Education: The Report of the Pew Health Professions Commission. *Journal of Nursing Education* 31:296–301, 1992.

de Tornyay, R. Creating the Teachers of Tomorrow's Professionals. *Inquiry* 31:283–288, 1994.

Dolan, J.A., Fitzpatrick, M.L., and Herrmann, E.K. *Nursing in Society. A Historical Perspective* (15th ed.). Philadelphia: W. B. Saunders, 1983.

Donaldson, M.O., and Sox, H.C., eds. *Setting Priorities for Health Technology Assessment.* Washington, D.C.: National Academy Press, 1992.

Downs, F.S. Differences between the Professional Doctorate and The Academic/Research Doctorate. *Journal of Professional Nursing* 5:261–265, 1989.

Drucker, P.F. *Knowledge Work and Knowledge Society. The Social Transformations of This Century.* Cambridge, Mass.: John F. Kennedy School of Government, Harvard University, 1994.

El-Khawas, E. *Campus Trends 1994. A Time of Redirection.* Washington, D.C.: American Council on Education, 1994.

Fagin, C.M. Collaboration between Nurses and Physicians. No Longer A Choice. *Nursing and Health Care* 13:354–363, 1992.

Fagin, C.M., and Jacobsen, B.S. Cost-Effectiveness Analysis in Nursing Research. Pp. 215–238 in:

H.H. Werley and J.J. Fitzpatrick, eds. *Annual Review of Nursing Research* (vol. 3). New York: Springer, 1985.

Fagin, C.M., and Lynaugh, J.E. Reaping the Rewards of Radical Change: A New Agenda for Nursing Education. *Nursing Outlook* 40:213–220, 1992.

Feldman, H.R. Preparing the Nurse Executive of the Future. *Nursing Leadership Forum* 1:18–22, 1995.

Fenton, M.V., and Brykczynski, K.A. Qualitative Distinctions and Similarities in the Practice of Clinical Nurse Specialists and Nurse Practitioners. *Journal of Professional Nursing* 9:313–326, 1993.

Fineberg, H.V., Green, G.M., Ware, J.H., and Anderson, B.L. Changing Public Health Training Needs: Professional Education and the Paradigm of Public Health. *Annual Review of Public Health* 15:237–257, 1994.

Flaherty, M.J. The Doctor of Nursing Science Degree: Evolutionary and Societal Perspectives. Pp. 17–31 in: S.E. Hart, ed. *Doctoral Education in Nursing: History, Process and Outcomes.* New York: National League for Nursing, 1989.

Fondiller, S.H. *The Entry Dilemma.* New York: National League for Nursing, 1983.

Friss, L. Nursing Studies Laid End to End Form a Circle. *Journal of Health Politics, Policy and Law* 19:597–631, 1994.

Garcia, M.A., Niemeyer, D.B.J., and Robbins, J. Collaborative Practice: A Shared Success. *Nursing Management* 24(5):72–78, 1993.

Goodnow, M. *Outlines of Nursing History* (5th ed.). Philadelphia: W.B. Saunders, 1937.

Gordon, S. Cutbacks on Caregivers. Is There a Nurse in the House? *The Nation* 260(6):199–202, February 13, 1995.

Grace, H. The Development of Doctoral Education in Nursing: An Historical Perspective. *Journal of Nursing Education* 17(4):17–27, 1978.

Hanner, M.B., Heywood, E.J., and Kaye, M.J. The Curriculum Revolution: Implications for Associate Degree Nursing Education. Pp. 61–68 in: J. Simmons, ed. *Prospectives. Celebrating 40 Years of Associate Degree Nursing Education.* New York: National League for Nursing Press, 1993.

Hart, S.E., ed. *Doctoral Education in Nursing: History, Process and Outcome.* New York: National League for Nursing, 1989.

Hartz, A., Krakauer, H., Kuhn, E., et al. Hospital Characteristics and Mortality Rates. *New England Journal of Medicine* 321:1720–1725, 1989.

Hegyvary, S.T. Education. Calculating the Stakes. *Journal of Professional Nursing* 7:325, 1991.

Hegyvary, S.T. Education. Nursing Education for Health Care Reform. *Journal of Professional Nursing* 8:3, 1992.

Hines, P.A.P., Smeltzer, C.H., and Galletti, M. Work Restructuring: The Process of Redefining Roles of Patient Caregivers. *Nursing Economic$* 12:346–350, 1994.

Iliffe, S., and Zwi, A. Beyond 'Clinical'?: Four-Dimensional Medical Education. *Journal of the Royal Society of Medicine* 87:531–535, 1994.

Inglis, A.D., and Kjervik, D.K. Empowerment of Advanced Practice Nurses: Regulation Reform Needed to Increase Access to Care. *The Journal of Law, Medicine and Ethics* 21:193–205, 1993.

IOM (Institute of Medicine). *America's Health in Transition. Protecting and Improving Quality.* Washington, D.C.: National Academy Press, 1994.

IOM. *Dental Education at the Crossroads: Challenges and Change.* M.J. Field, ed. Washington, D.C.: National Academy Press, 1995.

Joel, L.A. Viewpoints: Changes in the Hospital as a Place of Practice. Pp. 220–225 in: J.C. McCloskey and H.K. Grace, eds. *Current Issues in Nursing* (4th ed.). St. Louis, Mo.: Mosby Year Book, 1994.

Kirchhoff, K.T. The Role of Nurse Researchers Employed in Clinical Settings. Pp. 169–181 in: J.J.

Fitzpatrick and J.S. Stevenson, eds. *Annual Review of Nursing Research* (vol. 11). New York: Springer, 1993.

Knaus, W.A., Draper, E.A., Wagner, D.P., and Zimmerman, J.E. An Evaluation of Outcome from Intensive Care in Major Medical Centers. *Annals of Internal Medicine* 104:410–418, 1986.

Knuteson, C.J., and Wielichowski, L.M. A Unique Approach to Designing Specialty Clinical Rotations. *Journal of Nursing Education* 33:167–168, 1994.

Koerner, J. Differentiated Practice: The Evolution of Professional Nursing. *Journal of Professional Nursing* 8:335–341, 1992.

Koerner, J. *Values: A Foundational Factor in Role Selection, Corporate and Curriculum Design for Professional Nurses.* Santa Barbara, Calif.: The Fielding Institute, 1993.

Larson, P.F., Osterweis, M., and Rubin, E.R., eds. *Health Workforce Issues for the 21st Century.* Washington, D.C.: Association of Academic Health Centers, 1994.

Lenburg, C.B. Nontraditional Nursing Education. Pp. 195–215 in: H.H. Werley, J.J. Fitzpatrick, and R.L. Taunton, eds. *Annual Review of Nursing Research* (vol. 4). New York: Springer, 1986.

Lowry, L.W. Is a Baccalaureate in Nursing Worth It? *Nursing Economic$* 10(1):46–52, 1992.

Lynton, E.A., and Elman, S.E. *New Priorities for the University.* San Francisco: Jossey-Bass, 1987.

Magrath, C.P. *The Future of Public Universities in the 21st Century.* Bloomington, Ind.: Indiana University, 1995.

Mallison, M. Nurses as House Staff. *American Journal of Nursing* 93:7, 1993.

Martin, E.J. The Doctor of Philosophy Degree: Evolutionary and Societal Perspectives. Pp. 1–16 in: S.E. Hart, ed. *Doctoral Education in Nursing: History, Process and Outcome.* New York: National League for Nursing, 1989.

Mathews, M.B., and Travis, L.L. Research on the Baccalaureate Completion Process for RNs. Pp. 149–171 in: J.J. Fitzpatrick and J.S. Stevenson, eds. *Annual Review of Nursing Research* (vol. 12). New York: Springer, 1994.

McBride, A.B. The National Center for Nursing Research. *Social Policy Report* (a publication of the Society for Research in Child Development) 2(2):1–11, 1987.

McBride, A.B., and Burgener, S. Strategies to Implement Geropsychiatric Nursing Curricula Content. *Journal of Psychosocial Nursing* 32(4):13–18, 1994.

McClure, M.L. The Nurse Executive. Nursing and Hospital Cost Containment. *Journal of Professional Nursing* 7:4, 1991.

Merritt, D.H. The National Center for Nursing Research. *Image: Journal of Nursing Scholarship* 18:84–85, 1986.

Moccia, P. Toward the Future: How Could 2 Million Registered Nurses Not Be Enough? *Nursing Clinics of North America* 25:605–612, 1990.

Montag, M. *The Education of Nursing Technicians.* New York: G.P. Putnam's Sons, 1951.

Morris, D.L., and Wykle, M.L. Minorities in Nursing. Pp. 175–189 in: J.J. Fitzpatrick and J.S. Stevenson, eds. *Annual Review of Nursing Research* (vol. 12). New York: Springer, 1994.

Moore, G.T., Inui, T.S., Ludden, J.M., and Schoenbaum, S.C. The "Teaching-HMO": A New Academic Partner. *Academic Medicine* 69:595–600, 1994.

Moses, E.B. *The Registered Nurse Population. Findings from the National Sample Survey of Registered Nurses, March 1992.* Washington, D.C.: Division of Nursing, Bureau of Health Professions, Health Resources and Services Administration, U.S. Department of Health and Human Services, 1994.

Mullinix, C.F. The Next Shortage: The Nurse Educator. *Journal of Professional Nursing* 6:133, 1990.

Murphy, J.F. Doctoral Education of Nurses: Historical Development, Programs and Graduates. Pp. 171–189 in: H.H. Werley and J.J. Fitzpatrick, eds. *Annual Review of Nursing Research* (vol. 3). New York: Springer Publishing, 1985.

Murphy, M.I. The Evolution of Professional Degrees and Roles in Nursing. Pp. 1–12 in: *Changes* in *Nursing Education. Implications for Practice.* Washington, D.C.: American Association of Colleges of Nursing, 1979.

NLN (National League for Nursing). *A Vision for Nursing Education.* New York: NLN, 1993.

NLN. *Nursing Data Review.* New York: NLN, 1994.

Noer, D.M. *Healing the Wounds. Overcoming the Trauma of Layoffs and Revitalizing Downsized Organizations.* San Francisco: Jossey-Bass, 1993.

Oermann, M. Professional Nursing Education in the Future: Changes and Challenges. *JOGNN (Journal of Obstetric, Gynecologic and Neonatal Nursing)* 23:153–159, 1994a.

Oermann, M. Reforming Nursing Education for Future Practice. *Journal of Nursing Education* 33:215–219, 1994b.

Office of Technology Assessment, U.S. Congress. *Health Technology Case Study 37: Nurse Practitioners, Physician Assistants and Certified Nurse Midwives: A Policy Analysis* (Pub. no. 224-8996). Washington, D.C.: Office of Technology Assessment, 1986.

Page, N.E., and Arena, D.M. Rethinking the Merger of the Clinical Nurse Specialist and the Nurse Practitioner Roles. *Image: Journal of Nursing Scholarship* 26:315–318, 1994.

Pew Health Professions Commission. *Healthy America: Practitioners for 2005.* Durham, N.C.: The Commission, 1991.

Pew Health Professions Commission. *Health Professions Education for the Future: Schools in Service to the Nation.* San Francisco: University of California Center for the Health Professions, 1993.

Pew Health Professions Commission. *Nurse Practitioners—Doubling the Graduates by the Year 2000.* San Francisco: University of California Center for the Health Professions, 1994a.

Pew Health Professions Commission. *Primary Care Workforce 2000—Federal Policy Paper.* San Francisco: University of California Center for the Health Professions, 1994b.

Pew Health Professions Commission. *State Strategies for Health Care Workforce Reform.* San Francisco: University of California Center for the Health Professions, 1994c.

Pike, A.W., McHugh, M., Canney, K.C., et al. A New Architecture for Quality Assurance: Nurse-physician Collaboration. *Journal of Nursing Care Quality* 7(3):1–8, 1993.

Prescott, P. Nursing: An Important Component of Hospital Survival under a Reformed Health Care System. *Nursing Economics* 11:192–199, 1993.

Rheingold, H. *The Virtual Community: Homesteading on the Electronic Frontier.* Reading, Mass.: Addison-Wesley, 1993.

Rice, R.E. The New American Scholar. *Metropolitan Universities* 1(4):7–18, 1991.

Rosenfeld, P. Recent Trends in Nursing Education. Pp. 11–19 in: A. Graubard, ed. *Perspectives in Nursing 1991–1993.* New York: National League for Nursing Press, 1992.

Rothert, M.L., Talarczyk, G.J., and Awbrey, S.M. Partnerships in Nursing Education. Expanding the Boundaries. Pp. 170–176 in: J.C. McCloskey and H.K. Grace, eds. *Current Issues in Nursing* (4th ed.). St. Louis, Mo.: Mosby Year Book, 1994.

Safriet, B. Health Care Dollars and Regulatory Sense: The Role of Advanced Practice Nursing. *Yale Journal on Regulation* 9:417–497, 1992.

Salmon, M.E. *Report to the American Association of Colleges of Nursing.* Washington, D.C.: Bureau of Health Professions, Health Resources and Services Administration, March 21, 1995.

Shalala, D.E. Nursing and Society—The Unfinished Agenda for the 21st Century. Pp. 3–8 in: A. Graubard, ed. *Perspectives in Nursing 1991–1993.* New York: National League for Nursing Press, 1992.

Shulman, L. Knowledge and Teaching: Foundation of the New Reform. *Harvard Educational Review* 57(1):1–22, 1987.

Simmons, J., ed. *Prospectives. Celebrating 40 Years of Associate Degree Nursing Education.* New York: National League for Nursing Press, 1993.

Smeltzer, C.H., Formella, N.M., and Beebe, H. Work Restructuring: The Process of Decision Making. *Nursing Economic$* 11:215–222, 1993.

Starck, P.L., Duffy, M.E., and Vogler, R. Developing a Nursing Doctorate for the 21st Century. *Journal of Professional Nursing* 9:212–219, 1993.

Tanner, C.A. Teaching Clinical Judgment. Pp. 153–123 in: J.J. Fitzpatrick and R.L. Taunton, eds. *Annual Review of Nursing Research* (vol. 5). New York: Springer, 1987.

Tanner, C.A. Rethinking Clinical Judgment. Pp. 153–123 in: N.L. Dickelmann and M.L. Rather, eds. *Transforming RN Education: Dialogue and Debate.* New York: National League for Nursing Press, 1993.

Tresolini, C.P., and the Pew-Fetzer Task Force. *Health Professions Education and Relationship-centered Care.* San Francisco: Pew Health Professions Commission, 1994.

Valberg, L.S., Gonyea, M.A., Sinclair, D.G., and Wade, J. *Planning the Future Academic Medical Centre.* London, Ont.: Canadian Medical Association, 1994.

VanOrt, S., Woodtili, A., and Williams, M. Prospective Payment and Baccalaureate Nursing Education: Projections for the Future. *Journal of Professional Nursing* 5:25–30, 1989.

Wald, F.S., and Leonard, R.C. Towards Development of Nursing Practice Theory. *Nursing Research* 13:309–313, 1964.

Watson, J., and Phillips, S. A Call for Educational Reform: Colorado Nursing Doctorate Model as Exemplar. *Nursing Outlook* 40(1):20–26, 1992.

Wolf, G.A., Boland, S., and Aukerman, M.A. A Transformational Model for the Practice of Professional Nursing. Part 1, The Model. *JONA (Journal of Nursing Administration)* 24(4):51–57, 1994a.

Wolf, G.A., Boland, S., and Aukerman, M. A Transformational Model for the Practice of Professional Nursing. Part 2, Implementation of the Model. *JONA (Journal of Nursing Administration)* 24(5):38–46, 1994b.

Nursing Staff and Quality of Care in Nursing Homes

Meridean Maas, Ph.D., R.N., F.A.A.N., Kathleen Buckwalter, Ph.D., F.A.A.N.,and Janet Specht, M.A., R.N.

This paper focuses on a review of literature and research regarding nurse staffing and quality of care in nursing homes. Background information for this review was obtained through computerized literature searches, through solicited contributions and personal communications from nurse researchers and long-term-care scholars, and from presentations at a special panel session convened at the Gerontological Society of America meeting in Atlanta, Georgia, in November of 1994. The first section of the paper reviews the background and historical development of nursing homes in the United States, while the second section describes the current status of institutional long-term care. The next two sections discuss the future demand for nursing home care and some selected issues in long-term care. The fifth section presents a detailed review of research relevant to the linkage of staffing and quality of care. The final three sections outline research questions and areas that need to be studied, present a case study of staffing and quality in an exemplary nursing home, and set forth recommendations for policy initiatives.

Dr. Maas is professor, Dr. Buckwalter is distinguished professor, and Ms. Specht is research program assistant and doctoral candidate at the University of Iowa College of Nursing.

BACKGROUND AND HISTORICAL DEVELOPMENT OF NURSING HOMES IN THE UNITED STATES

From Almshouses to Nursing Homes

Nursing home policy was developed from social welfare issues regarding care of the poor. A strategy known as "indoor relief" was developed in Elizabethan England when social planners used almshouses to care for the poor, who were divided into the "deserving poor" (those who were unable to work) and the "undeserving poor" (those who were perceived as morally corrupt because they were able to work). The poor elderly were housed in almshouses and exempt from moral judgments because of their age and inability to work (Hall and Buckwalter, 1990).

In the United States in the 1920s, almshouses were funded by the states and were used to continue the policy of providing indoor relief for the deserving poor who were unable to be employed in the factories, as well as providing care for the blind, chronically ill, mentally ill, and frail and old individuals. In 1923, about half of the 78,000 residents of almshouses were elderly and infirm. Society began to protest the housing of the infirm elderly with the poor and insane and Congress, because of this public pressure, stipulated that persons in public institutions should not receive old age funds; people in boarding houses, however, were eligible. Not surprisingly, this legislation prompted a sharp increase in the number of boarding homes in which nurses were hired to care for the frail and chronically ill. Thus, many boarding homes became known as nursing homes (Kalisch and Kalisch, 1978; Vladeck, 1984). Also in the early 20th century, private care homes emerged for elderly widows of various ethnic or religious groups (e.g., Lutheran homes, Jewish homes), which served as the precursors for today's charitable and nonprofit nursing homes (Vladeck, 1984).

Nursing homes really began to develop following passage of the Social Security Act of 1935, which provided payment to individual beneficiaries and thus turned indoor relief into "outdoor relief." That is, community-based services began to emerge that prevented the need for almshouse placement (Kalisch and Kalisch, 1978; Vladeck, 1984). With passage of the Kerr-Mills Medical Assistance to the Aged Act in 1950, which allowed for direct payment to care providers, and with increases in the number of older adults in the population, the nursing home industry boomed.

In 1954, the American Nursing Home Association lobbied for and won the right for nonprofit nursing homes to be built in conjunction with hospitals using Hill-Burton funds. Thus, nonproprietary homes were moved into the medical-surgical domain where, after passage of the Medicaid and Medicare Acts in 1965, they were required to meet strict federal nursing standards, creating the skilled-level facilities of today. Standards of care relaxed somewhat during the Nixon administration, and proprietary homes could apply for small business development loans, which excluded them from the strict federal nursing criteria and led to the creation of intermediate-level care facilities with criteria developed by individual states for reimbursement under Medicaid (Vladeck, 1984).

Altogether, between 1980 and 1990, there was a 24 percent increase in nursing home occupancy rates (*McKnight's Long-term Care News,* 1993). The percentage of residents requiring more hours of care, more services on a daily basis, and having higher acuity levels has also risen over the past few years. Indeed, 43 percent of all Americans who passed their 65th birthday in 1990 are expected to use a nursing home at least once in their lives (Murtaugh et al., 1990).

Development of Long-Term Care for the Mentally Ill Elderly

For the first half of the 20th century, the mentally ill elderly were systematically admitted to state hospitals, which provided them with custodial care (Kermis, 1987). By the late 1950s and early 1960s, however, the indoor relief policy regarding care of the mentally ill began to change as mental health programming was reoriented to a system of outpatient psychiatric treatment, rehabilitation, and prevention. Both the Kennedy and Johnson administrations supported de-institutionalization of mental patients in the large state hospitals and the creation of community mental health centers to provide outpatient treatment. Thus, the population of the state mental hospitals, which included many elderly, decreased by as much as 66 percent (Kane, 1984), and those elderly who continued to require institutionalization were most often placed in nursing homes to receive care (Mechanic, 1980).

Unfortunately, the medical focus of most nursing home administrators and personnel left them unprepared to care for those elders with cognitive, behavioral and affective disorders, and nursing homes were faced with large numbers of residents who failed to respond to programming in a conventional manner, did not sleep at night, and became violent when confronted with other residents (Hall and Buckwalter, 1990). Research by Zimmer and colleagues (1984) found that 64 percent of elderly residents of skilled nursing homes had significant behavioral problems, of which nearly 23 percent were classified as "severe." Despite the fact that 58 percent of these patients were receiving psychoactive drugs, both psychiatric diagnoses and consultations were absent. Similarly high rates of mental illness and cognitive disorder (70 to 80 percent) in the absence of active treatment were reported by Roybal (1984) and Rovner and Rabins (1985). By and large, health planners and economists failed to recognize the additional staffing and financial burdens these mentally ill and cognitively impaired residents placed on the nursing home system (Vladick and Alfano, 1987). The current trend, however, is for integrated interdisciplinary treatment teams to provide psychiatric care in nursing homes, an approach that allows for the use of psychopharmacologic, psychoeducational, behavioral, and family or social interventions. Preliminary outcome data suggest, moreover, that this more comprehensive approach results in the use of fewer psychotropic medications, more effective resolution of behavioral problems, and decreased costs related to the need for hospitalization (Dey, 1994).

CURRENT STATUS OF INSTITUTIONAL LONG-TERM CARE

Institutional long-term care can be viewed from several vantage points. This section presents data on the number and types of facilities and on the mix of residents cared for in those facilities. Federal and state regulations affecting long-term care and how those regulations affect reimbursement for care are discussed. Finally, staffing issues, including staffing requirements, staff mix and qualifications, the nature of nursing home work, and staff salaries, are described.

Numbers and Types of Homes

Long-term institutional care of elderly residents falls into two major categories: (1) traditional nursing homes, which primarily are facilities that provide either intermediate-level nursing care or skilled nursing care, but might also include "board-and-care" residential homes, and (2) recent alternatives to the traditional nursing homes, such as foster care homes, family homes, or assisted-living homes. Numbers of homes are presented to illustrate trends in the availability of institutional long-term-care options.

Traditional Nursing Homes

Today, the primary providers of institution-based care for dependent elders are the more than 20,000 intermediate and skilled nursing homes. Although the Omnibus Budget Reconciliation Act of 1987 (OBRA 87) eliminated the distinction between skilled and intermediate nursing homes, Title XIX continues to distinguish the two types for reimbursement. According to the 1985 National Nursing Home Survey (NCHS, 1987), 75 percent of nursing homes were proprietary, 20 percent voluntary nonprofit, and 5 percent government operated. Forty-one percent were operated by nursing home chains and about 50 percent were independently operated. Proprietary homes provided 69 percent of the nursing home beds, voluntary nonprofit homes provided 23 percent of the beds, and public homes 8 percent. Eighteen percent of the available beds were skilled nursing, 30 percent were skilled nursing and intermediate level, 28 percent were intermediate level only, and 25 percent were not certified. One-third of the nursing homes had fewer than 50 beds, about another third had between 50 and 99 beds, 28 percent had 100 to 199 beds, and only slightly more than 6 percent had 200 or more beds.

Another type of traditional nursing home is the board and care home. A board and care home differs from intermediate- or skilled-level nursing homes in that continuous care provided by licensed nurses is not required. Board and care homes outnumber skilled and intermediate nursing homes by more than 2 to 1 in the United States and have an average size of 15 beds (*Brown University Long-Term Care Quality Letter*, 1994).

Both nursing homes and board and care homes have high occupancy rates, 91.5 percent and 85.6 percent respectively. However, the 1991 National Health Provider Inventory, mailed to providers and analyzed by the National Center for Health Statistics (NCHS), found wide geographic variations in the prevalence of nursing homes versus board and care homes or home care (*Brown University Long-Term Care Quality Letter*, 1994). The Midwest relied heavily on regular nursing homes, little on board and care, and moderately on home care. The Northeast relied heavily on all three, with much more home health care use than in the other regions. The South showed moderate usage of all three types of care, and the West relied on board and care more than any other region. Nationwide, the study counted 15,511 nursing homes, with 1.6 million beds and 1.5 million residents. While the number of free-standing nursing homes has dropped by 1,644 since 1986, the number of nursing home beds has increased by 60,000—meaning that existing nursing homes are becoming larger.

Recent Alternative Long-Term-Care Models

A number of residential care models have recently arisen in response to the need to develop alternatives to the medical model emphasis in most traditional long-term-care facilities. These alternatives include a range of state-licensed residential living environments such as foster care, family homes, residential care facilities, and assisted-living arrangements (Wilson, 1994).

These variations in facilities are possible because there are no federal guidelines standardizing long-term residential care, and state regulations vary widely regarding environmental, programming, and nursing care standards, with minimum staffing ratios ordinarily set quite low. Although residential care settings vary in size (ranging from small private homes accommodating up to 4 residents, to large congregate care facilities that may care for more than 100 residents), all offer assistance or care and share with the residents the responsibilities for activities of daily living. Ideally, the care provided is flexible, resident and family oriented, and intended to optimize individual dignity, functioning, health, and well-being. Because these alternative facilities also provide care for demented residents, the physical environment and design features of the facility should support the functioning of the impaired older adult and accommodate difficult behaviors and diminished abilities (Alzheimer's Association, 1994).

Assisted living, for example, is a model of supportive housing that is growing rapidly because of consumer preferences and lower costs than those associated with traditional models of long-term care (Wilson, 1994). The state of Oregon has been a leader in developing standards of assisted-living care for the purposes of licensure and evaluating resident outcomes. Residents are entitled to a private apartment (shared only by choice) that includes a kitchen, a bath with roll-in shower, locking doors, and temperature control capability. Routine nursing services and case management for ancillary services are provided. Data show that residents in these Oregon assisted-living facilities have a remarkably high level of disability: 84 percent have some mobility impairment, 75 percent require assistance with medications, and 63 percent require assistance with bathing. Most importantly, the orientation of staff toward the residents is to empower them by sharing responsibilities, enhancing choices, and managing risks (Wilson, 1994). Because of the lack of regulations and standards, consumers need to question providers about all aspects of services, including the philosophy of care, number and type of staff, staff training, staff supervision, and costs, to determine if resident and family needs will be met.

The sub-acute unit is another alternative long-term-care model. With the advent of the Medicare prospective payment system and use of diagnosis-related groups (DRG) as the basis for payment in hospitals, older adults began to be discharged "quicker and sicker" to nursing homes. In the United States, this early discharge of older adults from hospitals has led to a movement to create sub-acute care units in nursing homes, discussed more fully below in "Future Demand for Institutional Long-term Care." These units do not necessarily focus on frail older adults in the latter stages of life, but are in response to the economic changes affecting hospitals and tend to reinforce a medical model of care (Lyles, 1986; Ganroth, 1988; Swan et al., 1990).

Case-Mix Data

According to Fries (1994), case-mix refers to distinctions of residents related to resource use where resource use is primarily defined as a ratio of nursing time to costs. Nursing home residents are a heterogeneous mix of vulnerable adults whose ages may span more than 50 years. Residents are also getting older; those over the age of 85 years constitute about 42 percent of nursing home residents, up from 34 percent in 1980. Despite the dramatic increase in the number of nursing home residents who are age 85 or older, there are more than 181,000 (12 percent) residents under the age of 65 in nursing homes (*McKnight's Long-term Care News*, 1993). As noted earlier, a high percentage (around 75 percent) of persons who reside in nursing homes are reported to suffer from a chronic dementing process or some form of mental health or behavioral alteration. Most of these residents also have medical and personal care needs that require ongoing staff intervention and support. For example, about half (51 percent) of residents are incontinent of urine. Physical care issues, low staff ratios, regulatory issues, and inadequate staff preparation and training often mean that residents with behavioral impairment are still poorly understood and tolerated in the long-term-care environment (Hall, 1995).

Regulations and Reimbursement

Over the past few years, a paradigm shift has occurred in long-term care—from a biomedical treatment orientation and custodial care approach to a more social-behavioral model of care with a rehabilitative focus (Burgio and Scilley, 1994). However, implementation of a social-behavioral model of care has been constrained by regulations and reimbursement that are still guided by a medical model and by tensions between federal and state jurisdictions for regulating and reimbursing nursing homes.

Issues of staffing and care policies in traditional long-term-care facilities are influenced by a combination of federal and state regulations. Because the federal government is the only payer for Medicare and shares the rapidly increasing payment with states for Medicaid, and because consumer concerns intensified, federal interest in regulation increased and resulted in the passage of OBRA 87. Yet state regulatory groups did not control the development of OBRA regulations and do not have the option to not implement them. The OBRA 87 regulations mandated higher standards for quality care, but federal and individual state reimbursement formulas have not necessarily changed to enable nursing homes to better meet the higher standards.

Enactment of OBRA 87 resulted in regulations that required nursing homes to adopt a more active social-behavioral treatment model for residents. In contrast to an earlier emphasis on facility cleanliness and the physical plant, the new regulations are more resident focused, emphasizing systematic assessment and individual plans of care that foster the highest achievable level of resident well-being. In addition to restricting the use of antipsychotic medications for the treatment of behavioral problems, OBRA also mandated more training for each nurse's aide (a minimum of 75 hours of initial training that addresses psychosocial as well and physical health care, and 12 hours of in-service education annually), as well as assurance of skill competency (Burgio and Scilley, 1994).

Thus, with OBRA 87 setting the standard for quality of care in long-term-care facilities, the nursing home industry today is among the most highly regulated businesses in America. Beset with regulations developed in response to perceived abuses and poor quality care, licensed nursing homes are charged with providing care that meets the vast needs of diverse residents, yet often they must try to meet that charge with only minimum reimbursement and inadequate staffing (Hall, 1995). Success or failure to meet the government mandates is evaluated by the facility's own quality assurance programs, as well as surveys conducted by multiple agencies, care review boards, and state ombudspersons who investigate complaints (Hall, 1995). A report by the Department of Health and Human Services Office of the Inspection General indicates that most states are doing an adequate job of carrying out their survey responsibilities as outlined under OBRA 87. However, survey staff issues, enforcement, and inspections remain problematic, and there is need for improved training of state surveyors and better communication between state and federal surveyors in terms of consistent application of guidelines for quality of care (*McKnight's Long-term Care News*, 1993). In addition to the surveying difficulties, the lack of attention to how reimbursement affects the ability of homes to meet quality standards is a serious concern.

Nationally, there is some movement toward case-mix reimbursement for nursing home care, although most states continue currently to reimburse by capitated cost-based systems—systems that are limited by a cap regardless of the cost to provide the care. Use of this system tends to encourage nursing homes to preferentially accept private pay and minimal care persons, rather than persons whose care is reimbursed by Medicaid.

The lack of federal regulation coupled with wide variation in state regulations also affects alternative forms of long-term-care facilities and the level of reimbursement available to those facilities. Currently there are few regulations for assisted-living facilities, and reimbursement under Title XIX for assisted living is limited to a few states. Public expenditures for community-based services are relatively small compared to those for nursing home care (O'Shaunessy and Price, 1987). Medicaid, which is the principal source of funding of health care services for low income persons, finances mostly nursing home care and was not designed to support a full array of social and other long-term-care community-based services. A few states provide some reimbursement, but because of a lack of Medicaid reimbursement most deny persons who cannot privately pay for this option. Some, but not all, long-term-care insurance policies cover assisted living and other arrangements alternative to nursing home care. There also is some controversy surrounding reimbursement rates for special care units, because of a lack of data to support whether or not a higher cost of care is justified on these units.

Staffing, Staff-Mix, and Qualifications

Over 1.5 million residents are cared for in nursing homes by 1,200,000 full-time equivalent (FTE) employees each day, of whom 700,000 FTEs provide some form of nursing or personal care. Nursing aides (designated by the acronym NAs and also referred to in this paper as nurse aides, nurse assistants, and nursing assistants) and orderlies account for over 40 percent of a home's total FTEs. Registered nurses (RNs), on the other hand, make up less than 7 percent of a nursing home's total FTEs and less than 20 percent of a facility's total nursing staff. Of the estimated 1.5 million employed RNs in the United States, fewer than 100,000 are employed in nursing homes (NCHS, 1988). And yet nothing is more important than the characteristics of the nursing staff in terms of determining the residents' quality of life. Staff interaction with residents and the nature of the relationship that develops between them is what matters most to residents, far more than the administrative philosophy or decor of the facility (Kayser-Jones, 1989).

Data from the 1985 National Nursing Home Survey (NCHS, 1988) indicated that nursing homes had an average of 71.4 FTE staff per 100 beds, with an average of 5.2 RN FTEs, 7.4 LPN FTEs, and 30.8 NA FTEs per 100 beds. Proprietary homes averaged 4.3 RN FTEs per 100 beds, while voluntary non-profit homes averaged 6.7 RN FTE per 100 beds and government-operated homes 7.4 RN FTEs per 100 beds.

Regulations are such that very few nursing homes (5.6 percent) have an RN on duty 24 hours a day (Jones et al., 1987). Because available staff are distributed over a 24-hour period, for every 100 beds the average staffing is 1 RN, who is most likely to be the director of nursing, 1.5 LPNs, and 6.5 nurse aides, as compared to a ratio of 1 RN for every 4 patients in a hospital (Mezey, 1992). The median amount of RN time per resident, per day, across all nursing homes in 1985 was 12 minutes or less, and nearly 40 percent of nursing homes reported 6 minutes or less of RN time per resident per day (Jones et al., 1987).

Similarly, the American Nurses Association (ANA) found staffing ratios of nursing assistants to patients in intermediate-level care facilities to be 1:11, whereas the ratio for licensed nurses was 1:100 (ANA, 1991). Nursing assistants are the primary care givers in long-term care. Consequently, the care that they provide is an important determinant of the quality of life and quality of care for nursing home residents. The typical NA is a 20- to 40-year-old female; about half are members of a minority group, with low socioeconomic status and a high school education or less. Typically, they are paid little more than the minimum wage.

Nurse vacancy rates are higher in nursing homes than in other practice settings. Despite recent improvements (in 1993, 70 percent of state nursing home association executives indicated that vacancy rates in their states had dropped to 10 percent or less) (*McKnight's Long-term Care News*, 1993), nurses still find hospitals a more attractive setting in which to work. RN salaries in nursing homes are about 15 percent lower than salaries for hospital RNs (Maraldo, 1991). While this situation may have changed somewhat, due to greater concerns about hospital costs in recent years, nursing homes continue to compete poorly for RNs because of wages and working conditions. Unfortunately, caring for the elderly is still not considered prestigious or financially rewarding when compared to other areas of nursing practice.

The OBRA 87 regulations contain no staffing standards except that an RN is to be on duty for 8 of the 24 hours each day. Some homes have obtained waivers that permit them to substitute LPNs. Thus, staffing requirements for nursing homes vary from state to state. In Iowa, for example, two hours of nursing care hours per patient day are required for certified Medicaid residents. This breaks down to only about five minutes per hour, even though the average resident who is unable to feed him- or herself requires about one hour of assistance for each meal provided. If these Medicaid residents who are dependent on receiving help to eat should lose weight continuously over a period of several months, the facility may receive a citation for poor quality care—a real "Catch 22." Some long-term-care providers have successfully sued to become eligible for staffing levels greater than those reimbursed by the Medicaid statute, as was the case with an Atlantic City, New Jersey, nursing home, which argued that the unusual configuration of the facility (three buildings connected by ramps and walkways) required additional Medicaid funds so it could provide adequate staff (*McKnight's Long-term Care News*, 1993).

According to the Select Committee on Aging (1992) in the U.S. House of Representatives, without changes in staffing regulations, the needs of the elderly will remain largely unmet through the year 2020. In their report to the chairman, the committee listed several reasons for a lack of health care personnel trained in geriatrics and gerontology: difficulty recruiting and retaining qualified personnel for direct care in nursing homes, poorly trained workers, little training of family and friend care givers, vague job descriptions, shortages of qualified faculty to teach the needed knowledge and skills to physicians, nurses, and other health professionals, and the lack of appropriate training sites. Clearly, low salaries for nursing home personnel contribute to recruitment and retention problems and low reimbursement rates affect nursing home providers' interest in paying higher salaries.

Nature of the Work in Nursing Homes

Nursing home work is often difficult, stressful, frustrating, and labor intensive, especially for NAs, who have the most direct contact with residents. Nursing home staff have to confront aging, disability, and dying. Much of the care of the elderly is not pleasant, such as caring for urinary and bowel incontinence or dealing with a cognitively impaired elder who is agitated and combative. Combined with low wages, minimal benefits, hard physical work, and the often progressively deteriorating abilities of the residents, the nature of the work for nursing staff is often characterized as tedious, unpleasant, and unrewarding. Furthermore, because concern for costs is likely to continue while resident acuity increases, the workload of NAs and nurses in nursing homes may very well get heavier.

Research related to the actual nature of the work role of NAs documents that the complexity level of most tasks is low (suggesting a routinized approach), and that even when NAs carry out direct care tasks, their attention is not always directed toward residents. The highest level of psychosocial quality interaction was found to occur in the process of socializing, an informal component of care, suggesting the need for alternative task structuring and more resident-centered models of care (Brannon et al., 1992). Other studies support the notion that staff-to-staff interactions are much more frequent than staff-to-resident interactions (Burgio et al., 1990).

In general, RNs in nursing homes suffer from a lack of prestige within the total health care delivery system. They are not only victims of financial disparity, but they are also subjected to humiliation and professional degradation, and their work role is often tied up exclusively with administrative functions. While the reasons are many, the lack of respect for nurses who choose to care for the elderly in nursing homes is at least in part because nurses and other health professionals often share the negative attitudes of society toward the elderly (Harrington, 1984).

The work of nursing home personnel is not without rewards, however. These rewards are largely intrinsic and evolve from the relationships formed with the elderly residents and the satisfaction gained from feeling that one has contributed to the quality of their lives, if only in a small way. For some, there are also the rewards of personal development that come from learning about aging and the opportunity to gain clinical skills. Nonetheless, extrinsic rewards for nursing staff remain problematic and this is largely responsible for the frequent turnover of staff and inability to recruit and retain qualified staff.

Staff Salaries and Incentives

As already mentioned, salaries and other incentives are problematic for all nursing staff in long-term care. One of the major reasons for the dearth of RNs in nursing homes is economic, and retention rates among long-term-care staff have been shown to increase concurrently with increases in average weekly salary. In 1988 they received 88 percent of the typical acute care wage, and by 1990 the percentage had dropped to 86 percent. For RNs, the highest hourly rate was $18.91 in hospitals, followed by $16.82 for home care, and $15.26 for nursing home RNs (Hospital and Healthcare Compensation Service, 1994). Since 1990, there is some evidence that salaries for some staff in nursing homes may be increasing, although they continue to lag behind salaries in hospitals. Annual salaries for Directors of Nursing (DON) were recently reported to have increased by 6 percent to $41,200 (*McKnight's Long-term Care News,* 1995). The salaries and benefits of nursing assistants, however, provide little incentive and lag behind those for hospital aides and home care aides. The median hourly wage reported by hospital aides was $7.12 between 1987 and 1989, compared to $5.29 for nursing home aides and $4.22 for home care aides.

Noting that RNs are a critical component of the rural health care delivery system and in some areas the sole providers of care, the Select Committee on Aging (1992) reported a shortage of 45,382 FTE RNs in nonmetropolitan areas of the United States. The $3,000 discrepancy in annual salary between nurses employed in small hospitals and those employed in large hospitals probably played a role in the shortage (Movassaghi et al., 1992). According to Kayser-Jones (1981b), often the only nurses willing to work for the low wages offered are those who cannot get employment in other types of health settings because of poor qualifications.

SELECTED ISSUES IN LONG-TERM CARE

Cultural Diversity Among Staff and Residents

Issues Regarding Minority Care Providers

Increasing the numbers of minority and disadvantaged persons in the health and allied health professions to care for the underserved, such as the elderly, is an important component of health care reform. Shortages of minority providers may adversely affect access, cost, and quality of care. At the same time, the background and characteristics of many nursing home staff may adversely affect their job performance (Burgio and Scilley, 1994). The lives of many nursing assistants, in particular, are beset with personal problems and tragedies that leave them with too few personal resources to respond effectively to residents and that interfere with their ability to provide quality care to the frail, dependent elderly (Tellis-Nayak and Tellis-Nayak, 1989). In their ethnographic study on quality of care, nursing homes, and nurse aides' cultures, Tellis-Nayak and Tellis-Nayak (1989, p. 312) concluded that the "institutional culture of the average nursing home not only ignores the affective needs of the nurse's aides, but it even assaults their self-esteem." They also assert that out of a concern for quality, advocates and policy makers have inappropriately reduced a complex problem to one of staffing and training issues alone, failing to appreciate the important role social history can play in staff apathy and lack of concern for residents.

Every individual carries a cultural heritage, and older people generally have more ties to their heritage than do many in the younger generations. Elders of particular ethnic or racial minority groups may have customs and beliefs that are important to them, but are no longer remembered or respected by the young. Although it is important for staff to respect and attend to the cultures of Black, Hispanic, Native American, and Asian minorities, it also should be remembered that many Caucasian persons are also members of ethnic groups that have distinct cultures, such as Jews, Poles, or Irish persons (Snyder, 1982). While it is neither practical nor necessary for staff to share the same ethnicity or cultural heritage as the residents, staff do need to learn about the usual lifestyles and backgrounds of the elders for whom they are caring. Even staff who share a common culture with residents may find that differences between generations present obstacles to understanding and respect. A clash of beliefs about health and illness and about appropriate remedies and treatments may be disconcerting to both staff and residents. When staff have some knowledge about the usual practices and beliefs of residents, there is a basis for communication that can optimize care and the residents' compliance with recommended treatment. To promote adjustment in the nursing home, staff need to know at least some of the basic vocabulary of the residents, and it is important that someone, either volunteer or staff, be available for translation when elders speak limited English (Snyder, 1982).

Problems related to cultural and racial diversity are particularly acute in urban nursing homes, where a majority of staff may belong to minority groups, whereas the residents are predominantly white. Preliminary findings from a study of ethnic and racial conflict between nursing home staff and residents in New York revealed a high prevalence of racially charged verbal abuse and name calling of aides by residents (Teresi et al., 1994).

Institutional Care Needs of Minority Elderly

There is a lack of research and thus an inadequate knowledge base about the long-term health care needs of minority elders and other age groups. The research that does exist strongly suggests some disparity of service use and inequity of access for ethnic and minority populations, despite increased need (Barresi and Stull, 1993). While the general growth of the elderly population in the United States is well known, the increase in racial and ethnic elderly populations is less well recognized. Yet the elderly population is increasing faster among ethnic and racial minorities populations (Hispanics, American Indians, African Americans, Asians, and Pacific Islanders) than among whites, and the total population of ethnic and minority elderly has doubled with each national census since 1960 (Harper and Alexander, 1990). In some parts of the country, these ethnic and minority elderly will soon be the majority among the population aged 65 years and older (Cuellar, 1990; Morioka-Douglas and Yeo, 1990; Richardson, 1990). In 1985, approximately 14 percent of the population 65 and over were persons of color (Elders of Color, 1991). A significant increase in the population 85 years of age and older and in the number of females is also occurring, and a substantial proportion of these elderly are of racial and ethnic minorities.

Despite having poorer health and less help from relatives than comparison groups of white elders, black elders are less likely to be institutionalized. At comparable rates of frailty, the likelihood of nursing home admission for blacks is less than half that of whites (Belgrave and Bradsher, 1994). Poverty, geographical isolation, and discrimination are now given more weight in this pattern than the previous characterization of personal preference.

Although the Indian Health Service (IHS) has a statutory responsibility to meet the health needs of American Indians, it tends to define its mission in terms of acute care. As a result, the rapidly increasing long-term-care needs of the growing numbers of aging tribal members are largely ignored. John (1991) points out that an additional problem confronting tribal elders is a policy of age discrimination in resource allocation within the IHS. Specifically, he notes that the IHS concentrates its resources on the health problems of younger tribal members through the Resource Allocation Method, which is based on a calculation of potential years of productive life lost. This strategy virtually ignores health issues for elders over age 65. For example, there are only ten reservation-based nursing homes in the United States, and they currently house 435 residents (Manson, 1989). A National Indian Council on Aging (1981) report indicated that 46 percent of older tribal members are assisted by extended family members to accomplish one or more activities of daily living.

Data regarding long-term care of the minority population are particularly lacking in respect to Hispanic elderly people, especially given the fact that Hispanics make up about 4 percent of the elderly population in the United States (AARP, 1985a) and are the fastest growing subgroup of the elderly (Lopez-Aqueres et al., 1984). More than 600,000 Hispanics are over the age of 65 (AARP, 1985b). What data do exist show that Hispanic populations report greater utilization of informal support systems than of professional health care providers (Greene and Monohan, 1984). As with Asians and Pacific Islanders in the United States, elder Hispanics face hypertension, tuberculosis, and cancers as their major health concerns. These elderly are less likely to use formal health care services, including nursing homes, due to lack of knowledge of available services (Holmes et al., 1983), cultural and language differences, and reliance on traditional medicine (Espino et al., 1988; AARP Minority Affairs, 1990).

In a study of nine nursing homes in San Antonio, Texas, Chiodo and colleagues (1994) found strong evidence that Mexican American nursing home residents are more cognitively and functionally impaired, after controlling for age and education, than non-Hispanic white residents. They also were significantly more likely to be funded by Medicaid, and they were more likely to have lived with relatives prior to institutionalization.

Major differences between Puerto Rican Hispanics and non-Hispanics admitted to nursing homes were identified in a study by Espino and coworkers (1988). The Puerto Rican Hispanics were significantly younger and functionally more impaired, both physically and mentally, than their non-Hispanic counterparts and more similar to chronologically older non-Hispanic nursing home residents.

Some research documents the need for nurses to be aware of the implications of ethnicity in caring for the elderly. In a study of immigrant, Canadian-born, and Anglo-born elderly in long-term-care facilities, Jones and Van Amelsvoort Jones (1986) found significant differences in the observed interactions among the groups. Although the elderly as a whole had minimal verbal interaction directed to them during morning and evening care, overall, male residents were spoken to less than female residents, and ethnic females had the least number of commands, the fewest statements, and the least number of questions spoken to them by staff.

Violence, Abuse, and Conflict

"Granny battering" and "slow euthanasia" are heard about quite often by nurses (Bahr, 1981), and it is usual to find daily reports in the news of elder abuse perpetrated by criminals, family members, or care givers. Because the numbers of dependent and vulnerable elderly in the population are increasing, abuse and crimes against the elderly will likely continue to occur in proportionate numbers in the future. Elder abuse is identified in the literature as rights violations, physical abuse, material abuse, and psychological abuse (Pollick, 1987). Rights violations are the denial of the basic rights of the elderly person as defined by the 1961 and 1971 White House Conferences on Aging (Beck and Ferguson, 1981). Material abuse is monetary or material theft or misuse (DHHS, 1980). Physical abuse includes acts of omission or commission that result in physical harm, with omission being the most common (Beck and Ferguson, 1981). Psychological abuse is behavior that demeans or diminishes the dignity or self-worth of the elderly person (Hickey and Douglass, 1981). Accurate documentation of elder abuse is problematic because the elderly are often unreliable witnesses or fear retaliation, and because observable physical signs are easily explained as caused by falls and injuries. Most professionals agree that elder abuse is a common and serious public health problem, with 1 study documenting 60 percent of 228 professionals (police officers, social workers, adult protection workers, mental health workers, legal services providers, clergy members, morticians, and coroners) reporting that they deal with elder abuse at least once per week (Hickey and Douglass, 1981). Typically, the abused elder is female, more than 70 years old, physically or mentally impaired or both, and living in the community with an adult child or some family member (DHHS, 1980).

Abuse also occurs, however, in institutional settings. Research conducted in one 200-bed nonprofit nursing home suggests that the majority of nursing assistants are kind and helpful most of the time, although abuse (primarily psychological abuse such as yelling, swearing, and being insulting) does occasionally occur. The investigator suggests that the stressful work role of NAs leads to exhaustion and burnout that may precipitate abuse, and argues that mechanisms are needed to help nonprofessional staff deal with their work-related stress (Foner, 1994). Others (Kayser-Jones, 1990) have characterized the behavior of NAs as rude, neglectful, uncaring, and sometimes verbally and physically abusive.

Although most nursing homes take care to observe residents' rights, no nursing home can guarantee that every right of every individual will be respected. Problems and conflicts are bound to occur occasionally. Usually complaints are equitably and amicably resolved within the facility. But when a problem cannot be resolved internally, a resident or family member may contact the local office of the long-term-care ombudsman program. Examples of problems and conflict between a family member and staff are feelings of being depreciated or belittled, perceptions that a loved one is not receiving all available services or treatments, concerns about financial matters that are not fully explained or accounted, feelings of discrimination, or concerns that the facility staff does not adequately discuss treatment, transfer, or discharge options.

Physical abuse resulting from poor care, such as skin breakdown, rough handling, or inattention to bowel and urinary elimination needs, is another serious problem that can occur in institutions. This type of physical abuse may be inflicted by health care personnel who are not well qualified (Baker, 1977). Citing the dearth of research regarding maltreatment of residents of nursing homes, Pillemer (1988) provides a theoretical model of maltreatment as the outcome of staff members' and patients' characteristics as these are influenced by aspects of the nursing home environment and by certain factors exogenous to the facility. As highlighted in the model and supported by a review of the literature, staff who are at more risk for abusive behaviors toward the institutionalized elderly are more likely to be young (Penner et al., 1984), have lower levels of education (Baltz and Turner, 1977; White, 1977), be male (U.S. Department of Justice, 1985; Straus, 1986), have the least experience (Penner et al., 1984), and be under more stress (Heine, 1986). More recently, Pillemer and Hudson (1993) report an evaluation of a model abuse prevention curriculum for nursing assistants, showing high satisfaction with the program and reduced conflict and abuse of residents. Cassell (1989) also suggests that physicians sometimes abuse their elderly patients when they employ their power in a manner they believe to be in the best interests of the sick.

Just as residents can suffer at the hands of staff, nursing staff are also subject to abuse by residents. Studies about the incidence of aggressive resident behavior in nursing homes are sparse, but the few available studies suggest that the presence of behavioral problems warrants concern (Zimmer et al., 1984; Beck et al., 1991). Sometimes aggressive resident behaviors are violent and may cause fear in nursing staff as well as harm. Management of aggressive resident behaviors presents difficult care problems for nursing staff. In a study of 101 nursing home and intermediate care residents in Veterans Administration (VA) facilities, Winger and colleagues (1987) found 9 percent of nursing home and 34 percent of intermediate care residents had no aggressive behaviors, while 84 percent of nursing home residents and 57 percent of intermediate care residents had behaviors that endangered themselves or others. A study by Everitt and coworkers (1991) documented that the three most distressing resident behaviors nursing staff encountered were physical abuse, verbal abuse, and wandering. Lusk (1992), in an exploratory study, found NAs reporting a variety of injuries (e.g., black eye, torn shoulder cuff requiring surgical repair) from residents' aggressive behaviors, while another study comparing physically aggressive behavior in two Department of Veterans Affairs nursing homes found more instances of aggressive behavior in the home with a greater percentage of neurologic and psychiatric patients (Rudman et al., 1993). Meddaugh (1987) reviewed chart and incident reports to investigate the aggressive behavior of 72 residents in a skilled nursing facility. Twenty-six staff members (27 percent) were abused by a resident 1 to 2 times in a 3-month period. In a study of 124 residents in 4 nursing homes, Ryden and colleagues (1991) found that 51 percent of aggressive behavior was physical,

48 percent was verbal, and 4 percent sexual. Aggression was correlated with functional dependence, although no category correlated with cognitive impairment.

Perhaps most difficult to deal with in nursing homes are the interactions among residents, some of which are positive and encourage friendships, while others are negative and involve violent arguments and even physical fights. Jones (1975) studied 441 residents in 10 intermediate care nursing homes and found that spatial proximity is an important consideration in the analysis of social interaction between residents. Arguments and fights occurred more frequently in fairly restricted spatial arrangements (e.g., 4-bed rooms), while friendship interactions were more likely to occur between residents who resided at least 2-rooms' distance from one another. The results suggest that in the limited environment of the nursing home both closeness and distance are needed for positive interactions among residents.

Access

It is estimated that 22 percent of the elderly long-term-care population live in nursing homes and other facilities, whereas 40 percent or more live at home with a spouse. The elderly are at higher risk for physical and mental health problems, impaired coping, functional decline, and premature institutionalization than the general population (Preston and Mansfield, 1984). These risks are even greater for the elderly who live alone and in poverty, particularly women (Krout, 1986).

Public expenditures for community-based services are relatively small compared to those for nursing home care (O'Shaunessy and Price, 1987). Medicaid, which is the principal source of funding of health care services for low income persons, finances mostly nursing home care. Expenditures for institutional long-term care in 1993 are estimated to be $74.9 billion. (Of that amount $36.9 billion were from Medicaid and $4.8 billion were from Medicare.) (DHHS, 1993).

Nevertheless, there is concern about underuse of nursing home care by some elderly, especially in areas where there are fewer nursing home beds per capita of elderly in the population. In general, rural areas have a higher concentration of the elderly and higher rates of chronic illness and disability. The growing number of older citizens in rural areas is especially pronounced in the Midwest and South. Yet the number of available nursing home beds—whether in traditional nursing homes or alternatives such as in-home care—is less per capita in these areas than in urban areas, and the shortage of RNs is greater in rural areas and in areas where the more impoverished elderly reside (Select Committee on Aging, 1992). Although Medicaid pays at least some of the costs of care for about 60 percent of nursing home patients, efforts by states to control costs of Medicaid have tended to limit the supply of nursing home beds. Further, the lack of Medicare reimbursement and the spend-down requirements to qualify for Medicaid assistance discourage some elderly from the use of nursing home care when it is needed (O'Shaunessy and Price, 1987).

FUTURE DEMAND FOR INSTITUTIONAL LONG-TERM CARE

Effect of Demographic Trends

As mentioned earlier, the population of older adults with complex and chronic conditions that require long-term care is growing. In 1985 there were about 1.4 million elders (people over age 65) residing in nursing homes; by the year 2050 this number is expected to increase fourfold (Andreoli and Musser, 1991). Current demographic predictions suggest that although the proportion of the U.S. population aged 65 and older will remain fairly constant, the proportion aged 85 and older will continue to rise in the next 30 years to about 2.1 percent of the population. With a stable population, these increases in proportion reflect the increase in the absolute numbers of elderly persons, particularly those 85 and older, who will increase in number from about 200,000 in 1951 to an estimated 1.2 million in 2011 (Bond and Bond, 1987). Over the next several decades, the proportion of nursing residents who are "old-old" (i.e., over age 85) is also expected to increase to somewhere around 50 percent.

Recent estimates indicate that one-half of the women and almost one-third of the men who turned 65 in 1990 will require nursing home care during their life. By the year 2010, an estimated 76 percent of the elderly are expected to be completely independent, but 24 percent of the elderly—about 7 million elderly persons—are projected to have some impairment that requires them to seek assistance with one or more activities of daily living (Scanlon, 1988; Kane and Kane, 1991). The number of dependent elders is expected to grow as the proportion of elderly in the population, especially those over age 75, increases (Griffin et al., 1989; Strumpf and Knibbe, 1990). Dependencies for assistance range from instrumental activities of daily living (IADL), such as cooking, shopping, and cleaning, to personal care activities of daily living (ADL), such as toileting, dressing, bathing, transfer and ambulation, and eating. Of the 7 million elderly needing long-term care by the year 2010, 1.75 million will be in nursing homes or other institutions; 1.4 million out of the total 7 million will need assistance with almost every ADL and IADL. Further, as a result of the aging population and increasing life expectancy, by the year 2020 the number of elderly residents in nursing homes could nearly double (Kemper and Murtaugh, 1991).

Trends in Case-Mix and Characteristics of Nursing Homes

By 2030, the elderly will comprise 20 percent of the population and use 30 percent of health care resources (Select Committee on Aging, 1992). The majority of residents in nursing homes will be 80 years and older, functionally dependent in multiple ADLs, have multiple chronic illnesses, and be cognitively impaired. Because of continued short hospital stays for acute illnesses and increased use of home care services where possible, residents in nursing homes will tend to be sicker and more acute illnesses will be treated in the nursing home. At the same time, alternative settings, such as assisted living and group home facilities, will be more available and will house more of the younger elderly with fewer or less severe impairments (O'Connor, 1995). More emphasis in these facilities will be placed on rehabilitation to maintain and improve function. Convalescent nursing homes are also expected to be more prevalent, with many elderly discharged to their own home after a short stay for recovery and rehabilitation.

Nursing homes will also include greater numbers of residents with AIDS, more residents with infections like methacycline-resistant *Staphylococcus aureus* and tuberculosis, elderly who are developmentally disabled, residents requiring rehabilitation, and hospice residents. Special units devoted to the care of residents with these conditions, as well as residents on ventilators and with pressure sores, are expected to increase.

Although it is positive that more alternatives to nursing homes will be available for the elderly, the downside is that the majority, if not all, of the residents of nursing homes will require more complex and intensive nursing care, and most will be highly functionally debilitated both cognitively and physically. Logically, this changing case-mix has clear implications for the types and numbers of staff that will be required to deliver quality care. More professional nursing staff (registered nurses) with gerontological training and greater use of gerontological nurse practitioners will be needed, both to plan and provide care and to direct and supervise the care provided by assisting staff. The nature of the work with mostly "old old," highly debilitated residents will provide quality-of-care challenges for assisting staff that they will not be able to meet without professional leadership and direction, and it will exacerbate stress, burnout, and turnover problems that are already of great concern.

Subacute Care

As home- and community-based long-term-care options (e.g., assisted-living facilities, continuing care retirement communities) erode the market share served by traditional nursing homes, subacute medical and rehabilitation services are emerging as a viable discharge option for patients who are suffering from cardiac conditions and cancer, recovering from surgical procedures and transplants, who require wound management, or who are ventilator dependent. More than 50 percent of nursing home admissions currently come from hospitals, with most needing care for unstable medical conditions.

According to a report on a subacute care demonstration project in Illinois (*McKnight's Long-term Care News*, 1993), subacute care includes physician supervision and RN care and physiological monitoring on a continuous basis. Facilities will be responsible for developing for every admission a comprehensive plan of care that includes measurable objectives and timetables designed to meet a broad range (e.g., medical, psychosocial) of patient care needs. Rules related to quality assessment and quality improvement, personnel requirements, and admissions practices have been set forth by the Joint Commission on Accreditation of Healthcare Organizations (JCAHO), which has recently incorporated subacute care into its survey process. Increased staff levels will be necessary to accommodate patients receiving subacute medical, nursing, and rehabilitation services. Outcomes, physical plant, and physician credentials are three major areas addressed in JCAHO accreditation standards for subacute units (Stahl, 1995). It is noted that RN credentials are not included, a curiosity since RNs will obviously play a large role in the care of residents in subacute units in nursing homes. A further concern is that the medical focus will continue to compromise implementation of a social-behavioral model of care in nursing homes.

Special Care Units for Dementia

Special care units (SCU) emerged as an important environmental intervention for care of persons with dementia in the 1980s. Today more than 1 in 10 nursing homes has a special unit or program for people with dementia, with more than 1,500 SCUs providing in excess of 50,000 special care beds. Data indicate that the number of SCUs is continuing to grow rapidly, with more than 2,500 units projected to be in operation by 1995 (NIA, 1994). Although there is much diversity among SCUs, most incorporate some type of physical modification, including security measures to limit egress, specialized activity programming for residents, and special training for staff, who are often permanently assigned to the unit.

There are several reports of studies to evaluate the effects of SCUs; however, most have not employed designs with sufficient control to rule out competing explanations (Greene et al., 1985; Hall et al., 1986; Cleary et al., 1988; Matthew et al., 1988). Experimental research by Maas and Buckwalter (1990) is one exception. Analysis revealed no significant changes in cognitive or functional abilities over time and no significant differences in these abilities between Alzheimer's disease patients on the SCU and on traditional integrated nursing home units (Swanson et al., 1994). Patients on the special unit were restrained less than those living on traditional units, but the SCU patients fell significantly more, on the average. The total number of medications for each patient was not significantly different for SCU versus traditional unit patients, and the number per patient did not increase over the 1-year study period. A multicenter collaborative initiative, funded by the National Institute on Aging and designed to explore the effectiveness of SCUs, evaluate specific interventions and family involvement in care, and compare SCU outcomes to those of traditional nursing home care, is currently under way.

Projected Staffing Requirements

The projected demand for nursing home care has sparked debate over costs and the adequacy of homes to deliver quality care. The anticipated need for qualified care givers in nursing homes is expected to increase anywhere from two- to fivefold by the middle of the next century (DHHS, 1991). Projections of the number of FTE registered nurses needed to supervise care by the year 2000 range from 260,000 to slightly over 1 million (NIA, 1987). There were only 92,000 FTE RNs employed in nursing homes in 1984 (Sheridan et al., 1992). The House of Representatives Select Committee on Aging (1992) forecast that by 2030, at least 36,000 geriatricians and 1.1 million RNs will be required to provide adequate health care for the elderly population in 2020. According to the Select Committee's estimate, 223,900 RNs will be needed in nursing homes compared to 94,900 in 1990. Current RN-to-resident ratios for nursing homes are estimated to be 6.3 nurses per 100 residents, while the projected need for the decade of the 1990s, due to the anticipated changes in case-mix, is from 10.2 to 16.2 RNs per 100 residents. In addition, 671,100 NAs will be needed in nursing homes compared to 421,900 in 1990, and 167,000 licensed practical nurses (LPN) compared to 112,100 in 1990 (Select Committee on Aging, 1992). Although estimates of current and projected staffing vary according to time frame and perspectives on the appropriate staff mix in nursing homes, it is apparent that the demand for nursing staff in nursing homes is rising dramatically. The rising demand may influence recommendations for staffing numbers and staff-mix in nursing homes, despite a lack of research evidence directly linking quality and staffing.

Regulatory and Reimbursement Projections

There is no doubt that OBRA has done a great deal to improve the quality of care in nursing homes by placing new emphasis on outcomes evaluation, staff training, residents' rights and quality of life, and the decreased use of restraints and psychoactive drugs. In regard to RN staffing, OBRA requires a licensed nurse to be on duty at all times, and for 8 hours each day that nurse must be an RN. Further, OBRA requires a full-time director of nursing who must be an RN.

In our view, the OBRA regulations are minimal and do not go far enough in requiring 24-hour RN coverage with specific numbers of assisting staff for a specific number of residents to assure quality of care and reasonable work expectations for staff. The American Nurses Association has advocated for quality nursing home care by promoting RN coverage around the clock, nurse aide training and certification, and opposing waivers of OBRA licensed nurse requirements. The Institute of Medicine's Committee on Nursing Home Regulation recommended that "nursing homes should place their highest priority on the recruitment, retention, and support of adequate numbers of professional nurses who are trained in gerontology and geriatrics to ensure an adequate number and appropriate mix of professional and nonprofessional nursing personnel to meet the needs of all types of residents in each facility" (IOM, 1986). Despite such recommendations, the nursing home industry has sought waivers even of OBRA's minimal increases in staffing standards (Francese and Mohler, 1994). The industry cites a shortage of RNs and inadequate reimbursement to pay their salaries as reasons for not being able to meet the OBRA staffing standards. Thus the nation's ability to meet the future demand for long-term care will continue to be affected by government reimbursement policies that are not commensurate with government regulations regarding the quality of care.

REVIEW OF RESEARCH RELEVANT TO LINKAGE OF STAFFING AND QUALITY OF CARE

This section undertakes a review of the literature that investigates the quality of care provided in long-term-care facilities and examines linkages between quality of care and various aspects of nurse staffing. Following an initial discussion of definitions of quality and how it is measured, we discuss the relationship between cost and quality of care. Studies are then presented that focus on aspects of staffing (staff attitudes, level of training, level of stress and turnover rates, number of staff and staff mix) and that consider the effect of the variables on quality of care. Finally, we review research that examines the relationship between quality of care and environmental factors such as reimbursement policies, type of facilities, and management systems or organizational climate.

Definitions and Measurement of Quality

Few concepts have been more elusive, controversial, or politically volatile than nursing home quality of care. Perhaps this is because as individuals we all fear functional impairment, loss of independence, and impoverishment, but as citizens we do not have the will to provide the financing for quality of care in nursing homes. Quality of care in nursing homes is a complex concept confounded by regulations and debates about what should be measured to assess quality, case-mix, facility characteristics, and methods of measurement (Mezey, 1989; Mezey and Lynaugh, 1989). Moreover, quality of care has been defined both as an input measure and as an outcome (Kruzich et al., 1992). But perhaps most confounding has been the continued reliance upon a medical model in defining standards of care and reimbursement formulas. Quality in long-term care requires different strategies than in acute care. In long-term care the focus is on replacing the patient role with a self-care role, emphasizing the individual's abilities to function with remaining abilities despite chronic disease, impairment, or both. Nursing homes are "nursing" homes so, clearly, quality of care is dependent upon the quality of nursing. Yet professional RNs are so scant in nursing homes as to be almost a novelty (Maraldo, 1991).

Prior to OBRA 87, quality of care in nursing homes was largely evaluated and regulated according to structure and process standards rather than the achievement of patient outcomes. Traditional reliance on structural measures failed to capture the essence of nursing home quality (Braun, 1991), although Stein and colleagues (1986) found that resident perceptions of quality and level of satisfaction were strongly related to objective surveyor ratings of nursing home quality. In Kurowski and Shaughnessey's (1985) review of studies comparing quality of homes with regulator surveys, many aspects of quality were not sensitive to the surveys and adding observation to surveys did not adequately measure quality (Fackelmann, 1986). Davis (1991) reviewed a number of studies that have examined macro-organizational and structural variables and quality and noted the paucity of empirical evidence to support these linkages. Thus, research findings in general have shed little light on the characteristics of nursing homes (such as size, ægis, age, and rural or urban location) that inform our understanding of what factors contribute to quality care.

The Omnibus Budget Reconciliation Act of 1987 provided a starting point for a new definition of quality in long-term care and focused measurement of quality on patient outcomes (Wilging, 1992). According to OBRA, a nursing home's purpose is to "bring each resident to the highest practicable level of mental, physical, and psychosocial well-being, and to do so in an environment that emphasizes resident's rights" (Wilging, 1992, p. 22). Quality care begins with a standardized, comprehensive patient assessment coordinated by an RN, which requires that specific attention be given to activities of daily living, vision and hearing, pressure sores, urinary incontinence, range of motion, psychosocial functioning, use of nasogastric tubes, accidents, nutrition, hydration, antipsychotic and other drug use, and special services such as respiratory therapy. (Bowel elimination was ignored as an outcome to be monitored, but has been added in version 2.0 of the minimum data set.) The OBRA legislation proved to be the impetus for improving the quality of care in nursing homes. The requirement that specific fields be included in a minimum data set (MDS) on all residents in nursing homes provides a valuable source of data for evaluating quality on the basis of resident outcomes (Zimmerman, 1991). From the data on resident outcomes included in the MDS, quality indicators have been proposed and are being tested for how well they measure quality for aggregates of residents in nursing homes (Rantz and Miller, 1994).

The "highest practicable level of functioning," however, is in reality defined by what is fiscally appropriate within each facility. Whether or not adequate resources are available to provide quality care is still an issue, and many would agree that resources are often not adequate. For example, the study conducted by the Institute of Medicine's Committee on Nursing Home Regulation supported higher nursing staff standards as a major means for assuring quality of care in nursing homes, along with new staffing, training, and registry requirements for nursing staff (IOM, 1986). Unfortunately, the goal of requiring 24-hour RN coverage in nursing homes was not achieved in OBRA because of political pressures touting a nursing shortage and higher costs. Although OBRA increased staffing requirements, the facts are that nursing assistants make up 85 percent of nursing staff in nursing homes and provide the majority of direct care to residents, with residents receiving on average only 12 minutes per day of care from RNs (Maraldo, 1991). As noted earlier, the issue of staff-to-resident ratios is also of concern. In acute care, there are an estimated 98 RNs for every 100 patients, while in nursing homes there are 5.2 RNs for every 100 residents (Wilging, 1992). This marked discrepancy is not likely due to a true corresponding difference in the needs of patients for nursing care in the two settings, but is rather due to how "highest practicable" is being defined by economic and political realities.

The concept of quality in the practice setting has, to date, included only limited attention to outcome assessments and public input (DHHS, 1993). Traditional paradigms of quality thus need redefinition to assure an excellence in health care that is responsive to the changing needs of the public. The movement to continuous quality improvement (CQI) is seen as one way of focusing on processes and systems, rather than individual efforts, in quality management applications (DHHS, 1993). When residents are asked what constitutes quality of care and what factors are most important in creating a good environment, they emphasize kindness, consideration, friendliness, and empathetic listening on the part of staff, suggesting that staff attitudes have a major impact on resident quality of life (Goodwin and Trocchio, 1987).

Although families continue to be involved in care following placement of their loved one in a nursing facility, relatively little is known about the relationships among families and nursing home staff, especially from the perspective of family members (Duncan and Morgan, 1994). What research has been conducted in this area indicates that families equate good quality nursing home care with care that is affectively appropriate, emotionally sensitive, respectful, and professional, and that emphasizes a personal relationship with the resident. Families tend to base their evaluations of care as much on social and emotional factors as they do technical competence in performing care tasks (Bowers, 1988; Duncan and Morgan, 1994), whereas staff often give priority to the smooth functioning of the organization. What this means is that nurse aides, in particular, often get caught between the desires of the organization and those of family members (Duncan and Morgan, 1994). To address these differences, Bowers (1988) proposed a collaborative approach to care that would encourage families to become more involved in technical aspects of care while facilitating staff's emotional involvement with residents. Interestingly, in those facilities where families found little respect for the work of the nonprofessional staff, they also enjoyed little support for their goal of having their loved one treated in a personal manner by the staff. As noted in a study using focus groups and interviews with families of patients with dementia, families concluded that "the demands and rewards of the nursing home as a system were often detrimental to quality care" (Duncan and

Morgan, 1994, p. 241). In another study, which examined the use of nasogastric feeding tubes in nursing homes, two themes of interest emerged in the family interviews. First, there was little or no communication among health care providers, patients, and their families regarding the use of nasogastric tubes. Second, some families perceived that the tubes were used for the convenience of the staff who did not want to take the time, or did not have the patience, to feed residents (Kayser-Jones, 1990).

Cost of Quality

The cost and financing of institutional long-term care to achieve the highest practicable functioning and well-being of patients is one of the biggest issues facing the assurance of quality care in nursing homes. Since OBRA, the average increase in reimbursement rate reported across the country has been about $1.50 per resident (Wilging, 1992). Few would argue that this is adequate to implement all that OBRA requires for assuring quality of care for nursing home residents, let alone to move beyond minimum standards. Without increased reimbursement, the nursing home industry will likely continue to seek ways to compromise OBRA standards, especially regarding RN staffing. "We get what we pay for" remains a truism that is no less applicable to nursing home quality of care than it is elsewhere.

As noted earlier, nursing homes are the major cost center for long-term care, with expenditures of more than $70 billion dollars in 1993 (DHHS, 1993). Data from the 1987 Medicare and Medicaid Automated Certification Survey (covering 14,000 nursing homes in 525 counties and 46 states) suggest that cost-saving decisions that lead to substituting less expensive staff and using more laborsaving techniques may lead to bad patient outcomes. That is, cost minimization may be achieved, but quality of care suffers. Where RN wages are high, nursing homes tend to use larger numbers of less expensive staff, whereas when LPN wages are higher, nursing homes use more RNs and NAs (Zinn, 1993). In addition, when the market price for nursing services is high, nursing homes use more laborsaving techniques such as catheterization, restraints, tube feedings, and nontoileting of residents, which may not necessarily represent good care strategies. However, where Medicaid per diem reimbursement rates are higher, and where there is more competition among facilities for patients, nursing homes use more licensed (RN and LPN) staff and have lower rates of catheterizations and nontoileting of residents. Spector and Takada (1991) also found that more RNs were employed when per capital income was higher, while more LPNs were used with higher Medicaid levels and in urban areas. When there was cost-based reimbursement, more RNs and LPNs were employed. These data suggest that nursing homes have not yet found consistent and effective ways to save money without sacrificing professional leadership and quality (Zinn, 1993).

Some have argued that families are a neglected resource for the delivery of care in nursing homes. In a study to evaluate the effects of a special care unit for residents with Alzheimer's disease on resident, staff, and family member outcomes, Maas and colleagues (1991) found that family members were dissatisfied with their lack of involvement in the care of their relatives, with the activities provided for the residents, and with the amount of resources devoted to the provision of care. Based on these troubling results, Maas and colleagues (1994) are currently conducting a study funded by NINR. The study will test the effects on family and staff satisfaction and stress, as well as on resident outcomes, of an intervention designed to create a family-staff partnership for the care of institutionalized persons with Alzheimer's disease.

Factors that Influence Staff Performance

Job Satisfaction and Turnover

Staffing problems are expected to continue at least through the end of this century (Caudill and Patrick, 1991). In light of the growing demand for qualified personnel in long-term-care facilities and concern over the nursing shortage, however, surprisingly little research (aside from state and national surveys) has been conducted in the area of staff turnover, and the important other side of the coin, staff retention (Robertson et al., 1994).

Turnover in nursing staff is generally affected by a variety of factors leading to low job satisfaction, including low compensation and benefits, poor working conditions and quality of the nursing home, few opportunities for advancement, and problems with staff relationships (Birkenstock, 1991). Studies specifically focusing on NAs in long-term-care settings have cited numerous individual characteristics (e.g., age, education, background) as well as management factors (e.g., inadequate in-service education, supervision and orientation; few opportunities for advancement, performance appraisal, and compensation) as contributing to the high rate of turnover and dissatisfaction (Reagan, 1986; Wagnild and Manning, 1986). A study by Wagnild identified a "cycle of turnover" and found that NA turnover can be reduced by careful analysis of management practices, starting with the recruitment and selection of applicants and extending through orientation, staff development, supervisory skills, employee compensation, and involvement of aides in management decisions (Wagnild, 1988, p. 22).

Comparing levels of job satisfaction in social care homes, Willcocks and colleagues (1987) found the lowest levels in homes where the ratio of staff hours to residents was below the average. Low levels of staff satisfaction were particularly prevalent where staff had less autonomy and time constraints allowed only the essentials of care to be carried out. Although staff tended to rate their overall job satisfaction highly, negative elements noted were in regard to working conditions, staff shortages perceived to result in poor care, inadequate involvement in decisions, and inadequacies of training and consultation.

A recent study by Robertson and colleagues (1994) identified factors that affected RN retention in long-term care, focusing on what nurses reported as enhancing their job satisfaction and commitment to this area of practice. Briefly, the three highest rated factors related to satisfaction were recognition from patients, challenge of the work, and the authority to exercise judgment for patient care. The most important factors seen as contributing to retention were relationships with colleagues, available support staff, authority to exercise judgment in patient care, challenge of the work, adequate nurse-to-resident ratio, support from administration, and adequate supplies and equipment. The investigators also calculated mean difference scores for all items, indicating that importance was greater than satisfaction in these areas for the nurse respondents. The largest mean differences found were in the areas of paperwork, salary and benefits, and staffing. Further analysis and synthesis of the data revealed, consistent with previous findings in the literature, five main areas in which issues associated with retention of nurses in long-term care arise: (1) relationships, (2) patient care factors, (3) money and benefits, (4) levels of staffing and supplies, and (5) amount of paperwork. Difficulties in these areas represent serious problems in long-term care that threaten the quality of care provided in these settings (Robertson et al., 1994). Thus, to promote staff retention in long-term care and to make nursing homes a more attractive and satisfying practice setting, administrators must recognize both the importance to nurses of patient care factors and the authority to manage patient care issues and make clinical decisions, and the need to provide RNs with attractive compensation and benefits, recognition, training, and participation in decision making about their work.

Stress and Burnout

Nurses who work with the elderly confront many complex and potentially stressful care situations. Nowhere is this more true than for nursing home staff who work in highly demanding, labor- and client-intensive jobs. High stress at work can create morale problems that ultimately detract from the staff member's job performance (Sheridan et al., 1990). The causal model depicted below (see Figure 1), derived from research on work stress and morale among nursing home employees, highlights both antecedents and outcomes of work-related stress (Weiler et al., 1990, p. 321).

The antecedent conditions include objective organizational characteristics such as: (1) the variety of tasks in nursing positions, (2) the degree to which supervisory authority is delegated, (3) the closeness of supervision, (4) the degree of specialization, (5) the skill level of the work, (6) the quantity of the work, and (7) the pace of the work. Subjective organizational characteristics include: (1) task routinization, (2) communication, and (3) distributive justice. Social support includes perceived support from supervisors, coworkers, spouse, friends, and relatives. Personal characteristics refer to variables such as age, sex, educational

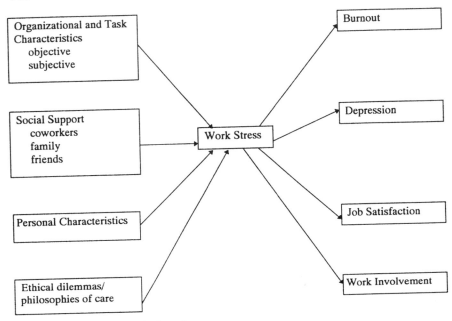

FIGURE 1   Causal model of work stress.

attainment, length of nursing service, occupational position or title, work status (e.g., full- or part-time), marital status, and number of relatives living nearby. Ethical dilemmas are situations in which no choice is clearly correct and the alternatives are equally unsatisfactory, while a philosophy of care incorporates ANA standards of care and the nurses' personal beliefs regarding the residents' right of autonomy, their role in the decision making process, and their right to respectful treatment (Weiler et al., 1990).

A large body of literature has examined the outcomes of work-related stress, revealing a strong link between stress and adverse physical and psychological consequences (LaRocco et al., 1980). There is equally compelling evidence, however, that social support serves to mitigate against these adverse effects and reduces burnout among nurses (Constable and Russell, 1986). Burnout, a phenomenon characterized by loss of concern for residents, and physical, emotional and spiritual exhaustion, may lead to indifference or negative feelings toward elderly residents, overuse of chemical or physical restraints, and heightened potential for abuse (Heine, 1986). Burnout has also been shown to result in administrative difficulties such as high rates of tardiness, absenteeism, and attrition (Goldin, 1985).

The outcomes of work-related stress, according to the above model, include: (1) burnout, defined as a syndrome of emotional exhaustion, depersonalization, and lack of personal accomplishment; (2) depression, which is the degree of negative affect experienced by nursing personnel; (3) job satisfaction, which is the affective orientation of nursing personnel toward the work situation; and (4) work involvement, defined as the degree to which nursing personnel identify with the job (Weiler et al., 1990).

It has been suggested that nursing personnel who work with patients with Alzheimer's disease are especially vulnerable to the effects of stress and burnout. Alzheimer's disease patients present many difficult care and management problems because of their progressive cognitive, functional, and psychosocial deterioration, which can result in bizarre and combative behaviors, emotional outbursts, and wandering. Moreover, nursing home staff are often poorly trained to cope with the disruptive behaviors of residents, and they are therefore repeatedly frustrated by their inability to manage recurrent problems (Stolley et al., 1991). Many nursing homes are also not equipped with environmental structures or the support and service systems required to care appropriately for the person with Alzheimer's disease (Peppard, 1984). A recent study, using a quasi-experimental design with repeated measures, examined whether staff who cared for Alzheimer's disease patients on a special care unit were less stressed and less burned out than staff who cared for such patients on traditional (integrated) units. Findings revealed that the principal area of stress reduction for nursing personnel working on the SCU occurred with respect to staff knowledge, abilities, and resources. Subscale analysis indicated significantly less stress for staff who worked in the SCU with respect to residents' verbal and physical behavior. The SCU was designed specifically to provide the special environmental structures and support and service systems for the care of Alzheimer's disease patients that would enhance functioning and decrease associated behavioral problems. These may be important factors in reducing stress and burnout for staff caring for residents with Alzheimer's disease (Mobily et al., 1992). The investigators also recommended that whenever possible, staff who work with residents who have Alzheimer's should be carefully screened and selected for their ability to be sensitive to the needs of these residents, their flexibility, and their imagination, as well as ability to respond to persons with impaired communication and ever-changing moods (Coons, 1991). Specialized training in the care of residents with Alzheimer's disease is also a critical factor (see next section, "Education and Training").

In an effort to manage stress among nursing personnel in long-term-care facilities, it seems logical to examine those antecedent conditions in the model depicted above that are amenable to change. Research by Hare and Pratt (1988) has shown that higher levels of nursing burnout in both acute and long-term-care settings may be related to the nature of the physically and emotionally strenuous work tasks, low status in comparison to other positions in the health care system, limited training, low wages and benefits and, of interest to this report, poor staffing-to-patient ratios. Further, problems with support in the work environment, especially from peers and supervisors, have repeatedly been shown to be a primary source of stress among nurses (Cronin-Stubbs and Rooks, 1985). It has also been suggested that nursing personnel who elect to work with clients who have a poor chance of survival (as opposed to nursing personnel who do not work with these patients by choice) have reduced vulnerability to burnout because their work provides them with a sense of meaning (Hare and Pratt, 1988). The interventions summarized below have been set forth to address organizational sources of stress in the long-term-care setting (Weiler et al., 1990, pp. 333–334):

- Improved in-service training, especially in multidimensional problems of the elderly, that emphasizes psychosocial and behavioral problems common in this population.
- Increased variety in job tasks.
- Improved supervision.
- Implementation of a management style that allows for feedback, flexibility, and sensitivity.
- Clear and realistic objectives for resident care.
- Higher wages and better benefits for staff.
- Adequate staffing levels.

Although the latter two recommendations may be considered nonnegotiable by some administrators because of the cost implications associated with their implementation, it should be noted that the costs related to staff burnout, absenteeism, and turnover can far outweigh the costs associated with adequate staffing and compensation (Weiler et al., 1990).

Another source of work-related stress that may be amenable to change has to do with the effect of the physical environment and structural factors. Although very little research has been done in this area, work by Lyman (1987) suggests that physical and architectural features, such as adequate space, separate activity rooms, staff offices and toilet facilities, resident care facilities, barrier-free hallways, visible exits with amenities such as wide entry doors and ramps, and emergency exits, may decrease caregiver burden and stress. Enhancing social support networks is another important strategy that can serve as a buffer against the stresses inherent in working with the elderly. Interventions designed to strengthen supportive relationships among staff, staff training related to stress management, and work-related counseling and support groups have all been shown to reduce vulnerability to burnout, depression, and job dissatisfaction (Weiler et al., 1990).

Education and Training

Although previous research has provided inconclusive evidence of a strong relationship between the care provider's attitudes toward the elderly and the quality of resident care (Wright, 1988), Storlie (1982) argued that dedicated and compassionate nursing staff are essential for maintaining high quality care on a day-to-day basis. Further, few would disagree that nurse aides need to be skilled in providing care, given that they make up about 85 percent of nursing home personnel and provide the majority of direct care. Yet many nurse aides are functionally illiterate, untrained, and inadequate to the tasks at hand (Maraldo, 1991). With the number of cognitively impaired and functionally dependent residents in nursing homes, sophisticated approaches for care are required that are beyond the knowledge and skill of persons with one year or less of training. The need for competent professionals who are caring, qualified, and compassionate caregivers has been documented by research on residents in long-term-care settings (NCCNHR, 1985). However, the reality is that the majority (96 percent) of directors of nursing in long-term-care facilities are not academically prepared for their positions (Bahr, 1991), having little or no specific education about the aging process, gerontological nursing principles, or managerial skills. The lack of educationally prepared RNs who understand the unique health and social needs of older adults and who are effective managers of assisting nursing staff is a critical problem. Combined with the small number of RNs employed in nursing homes and the reported vacancy rate of about 10 percent for RNs, the problem takes on gargantuan proportions (Bahr, 1991).

Much of the published literature on education in long-term care discusses the need for more training and adequate supervision of staff, especially for NAs. Methods most commonly used in staff training are didactic, using both verbal and written instruction, but there has been relatively little effort to study systematically the success of these methods with long-term-care staff, or to evaluate their ability to maintain therapeutic staff behaviors over time (Burgio and Burgio, 1990). In a review of the literature on this topic, Burgio and Burgio (1990, p. 289) urge the development of efficient training procedures "to teach nursing assistants basic therapeutic principles and skills," and argue that "management systems must be designed and implemented to assure that these skills will be performed appropriately and consistently in the natural environment." They also outline a number of strategies to overcome organizational resistance to staff-management interventions.

Burgio and Burgio (1990) suggest that an important step in motivating staff to perform patient-related tasks is effective in-service training, which should include: (1) didactic instruction presented both in verbal and written formats, (2) modeling of the procedure by a trainer, and (3) role playing by the trainees coupled with immediate trainer feedback regarding their performance. The attitudes of staff affect not only their own expectations about their working lives, but also the way in which they approach residents. Thus an important aspect of in-service training is to correct the tendencies to view residents as childlike, unreliable, and manipulative, and to reduce depersonalization of physical care and the neglect of psychosocial needs.

Assessment of training outcomes includes more than simple paper and pencil tests to determine knowledge of the procedure; rather, assessment should also include a checklist assessment of skill performance in a situation that permits immediate corrective feedback and praise, followed by assessment of the trainee's skill performance on the nursing unit. Burgio and Burgio (1990) argue that these assessments should take place immediately following the in-service training, as well as at regular intervals thereafter, with remedial training sessions required in the event of poor performance.

Consultation

As noted earlier in the section on staffing qualifications and preparation, most RNs employed by long-term-care facilities have associate degrees, that is, two years of training that includes little specialized training in gerontology or psychiatry. Thus, liaisons with advanced practice nurses (e.g., geriatric and psychiatric nurse practitioners) who possess skill in these areas can provide an invaluable resource to the long-term-care team, especially when dealing with behaviorally impaired residents. The liaisons can thus improve the quality of care for residents and the quality of life for visitors and staff (Hall, 1995).

Psychiatric nurses, in particular, can play a critical role in meeting the mental health and behavioral needs of nursing home residents through consultation and education efforts, which have been found to improve care through the reduction of symptoms and negative behaviors and the achievement of optimal resident functioning (Samter et al., 1994). Assessment and management of emotional problems require specialized knowledge, skill, and creativity (Stevens and Baldwin, 1988). Currently, the vast majority of nursing home personnel are nonprofessionals in whom these attributes are underdeveloped. The lack of skilled care givers and adequate resources to meet the mental, emotional, and behavioral problems of nursing home residents suggests that without specialized psychiatric interventions the mental health needs of the elderly residing in nursing homes will remain unmet or be treated inappropriately (Stevens and Baldwin, 1988).

Consultations with skilled mental health professionals is thus an important and effective intervention (Parsons et al., 1988; Smith et al., 1994). Effective psychiatric consultation can influence staff attitudes and behaviors toward residents by helping long-term-care staff to develop systematic approaches to the assessment and management of disturbed residents, and to focus on specific behaviors and plans of action related to those behaviors (Parsons et al., 1988). Such consultations are among the many vital factors that can ensure that the nursing homes of today will truly provide better quality of care to behaviorally impaired residents than did the almshouses and state mental hospitals of yesteryear.

Quality and Number of Staff

As noted above, the nursing shortage still exists in many long-term-care settings. Difficulty recruiting and retaining qualified personnel to provide direct care in nursing homes remains a crucial problem, although the number of staff per se may not be the whole answer to the provision of quality care in nursing homes. Research by Fries (1994) has documented that much of staffing is driven by the type of resident. Resident characteristics (case-mix) explained 55 percent of the variance in resource use, with facility characteristics (including staffing levels) adding another 13 percent. The remaining one-third of the variance in resource use was accounted for by differences in residents across days (e.g., number of baths per week). Case-mix also explained about 35 percent of the variance in RN costs.

According to Fries (1994), different states have different staffing levels, but the relative use for types of residents remains constant. Much of staffing is also driven by the type of resources and use of the available staff time is discretionary (Fries, 1994). Thus, adding additional staff may result in some more staff time for all residents and not more time for those who really need it. At the special panel session on "Quality and Staffing in Nursing Homes" held at the 1994 Gerontological Society of America meeting, Fries argued the need, based on his data, to be more efficient in the use of current numbers of staff before it is assumed that higher staffing numbers are needed in nursing homes. He questioned whether some residents in nursing homes truly need that level of care, but rather are encouraged to be in nursing homes by flat rate reimbursement systems. Further, Fries (1994) suggested that higher quality may be possible by changing some staff practices in nursing homes without substantially greater resource investment. For example, use of fewer chemical and physical restraints was found to save staff time. Schnelle (1994) argued that despite the considerable experience of his research team in implementing highly specific protocols for managing incontinence, 100 percent compliance was never achieved. Thus, while nursing staff in nursing homes should have higher salaries and more help, just giving them more money and adding more staff is not the total answer. More specific protocol and management technologies also are needed in order to actually achieve higher quality care. Finally, consistent administrative support and RN leadership are also needed to guide staff performance so that it will result in quality outcomes.

Others also report that staffing shortages include insufficient numbers of NAs to provide the "hands on" care, as well as too few geriatrically prepared professional nurses to supervise care and provide leadership and guidance to the staff (Kayser-Jones, 1994). Current staffing patterns contribute to meeting resident needs through functional routines rather than individual care needs or resident preferences (Wright, 1988). Truly individualized care requires that a professional nurse, with specialized training, not only supervises the work of nonprofessional staff but also participates in and directs that care.

Although there are mixed results from research comparing quality to nursing hours, several studies have found nursing hours significantly related to quality indicators (Linn et al., 1977; Mech, 1980; Fottler et al., 1991). Disturbing data from a national survey conducted by the ANA suggest that those nursing homes with higher nurse vacancy rates experience more problems in areas such as medication errors and resident falls (McKibbin, 1990). Further, research by Kayser-Jones and colleagues (1989) indicated that insufficient and inadequately trained nursing staff was a contributing factor to the deterioration and eventual hospitalization of nursing home residents.

Other research supports the notion that staffing is an important variable that influences eating behavior (Kayser-Jones, 1994). The consequences of inadequate staffing can include: (1) the feeding of residents in a hurried manner that does not preserve their dignity (e.g., giving residents a large amount of food with each bite, feeding several residents at once, mixing food), and (2) inadequate nutritional intake, resulting in weight loss in residents and necessitating the use of liquid supplements and sometimes tube feedings. These finding are supported by research conducted by Blaum and colleagues (in press), which shows low nutrition of residents associated with their being fed by staff.

Willcocks and colleagues (1987) also found that staff-oriented rather than resident-oriented practices were strongest in homes with the lowest staffing levels. Staff shortages resulted in dispensing with flexibility for both residents and staff and opting for formalization of the care regime in order to complete what was regarded as essential work. Homes with higher ratios of staff-to-resident hours and a higher proportion of part-time staff rather than full-time staff were more likely to have resident-oriented practices as well as higher levels of agreement between staff and residents about what constitutes ideal environmental features.

Many gerontologists have proposed that ombudsman programs and other forms of community presence could improve nursing home quality of care. Cherry (1991) compared the effects of community presence programs on quality of nursing care with a random sample of 134 Medicare- and Medicaid-certified long-term-care facilities in Missouri. The presence of an ombudsman program was found to be the most important factor associated with quality for intermediate care facilities and also was significantly associated with quality for skilled nursing homes where there was ample staffing of RNs.

Quality and Staff-Mix

Type of staff may be more important than the available staff hours. Willcocks and colleagues (1987) found that management staff in homes with a social model of care, as opposed to a medical model of care, had more resident-oriented views on features of residential life, while care staff were more likely to express views that spring from organizational needs for routine. Since ideas about the provision of quality care are likely to flow from management and professional staff, available hours and organizational practices that permit them to demonstrate skilled care and supervise nonprofessional staff are necessary. Otherwise, supervisory staff can only carry out inspections to ensure that the worst practices are avoided.

Some experts believe that nursing homes that rely on predominately unskilled nursing staff jeopardize the quality of nursing home care (Shields and Kick, 1982). In a landmark study by Linn and colleagues (1977), higher levels of RN hours per patient were associated with improved functional status, survival, and the discharge of residents to the community. Other variables, however, such as higher cost, professional staff-to-patient ratios, better meal service, physical plant, and patient records were also associated with positive outcomes. Braun (1991), in an historical cohort study in which 390 veterans discharged to 11 nursing homes were followed for 6 months, found the quality variable "RN hours" was significantly and inversely related to mortality, while the quality variable "use of nursing process" was significantly related to probability of discharge. Using data from reports of 455 Medicare-certified skilled nursing facilities, Munroe (1990) found a positive, significant relationship between nursing home quality and the ratio of RN hours to licensed vocational nurse (LVN) hours per resident day. For every 25 percent increase in the ratio of RN hours to LVN hours, there was a decrease of 0.53 in the number of health-related deficiencies in the facilities.

In an analysis of data from the National Medical Expenditure Survey, Spector (1994) and a colleague found that higher per capita income and urban location led to more RNs employed in nursing homes. They also found that compared to for-profit homes, hospital-based and government nursing homes had more RNs and LPNs, but nonprofit homes had more RNs and fewer LPNs. In terms of outcomes, having a greater number of RNs was associated with fewer deaths annually, having more LPNs was associated with an increase in ADLs, and having more nurse aides had no impact. Spector reported less variation in nurse aide numbers across nursing homes than in RNs and LPNs, which may explain the failure to observe a nurse aide staffing effect on quality. Spector also found that states with higher Medicaid reimbursement levels had more LPNs per 100 residents, adjusted for case-mix. Although these states also tended to have more RNs, the relationship was not significant. Further, Spector found that in states where reimbursement was cost-based, more RNs were used but at the expense of LPNs. The implications of these findings for quality, however, were not straightforward. In a study of nursing homes in Rhode Island, Spector and Takada (1991) found that low RN and LPN turnover was related to greater functional improvements among residents. Spector (1994) noted that his findings support the notion that consistent RN leadership leads to better resident outcomes.

Attempts have been made to establish staff requirements for particular groups of residents (Senior, 1978) or in accordance with prescribed tasks (Rhys-Hearn, 1979), but without regard for the quality of care or resident outcomes. When staff were allocated in accordance with nurses' identification of patients' optimal nursing requirements, Rhys-Hearn (1979) found that in no case was the care given equivalent to the care prescribed. Norwich (1980) noted that when "extra" time was available, it was spent in physical care activities rather than psychosocial or therapeutic support, a finding supported in research by Savage and coworkers (1979) about psychogeriatric wards. In an observational study of staff behaviors in a nursing home, Burgio and colleagues (1990) found that LPNs displayed significantly more patient care behaviors and nurse aides significantly more nonwork behaviors than other nursing staff. RNs displayed the least nonwork behavior. Although all staff used most of their time for work, the study results may support the need for more licensed staff for greater productivity and for supervision of assisting staff. However, more than a decade ago Eliopoulos (1983) presented mathematically derived staff models to argue that higher RN staffing would be financially insupportable, in that the cost per patient would almost double with an all RN staff.

Staffing level and mix provide important information about the organizational climate of a nursing home and the way in which care is provided, and may help to explain agitated psychomotor behaviors of residents as related to environmental and personal variables (Kolanowski et al., 1994). Specifically, in a study conceptually grounded in Kayser-Jones' (1989) model of environment and quality of life in nursing homes, Kolanowski and colleagues (1994) found that the addition of staff mix as an organizational variable significantly increased the amount of variance explained, over and above that contributed by personal variables of the residents such as functional ability, cognitive and health status, mood, sensory deficits, and psychotropic drugs prescribed. Residents on those units with a higher ratio of licensed personnel had fewer instances of problematic behaviors, suggesting that staff who have the knowledge to care for frail elders are less likely to use restraints to manage behavior. Findings in a study by Bleismer (1994) of nursing homes in Minnesota also support the positive relationship between licensed nursing staff and quality of care and the idea that licensed nurse leadership needs to be doing more than completing paper work and assuring recorded compliance with regulations. The study found that in the first year after patient admission, higher licensed nursing hours were significantly related to improved functional ability in the patient, decreased probability of patient death, and increased probability of discharge home. Thus the data suggest that licensed nurse leadership needs to be directly involved with resident care and staff guidance.

Even among the licensed staff, research has shown that nurses' perceptions and attitudes about problem behaviors in residents vary according to educational background and preparation (e.g., LPNs vs. RNs) (Burgio et al., 1988). Most RNs employed by long-term-care facilities have associate degrees, that is, two years of training that includes little specialized training in gerontology or psychiatry. As noted earlier, in contrast to hospitals, where is it rare that DONs have less than a bachelor's degree and more often are at least master's prepared, DONs in nursing homes are often graduates of associate degree and diploma programs. Leadership and management are not part of the basic preparation offered by these programs and these DONs rarely have advanced training in gerontology. Turnover among DONs is also high, amounting to over 30 percent annually in Minnesota (Ryden, 1994).

"Nursing homes are beginning to use advanced practice nurses (gerontological nurse practitioners and specialists) to deal with the complex and multiple care needs of older persons in nursing homes. Their expert knowledge and skill in gerontological nursing has had a positive impact on reducing admissions to hospitals and reducing emergency room visits. Researchers at the University of Minnesota School of Nursing are currently involved in a 4-year study to look at clinical and cost outcomes with using advanced practice nurses in nursing homes" (C. Heine, personal communication, 1995).

Studies of advanced practice nurses, such as clinical nurse specialists and geriatric nurse practitioners, in nursing homes have shown that they can improve resident outcomes and contribute to quality by changing the focus from custodial to rehabilitative care (Kane et al., 1976, 1988), and by increasing the ability of facilities to care for more complex and acutely ill patients (Mezey and Scanlon, 1988). Nurse practitioners (NP) can enhance care and revenues by developing specialty services (e.g., bowel and bladder training programs, diabetes and wound management centers) that can be staffed by the general nursing staff and members of interdisciplinary teams. NPs can also serve as nurse managers in Medicare skilled units so that those units can develop higher quality, more technologically advanced subacute programs, and increase Medicare skilled care occupancy rates (Knapp, 1994).

Research by Evans and Strumpf (1994), investigating the relative effects of two experimental interventions delivered by GNSs on the use of physical restraints and resident and staff outcomes, found that staff mix and resident personal competence were important factors in the occurrence of disturbing behaviors likely to be managed by restraint. These disturbing behaviors occurred more frequently in situations where the availability of licensed nurses was low and resident frailty high. Further, although staff increased their assessment and intervention skills, the investigators noted the need for a "consistent professional presence" by a clinician with geriatric expertise to maintain minimal restraint use in the facility. Findings suggest that quality outcomes (e.g., restraint reduction) do not necessarily require more staff, but do require staff who have the requisite knowledge base and access to gerontological expertise, education, resident-centered assessment, monitoring, care planning, evaluation, and support in their efforts to provide quality individualized care (Evans and Strumpf, 1994; Strumpf, 1994).

A number of demonstrations have provided convincing evidence that GNPs and GNSs are effective in nursing homes. The Health Care Financing Administration (HCFA) supported the evaluation of two demonstration projects, the Robert Wood Johnson Foundation Teaching Nursing Home Program and the Nursing Home Connection, while the Kellogg Foundation supported the Mountain States program to place GNPs in nursing homes. These evaluations confirmed that nurses with advanced preparation in care of the elderly decrease unnecessary hospitalizations and use of emergency rooms, improve admission and ongoing patient assessments, provide better illness prevention and case finding, decrease incontinence, lower the use of psychotropic drugs and physical restraints, and generally improve the overall management of chronic and acute health problems. These improvements in care occurred without incurring additional costs, and in some instances at a reduced cost.

The experience of the Teaching Nursing Homes (TNH) provides further evidence of the need for professional gerontological nurses in nursing homes (Mezey, 1994). In comparing the TNHs with matched nursing homes in the same state, with the only difference being the presence of an advanced practice nurse in the TNHs, the TNHs had significantly fewer hospitalizations than the comparison homes and fewer emergency room visits. There also were notable improvements on a variety of quality indicators, such as management of urinary incontinence, decreased use of psychotropic medications including long-acting benzodiazepines and other such medications related to poor quality outcomes in nursing homes, and less use of restraints. Mezey (1994) noted that quality in some of the nursing homes was improved by increasing the number of RN FTEs, an observation that is not at all counterintuitive to the relationship between increased professional staff and improved practice. Ryden (1994) supports the assertion that RN leadership is a key to achieving quality outcomes in nursing homes.

Other research that tests interventions in nursing homes also supports the need for a continuous professional nurse presence to provide leadership and direction for assisting staff (Evans and Strumpf, 1989). For example, several researchers (Schnelle, 1990; Schnelle et al., 1990; Hawkins et al., 1992) tested management systems for nursing assistants to carry out interventions for incontinence that have shown significant improvements in resident dryness. According to Schnelle (1994), the interventions had a positive effect until the controlled conditions were withdrawn, when staff reverted to previous practices. In a multisite study, after the controlled conditions ceased, the management system and incontinence protocol were continued in only one of the sites. In this site the DON was particularly interested and involved. Schnelle (1994) concluded that it was the interest and leadership of this RN that resulted in the sustained use of the management system and intervention. Fries (1994) suggests, however, that with staff being forced to use the National Resident Assessment Instrument on a regular basis, it is hard to believe that staff will regress from the use of such interventions.

Some facilities use level of care or case-mix systems to allocate numbers and type of staff, with clinical nurse specialists available throughout the facility (Morris, 1994). According to Morris (1994), this systems approach allows for better decisions regarding number and type of staff needed, produces a better match between patient's need for care and the care provided, and improves resident outcomes. Thus, different categories of residents (e.g., short stay convalescent or rehabilitation, hospice residents, long stayers who have severe chronic mental and physical impairments) require very different staff numbers and skills.

Quality, Staff Satisfaction, and Turnover

There is no simple relationship between how staff regard the quality of their working life, staff turnover, and the quality of resident care, although most agree that dissatisfied staff are more likely to produce poor quality of care (Bond and Bond, 1987).

The behavior and attitudes of NAs can play a critical role in the quality of life of nursing home residents, and yet high attrition rates and alienation have been reported by nursing assistants. Mor (1995) noted that if aides are treated like "replaceable parts," then they are more likely to treat the residents in their care as "objects" as well, whereas active NA involvement in the care planning process may be related to quality of care. Research has demonstrated that long-term-care facilities that have lower bed-to-aide ratios, include NAs as part of the care team, value NAs' opinions, and acknowledge their important role in the provision of quality care, have lower turnover rates (Mor, 1995). Factors not related to NA turnover were: case-mix severity, payer source mix, facility size and ownership, and hours of aide training.

Survey data examining staff turnover rates in nursing homes have documented rates ranging from 55 to 65 percent for RNs. Turnover rates for NAs go up to 400 percent, with an average of around 99 percent. According to the Institute of Medicine (IOM, 1986), 45 percent of NAs left their jobs within the first three months and another 30 percent left within the first year of employment. Munroe (1990) reported an average of 107 percent turnover for the entire staff of 455 California nursing homes, with turnover significantly greater in proprietary homes. Thus, nurse aides, who provide somewhere between 80 percent and 90 percent of personal care, have the highest turnover of any nursing home staff (IOM, 1986).

Kane (1994) has argued persuasively that the frontline workers, including NAs, who most directly affect the daily experiences of nursing home residents receive the "least social investment" in terms of job training, wages, benefits, and social support. Because they have little autonomy in terms of altering their daily routine, these frontline workers may tend to focus more on the tasks than on the resident for whom the tasks are being performed, resulting in poor quality care.

A review of the research literature finds several studies suggesting that an adequate number of well prepared and stable personnel is essential for quality care. The reciprocal relationship between quality of care and levels of staff turnover has been referred to since Revans (1964) found that high turnover of nurses in acute hospitals was related to length of patient stay. Garibaldi and colleagues (1981) found that the physical care of nursing home residents in the United States deteriorated during periods of high staff turnover, while Stryker (1981) hypothesized that depression, disengagement, disorientation, and isolation among long-term-care residents is likely to increase when staff-resident relationships are disrupted by high turnover. Thus, staff hours available, the relationships between full-time and part-time staff, and staff turnover are likely to be relevant to the quality of care. Further, staff turnover may be related to other circumstances associated with quality care. Mor (1994) found, for example, that in facilities where value was placed on involvement of nurse aides in the care planning process, there was a substantially lower turnover rate after controlling for a number of other theoretically relevant factors.

Job turnover can be costly in terms of hiring, training, and facility productivity losses, but perhaps most importantly high attrition rates can adversely affect sensorially impaired residents who do not cope well with frequent changes in staff (McDonald, 1994). Further, the effect of high turnover rates among nonprofessional staff is such that they fail to be assimilated into a sociocultural environment that fosters positive attitudes toward quality of care (Wright, 1988). Because residents value the relationship between the nursing assistant and themselves and consistency in the persons who deliver their care, high turnover, heavy use of part-time staff, and use of float or agency staff negatively impact the quality of care (Erickson, 1987). High turnover of RN and LPN staff compromises the continuity of leadership and supervision of staff as well as the treatment and care of residents.

Quality, Reimbursement, and Staffing

The relationship between reimbursement and staffing is complex, and the implications for quality are not straightforward. Cost-based and case-mix-based are two types of reimbursement schemes used for nursing homes. In cost-based reimbursement, a facility may supply services as needed and submit the resulting cost to the state for reimbursement. To control expenditures, some states place advance limits on each facility's rate, based on the prior year's cost per resident. Some states even "cap" the number of staff hours or the number of dollars per resident day, regardless of differing care needs. Such reimbursement limits can put a chilling effect on a nursing home's willingness to change its mix of residents by admitting residents supported by Medicaid or residents who require much care. In case-mix-based reimbursement, each resident is categorized according to a classification system that reflects the staff time and costs required for care of the residents in each category. The state determines a reimbursement rate for each facility based on the number of residents it serves in each category. Case-mix formulas deserve careful scrutiny and a number of questions warrant further investigation. For example, are staff values derived from valid counts of time for care of each category of resident? Was the timed care what the resident needed, and was it performed by appropriately qualified staff? Does the reimbursement formula also include realistic time for assessments, care planning, and documentation? Does it allow for professional observation and evaluation of care, decision making and planning of care, and coordination with families and other disciplines involved in the care? Are compensation factors for each kind of nursing personnel realistic?

When reimbursement does not fully provide for the cost of care, nursing homes respond in a number of ways. They may increase private pay rates or seek to cut costs by increasing efficiency or reducing expenditures for services, including nurse staffing. Some nursing homes have been known to cut nourishment or supplies for the care of incontinent residents (Harrington, 1984). Changes in staffing may take the form of fewer full-time personnel and a greater proportion of less qualified personnel. Either of these "solutions" can have negative effects on work conditions and the quality of resident care.

Spector (1994) reported results from analysis of data from the 1987 National Expenditure Survey. Spector noted that if a state had a higher Medicaid reimbursement level, the higher level was associated with more LPNs per 100 residents adjusted for case-mix, but it was not related to the number of nurse aides. There were more RNs with higher Medicaid reimbursement, but the relationship was not significant. As discussed earlier, in states where there was a cost-based reimbursement system the nursing homes had more RNs, but fewer LPNs. Overall, Spector (1994) reported that while no relationship was found between reimbursement and outcomes, reimbursement had an effect on staffing and staffing had an effect on outcomes.

Current institutional long-term-care classification systems, such as the Resource Utilization Groups System (RUGS), separate persons with severe behavioral problems from those with primarily physical problems (Fries and Cooney, 1985). The RUGS-II revision continued to assume that emotional and cognitive problems do not complicate the care of the elderly person's physical problems, or the care of persons who can independently perform ADLs, in a way that adds appreciably to their care requirements or consumption of nursing resources (Rohrer et al., 1989). This assumption is not in keeping with data indicating, based on time records, that nursing home staff spend 36 percent of their time caring for residents with cognitive impairment (Hu et al., 1986).

Thus, case-mix-based reimbursement systems may actually discourage the delivery of therapeutic care by failing to fully account for the impact of mental illness or cognitive impairments on requirements for care (Rohrer et al., 1989). A study of 285 nursing home residents found that their behavioral problems influenced the care they received. Lack of cognitive ability caused staff to spend more time in the delivery of personal care and medications, even when extent of physical disability was controlled for. Negative affect was found to increase the quantity of psychosocial care received, while aggressive behaviors had no effect on the types of nursing time studied. This interesting latter finding may reflect the lack of mental health therapy provided by nursing staff at the time the study was conducted (pre-OBRA), many of whom relied on restraints and/or sedation to manage aggressive residents (Rohrer et al., 1989). These data, together with other supporting literature, indicate that mental health problems clearly affect the amount of nursing time that elderly long-term-care residents require. This suggests that nursing homes must be reimbursed in a way that permits and encourages mentally ill and cognitively impaired residents to receive needed psychosocial services.

In 1989, the Health Care Financing Administration formally began a project to develop and test the RUGS classification in nursing homes on a national level. The Multi-State Nursing Home Case-Mix and Quality Project involved the design of a resident-level resource use classifications system for the prospective payment of Medicare and Medicaid nursing facility services. Kansas, Maine, Mississippi, and South Dakota participated in the project, with additional data contributed by Nebraska and Texas. A total of 6,660 resident assessments were used in the study. The analysis resulted in a 43-group classification system called Resource Utilization Groups System, Version III (RUGS-III) (Fries et al., 1994). The classification model will be used for a Medicare prospective payment system across all six states and New York and as the basis for Medicaid reimbursement to nursing homes in the first four project states.

Like RUGS-I and -II, RUGS-III is a category-based classification system. Nursing home residents are classified into one of the mutually exclusive groups of the system. Placement into a group is done by evaluating the fit with a sequence of three hierarchically arranged levels. The first major dimension is five categories of resident type: rehabilitation, special care, clinically complex, "impaired cognitive/behavior problem," and "physical functioning (reduced)." The second level looks at either intensity of care, extensive and special needs, or activities of daily living. Bed mobility, eating, toileting, and transfer are activities of daily living that are measured. A third level evaluates and rates activities of daily living, treatment count, additional nursing attention required for depression, and nursing rehabilitation. For the first time, nursing rehabilitation has been added as the third level for "impaired cognitively/behavior problem" and "physical functioning (reduced)." A toileting program performed by nurses is added to rehabilitation measures. Categories are listed hierarchically in order of cost from the highest, rehabilitation, to the lowest, physical functioning (reduced). Thus RUGS-III expands the number of categories in the classification and included the need for nursing resources for rehabilitation and treating depression, both of which were frequent criticisms of RUGS-I and -II. With RUGS-III revisions, the RUGS case-mix system, which recognizes the differences in the costs of caring for distinct residents, currently appears to offer the best compromise between appropriate resources for each resident's needs and administrative feasibility, providing appropriate incentives and equitable reimbursement.

Quality and Type of Facility

Most research on the relationship of nursing home characteristics to quality of care has targeted two main areas: (1) the interrelationships among organizational characteristics, and (2) the relationship of organizational characteristics to resident functioning (Kruzich et al., 1992).

Research relating type of ownership to quality of care is equivocal. Although Elwell (1984) found that nonprofit homes are more likely to spend more money on direct patient care and have higher staff-to-patient ratios than proprietary homes, Kosberg and Tobin (1972), and more recently Kruzich and colleagues (1992), found no relationship between facility ownership and quality of care. Spector (1994) was unable to link type of facility with quality of care.

Little relationship has been found between type of ownership (e.g., for-profit vs. nonprofit) and RN and LPN nurse staffing ratios in a recent Massachusetts study (Kaffenberger, 1994). That is, for-profit homes did not use more LPNs instead of more highly trained RNs. The investigators speculate that the limited effect of ownership type may be due to many factors, such as the demanding regulatory environment, cost-based public payment, and the importance of quality to the private market.

Quality, Management Systems, and Organizational Climate

Management Systems

Management procedures are noted to play a critical role in the maintenance of staff performance (Sheridan et al., 1992). Direction, delegation, assertiveness, recognition, reprimand, liaison, and sensitivity are leadership dimensions that have been found to have significant effects on the job attitudes and job performance of nursing staff in nursing homes and hospitals (Sheridan et al., 1984; Sheridan et al., 1990). Mor (1994), however, found huge variation in the degree to which the authority and the management perspective of the DON in nursing homes is actually implemented.

Clear guidelines and monitoring systems, including contingent, supervisory feedback and praise, have been shown to effectively maintain staff behavior change and diminish the need for disciplinary procedures (Burgio and Burgio, 1990). Most staff management systems employ some type of ongoing performance monitoring and feedback, although they vary in terms of incentives and consequences related to staff performance (Burgio and Scilley, 1994). A study by Burgio and colleagues (1990), which compared the use of individual staff performance feedback and group staff performance feedback, showed significantly greater compliance with prompted voiding regimens when individual staff performance feedback was used.

Permanent assignment of staff to residents results in more quality outcomes for residents and more satisfaction and feelings of accountability for employees. Evaluation of a primary care model of delivery of nursing aide care (e.g., permanent aide assignment, a team approach, and enhanced communication) in nursing homes demonstrated increased quality-of-care indicators such as improved behavior, affect, and social activities among residents (Teresi et al., 1993).

The importance of a staff management system was illustrated in research by Schnelle and colleagues (1990) that evaluated a prompted voiding procedure for urinary incontinence. The investigators found that the staff did not maintain the prompted voiding program without the Industrial Quality Control procedure in place. This procedure had three components: (1) a performance standard; (2) staff monitoring (by self and supervisors), and (3) quality control sampling. As noted above, Schnelle (1994) reported only one site where the protocols were continued. This occurred at a site where the DON provided leadership and direction to staff.

The work of Tellis-Nayak and Tellis-Nayak (1989, p. 312) suggests that those nursing homes that successfully break the hopeless cycle of high staff attrition, low morale, and indifferent care have managed to "create an institutional structure that remains sensitive to the nurse's aides needs, nurtures their idealism, and values their central role." The relationships between social climate, quality of care, and resident health and well-being are increasingly being recognized. Indeed, while the recreational and physical environments have been shown to be important, nothing is more central to determining quality of life for residents than the social contacts and human relationships that emerge in the long-term-care setting (Kayser-Jones, 1989). Research supports the notion that social-environmental factors such as cohesion (the degree to which staff are perceived as being supportive) are significantly related to life satisfaction in residents (Gould, 1992), and that the sociocultural environment shapes staff attitudes, which then get translated into actions (Wright, 1988).

Organizational Climate

A typology of social climates in group residential facilities for older adults was developed by Timko and Moos (1991). Six distinct types of social climate were identified, including: supportive, self-directed; supportive, well-organized; open conflict; suppressed conflict; emergent-positive; and unresponsive. Those facilities with social climates in the first two categories—supportive, self-directed and supportive, well-organized—had residents who rated higher in well-being and levels of self-initiated activities and who used fewer health services.

Sheridan and colleagues (1992) argued that the climate the administrator builds is key to the delivery of quality care, and that OBRA will likely fail because it restricts management initiatives and emphasizes punitive consequences of staff shortcomings. A study by Kayser-Jones (1989) reported that rehospitalization rates were affected as much by social-structural factors as by clinical factors, although Booth (1986) found no relationship between restrictiveness of the environment and rates of mortality and functional dependency. In their study of 530 nursing staff working in 25 for-profit and nonprofit nursing homes, Sheridan and colleagues (1992) found that staff members' job attitudes, opinions regarding elderly residents, and perceptions of the organizational climate varied between successful for-profit and nonprofit homes, but the human relations-oriented organization and cohesion climate in the unsuccessful homes was significantly lower than the climate in either the successful for-profit or nonprofit homes. There is also some evidence that involvement of staff in an interdisciplinary process for assessing and planning care is related to the psychological well-being of residents (Mor, 1994).

Case Study: The Iowa Veterans' Home

The following case study is presented as additional evidence that a higher ratio of RNs with specific gerontological preparation to assisting staff is related to improved quality of care in nursing homes. The case study also illustrates the importance of professional nurse involvement in resident assessment, delivery of care, and the direction and supervision of care delivered by assisting staff (Maas, 1989). A key to the delivery of quality care is that each resident has a specific RN who has authority and accountability for his or her care, 24 hours each day, and over an extended period of time. Formal and continuing education in geriatric and gerontological nursing for all nursing staff is another key to the achievement of quality outcomes for residents.

A model of professional nursing practice in a nursing home is demonstrated at the Iowa Veterans Home (IVH) in Marshalltown, Iowa (Maas, 1989). This model was developed in the late 1960s and early 1970s and has been in the process of implementation since that time. The professional governance model includes an RN nurse organization that determines all standards for nursing practice, policies governing practice, and nursing clinical programming.

The IVH is a state-owned long-term-care facility that provides nursing care to more than 800 mostly elderly veterans and spouses. Three levels of care are provided: residential, intermediate, and skilled. In 1988, about 12 percent of the residents required residential care, with the remainder nearly equally divided between intermediate and skilled care. In 1988 there were 70 RNs, 330 ancillary personnel, and 50 other health professionals. From 1983 through 1988, the average annual turnover among RNs was 5 percent, and the average length of employment for nurses who were on staff for this period was 7.5 years. Furthermore, in 1988 at the height of the nurse shortage, 50 RN applications were on file.

In contrast, an average length of stay of 1 year for RNs in nursing homes has been reported (Kayser-Jones, 1981a).

An interdisciplinary model is used to plan, implement, and evaluate health services for each resident. Core members of each interdisciplinary team are the resident's primary RN, social worker, dietitian, physician, and recreation therapist. Each RN has 24-hour, seven-days-a-week authority and accountability for a caseload of residents.

Before the professional model of practice was implemented, the philosophy of care was mostly custodial in nature. Registered nurses were assigned to shifts and patient care units as supervisors of the care delivered by the assisting staff, with little authority to decide matters that affected the quality of the residents' lives or health.

As the RNs progressed in the conceptualization and implementation of the professional practice model, they were aware of the need for additional nursing knowledge. The nurses determined that practice should be data-based whenever possible, that each nurse should specialize in the treatment of one or more of the nursing diagnoses of the long-term-care residents, and that the knowledge needed for accountability should be organized by the nursing diagnoses of the residents. The incidence of nursing diagnoses and interventions for the elderly and long-term-care clients determines priorities for continuing education and research. One illustration of the nurses' emphasis on knowledge and continuing education was the number who were certified by the ANA. In 1989, 33 nurses had been certified by the ANA as gerontological nurses, 1 as a mental health nurse, and 1 in community health. Thirty of the certified nurses were employed at IVH; five more nurses were preparing for the 1989 certification test. Thirty-five nurses had continued formal education in baccalaureate and master's programs. Since 1989, between five and eight RNs have been certified as gerontological nurses each year and five or six are enrolled in advanced education programs at any given time.

The nurses discovered that the results of interventions for nursing diagnoses included increased patient welfare and favor from families, administrators, and other health disciplines. There are a number of indicators of increased quality of nursing care. For example, the number of indwelling catheters and decubiti was much lower after the model of practice was implemented, even though the proportion of residents with complex nursing care problems increased. The rates of monitors of poor quality care also were consistently below the average rates for comparable long-term-care institutions. A descriptive study, "Nurse Autonomy and Patient Welfare," funded by the Division of Nursing in the National Institutes of Health, was conducted from 1972 to 1976 to document the process whereby nurses collectively developed professional governance and the consequences of this for residents. Data for a number of patient welfare measures (self-care scale, nurse- and resident-rated; well-being scale, resident-rated; problems inventory, resident-rated; resident interviews) were collected at regular intervals throughout the study period. The trend for all measures was that resident welfare increased throughout the study period. The discrepancy between actual self-care and capacity to perform self-care decreased as rated by both nurses and residents, total scores for the well-being scale increased, and the problems inventory total scores decreased. Results of the resident interviews were consistent with the findings using the standardized measures, with more residents reporting satisfaction with their care and increased control over their lives at the end of the study (Maas and Jacox, 1977).

In addition, the IVH Nursing Department reports show that in the late 1960s and early 1970s, the monthly rate of skilled care residents with Foley catheters averaged 25 percent, whereas in the 1980s the average monthly rate of indwelling catheters was 7 percent for a larger group of skilled-care patients. Similarly, the average monthly decubitus rate was 8 percent in the early 1970s but in the 1980s averaged 4 percent, despite an increase in the numbers of debilitated, at-risk residents. The 1987 Iowa Department of Health and Iowa Foundation for Medical Care reports contain statistics for quality-of-care indicators for intermediate care facilities in Iowa. These statistics support the improved quality-of-care indicators at the IVH in contrast to all other intermediate care facilities in Iowa. Measures of the quality of the residents' lives also reflect achievement of high standards; for example, in the extent to which residents' rights to determine their care and to control other circumstances of living are protected and enabled.

PRIORITY QUESTIONS NEEDING FURTHER RESEARCH

Who Should Be in a Nursing Home?

Some researchers question whether or not certain residents currently in nursing homes should really be there. Morris and coworkers (1990) found a number of light care residents, according to the National Resident Assessment Instrument, in their data base. These data suggest that perhaps a substantial number of residents should have been discharged. Analysis of residents in facilities reimbursed using a case-mix formula indicated that the percentage of light care residents is less under these incentives.

• There is still a critical need for research to examine the role that nursing homes should play in long-term care, including what residents are best served by what types of facilities.

How Can Quality Best Be Measured?

Schnelle (1994) suggests that there is a myth associated with chart-based review of quality. Because of high regulatory pressure and specific standards for documentation, but little specificity as to how to actually meet regulations, chart documentation systems are created that are largely fictional. Technology that provides specific directions for nurse aide behaviors, so as to meet regulations regarding the management of restraint use, has been developed. In research testing the effects of this technology, the actual release of restraints was monitored unobtrusively. Findings revealed that, as opposed to the "release every 2 hours and exercise" regulation, 60 percent of the residents who were restrained actually stayed restrained for 6 hours or longer. Yet on the chart there was very consistent documentation of release every 2 hours (Schnelle, 1994). Because most of the effort is put into compliance on paper, Schnelle argues that this creates a situation where both policy researchers and nursing home providers avoid real problem solving. OBRA, however, has placed more emphasis on monitoring actual patient outcomes in conjunction with chart review.

Based on her research, Baldwin (1994) believes that some outcome measures, such as quality-of-life and quality assurance measures used in other settings, may have to either be modified or developed specifically for nursing homes. Baldwin further suggests that qualitative data may convey more information about quality outcomes than the more traditionally used quantitative measures.

There are concerns about the reliability and validity of MDS data because of emphasis on regulations and the use of chart review to assess quality. Correlations between direct observation of quality indicators and MDS rating have been found to range between 0 to 0.75 (Schnelle, 1994). The use of consultant RNs, who are hired by some nursing homes to come in specifically to fill out the MDS, adds to concern about the reliability and validity of the data for measuring quality of care.

- Investigations to assess the reliability and validity of MDS data and to test other strategies for assuring the reliability and validity of quality care data in nursing homes are needed.

Wright (1988) has argued that the attitudes of nursing home personnel have been measured inappropriately, with scales based on negative stereotypes and inaccurate knowledge about the aged. She recommends reconceptualizing attitudes from those toward older people in general to attitudes toward behavior that is essential to the care of residents in nursing homes, including concepts of individualized care, rehabilitation potential, and choice. Wright also sets forth a proposed research model for examining staff attitudes and quality of care.

According to Burgio (1994), there are good, reliable quantitative measures of quality being used with developmentally disabled populations that are not being used in nursing homes. In general, Burgio asserts that the quality of care in nursing homes has been measured poorly.

- Additional research efforts should focus on reconceptualizing and evaluating measures of quality and staff characteristics that are hypothesized to be related to quality outcomes.

What Are the Effects of Organization, Staff, and Staffing Characteristics on Quality?

Results from a recent survey conducted by Decision Data Collection, Inc., for the ANA (ANA, 1995) indicate that reduction of the RN work force by cutting nursing budgets in hospitals is causing unsafe conditions for patients and massive increases in the workload of the remaining RNs. The survey found more medication errors, accidents resulting in patient falls and fractures, and unnecessary inconveniences for patients. Concerns expressed were primarily in the areas of insufficient time to spend with patients and to monitor their conditions adequately. In light of 1990 data from the ANA, which indicated that 66 percent of nursing homes reported increased nurse workloads and more nurse hours worked (McKibbin, 1990), there is some cause for concern about increased workload having a similar impact on quality of care in the long-term-care industry. According to Close and colleagues (1994, p. 26), "Patterns of workload increases and staff turnover may indicate unintended and unanticipated responses in the long-term care labor arena to policies intended to control acute care costs and to improve the quality of care to long-term care recipients." Therefore, the following areas of research need to be addressed.

• There is a critical need to study causes and circumstances of employment, staff relations, and work that promote staff job satisfaction and retention, and to test strategies for retention of NAs, LPNs, RNs, and DONs in nursing homes.

• Additional needs are to systematically study the effects of different numbers of staff, staff mix, and staff-to-resident ratios on resident outcomes, including resident and staff abuse and controlling for case-mix and organization structure variables.

• More research also is needed to assess and test the effects of staff's abilities to manage patients with varying levels of professional nurse consultation, direction, and oversight.

• The advantages and disadvantages of part-time versus full-time staff for achieving quality outcomes should be systematically examined.

• Clearly, the etiology and appropriate management of aggressive behaviors of nursing home residents against staff, and vice versa, is an area deserving of more research.

• Further studies also are needed to better understand the specific causes of elder abuse and to test interventions for institutional staff and families that are designed to prevent instances of abuse.

• Experimental research focusing on relationships between nurses and residents and on the effectiveness of interventions designed to control resident behavior, other than chemical and physical restraints, are especially needed.

Efforts to improve nursing home care through training and job redesign have had mixed results (Smyer et al., 1991). Job redesign was implemented by a team of Penn State investigators to enhance motivation and change the nature of the work itself by making it the focus of a guided staff process. Findings revealed that improvements in staff knowledge had little impact on NA job performance as reflected in the ratings of supervisors, suggesting that training alone will not dramatically improve the quality of care and quality of life in nursing homes (Smyer et al., 1991).

- Research needs include: (1) descriptive studies of what licensed nurses and other staff do in nursing homes, distinguishing among advanced practice nurses (e.g., GNPs, GCNs, RNs, and LPNs); (2) studies that examine how DONs and RNs provide effective leadership and direction of staff; (3) studies that evaluate and compare the most effective use of RNs and LPNs in nursing home settings; (4) studies to test a variety of management interventions on staff satisfaction and performance and resident outcomes; and (5) studies to design and test technologies that specify clinical interventions and assist staff with their implementation.

Few studies have examined the relationship between macro-organizational and structural variables and quality; thus, there is a paucity of empirical evidence to support these linkages. To date, research findings have shed little light on the characteristics of nursing homes (such as size, ægis, age, and rural or urban location) that might inform our understanding of what results in quality care.

- More research assessing the relationships among organization characteristics and quality outcomes should be conducted.

How Are Families Involved in Care and What Do They Understand About Quality and its Cost?

Questions about family member involvement in the care of their institutionalized relatives continue to be of interest. Some argue that there is the potential to augment staff resources and improve the quality of care in nursing homes by involving families more in the care of residents (Brubaker, 1987; Buckwalter and Hall, 1987; Bowers, 1988; Maas et al., 1994).

- Based on the current literature and research findings, more research is needed to document: (1) how families and nursing home staff can best work together to achieve quality care outcomes, (2) what families and the public understand about quality and its costs, and (3) at what level of quality are families and the public willing to assume costs?

What Are the Effects of Cultural Differences Among Residents and Staff in Nursing Homes and What Strategies Are Needed to Ensure Quality?

• Based on the review of cultural diversity issues in nursing homes, research is needed to describe: (1) the ability of racial and ethnic minority elderly and their families to mobilize community resources; (2) the access of these elderly to informal caregivers; (3) perceptions of alienation experienced by minority elderly residents and their families; and (4) minority families' perceptions of social, medical, and functional factors resulting in nursing home admission.

• More research related to ethnicity and race is needed to help determine the approach and perspective older persons take toward the problems they encounter in adapting to institutionalization.

• Research also is needed to describe cultural differences: (1) among elderly residents and staff who are members of the same ethnic and racial groups; (2) among staff who are members of different age, ethnic, and racial cultures; and (3) among residents of different racial and ethnic groups. In addition, strategies must be tested for: (1) educating staff and residents about cultural differences, and (2) incorporating the appropriate cultural practices into care and staff-resident relationships so that care is culturally competent.

POLICY RECOMMENDATIONS

Long-term care must be part of any health care reform in order to ensure funds, care, and dignity for the elderly served. The predominance of chronic conditions requires the development and testing of new models of care that effectively bridge acute and long-term-care services. The relationship of staffing and quality of care is a primary concern in policy reforms. Based on the review of the historical background of nursing homes, the current status and future demand for nursing home care, and research relevant to the linkage of staffing and quality care, the following policy recommendations are set forth.

Recommendation 1: The minimum standards for the number of RNs in nursing homes should be increased.

Recommendation 2: At least one RN for every 50 residents, in addition to the DON, should be required to be present daily over each 24-hour period of care.

Recommendation 3: Every RN employed by a nursing home should be required to have specific formal education in gerontological nursing and in the management and supervision of assisting staff. At least 50 percent of continuing education credits for relicensure should be in these content areas as well.

Recommendation 4: The minimum qualification for a DON in a nursing home should be a bachelor's degree in nursing.

Recommendation 5: Every nursing home should be required to have at least one advanced gerontological nurse practitioner in their employ to provide both direct resident care and leadership for other nursing staff in caring for residents and monitoring quality outcomes.

Recommendation 6: Compensation for qualified RNs and all nursing staff in nursing homes should be required to be more competitive with that provided by hospitals.

Recommendation 7: Medicaid, Medicare, and other third party payers should be required to reimburse master's and doctorally prepared advanced practice nurses (GNPs and GCNs) for their clinical services.

A recurrent theme throughout this review was the need for a consistent professional nurse (RN, NP) presence in nursing homes for the provision of quality care. This paper emphasized the need for RN leadership, direction, and supervision of assisting nursing staff because: (1) there is high turnover among assisting staff; (2) assisting staff have minimal training; (3) nurse aide work is difficult, often unpleasant, and rewards are few—circumstances that will likely worsen with the trend toward more acutely ill and frail future nursing home residents; (4) assisting staff need help coping with stress and maintaining quality, individualized care of residents; (5) salaries and benefits lag behind those in hospitals and home care, compromising the recruitment and retention of quality staff; (6) adding assisting staff without increased direction and supervision is likely to result in an inappropriate use of time and resources; (7) while mandated standardized assessment (e.g., MDS, RAI) does help to get resident problems identified, it does not provide for solutions to the problems or get the care provided; (8) there is some empirical evidence that the number of RNs in nursing homes is linked with positive resident outcomes; and (9) there is need for supportive and motivating systems to manage staff performance. Administrators also must recognize the importance to nurses of the authority to manage patient care issues and make clinical decisions.

Recommendation 8: Require case-mix reimbursement with higher levels of reimbursement and higher minimum staffing standards.

To promote recruitment and retention of qualified staff in long-term care and to make nursing homes a more attractive and satisfying practice setting, salaries need to be more competitive with those for comparable positions in other settings. Nursing homes also must be reimbursed in a way that permits and encourages all residents, including the mentally ill and cognitively impaired, to receive needed physical and psychosocial services.

A goal in long-term care is to move from a custodial to a rehabilitative model of care. With the majority of direct care provided by nurse aides, this cannot be accomplished when staff-to-patient ratios are high (e.g., 1 staff person to 20 residents). However, it is known that nursing homes can have low staff-to-resident ratios and still have poor quality care. Thus, greater staff numbers must be combined with the recommendations for increased staff training, strategies to decrease turnover rates, and more intensive supervision and direction of nurse aides by qualified RNs. One aspect of training that must be improved is that provided by effective role models who supervise and consult with staff, as well as unit delivering resident care, when they are on the unit.

Recommendation 9: Require improved training of nursing home surveyors as consultative overseers who interpret and apply standardized state and federal mandated guidelines for quality-of-care assessment.

Because of the variation in the quality of surveyors and the interpretations of guidelines, combined with the increase in surveyors for different regulators, nursing homes deserve to be assured that all surveyors have comparable skills and are applying standards correctly, judiciously, and equitably toward the goal of improved resident care.

Recommendation 10: Require nursing homes to provide a minimum of three hours of didactic and three hours of supervised practicum education annually for staff and family members on techniques for managing and preventing disruptive and aggressive resident behaviors.

Recommendation 11: Require nursing homes to educate families and staff, both at the time of resident admission and with periodic reinforcement, about how to interact with each other to be mutually supportive and to recognize quality care outcomes.

Staff and family members need to have the knowledge and skills that best prepare them to understand and recognize quality resident outcomes, to be better able to establish cooperative relationships, and to share decisions so that the optimal resources of both staff and families are used to achieve quality outcomes. Staff and families need to recognize families as allies and resources in the care of elderly residents, and acknowledge the need for staff to involve family members in decisions about the care of their loved ones. Staff also should encourage the negotiation of family-staff partnerships in the care of residents, which may be an important aspect of delivering quality nursing home care.

Recommendation 12: Require nursing homes to provide education programs for staff on the cultural beliefs, values, and practices of ethnic and racial minority residents.

Recommendation 13: Require nursing homes to attempt to hire staff representatives of ethnic and racial minority groups of which residents are members.

With increasing cultural diversity among elderly residents and staff in nursing homes, the achievement of quality outcomes requires that staff have an understanding of the values and practices that are important to the quality of life of residents and to satisfying and effective work relationships among staff. Minority elders need available gerontological services that are affordable, accessible, and culturally competent.

Recommendation 14: More opportunities for formal educational preparation in gerontological nursing should be provided by: (1) enhancing opportunities for mid-career nursing faculty to continue learning and to obtain gerontological content through the provision of faculty development awards, fellowships, short term courses, certificate programs, continuing education, and opportunities to work with master teachers in gerontology; (2) development of gerontological nursing education related to special populations of the diverse elderly; (3) merging the categories of geriatric nurse clinical specialists and geriatric nurse practitioners, and preparing geriatric nurses in advanced practice roles to provide primary and comprehensive care to the elderly in nursing homes; (4) developing model geriatric nursing curricula that incorporate advanced information technologies at both undergraduate and graduate levels; (5) offering freestanding undergraduate gerontological nursing courses that are available to all undergraduate students; (6) mandating continuing education credits (a minimum of 1 credit per year in gerontological nursing for re-licensure); (7) providing traineeships for faculty and student training in gerontological nursing; (8) continuing to emphasize the need to increase numbers of minorities in gerontological nursing; and (9) promoting interdisciplinary training and consultation.

Nursing faculty who have learned gerontological and geriatric content and skills are more likely to support the introduction of gerontological content in curricula and improve the quality of education in both undergraduate and advanced practice programs. Education in gerontology must recognize the specific characteristics and needs of various populations in America such as rural Americans, aging women, and older adults with mental health problems. Thus it is no longer relevant to discuss persons over 65 as a homogenous group. More advanced nurse practitioners are needed to meet the complex and growing future needs of the aging population, and to lead, teach, and provide patient care in nursing homes. For nursing to prepare sufficient numbers of expert gerontological clinicians, appropriate curricula must be implemented at all levels of the educational process and evaluated to ensure they meet minimum standards. Funding for enhanced training opportunities for faculty and graduate students will increase the knowledge base that supports geriatric nursing practice. There also is a need to prepare more nurses with geriatric knowledge to meet the demands for the future, including an increased number of persons from minority groups. All gerontological and geriatric nurses, educators, and clinicians will need to regularly update their knowledge base in gerontology. Adequate compensation for nurses who work with the elderly needs to be assured to provide incentives for increased recruitment and retention of qualified nurses in nursing homes.

Advanced information technologies (i.e., fiber optic and digital networks) will increasingly be used in settings remote from educational institutions. Nurses will need to be proficient in the use of such technologies in order to provide care to elders and education to staff. Finally, because geriatric care in the next century will be increasingly interdisciplinary, students from a variety of disciplines should be exposed to interdisciplinary care in their training if they are to be expected to practice in a cooperative, collegial manner.

Recommendation 15: Increased funding for gerontological nursing research should be provided by: (1) increasing the number of postdoctoral opportunities in gerontological nursing to prepare future researchers, (2) increasing the level of funding to NINR for gerontological research, (3) encouraging GECs and Centers on Aging to hold geriatric nursing faculty training workshops in grantsmanship and proposal development, and (4) increasing funding for faculty and doctoral student training in gerontological research.

Geriatric nursing research has benefited older persons by improving care practices and quality of life, and yet nurses have not fared well in terms of successfully competing for NIH monies in aging-related research. In some cases it is because the quality of the proposals submitted (especially with regard to methodological rigor) is not sufficient to merit consideration for funding. Those gerontological nurse researchers who are fully qualified and produce competitive research proposals are disadvantaged by the disproportionately low level of funding for NINR, which must fund all nursing research, and the competition for limited funds from other NIH agencies. This situation is particularly unfortunate in that the relationship between education, research, and practice should be a dynamic one, with research informing practice and teaching and with more curricula being research driven.

Recommendation 16: A provider number for the accountable RN and standardized nursing interventions should be added to the long-term-care minimum data set so that practice pattern variations and outcomes effectiveness can be assessed for specific interventions and nurse providers with MDS data.

REFERENCES

AARP (American Association of Retired Persons). *A Portrait of Older Minorities*. Washington, D.C.: AARP, 1985a.

AARP. *A Profile of Older Americans 1985*. Washington, D.C.: AARP, 1985b.

AARP Minority Affairs. *A Portrait of Older Minorities*. Washington, D.C.: AARP, 1990.

Alzheimer's Association. *Residential Settings: An Examination of Alzheimer Issues*. Chicago: Alzheimer's Association, 1994.

ANA (American Nurses Association). *Report on Long Term Care Staffing*. Kansas City: ANA, 1991.

ANA. The Report of Survey Results: The 1994 ANA Layoffs Survey. *The American Nurse* (March):1 and 7, 1995.

Andreoli, K.G., and Musser, L.A. Trends That May Affect Nursing's Future. Pp. 71–80 in: B.W. Spradley, ed. *Readings in Community Health Nursing*, 4th ed. Boston: Little, Brown, 1991.

Bahr, R.T. The Battered Elderly: Physical and Psychological Abuse. *Family and Community Health* 4(2):61–69, 1981.

Bahr, R.T. Reaction to the Invitational Conference: "Mechanisms of Quality in Long Term Care: Service and Clinical Outcomes." Pp. 103–109 in: *Mechanisms of Quality in Long Term Care: Service and Clinical Outcomes*. Pub. no. 41-2382. New York: National League for Nursing Press, 1991.

Baker, A. Granny Battering. *Nursing Mirror* 144:65–66, 1977.

Baldwin, B. Presentation at special session on staffing and quality care in nursing homes, at the annual meeting of The Gerontological Society of America, Atlanta, Georgia, November 1994.

Baltz, T.M., and Turner, J.G. Development and Analysis of a Nursing Home Aide Screening Device. *The Gerontologist* 17:66–69, 1977.

Barresi, C.M., and Stull, D.E., eds. *Ethnic Elderly and Long Term Care*. New York: Springer Publishing, 1993.

Beck, C.M., and Ferguson, D. Aged Abuse. *Journal of Gerontological Nursing* 7(6):333–336, 1981.

Beck, C., Rossby, L., and Baldwin, B. Correlates of Disruptive Behavior in Cognitively Impaired Elderly Nursing Home Residents. *Archives of Psychiatric Nursing* 5(5):281–291, 1991.

Belgrave, L.L., and Bradsher, J.E. Health as a Factor in Institutionalization: Disparities Between African Americans and Whites. *Research on Aging* 16(2):115–141, 1994.

Birkenstock, M. From Turnover to Turnaround. *Geriatric Nursing* 12(4):194–196, 1991.

Blaum, C.S., Fries, B.E., and Fiatarone, M.A. Factors Associated with Low Body Mass Index and Weight Loss in Nursing Home Residents. *Journals of Gerontology: Medical Sciences*, in press.

Bleismer, M. Outcomes of Minnesota Nursing Home Residents and Their Relationship to Structural and Process-Related Attributes (Doctoral dissertation, Rush University, 1994). *Dissertation Abstracts International*, 1994.

Bond, J., and Bond, S. Developments in the Provision and Evaluation of Long Term Care for Dependent Old People. Pp. 47–85, in: P. Fielding, ed. *Research in The Nursing Care of Elderly People*. New York: John Wiley and Sons, 1987.

Booth, T. Institutional Regimes and Induced Dependency in Homes for the Aged. *The Gerontologist* 26:418–423, 1986.

Bowers, B. Family Perceptions of Care in a Nursing Home. *The Gerontologist* 28:361–368, 1988.

Brannon, D., Streit, A., and Smyer, M. The Psychosocial Quality of Nursing Home Work. *Journal of Aging and Health* 4(3):369–389, 1992.

Braun, B.I. The Effect of Nursing Home Quality on Patient Outcome. *Journal of American Geriatric Society* 39:329–338, 1991.

Brown University Long-term Care Quality Letter. National Center for Health Statistics Studies Nursing, Board and Care Homes. 6(12):8, 1994.

Brubaker, T.H., ed. *Aging, Health and Family*. Newbury Park, Calif.: Sage Publications, 1987.

Buckwalter, K.C., and Hall, G.R. Families of the Institutionalized Older Adult: A Neglected Resource. In: T.H. Brubaker, ed. *Aging, Health and Family*. Newbury Park, Calif.: Sage Publications, 1987.

Burgio, L.D. Presentation at special session on staffing and quality care in nursing homes, at the annual meeting of The Gerontological Society of America, Atlanta, Georgia, November 1994.

Burgio, L.D., and Burgio, K.L. Institutional Staff Training and Management: A Review of the Literature and a Model for Geriatric, Long-term Care Facilities. *International Journal of Aging and Human Development* 30(4):287–302, 1990.

Burgio, L.D., and Scilley, K. Caregiver Performance in the Nursing Home: The Use of Staff Training and Management Procedures. *Seminars In Speech and Language* 15(4):313–322, 1994.

Burgio, L.D., Butler, F., and Engel, B. Nurses' Attitudes towards Geriatric Behavior Problems in Long Term Care Settings. *Clinical Gerontologist* 7(3/4):23–34, 1988.

Burgio, L.D., Engel, G.T., Hawkins, A., McCormick, K., and Scheve, A. A Descriptive Analysis of Nursing Staff Behaviors in a Teaching Nursing Home: Differences Among NAs, LPNs, and RNs. *The Gerontologist* 30:107–112, 1990.

Cassell, E.J. Abuse of the Elderly: Misuses of Power. *New York State Journal of Medicine* (March):159–162, 1989.

Caudill, M.K., and Patrick, M. Costing Nurse Turnover in Nursing Homes. *Nursing Management* 22(11):61–64, 1991.

Cherry, R.L. Agents of Nursing Home Quality of Care: Ombudsmen and Staff Ratios Revisited. *The Gerontologist* 31:302–308, 1991.

Chiodo, L.K., Kanten, D.N., Gerety, M.B., Mulrow, C.D., and Cornell, J.E. Functional Status of Mexican American Nursing Home Residents. *Journal of The American Geriatrics Society* 42:293–296, 1994.

Cleary, T.A., Clamon, C., Price, M., and Shullaw, G. A Reduced Stimulation Unit: Effects on Patients with Alzheimer's Disease and Related Disorders. *The Gerontologist* 28:511–514, 1988.

Close, L., Estes, C.L., Linkins, K.W., and Binney, E.A. A Political Economy Perspective on Front-line Workers in Long Term Care. *Generations* XVIII(3):23–27, 1994.

Constable, J.F., and Russell, D.W. The Effect of Social Support and the Work Environment upon Burnout Among Nurses. *Journal of Human Stress* 12:21–26, 1986.

Coons, D. Training Direct Service Staff Members to Work in Dementia Care Units. Pp. 126–143 in: D. Coons, ed. *Specialized Dementia Care Units*. Baltimore: The Johns Hopkins University Press, 1991.

Cronin-Stubbs, D., and Rooks, C. The Stress, Social Support, and Burnout of Critical Care Nurses: The Results of Research. *Heart-Lung* 14:31–39, 1985.

Cuellar, J. *Aging and Health: American Indian/Alaska Native Elders*. Stanford, Calif: Stanford Geriatric Education Center, 1990.

Davis, M.A. On Nursing Home Quality: A Review and Analysis. *Medical Care Review* 48(2):129–166, 1991.

Dey, S.E. The Shift from Nursing Homes to Care at Home. *International Psychogeriatrics* 21–22, 1994.

DHHS (U.S. Department of Health and Human Services). *Elder Abuse*. Washington, D.C., U.S. Government Printing Office, 1980.

DHHS. *Health Personnel in the United States. Eighth Report to Congress*. Washington, D.C.: U.S. Government Printing Office, 1991.

DHHS. *An Agenda for Health Professions Reform*. Rockville, Md.: Bureau of Health Professions, 1993.

Duncan, M.T., and Morgan, D.L. Sharing the Caring: Family Caregivers' Views of Their Relationships with Nursing Home Staff. *The Gerontologist* 34:235–244, 1994.

Elders of Color. *Geriatric Care News* 17(9):1732–1733, 1991.

Eliopoulos, C. Nurse Staffing in Long Term Care Facilities: The Case Against a High Ratio of RNs. *Journal of Nursing Administration* 10:29–31, 1983.

Elwell, F. The Effects of Ownership on Institutional Services. *The Gerontologist* 24:77–83, 1984.

Erickson, J. Quality and the Nursing Assistant. *Provider* 13(4):4–6, 1987.

Espino, D.V., Neufeld, R.R., Mulvihill, M., and Libow, L.S. Hispanic and Non-Hispanic Elderly on Admission to the Nursing Home: A Pilot Study. *The Gerontologist* 28:821–824, 1988.

Evans, L.K., and Strumpf, N.E. Tying Down the Elderly. *Journal of the American Geriatrics Society* 37:65–74, 1989.

Evans, L.K., and Strumpf, N.E. *Reducing Restraints in Nursing Homes: A Clinical Trial.* Paper presented at special session on staffing and quality of care in nursing homes, at the annual meeting of The Gerontology Society of America, Atlanta, Georgia, November 1994.

Everitt, D.E., Fields, D.R., Soumerai, S.S., and Avorn, J. Resident Behavior and Staff Distress in the Nursing Home. *Journal of The American Geriatric Society* 39:792–798, 1991.

Fackelmann, K.A. Critics Cite Flaws in HHS' New System for Inspection of Nursing Homes. *Modern Healthcare* 16(3):27, 1986.

Foner, N. Nursing Home Aides: Saints or Monsters? *The Gerontologist* 34:245–250, 1994.

Fottler, M., Smith, H., and James, W. Profits and Patient Care Quality in Nursing Homes: Are They Compatible? *The Gerontologist* 21:532–538, 1991.

Francese, T., and Mohler, M. Long-term Care Nurse Staffing Requirements: Has OBRA Really Helped? *Geriatric Nursing* 15(3):139–141, 1994.

Fries, B.E. Presentation at special panel session on staffing and quality of care in nursing homes, at the annual meeting of The Gerontological Society of America, Atlanta, Georgia, November 1994.

Fries, B.E., and Cooney, L.M. Resource Utilization Groups: A Patient Classification System for Long Term Care. *Medical Care* 23:110–122, 1985.

Fries, B.E., Schneider, D.P., Foley, W.J., et al. Refining a Case-Mix Measure for Nursing Homes: Resource Utilization Groups (RUG-III). *Medical Care* 32(7):668–685, 1994.

Ganroth, L. Long-term Care Resource Requirements Before and After the Prospective Payment System. *Image* 20(1):7–11, 1988.

Garibaldi, R.A., Brodine, R.N., and Matsumiya, S. Infections Among Patients in Nursing Homes. *New England Journal of Medicine* 305:731–735, 1981.

Goldin, G.J. The Influence of Self-Image upon the Performance of Nursing Home Staff. *Nursing Homes* 34:33–38, 1985.

Goodwin, M., and Trocchio, J. Cultivating Positive Attitudes in Nursing Home Staff. *Geriatric Nursing* 8(1):32–34, 1987.

Gould, M. Nursing Home Elderly: Social-Environmental Factors. *Journal of Gerontological Nursing* 18(8):13–20, 1992.

Greene, J.A., Asp, J., and Crane, N. Specialized Management of the Alzheimer's Disease Patient: Does It Make a Difference? *Journal of The Tennessee Medical Association* (September):559–563, 1985.

Greene, V.L., and Monahan, D.J. Comparative utilization of community-based long term care services by Hispanic and Anglo elderly in a case management system. *Journal of Gerontology* 39, 730–735, 1984.

Griffin, K.M., Leftwich, R.A., and Smith, M.S. Current Forces Shaping Long-term Care in the 1990s. *The Journal of Long Term Care Administration* 17(3):8–11, 1989.

Hall, G.R. OBRA, MDS, and RAPS In NFs: Learning The Language of Long Term Care. Paper presented at Psychiatric Nursing Retreat, University of Iowa Hospitals and Clinics, Iowa City, March 1995.

Hall, G.R., and Buckwalter, K.C. From Almshouse to Dedicated Unit: Care of the Institutionalized Elderly with Behavioral Problems. *Archives of Psychiatric Nursing* VI(1):3–11, 1990.

Hall, G., Kirschling, M.V., and Todd, S. Sheltered Freedom: An Alzheimer's Unit in an ICF. *Geriatric Nursing* 7(3), 132–137, 1986.

Hare, J., and Pratt, C.C. Burnout: Differences Between Professional and Paraprofessional Nursing Staff in Acute and Long Term Care Health Facilities. *The Journal of Applied Gerontology* 7:60–71, 1988.

Harper, M.S., and Alexander, C.D. Profile of the Black Elderly. In: M.S. Harper, ed., *Minority Aging: Essential Curricula Content for Selected Health and Allied Health Professionals.* Washington, D.C.: U.S. Government Printing Office, 1990.

Harrington, V.L. Nursing Home Abuse: The Tragedy Continues. *Nursing Forum* 21(3):102–108, 1984.

Hawkins, A.L., Burgio, A.L., and Engel, B. The Effects of Verbal and Written Supervisory Feedback on Staff Compliance with Assigned Prompted Voiding in a Nursing Home. *Journal of Organizational Behavior Management* 13:137–150, 1992.

Heine, C.A. Burnout Among Nursing Home Personnel. *Journal of Gerontological Nursing* 12(3):14–18, 1986.

Hickey, T., and Douglass, R.L. Mistreatment of the Elderly in the Domestic Setting. *American Journal of Public Health* 71:502, 1981.

Holmes, D., Teresi, J., and Holmes, M. Evaluation of the Costs of Caring for the Senile Demented Elderly: A Pilot Study. *The Gerontologist* 26:158–163, 1983.

Hospital and Healthcare Compensation Service. *The 1994–1995 Home Care Salary and Benefits Report.* Oakland, N.J.: Hospital and Healthcare Compensation Service, 1994.

Hu, T., Huang, L., and Cartwright, W.S. Differences Among Black, Hispanic, and White People in Knowledge about Long Term Care Services. *Health Care Financing Review* 2:51–67, 1986.

IOM (Institute of Medicine). *Improving the Quality of Care In Nursing Homes.* Washington, D.C.: National Academy Press, 1986.

John, R. The Health of Research on American Indian Elders' Health, Income Security, and Social Support Networks. Pp. 38–50 in: Gerontological Society of America. *Minority Elders: Longevity, Economics and Health—Building a Public Policy Base.* Washington, D.C.: Gerontological Society of America, 1991.

Jones, D.C. Spatial Proximity, Interpersonal Conflict, and Friendship Formation in the Intermediate Care Facility. *The Gerontologist* 15:150–154, 1975.

Jones, D.C., and Van Amelsvoort Jones, G.M.M. Communication Patterns Between Nursing Staff and the Ethnic Elderly in a Long Term Care Facility. *Journal of Advanced Nursing* 11:265–272, 1986.

Jones, D.C., Bonito, A., Gower, J., and Williams, R. Analysis of the Environment for Recruitment and Retention of Registered Nurses in Nursing Homes. Washington, D.C.: Bureau of Health Professions, Health Resources and Services Administration, U.S. Department of Health and Human Services, 1987.

Kaffenberger, R. *Do Profit Oriented Ownership Decisions Lead to More Use of LPNs versus RNs in Nursing Homes?* Paper presented at the annual meeting of The Gerontological Society of America, Atlanta, Georgia, November 1994.

Kalisch, P., and Kalisch, B. *The Advance of American Nursing.* Boston: Little, Brown, 1978.

Kane, C. The Outpatient Comes Home: The Family's Response to Deinstitutionalization. *Journal of Psychosocial Nursing and Mental Health Services* 22:19–25, 1984.

Kane, R.A. Ethics and the Frontline Care Worker: Mapping the Subject. *Generations* XVIII(3):71–75, 1994.

Kane, R.L., and Kane, R.A. A Nursing Home in Your Future? *New England Journal of Medicine* 324(9):627–628, 1991.

Kane, R.L., Jorgenson, L.A., Teteberg, B., and Kuwahara, J. Is Good Nursing Home Care Feasible? *Journal of the American Medical Association* 235:516–519, 1976.

Kane, R.A., Kane, R.L., Arnold, S. et al. Geriatric Nurse Practitioners as Nursing Home Employees: Implementing the Role. *The Gerontologist* 28:469–477, 1988.

Kayser-Jones, J. A Comparison of Care in a Scottish and United States Facility. *Geriatric Nursing* 2:44–50, 1981a.

Kayser-Jones, J. *Old, Alone, and Neglected.* Berkeley and Los Angeles, Calif.: University of California Press, 1981b.

Kayser-Jones, J. The Environment and Quality of Life in Long Term Care Institutions. *Nursing and Health Care* 10(3):124–130, 1989.

Kayser-Jones, J. The Use of Nasogastric Feeding Tubes in Nursing Homes: Patient, Family and Health Care Provider Perspectives. *The Gerontologist* 30:469–479, 1990.

Kayser-Jones, J. Presentation at special session on staffing and quality of care in nursing homes, at the annual meeting of The Gerontological Society of America, Atlanta, Georgia, November 1994.

Kayser-Jones, J.S., Wiener, C.L., and Barbaccia, J.C. Factors Contributing to the Hospitalization of Nursing Home Residents. *The Gerontologist* 29:502–510, 1989.

Kemper, P., and Murtaugh, C.M. Lifetime Use of Nursing Home Care. *New England Journal of Medicine* 324(9):595–601, 1991.

Kermis, M.D. Equity and Policy Issues in Mental Health Care of the Elderly: Dilemmas, Deinstitutionalization, and DRGs. *The Journal of Applied Gerontology* 6(3):268–283, 1987.

Knapp, M. Nurse Practitioners: Expanded Role in Long Term Care. *The Brown University Long-term Care Quality Letter* 6(5):1–2, 1994.

Kolanowski, A., Hurwitz, S., Taylor, et al. Contextual Factors Associated with Disturbing Behaviors in Institutionalized Elders. *Nursing Research* 43(2):73–79, 1994.

Kosberg, J., and Tobin, S. Variability Among Nursing Homes. *The Gerontologist* 12:214–219, 1972.

Krout, J.A. *The Aged in Rural America.* New York: Greenwood Press, 1986.

Kruzich, J.M., Clinton, J.F., and Kelber, S.T. Personal and Environmental Influences on Nursing Home Satisfaction. *The Gerontologist* 32:342–350, 1992.

Kurowski, B.D., and Shaughnessy, P.W. The Measurement and Assurance of Quality. Pp. 103–132 in: R.J. Vogel and H.C. Palmer, eds. *Long-term Care: Perspectives from Research and Demonstrations.* Rockville, Md.: Aspen Systems, 1985.

LaRocco, J.M., House, J.S., and French, J.R.P., Jr. Social Support, Occupational Stress, and Health. *Journal of Health and Social Behavior* 21:202–218, 1980.

Linn, M, Gurel, L., and Linn, B.A. Patient Outcome as a Measure of Quality of Nursing Home Care. *American Journal of Public Health* 67:337–344, 1977.

Lopez-Aqueres, W., Kemp, B., Plopper, M., Staples, F.R., and Brummel-Smith, K. Health Needs of the Hispanic Elderly. *Journal of The American Geriatric Society* 32:191–198, 1984.

Lusk, S.L. Violence Experience by Nurses' Aides in Nursing Homes. *AAOHN (American Association of Occupational Health Nursing) Journal* 40(5):237–241, 1992.

Lyles, Y. Impact of Medicare DRGs on Nursing Homes in the Portland Oregon Metropolitan Area. *Journal of The American Geriatrics Society* 34(8):573–578, 1986.

Lyman, K.A. *Work-Related Stress For Staff In An Alzheimer's Day Care Center: The Effects of Physical Environments.* Paper presented at the 40th annual meeting of The Gerontological Society of America, Washington, D.C., 1987.

Maas, M. Professional Practice for the Extended Care Environment: Learning from One Model and its Implementation. *Journal of Professional Nursing* 5(2):66–76, 1989.

Maas, M., and Buckwalter, K. *Nursing Evaluation Research: A Special Alzheimer's Unit. A Final Report.* Funded under NR0689. The University of Iowa, Iowa City: National Center for Nursing Research, National Institutes of Health, 1990.

Maas, M., and Jacox, A. *Guidelines For Nurse Autonomy/Patient Welfare.* New York: Appleton-Century Crofts, 1977.

Maas, M., Buckwalter, K., Kelley, L., and Stolley, J. Family Members' Perceptions: How They View Care of Alzheimer's Patients in a Nursing Home. *Journal of Long Term Care Administration* 19(1):21–25, 1991.

Maas, M., Buckwalter, K., Swanson, E., et al. The Caring Partnership: Staff and Families of Persons Institutionalized with Alzheimer's Disease. *Journal of Alzheimer's Disease and Related Disorders* 9(6):21–30, 1994.

Manson, S.M. Long-term Care in American Indian Communities: Issues for Planning and Research. *The Gerontologist* 29:38–44, 1989.

Maraldo, P.J. Quality in Long-term Care. Pp. 1–11 in: *Mechanisms of Quality in Long-term Care: Service and Clinical Outcomes.* Pub. no. 41-2382. New York: National League for Nursing Press, 1991.

Matthew, L., Sloan, P., Kilby, M., and Flood, R. What's Different About a Special Care Unit for Dementia Patients? A Comparative Study. *American Journal of Alzheimer's Care and Related Disorders and Research* 21(2):16–23, 1988.

McDonald, C.A. Recruitment, Retention, and Recognition of Frontline Workers in Long Term Care. *Generations* XVIII(3):41–49, 1994.

McKibbin, R.C. *The Nursing Shortage and The 1990s: Realities and Remedies.* Kansas City, Mo.: American Nurses Association, 1990.

McKnight's Long Term Care News. Late Breaking News. 14(7):1, July 1993.

McKnight's Long Term Care News. Annual DON Salaries Increase 6% to $41,200. 16(3):1, 18, 1995.

Mech, A.B. Evaluating the Process of Nursing Care in Long Term Care Facilities. *Quality Review Bulletin* 6:24–30, 1980.

Mechanic, D. The Development of Mental Health Policy in the United States. Pp. 73–90 in: *Mental Health and Social Policy.* Englewood Cliffs, N.J.: Prentice-Hall, 1980.

Meddaugh, D.I. Staff Abuse by the Nursing Home Patient. *The Clinical Gerontologist* 6:45–47, 1987.

Mezey, M. Institutional Care: Caregivers and Quality. Pp. 155–166 in: *Indices of Quality In Long Term Care: Research and Practice.* Pub. no. 20-2292. New York: National League for Nursing Press, 1989.

Mezey, M. Care in nursing homes: Patients' needs; nursing's response. In Aiken, L., and Fagin, C. (eds.), *Nursing in the 90s.* Philadelphia: J.B. Lippincott Publishing Co., 1992.

Mezey, M.D. Presentation at special session on staffing and quality of care in nursing homes, at the annual meeting of The Gerontological Society of America, Atlanta, Georgia, November 1994.

Mezey, M.D., and Lynaugh, J.E. The Teaching Nursing Home Program: Outcomes of Care. *Nursing Clinics of North America* 24(3):769–780, 1989.

Mezey, M.D., and Scanlon, W. *Registered Nurses in Nursing Homes*: Secretary's Commission of Nursing. Washington, D.C.: DHHS, 1988.

Mobily, P.R., Maas, M.L., Buckwalter, K.C., and Kelley, L.S. Taking Care of the Caregivers: Staff Stress and Burnout on a Special Alzheimer's Unit. *Journal of Psychosocial Nursing* 30(9):25–31, 1992.

Mor, V. Presentation at special session on staffing and quality of care in nursing homes, at the annual meeting of The Gerontological Society of America, Atlanta, Georgia, November 1994.

Mor, V. Invest in Your Frontline Worker: Commentary. *The Brown University Long-term Care Quality Letter* 7(1):4–5, 1995.

Morioka-Douglas, N., and Yeo, G. *Aging and Health: Asian/Pacific Islander Elders.* Stanford, Calif.: Stanford Geriatric Education Center, 1990.

Morris, J. Presentation at special session on staffing and quality of care in nursing homes, at the annual meeting of The Gerontological Society of America, Atlanta, Georgia, November 1994.

Morris, J.N., Hawes, C., Fries, B.E., et al. Designing the National Resident Assessment Instrument for Nursing Facilities. *The Gerontologist* 30:293–315, 1990.

Movassaghi, H., Kindig, D.A., Juhl, N., and Geller, J.M. *Nursing Supply and Characteristics in the Nonmetropolitan Areas of the United States: Findings from the 1988 National Sample Survey of Registered Nurses* (Grant No. HAR000004-03). Rockville, Md.: Health Resources and Services Administration, U.S. Department of Health and Human Services, 1992.

Munroe, D.J. The Influence of Registered Nurse Staffing on the Quality of Nursing Home Care. *Research in Nursing and Health* 13:263–270, 1990.

Murtaugh, C.M., Kemper, P., and Spillman, B.C. The Risk of Nursing Home Use in Later Life. *Medical Care* 28(10):952–962, 1990.

National Indian Council on Aging. *American Indian Elderly: A National Profile.* Albuquerque, N.M.: National Indian Council on Aging, 1981.

NCHS (National Center for Health Statistics). Nursing Home Characteristics: Preliminary Data from the 1985 National Nursing Home Survey. G. Strahan. *Advance Data from Vital and Health Statistics.* No. 131. Pub. No. (PHS) 87-1250. Hyattsville, Md.: NCHS, U.S. Public Health Service, 1987.

NCHS. Characteristics of Registered Nurses in Nursing Homes: Preliminary Data from the 1985 National Nursing Home Survey. G. Strahan. *Advance Data from Vital and Health Statistics.* No. 152. Pub. no. (PHS) 88-1250. Hyattsville, Md.: NCHS, U.S. Public Health Service, 1988.

NCCNHR (National Citizens' Coalition for Nursing Home Reform). *A Consumer Perspective on Quality Care: The Residents' Point of View.* Washington, D.C.: NCCNHR, 1985.

NIA (National Institute on Aging). *Personnel Needs for Health Needs of the Elderly Through the Year 2020.* Administrative Document. Committee on Personnel for Health Needs of the Elderly. Bethesda, Md.: NIA, 1987.

NIA. *Progress Report on Alzheimer's Disease: Research Is the Key to Unlocking the Mysteries of Alzheimer's Disease.* Pub. no. (NIH) 94-3885. Silver Spring, Md.: NIA, 1994.

Norwich, H.S. A Study of Nursing Care in Geriatric Hospitals. *Nursing Times* 76:292–295, 1980.

O'Connor, J. LTC Facilities Embrace Assisted Living. *McKnight's Long Term Care News* 16(3):1, 42, 1995.

O'Shaunessy, M.A., and Price, M.A. Financing and Delivery of Long-term Care Services for the Elderly. Pp. 191–224 in: C.J. Evashwick and L.J. Weiss, eds. *Managing the Continuum of Care.* Rockville, Md.: Aspen, 1987.

Parsons, W.A., Myrick, R.D., and Gunnoe, J. The Case of Mr. W. Mental Health Consultation. *Journal of Gerontological Nursing* 14(8):14–18, 1988.

Penner, L.A., Luderria, K., and Mead, G. Staff Attitudes: Image or Reality. *Journal of Gerontological Nursing* 10:110–117, 1984.

Peppard, N. Alzheimer's Special Care Nursing Home Units. *Nursing Homes* 34(5):25–28, 1984.

Pillemer, K. Maltreatment of Patients in Nursing Homes: Overview and Research Agenda. *Journal of Health and Social Behavior* 29:227–238, 1988.

Pillemer, K., and Hudson, B. A Model Abuse Prevention Program for Nursing Assistants. *The Gerontologist* 33:128–131, 1993.

Pollick, M.F. Abuse of the Elderly: A Review. *Holistic Nurse Practitioner* 1(2):43–53, 1987.

Preston, D.B., and Mansfield, P.K. An Exploration of Stressful Life Events, Illnesses, and Coping Among the Rural Elderly. *The Gerontologist* 24:490–494, 1984.

Rantz, M., and Miller, T. Pp. 26–28 in: *Quality Assurance for Long Term Care: Supplement #3.* Gaithersburg, Md.: Aspen Publications, 1994.

Reagan, J. Management of Nurse's Aides in Long Term Care Settings. *Journal of Long Term Care Administration* 14:9–14, Summer 1986.

Revans, R.W. *Standards for Morale: Cause and Effect in Hospitals.* London: Oxford University Press for the Nuffield Provincial Hospital Trust, 1964.

Rhys-Hearn, C. Staffing Geriatric Wards: Trials of a Package. *Nursing Times* 75:45–48, 52, 1979.

Richardson, J. *Aging and Health: Black American Elders.* Stanford, Calif.: Stanford Geriatric Education Center, 1990.

Robertson, J.F., Herth, K.A., and Cummings, C.C. Long-term Care: Retention of Nurses. *Journal of Gerontological Nursing* 20(11):4–10, 1994.

Rohrer, J.E., Buckwalter, K.C., and Russell, D.W. The Effects of Mental Dysfunction on Nursing Home Care. *Social Science and Medicine* 28(4):399–403, 1989.

Rovner, B.W., and Rabins, P.V. Mental Illness Among Nursing Home Patients. *Hospital and Community Psychiatry* 36(2):119–128, 1985.

Roybal, E.R. Federal Involvement in Mental Health Care for the Aged. *American Psychologist* 39(2):163–166, 1984.

Rudman, D., Alverno, L., and Mattson, D.E. A Comparison of Physically Aggressive Behavior in Two VA Nursing Homes. *Hospital and Community Psychiatry* 44(6):571–575, 1993.

Ryden, M. Presentation at special session on staffing and quality of care in nursing homes, at the annual meeting of The Gerontological Society of America, Atlanta, Georgia, November 1994.

Ryden, M.B., Bossenmaier, M., and McLachlan, C. Aggressive Behavior in Cognitively Impaired Nursing Home Residents. *Research In Nursing and Health* 14(2):87–95, 1991.

Samter, J., Braun, J.V., Culpepper, W.J., and Cohen-Mansfield, J. Description of a Program for Psychiatric Consultations in the Nursing Home. *American Journal of Geriatric Psychiatry* 2:144–156, 1994.

Savage, B., Widdowson, T., and Wright, T. Improving the Care of the Elderly. In: D. Towell and C. Harries, eds. *Innovation in Patient Care: an Action Research Study of Change in a Psychiatric Hospital.* London: Croom Helm, 1979.

Scanlon, W.J. A Perspective for Long-term Care for the Elderly. *Health Care Financing Review* (Annual Supplement):1–15, 1988.

Schnelle, J. Treatment of Urinary Incontinence in Nursing Home Patients by Prompted Voiding. *Journal of The American Geriatric Society* 38:356–360, 1990.

Schnelle, J. Presentation at Special Session on Staffing and Quality of Care in Nursing Homes, at the annual meeting of The Gerontological Society of America, Atlanta, Georgia, November 1994.

Schnelle, J.F., Newman, D.R., and Fogarty, T. Management of Patient Continence in Long Term Care Nursing Facilities. *The Gerontologist* 30:373–376, 1990.

Select Committee on Aging, House of Representatives, One hundred and second Congress session. *Shortage of Health Care Professions Caring for the Elderly: Recommendations for Change. A Report by the Chairman.* Pub. no. 102-915. Washington, D.C.: U.S. Government Printing Office, 1992.

Senior, O.E. *Nurse/Patient Dependency.* London: Management Services, 1978.

Sheridan, J.E., Vredenburgh, D.J., and Abelson, M.A. Contextual Model of Leadership Influence in Hospital Units. *Academy of Management Journal* 27:48–57, 1984.

Sheridan, J., Hogstel, M., and Fairchild, T.J. Organization Climate in Nursing Homes: Its Impact on Nursing Leadership and Patient Care. Pp. 90–94 in: L.R. Jouch and J.L. Wall, eds. *Best Papers Proceedings 1990.* San Francisco: Academy of Management, 1990.

Sheridan, J., White, J., and Fairchild, T.J. Ineffective Staff, Ineffective Supervision, or Ineffective Administration? Why Some Nursing Homes Fail to Provide Adequate Care. *The Gerontologist* 32:334–341, 1992.

Shields, E.M., and Kick, E. Nursing Care in Nursing Homes. Pp. 195–209 in: L. Aiken, ed. *Nursing In The 1980s: Crises, Opportunities, Challenges.* Philadelphia: J.B. Lippicott, 1982.

Smith, M., Mitchell, S., Buckwalter, K.C., and Garand, L. Geropsychiatric Nursing Consultation: A Valuable Resource in Rural Long Term Care. *Archives of Psychiatric Nursing* VIII(4):272–279, 1994.

Smyer, M., Brannon, D., and Cohn, M. Improving Nursing Home Care through Training and Job Redesign. *The Gerontologist* 32:327–333, 1991.

Snyder, P. Creating Culturally Supportive Environments in Long Term Care Institutions. *The Journal of Long Term Care Administration*, (Spring):19–28, 1982.

Spector, W.D. Presentation at special session on staffing and quality of care in nursing homes, at the annual meeting of The Gerontological Society of America, Atlanta, Georgia, November 1994.

Spector, W.D., and Takada, H.A. Characteristics of Nursing Homes that Affect Resident Outcomes. *Journal of Aging and Health* 3(4):427–454, 1991.

Stahl, D.A. 1995 Leadership Challenges for SNFs. *Nursing Management* 3:17–19, 1995.

Stein, L, Linn, M.W., and Stein, E.M. Patients' Perceptions of Nursing Home Stress Related to Quality of Care. *The Gerontologist* 26:424–430, 1986.

Stevens, G.L., and Baldwin, B.A. Optimizing Mental Health in the Nursing Home Setting. *Journal of Psychosocial Nursing* 26(10):27–31, 1988.

Stolley, J.M., Buckwalter, K.C., and Shannon, M. Caring for Patients with Alzheimer's Disease: Recommendations for Nursing Education. *Journal of Gerontological Nursing* 17(6):34–38, 1991.

Storlie, F.J. The Reshaping of the Old. *Journal of Gerontological Nursing* 8:555–559, 1982.

Straus, M.A. Domestic Violence and Homicide Antecedents. *Bulletin of The New York Academy of Medicine* 62:446–465, 1986.

Strumpf, N. Presentation at special session on staffing and quality of care in nursing homes, at the annual meeting of The Gerontological Society of America, Atlanta, Georgia, November 1994.

Strumpf, N.E., and Knibbe, K.K. Long Term Care: Fulfilling Promises to the Old Among Us. Pp. 217–225 in: J. McCloskey and H. Grace, eds. *Current Issues In Nursing* (3rd ed.). St. Louis, Mo.: C.V. Mosby, 1990.

Stryker, R. *How To Reduce Employee Turnover In Nursing Homes and Other Health Care Organizations.* Springfield, Ill.: Charles C Thomas, 1981.

Swan, J., Torre, A., and Steinhart, R. Ripple Effects of PPS on Nursing Homes: Swimming or Drowning in the Funding Stream? *The Gerontologist* 30:323–331, 1990.

Swanson, E., Maas, M., and Buckwalter, K. Cognitive and Functional Status: Unit Comparison. *Clinical Nursing Research* 3(1):27–42, 1994.

Tellis-Nayak, V., and Tellis-Nayak, M. Quality of Care and the Burden of Two Cultures: When the World of Nurse's Aide Enters the World of Nursing Home. *The Gerontologist* 29:307–313, 1989.

Teresi, J., Holmes, D., Benenson, E., et al. A Primary Care Nursing Model in Long Term Care Facilities: Evaluation of Impact on Affect, Behavior, and Socialization. *The Gerontologist* 33:667–674, 1993.

Teresi, J.A., Holmes, D., Ramirez, M., et al. Preliminary Findings: A Study of Ethnic/Racial Conflict Between Nursing Home Staff and Residents. Unpublished manuscript, 1994.

Timko, C., and Moos, R.H. A Typology of Social Climates in Group Residential Facilities for Older People. *Journal of Gerontology* 46(3):160–169, 1991.

U.S. Department of Justice. *Crime in the United States.* Washington, D.C.: U.S. Government Printing Office, 1985.

Vladeck, B. *Unloving Care: The Nursing Home Tragedy.* New York: Basic Books, 1984.

Vladeck, B., and Alfano, G. *Medicine and Extended Care: Issues, Problems, and Prospects.* Owings Mill, Md.: Rynd Communications, 1987.

Wagnild, G. A Descriptive Study of Nurse's Aide Turnover in Long Term Care Facilities. *The Journal of Long-term Care Administration* 16(Spring):19–23, 1988.

Wagnild, G., and Manning, R. The High Turnover Profile: Screening and Selecting Applicants for Nurse's Aides. *Journal of Long-term Care Administration* 14(Summer):1–4, 1986.

Weiler, K., Buckwalter, K.C., and Curry, J.P. Nurses, Work-Related Stress, and Ethical Dilemmas. Pp. 320–339 in: D.M. Corr and C.A. Corr, eds. *Nursing Care in an Aging Society.* New York: Springer Publishing Company, 1990.

White, C.M. The Nurse-Patient Encounter: Attitudes and Behavior in Action. *Journal of Gerontological Nursing* 3:16–20, 1977.

Wilging, P.R. OBRA as a Measure of Quality. Pp. 21–25 in: E.L. Mitty, ed. *Quality Imperatives In Long-term Care: The Elusive Agenda.* New York: National League for Nursing Press, 1992.

Willcocks, D., Peace, S., and Kellaher, L. *Private Lives in Public Places.* London: Tavistock Publications, 1987.

Wilson, K.B. Assisted Living: Model Program May Signify the Future. *The Brown University Long Term Care Quality Letter* 6(15):1–4, 1994.

Winger, J., Schirm, V., and Stewart, P. Aggressive Behavior in Long-term Care. *Journal of Psychosocial Nursing and Mental Health Services* 25:28–33, 1987.

Wright, L.K. A Reconceptualization of the "Negative Staff and Poor Care in Nursing Homes" Assumption. *The Gerontologist* 28:813–820, 1988.

Zimmer, J.G., Watson, N., and Treat, A. Behavioral Problems Among Patients in SNFs. *American Journal of Public Health* 74(10):1118–1121, 1984.

Zimmerman, D.R. Impact of New Regulations and Data Sources on Nursing Home Quality of Care. Pp. 29–42 in: *Mechanisms of Quality in Long-term Care: Service and Clinical Outcomes.* Pub. no. 41-2382. New York: National League for Nursing Press, 1991.

Zinn, J.S. The Influence of Nurse Wage Differentials on Nursing Home Staffing and Resident Care Decisions. *The Gerontologist* 33:721–729, 1993.

Quality of Care and Nursing Staff in Nursing Homes

Jean Johnson, Ph.D., C. McKeen Cowles, M.S., and
Samuel J. Simmens, Ph.D.

OVERVIEW OF PAPERS PREPARED FOR THE INSTITUTE TO MEDICINE

This paper is comprised of two sections for committee review. The first section presents a broad picture of issues related to nursing homes and staff. It describes the nursing home environment, characteristics of nursing homes using trend data since 1992, roles and education of nursing staff, the relationship of resident needs to staffing, and quality-of-care measures in nursing homes. The second section presents the results of a study undertaken specifically to provide new information related to nurse staffing and quality of care in nursing homes. Both papers need to be considered jointly since the first establishes the context for the research described in the second.

THE CONTEXT OF NURSING CARE IN NURSING HOMES

Background

The relationship between quality of care and the number and type of nursing staff in nursing homes is complex. At present there is no definitive information

---

Dr. Johnson is associate dean for health sciences programs, The George Washington University; Mr. Cowles is a consultant; and Dr. Simmens is an assistant research professor in the Department of Health Care Sciences, The George Washington University.

to determine what exact nursing inputs will relate to specified resident outcomes. There is information emerging, however, that will help establish a set of relationships between resident needs, staffing, and quality.

There has been considerable controversy over the past years about the minimum staff required to meet resident needs. A significant tension has existed between consumer and professional groups who propose increased numbers of registered nurses (RNs) and total staff, and payers, primarily state Medicaid agencies, who are concerned about the cost to the public of paying for additional staff. It is important to recognize that while minimum staffing levels are particularly tied to Medicaid payment, Medicare is an increasingly significant payment source through expansion to subacute services. It is likely, given the current funding crisis in the Medicaid and Medicare programs, that financing for nursing home care will be increasingly problematic, especially if these programs are cut. Financing of nursing home care will require potentially a new funding structure. If money were not an issue, there would be no need to constrain staff, and every nursing home resident could have their own RN care 24 hours a day.

Many states have established a minimum standard for nursing time per resident per day. Federal requirements state that an RN must be present in a facility for 8 hours a day, 7 days a week, regardless of the size of the facility. It is difficult to argue against the need for a minimum number of staff members with defined capabilities to carry out the basic functions of nursing home care. However, the notion of a minimum number applied uniformly to all facilities is complicated by the fact that nursing homes have differing case-mix populations needing different levels of nursing expertise and different amounts of care. The problem with the concept of minimum staff is that it becomes translated to mean the maximum staff for payment purposes. In addition to the actual minimum levels, there is a more general requirement that there be sufficient staff to provide the required care to residents. However, there has been little guidance as to what "sufficient" staff actually means. The definition of sufficient has been operationalized in conflicting ways. The regulatory agencies hold nursing homes to a standard of "highest practicable level" for resident care, yet the payment agencies provide funding for staffing at minimum levels.

Quality of care has received increasing attention over the past 5 years, yet there has been relatively limited research examining the relationship of staffing to quality. There is some consensus about a limited number of indicators of quality care, but in general there remain issues of definition of quality. For instance, should the emphasis on quality measurements be on process or outcome? Who should define quality: the regulators, residents, family, or staff? Is there a consensus about measures of quality among these groups of stakeholders?

Nursing Home Environment

As the lines between the hospital, nursing home, and home care blur, the definition of a nursing home has become less boundaried. The typical nursing home of the past provided care for primarily elderly individuals who needed assistance with some aspects of taking care of themselves or simply needed a sheltered place to live. The focus of care was generally custodial. If a resident had an acute problem they were promptly sent to the hospital.

Nursing homes today provide a range of services to persons who are more disabled with an increased number of unstable chronic conditions (Morrisey et al., 1988; Shaughessy and Kramer, 1990). Care provided in a nursing facility may range from provision of ventilator assistance to rehabilitation for individuals with, for instance, hip fracture or stroke. It also ranges from care of a resident with an emerging acute care crisis, to caring for a resident whose death is expected and imminent. The general philosophy of care has shifted from one of custodial care to one of maximizing each resident's well-being. Specifically stated in the long-term-care regulation, "each resident must receive and the facility must provide the necessary care and services to attain or maintain the highest practicable physical, mental, and psychosocial well-being." Rehabilitation is now a basic conceptual framework for care.

The types of services offered by nursing homes is changing as is the setting in which nursing home care is delivered. A nursing home may offer respite care or specialized care units such as an Alzheimer's unit. There are currently approximately 13,029 special care beds in nursing homes (Health Data Associates, 1994). A new category of care, subacute, is offered by many nursing homes. Subacute units provide care for residents with serious wound conditions, intravenous lines, rehabilitative needs including occupational therapy, physical therapy, and speech therapy, as well as medically complex patients. Traditional nursing home care is now offered in hospitals, life care communities, and residential care facilities.

For some residents the nursing home will be where they live out the remainder of their lives, while others will only be in the home for a brief period of rehabilitation or respite care. With the requirement for advance directives, a major challenge to nursing homes is to provide more end-of-life care. Fewer residents are sent to hospitals to die (Sager et al., 1989). In addition, based on anecdotal information, more acute care problems are being managed within nursing homes to prevent the need for hospitalization.

Characteristics of Nursing Homes

A review of nursing home characteristics may be helpful in defining the context of nursing care. The characteristics that are both relevant and for which national data are available are included in Table 1. The 1994 data are obtained from the *Nursing Home Yearbook* (Health Data Associates, 1994). Data for the remaining years were directly computed from the On-line Survey Certification and Reporting (OSCAR) data set for those years. Occupancy has been about 85

TABLE 1 National Nursing Home Characteristics

Characteristics	1992 (mean)	1993 (mean)	1994 (mean)
Occupancy	84.81	85.07	84.79
Percent Medicaid	68.33	68.61	68.79
Case-mix	10.48	10.56	10.61
Hours of staff			
RN	.31	.32	.34
LPN	.60	.61	.62
NA	2.09	2.09	2.08
Total	3.00	3.01	3.04
Deficiencies related to nursing care			
Level A	0.13	0.15	0.13
Level B	8.11	8.01	7.41
Total	8.24	8.16	7.54

percent over the past 3 years. As indicated, Medicaid plays a large role in financing nursing home care with approximately 68 percent of residents over the past 3 years being covered by Medicaid. The case-mix index has increased slightly each year from 10.48, to 10.56, then 10.61. Registered nurse time has also increased slightly over the past 3 years, with 0.31, 0.32, 0.34 hour per resident per day respectively. Licensed practical nurse (LPN) time has also very slightly increased. Nurse assistant (NA) time has remained stable at about 2.09.

The mean number of citations were calculated for nursing-care-related deficiencies. Expert nurse and ombudsman groups identified federal requirements that were most directly related to nursing care. Deficiencies in any of these requirements comprised the nursing care deficiencies (Johnson-Pawlson, 1993a). The mean number of level A deficiencies has been reasonably constant at 0.13. The mean number of level B deficiencies has decreased from 8.11 in 1992 to 7.41 in 1994.

Nursing Staff Characteristics, Retention, Roles, and Educational Preparation

Nursing Characteristics

Nursing staff in a nursing home are primarily comprised of RNs, LPNs, and NAs. According to data from the 1992 nursing survey, 7 percent of RNs work in nursing homes (Moses, 1994). The proportion has been virtually unchanged since 1986 (National Center for Health Statistics, 1988). Of the RNs currently in nursing homes, 45.5 percent are diploma prepared, 31.7 percent are associate degree prepared, 19.2 percent are bachelor's prepared, and 6 percent are master's prepared. The average turnover rate for nursing staff in 1994 was: RNs (56.3 percent); LPNs (52.5 percent); and NAs (100.4 percent) (American Health Care Association, 1995). The salary level for nursing staff in nursing homes is significantly lower than for hospital-based nurses. Based on the 1992 National Sample Survey of Registered Nurses, an RN in a staff position in a hospital earned $36,618, while staff nurses in a nursing home earned $31,298. The differential is greater at the supervisory level. The average salary of a supervisor in a hospital is $42,948, while in a nursing facility it is $32,569. The average nursing home LPN salary is comparable to the salary level of LPNs in hospital (American Health Care Association, 1994). Salary levels for NAs are lower in nursing facilities ($6.33 per hour) compared to the hospital setting ($7.31 per hour) (American Health Care Association, 1994).

Retention

As noted above, the average national turnover rate is very high for all levels of staff. A turnover rate of 100 percent for NAs and over 50 percent for RNs and LPNs indicates a major problem in continuity of care, which is an important factor in providing good care to residents with chronic conditions. Disruption of staff leads to residents having to constantly "train" staff, problems in carrying through care plans, inaccurate assessment because of failure to be familiar with the baseline status of a resident, and failure of a facility to fully develop a philosophy of caring. Inefficiency also exists because of the time needed for constant recruitment efforts. Staff are less productive as new staff spend time getting to know the residents and procedures of the facility, and stable staff spend time helping to orient new staff. It should be noted that even though NA staff turnover may be 100 percent, there is usually a reasonably stable group of NAs. The key issue is whether the stable core of NAs is large enough to create a critical mass to maintain stability of care.

Role

Licensed Nurses   Licensed nurses, including RNs and LPNs, have two major functional roles in nursing homes: clinical and management. The clinical role requires a broad knowledge of nursing because of the wide variation in resident problems and needs. A licensed nurse is responsible for the overall care of the residents. This includes being able to accurately assess the status of residents, define physical, psychological, and social problems and strengths, and develop plans of care that extensively incorporate rehabilitation as well as health promotion concepts. Registered nurses work with residents whose main interests may not be based on their health problems but on the management of everyday living, which may include concern about dying, relationships with family members, or what will happen to the house they have left.

It is extremely important that the nurse accurately and comprehensively assess all problems. Life threatening problems such as fever, trauma from a fall, or change in mental status carry a particular burden for timeliness and accuracy. Accurate assessment and management can save the life of a resident and may assist in avoiding unnecessary transfer to the emergency room. It has been noted that early detection and monitoring of a resident with a fever can prevent dehydration and the need for hospitalization (Weinberg et al., 1994).

Effective nursing interventions must be based on a broad range of competencies in the physical, psychological, and social realms. In order to provide consistent care to individuals, care that is planned by other health disciplines such as social work, physical therapy, or a consulting psychiatrist must be incorporated into the day-to-day care provided by nursing staff. In many cases nursing staff must substitute for health professionals that are not on site. An example is if a medical problem arises, most facilities have no daily on-site medical coverage (Karuza and Katz, 1994). One study reported that the mean response time between staff notification of an acute event and a physician response by telephone was 5.12 hours, which means the nurse is critical to the well-being of residents in these situations and requires a high level of nursing competency in clinical decision making (Brooks et al., 1994).

The clinical care is very complicated, given that residents are likely to have multiple chronic illnesses requiring complete understanding of each illness and the interacting effects. The nursing care problems include not only physical problems, but mental and behavioral problems as well. There is a high prevalence of depression in nursing homes. In addition, a major challenge to nursing is the care of residents with dementia. It has been estimated that over half of all nursing home residents have memory impairment. This is frequently accompanied by agitated and aggressive behavior which has significant implications for the well-being of other residents and staff. Residents are frequently on complicated medication and treatment regimens requiring extensive pharmacologic knowledge.

An RN or LPN may be the only licensed nurse on a particular unit or in the facility during evenings, nights, or weekends to ensure that the clinical needs of residents are met. Being the sole responsible clinician requires a nurse to have considerable clinical expertise. Whereas historically nurses in nursing homes were viewed more as house mothers than professionals, current resident care requires a highly qualified nursing staff, with licensed nurses needing a broad base of knowledge spanning basic nursing, rehabilitation, and psychiatric skills.

The management role of licensed nurses is neither very well understood nor recognized. Most nurses, whether RNs or LPNs, have significant management responsibilities. A major management responsibility is staff supervision. A licensed nurse must oversee the direct resident care that is provided by NAs as well as other licensed nurses. Given that NAs are minimally trained for resident care activities, oversight is crucial. Ensuring follow-through with therapeutic programs such as bladder training or behavioral management requires consistent staff performance and continual interaction between the supervising nurse and staff. In addition, establishing and reinforcing the expectation that all residents are treated with respect and caring is often a very challenging proposition.

Management responsibilities in addition to staff supervision include resolution of conflicts, conducting patient care conferences, organizing systems of care such as bladder training programs, and conducting quality assurance activities. It has been recognized that organization of bladder training and restraint reduction take significant organizational skills on the part of licensed nurses (Schnelle et al., 1991; Werner et al., 1994). In addition, nurse managers must be able to work within interdisciplinary groups to conduct care planning. Nurses are usually responsible for interdisciplinary care planning and coordination of care.

Nurse Assistants   The nurse assistant has provided the backbone of care in nursing homes. This individual is responsible for most of the day-to-day assistance with activities of daily living (ADL), providing direct care and comfort, noting abnormalities such as pressure sores or change in mental status, and participating in rehabilitative care such as bladder training, use of assistive devices for eating, and strengthening exercises. The communication skills of an NA are very important in being able to effectively work with and involve residents in their care, convey a caring attitude, and provide information to residents and other care providers. Given the level of direct care responsibilities and the minimal preparation required for NAs, it is critical that licensed nursing staff be available and work closely through constructive supervision with nurse assistants.

Education

Understanding the educational process that prepares the nursing work force is critical to evaluating the capacity of the current work force to meet the needs of residents. Up until 1990, there was no uniform requirement for nurse assistant training. Some states required 100 or more hours of training, while others required none. With the passage of the Omnibus Budget Reconciliation Act of 1987, nurse assistants are required to have 75 hours of training and must complete a written and performance competency exam within 4 months of hire. While this is a landmark requirement, there has been no effective evaluation as to whether or to what extent this has improved the quality of care in nursing facilities.

Licensed practical nurses provide a significant contribution to the care of residents and account for the majority of licensed nurses in nursing homes. Training of LPNs averages between 12 and 13 months, focusing predominantly on technical aspects of care such as medication distribution, wound care, and catheter care. A program may offer specific content in geriatrics. For instance, an LPN program in the District of Columbia offers approximately 108 hours of clinical experience and approximately 50 hours of classroom time in geriatrics. This same program also offers 1 week of leadership training. While the content of most LPN programs offer similar curricula, it is clear that LPN education prepares individuals for the technical role of nursing but is limited in its leadership and clinical decision making content, both of which are critical to effectively functioning in a leadership position in a facility.

Registered nurses include three major groups: those prepared at the diploma level, the associate degree level, and the bachelor's degree level. The vast majority of nurses in nursing homes are diploma or associate degree prepared. Information from a survey done by the Community College-Nursing Home Partnership suggests that there is a limited inclusion of gerontology in the associate degree nurse (ADN) curriculum (Hanson, 1992). While 66 percent of programs provide a nursing home experience in the first year, only 20 percent include one in the second year. This suggests that the nursing home is the site for basic skills development, rather than the more advanced course work. Since that report, considerable work has been done by the partnership to expand the gerontology curriculum at the ADN level.

Diploma programs are hospital based by definition. The number of these programs has decreased significantly over the past two decades with the rise of ADN and bachelor of science in nursing (BSN) programs. However, diploma nurses comprise a significant number of RNs in nursing homes. The hospital-based education of diploma graduates clearly limited their exposure to nursing homes.

A recent report on BSN curricula suggests that 78 percent of respondents to a survey have participated in clinical experiences in long-term care and 83 percent have clinical experiences in geriatrics (Johnson, 1995). This is consistent with earlier information from the American Association of Colleges of Nursing that 75 percent of schools integrated gerontology content into clinical courses and 74.8 respondent schools incorporated long-term care into clinical course work. It is not at all clear from curricula information for BSN programs, however, that the focus of the content is to prepare nurses to take a leadership role in nursing home care. Based on anecdotal information and personal observation, most clinical experiences in geriatrics, if in nursing facilities, relate to basic nursing skills and are not offered as required senior-level nursing management courses. In addition, gerontology content could easily be taught in an hospital. BSN nurses have the most extensive education in leadership and clinical decision making skills of any of the RN levels.

There are issues that affect all levels of licensed nurses. One is that there are no specific accreditation requirements related to experiences in nursing homes. Nursing homes have been more a setting of last resort than one that is valued as a legitimate practice site. Nurses from an intensive care background continue to receive greater recognition than nurses in nursing homes. Another concern is the scarcity of faculty who are expert in nursing home care. There are increasing (although limited) numbers of nurses who have some expertise in geriatrics, yet have no nursing home experience. Most nurses who have extensive clinical experience in nursing homes do not have the academic credentials to be on a faculty of nursing, nor perhaps the desire. With a shortage of faculty prepared to be a role model and teacher, it is very difficult to build a cadre of graduating students with the knowledge and skills to effectively provide clinical and management expertise in nursing homes.

Finally, few states have continuing education or re-examination requirements to maintain licensure. Health care information is changing at an ever more rapid pace, necessitating that nurses have current information. Without continuing education requirements for licensure, however, some nurses may be working with woefully outdated information. One might argue that the current regulations governing nursing homes that require continuing education for all staff address this issue. The quality and content of these programs, however, are extremely variable.

Case-Mix and Staffing Needs

Case-mix is an important factor in examining the relationship between resident needs and nursing staff required to meet those needs. Substantial and seminal work has been conducted as part of the Multistate Nursing Home Case-Mix and Quality Demonstration project sponsored by the Health Care Financing Administration (HCFA) beginning in 1989 (Fries et al., 1994). The goal of the project is development of a payment and quality monitoring system for nursing homes. The basic principle of the case-mix project is that resources should be allocated based on resident need and that sicker and more debilitated residents need more services, both in terms of amount of staff time as well as level of expertise. To date, work has included development of categories of resource need and measurement of staff time to meet those needs. The next step in the project is to link this with quality-of-care measures.

As a result of research into case-mix, the third iteration of a resource utilization grouping (RUGS-III) has been developed. RUGS-III development, like other methods of relating resident needs to resource use, relies heavily on measures of activities of daily living which have been recognized as the most important predictor of the cost of nursing home care (Butler and Schlenker, 1989; Weissert and Musliner, 1992; Williams et al., 1994). RUGS-III is based on several levels of categorization of resident need. The first categorization identifies resident types, reflecting patients with certain conditions. The levels are: rehabilitation, extensive services, special care, clinically complex, impaired cognition, behavior problems, and (reduced) physical functions. These categories of residents represent a hierarchy of groups with different needs, the rehabilitative group having the highest resource need. Each of these major categories are then further divided into subcategories which form 44 different RUGS-III groupings.

Based on the case-mix project, it is evident that the need for nursing time and skills varies significantly depending on the resident classification. The case-mix project measured actual nursing times needed for various levels of nursing. Nursing times were classified as either resident-specific time or non-resident-specific time. Resident-specific time included time spent performing services for an individual resident and interactive time. Non-resident-specific time included routine operations and procedures necessary for the day-to-day function of a nursing unit, including staff meetings, team conferences, routine charting and documentation, unit administration, supervision and the like.

Based on the case-mix data, there is evidence of a wide variation of total nursing time needed for different categories of RUGS. For instance, the category requiring the least care is the first level of the reduced physical function group. Based on minutes per resident per day, the nursing times calculated for the group are: RN, 13 minutes; LPN, 24 minutes; and NA, 67 minutes. This is a total of 104 minutes. This is contrasted with a resident in the highest resource need group requiring the following times: RN, 82 minutes; LPN, 63 minutes; and NA, 186 minutes, to total 331 minutes per day of nursing care. As the resource need increases, so does the need for more skilled nursing time as well increased total staff time.

There is evidence that case-mix has evolved toward a more debilitated resident population following implementation of diagnosis-related groups (DRG) (Morrisey et al., 1988; Shaughnessy and Kramer, 1990). Analysis of the OSCAR data set as presented above indicates a continuing increase in case-mix since 1992. The first surge in case-mix took place shortly after the implementation of DRGs. However, it is significant that the case-mix index is still increasing, which is consistent with what would be expected under continued pressures for hospitals to decrease length of stay.

Quality of Care

There has been considerable attention paid to the issues of how many staff and what types of staff are needed to meet the needs and expectations of nursing home residents as measured by outcomes. A review of current information on quality of care and nurse staffing suggests there is a relationship between staffing and resident outcomes. Mezey and Lynaugh (1989) reported a reduction in pressure sores, use of physical restraints, and falls when nursing school faculty participated in care at nursing homes. Munroe (1990) found a significant relationship between a higher ratio of RNs to LPNs and fewer deficiencies noted on surveys in California after controlling for several variables, including case-mix. A study of nursing homes in Maryland indicates that higher total staff levels are related to fewer nursing deficiencies (Johnson-Pawlson, 1993a). Another study found a relationship between higher staff levels and lower RN turnover and resident functional improvement (Spector and Takada, 1991). Cherry (1991) found RN staffing to be associated with better resident outcomes as measured through a composite of indicators, including number of resident developing decubitus ulcers per immobile resident, number of residents catheterized per incontinent resident, number of urinary tract infections per incontinent residents, and rate of antibiotic use per resident. Finally, a study of pressure sores in three Department of Veterans Affairs nursing homes concluded that better outcomes in preventing pressure sores was likely due to more favorable staffing (Rodman et al., 1993; Brandeis et al., 1994).

The measures relating to deficiency citations need to be carefully viewed. Federal nursing home requirements have been established using a very extensive and inclusive process to identify measurable criteria by which to determine whether or not a facility is providing adequate care, but there is evidence that the survey process is not applied uniformly. There are serious questions about whether the current survey process produces uniformly reliable and valid determinations of nursing home care (Abt Associates, 1993; Johnson-Pawlson, 1993b; Office of the Inspector General, 1993). It is likely, however, that surveyors are reasonably accurate at the extremes in identifying very good facilities and very bad ones.

The determination of quality cannot be left solely to health professionals and regulators. The resident and family perception of quality of care has not received much attention. The expectations of family members or surrogates may differ from those of the resident. A study of the ability of a surrogate to represent the resident's view of quality of care indicates that surrogates cannot accurately express the resident's perspective in all areas of nursing home care (Lavizzo-Mourey et al., 1992). There may also be a difference in what a family member considers quality of care for a resident with severe dementia as compared to a family member of a resident who has severe emphysema.

Information concerning what residents want is described in a study done by the National Citizen's Coalition for Nursing Home Reform. The findings of this study suggest that nursing home residents most value staff being nice to them, including smiling and treating them with dignity (National Citizens' Coalition for Nursing Home Reform, 1986). Focus groups conducted in Maine by DeSisto (1994) indicate that residents rarely identified clinical care, such as receiving medications, as being important. The areas they considered important included good food, privacy, being treated with dignity and respect, activities, and comfort. There is a study currently being conducted by the American Health Care Association on resident perceptions of quality. Data are not yet available from this study.

Conclusion

Based on the information presented above, it is likely that the current needs of residents require consideration of case-mix in determination of staffing. It also suggests that the needs of residents require highly capable staff, consistent with RN education, to accurately assess physical, psychological, and social problems; develop overall care plans; monitor implementation of those plans; provide direct care services; manage the work of the LPN and NA staff; and work with other disciplines. There is also evidence that quality-of-care needs to be viewed beyond the perspectives of care providers and regulators to include the most important perspective of all, the resident's perspective.

STUDY OF HIGH- AND LOW-QUALITY FACILITIES

Background

Based on questions related to staffing and quality, and after review of nursing home issues as presented above, a study was conducted to explore the characteristics of facilities that provide high- and low-quality care. Several indicators of quality identified as important criteria were used for facility selection and included prevalence of pressure sores, use of restraints, and medication errors (Institute of Medicine, 1986; Rodman et al., 1994). A constraint of facility selection was that information on indicators be available for all certified facilities in the OSCAR data set maintained by HCFA.

Identification of the high- and low-quality facilities allows for examination of differences between groups that are not as apparent among groups of facilities that are only slightly different. The hypothesis for this analysis is that high-quality facilities use higher levels of RNs and total staff, after controlling for case-mix, size, type of ownership, and percent Medicaid residents.

Method

An analysis was undertaken to explore staffing as related to quality and to examine the characteristics of each set of facilities.

Sample Selection

Facilities were selected from the 16,000 certified facilities using 3 indicators of quality of care that were accessible through the OSCAR data set. The characteristics were: (1) the number of residents with pressure sores per number of bedbound residents; (2) the percent of residents in restraints; and (3) the drug error rate. The low-quality facilities were those in the top 25 percent for each of the 3 characteristics. The high-quality facilities were those in the lowest quartile.

The deficiency rates for the samples selected were examined to provide construct validity for the criteria used to identify high- and low-quality facilities. To control for interstate variations in deficiency citation rates, the number of deficiencies for each facility was divided by the state average of citations. If high-quality facilities had a low rate of citations and low-quality facilities had a high rate of citations, the findings would provide evidence of construct validity.

Data Source

Data from the OSCAR include three categories: resident characteristics, facility characteristics, and survey deficiency citations. The data were obtained from the Health Care Financing Administration and included information through October 1994.

Variables

The dependent variable was quality of facility. The determination for this variable is described above. The main independent variable is nurse staffing. The levels of nurse staffing were obtained from the facility characteristics portion of the OSCAR data set. An edit was done to eliminate extreme staffing outliers from the data set. The numbers are based on a facility report of the hours worked for each level of nursing staff during a 2-week period. The hours include full- and part-time staff and contract workers. Other variables included in the analysis are the percent of Medicaid-covered residents; type of ownership including for profit (chain and nonchain), not-for-profit, and government; occupancy; size of facility; and facility case-mix. Geographic location was also considered in terms of urban or rural. Facilities were coded as urban if their zip code was in a metropolitan statistical area as defined by HCFA.

The facility case-mix was calculated using a classification system based on measures of activities of daily living deficits and need for special treatment. Scores for ADLs, namely toileting, transferring, and eating were calculated based on five levels ranging from (1) independent to (5) total dependence. Mobility was scored on a three level scale of (1) ambulatory, (2) chairbound, and (3) bedbound. Bathing was not included because of a distortion caused by some state requirements for full assistance with bathing, regardless of the resident's capabilities. Each of the levels were weighted using a system developed for the RUGS-III tool. A facility ADL index was then calculated. The facility case-mix index was obtained by adding the percent of residents receiving each special treatment to the ADL index.

Results

Classification of Facilities

The number of facilities selected which met the editing criteria were 210 in the low-quality category and 1,429 in the high-quality category. The imbalance in sample size supports the notion that facilities in general provide better than low-quality of care as defined by the study, either from internal commitment, certification requirements, or both.

As noted above, in order to validate this grouping into high- and low-quality facilities, the average number of deficiencies specifically related to nursing care were examined for both groups for the two most recent annual surveys. The nursing-related deficiency citations had been established through expert panels of nurses and ombudsmen as part of a prior study (Johnson-Pawlson, 1993a). Two consecutive surveys were used to provide a measure of consistency for deficiency citations. High-quality facilities received 68 percent and 72 percent as many deficiencies as their state average in the most recent and prior surveys, respectively. By contrast, low-quality facilities received 146 percent and 129 percent as many deficiencies as state averages in the two most recent surveys. The differences between the adjusted deficiency citation rate of the high- and low-quality facilities is statistically significant at the .01 level. These findings support the validity of the classification.

Relationship Among Predictor Variables

As shown in Table 2, comparison of the two groups of facilities indicate significant differences in facility characteristics. High-quality facilities have significantly fewer beds on average than low-quality facilities, 84 beds versus 132 beds. The high-quality facilities have a lower percent of residents who are Medicaid supported (62 percent vs. 70 percent), and the case-mix is significantly lower in high-quality facilities than low-quality facilities, 9.55 compared to 11.03.

Nursing staff data for high- and low-quality facilities indicate a significant difference among the two groups for RN staff. High-quality facilities staff at 0.42 hours per resident per day (25 minutes per resident per day) compared to low-quality facilities which staff at 0.29 hours per resident per day (17 minutes per resident per day). There is also a statistically significant difference between high- and low-quality facilities for total staffing. Total staffing is higher (3.16 hours per resident per day) in high-quality facilities compared to low-quality facilities (3.04 hours per resident per day). The overall greater number of staff in the high-quality facilities is due to more RN staff.

Based on Chi square test, there was a significant difference between high- and low-quality facilities based on ownership (see Table 3) and location (urban or rural) (see Table 4). The major difference for type of ownership was that for-

TABLE 2   Facility Characteristics by Quality of Care

Characteristics	Quality of Care	
	High Quality Mean (Standard deviation) (N = 1429)	Low Quality Mean (Standard deviation) (N = 210)
Total beds[a]	84.28 (60.72)	131.83 (64.30)
Occupancy	0.87 (0.17)	0.88 (0.12)
Medicaid[b]	0.62 (0.28)	0.70 (0.19)
Case-mix index[a]	9.55 (2.11)	11.03 (1.34)
Hours per resident per day		
RN[a]	0.42 (0.34)	0.29 (0.19)
LPN	0.64 (0.40)	0.64 (0.26)
NA	2.11 (0.66)	2.11 (0.53)
Total staff[b]	3.16 (1.10)	3.04 (0.75)

[a]Significant at $p < .0001$.
[b]Significant at $p < .05$.

profit, chain facilities had a higher than expected rate of low-quality facilities (18.3 percent) than other types of ownership. Government and for-profit, non-chain facilities had the least percent of facilities in the low-quality category. In addition, as shown in Table 4, a higher percent of high-quality facilities were in rural settings (91.8 percent) compared to urban facilities (83.2 percent).

Given that high- and low-quality facilities differed by type of ownership and urban or rural location, facility characteristics were further examined for these variables. Data related to type of ownership are presented in Table 5. The differences in RN staffing were significant even though there were no statistically significant differences in total staff for all types of ownership among the high- and low-quality facilities. There were higher levels of all staff in government and not-for-profit facilities than in for-profit chain and nonchain facilities. Total bed size was smaller in the high-quality facilities for all categories of ownership, and the percent of Medicaid-covered residents was significantly less in the for-profit

TABLE 3 Chi Square of High- and Low-Quality Facilities by Type of Ownership

Type of Ownership[a]	Quality of Care	
	High Quality (%) (number)	Low Quality (%) (number)
For-profit chain (N = 518)	81.7 (423)	18.3 (95)
For-profit, nonchain (N = 491)	97.3 (433)	2.7 (58)
Government-owned (N = 110)	97.3 (107)	2.7 (3)
Non-profit (N = 520)	89.6 (466)	10.4 (54)

[a]Significant at $p < .001$.

TABLE 4 Chi Square of High- and Low-Quality Facilities by Urban and Rural Location

Location[a]	Quality of Care	
	High Quality (%) (number)	Low Quality (%) (number)
Urban (N = 889)	83.2 (740)	16.8 (149)
Rural (N = 750)	91.8 (689)	8.1 (61)

[a]Significant at $p < .001$.

chain and not-for-profit, high-quality facilities. In addition, case-mix was significantly less in high-quality facilities for all classes of ownership. This finding is important when coupled with data indicating that even though case-mix was higher in poor quality facilities, there were fewer RNs. It should be noted that the sample size in the government-owned category was too small to test for statistical significance.

Facilities that differed by urban and rural classification showed the same general pattern for high- and low-quality facilities as with type of ownership. These data are presented in Table 6. Registered nurse staff in high-quality rural facilities had 0.36 compared to 0.27 hours per resident per day of time and high

TABLE 5 T Test of Type of Ownership for High- and Low-Quality Facilities

| | Types of Ownership | | | | | | | |
| | For-profit Chain | | For-profit Nonchain | | Not-for-Profit | | Government | |
	High Quality (N = 423)	Low Quality (N = 95)	High Quality (N = 433)	Low Quality (N = 58)	High Quality (N = 466)	Low Quality (N = 54)	High Quality (N = 107)	Low Quality (N = 3)
Staff								
RN	.35[a]	.28	.34[a]	.26	.53[a]	.34	.48	.34
LPN	.62	.64	.58	.58	.68	.67	.73	1.02
NA	1.96	2.07	2.01	2.01	2.25	2.25	2.41	2.45
Total staff	2.94	2.99	2.93	2.85	3.47	3.27	3.62	3.80
Total beds	85.67[a] (42.16)	118.79 (47.07)	83.30[a] (63.18)	138.14 (80.86)	83.07[a] (62.39)	144.44 (66.62)	88.10 (95.98)	195.67 (65.62)
Occupancy	87% (0.16)	89% (0.11)	88% (0.15)	87% (0.13)	87% (0.19)	89% (0.14)	83% (0.22)	82% (0.17)
Percent Medicaid	63%[a] (0.26)	73% (0.13)	73% (0.23)	70% (0.21)	51%[a] (0.30)	63% (0.23)	61% (0.29)	76% (0.02)
Case-mix	9.35[a]	11.15	9.41[a]	10.72	9.75[a]	11.11	9.99	11.66

[a]Significant at $p < .0001$.

TABLE 6 T Test of Facility Characteristics by Urban or Rural Location for High and Low Quality

	Rural		Urban	
	High Quality Mean (standard deviation)	Low Quality Mean (standard deviation)	High Quality Mean (standard deviation)	Low Quality Mean (standard deviation)
Staff				
RN	36[a] (0.28)	.27 (0.22)	.47[a] (0.37)	.31 (0.18)
LPN	.59 (0.38)	.63 (0.26)	.68 (0.42)	.64 (0.26)
NA	2.04 (0.58)	1.99 (0.38)	2.17 (0.73)	2.15 (0.58)
Total staff	3.00[b] (0.95)	2.89 (0.58)	3.32[b] (1.19)	3.10 (0.80)
Percent Medicaid	60[a] (0.25)	75 (0.15)	63[a] (0.31)	68 (0.20)
Case-mix	9.60[a] (1.65)	10.63 (1.38)	9.5[a] (2.47)	11.19 (1.29)
Percent occupancy	88 (0.15)	90 (0.12)	86 (0.19)	87 (0.13)
Total beds	70.00[a] (37.37)	103.98 (44.02)	97.59[a] (73.86)	143.22 (67.84)

[a]Significant at p < .0001.
[b]Significant at p < .001.

TABLE 7 Pearson Correlation Coefficients for Nursing
Staff and Facility Characteristics

	Hours per Resident per Day			
	RN	LPN	NA	Total Staff
Coefficients				
Probability				
Occupancy	−0.32	−0.31	−0.30	−0.39
Medicaid	−0.39	−0.18	−0.18	−0.30
Case-mix	−0.11	−0.15	−0.26	−0.25

NOTE: All of the coefficients in this table are significant at p < .0001.

quality urban facilities had 0.47 compared to 0.31 hours per resident per day of RN time. The percent of Medicaid-covered residents was significantly less in the high-quality rural facilities compared to low-quality facilities, 60 percent versus 75 percent respectively. This same relationship existed for Medicaid in urban facilities, with 63 percent of residents covered by Medicaid in high-quality facilities compared to 68 percent in low-quality facilities. Another consistent difference was that high-quality facilities have a statistically significant lower case-mix index, 9.6 in high-quality facilities versus 10.63 in low-quality facilities in rural areas, and 9.5 versus 11.16 respectively in urban facilities. Finally, high-quality facilities are smaller than low-quality facilities in both urban and rural areas. The average bed size in high-quality rural areas is 70.00 compared to 103.98. In urban areas, high-quality facilities have an average of 97.59 beds, compared to 143.22 beds.

Bivariate analyses of nursing staff and facility characteristics, displayed in Table 7, indicate a statistically significant relationship between hours per resident per day for each level of staff and occupancy rate, percent of Medicaid residents, and case-mix. As one would expect, an increase in occupancy is related to a decrease in nursing time. Also, as the percent of Medicaid residents increases, there are fewer hours per resident per day of nursing time. Contrary to what would be expected as case-mix increases, the amount of staff time decreases. Correlation coefficients for facility characteristics are presented in Table 8. These data indicate a significant positive relationship between occupancy and percent Medicaid. There is a negative relationship between total beds and occupancy suggesting that larger facilities have lower occupancy. There is also a positive relationship between total beds and both case-mix and Medicaid, suggesting that larger facilities fill their additional beds with Medicaid residents and residents who are more debilitated.

TABLE 8 Pearson Correlation Coefficients for Facility Characteristics

Coefficients Probability	Occupancy	Percent Medicaid	Case-Mix	Total Beds
Occupancy	—	0.26[a]	0.01	−0.39[b]
Percent Medicaid	—	—	0.11[a]	0.08[b]
Case-mix	—	—	—	0.13[a]
Total beds	—	—	—	—

[a]Significant at p < .0001.
[b]Significant at p < .01.

Results of logistic regression are displayed in Table 9. Controlling for all other variables, RN time was significantly related to whether a facility provided high- or low-quality care. The odds ratio indicates that a 15-minute increase in RN time per resident per day increased by 1.73 the odds of a facility providing high-quality care as opposed to providing low-quality care. Size of facility provides a powerful explanatory variable for quality. Facilities with fewer than 60 beds are 9.74 times as likely to be a high-quality facility and facilities with between 61 and 120 beds are 2.28 times as likely to be high-quality facilities than the reference group. Each unit increase in case-mix (3–18 scale) decreased the likelihood of a facility being a high-quality facility by .66. The relationship of type of ownership to high- and low-quality facilities is significant. The reference group for the ownership variable was the for-profit chain group. Based on the regression results, a nonprofit facility is 1.69 times as likely to be a high-quality facility as the reference group; government-owned facilities were 7.02 times as likely to be a high-quality facility as the reference group; and for-profit, nonchain facilities were 1.62 times as likely to be a good facility as the for-profit chain facilities. The government-owned group is a very small group and limited conclusions can be drawn from these data. Finally, rural facilities are 1.58 times as likely to be in the high-quality category.

Discussion

It is important to note that the high-quality facilities selected in this study are not facilities that are necessarily providing care beyond federal and state requirements. They are facilities that, based on the criteria used for selection, are doing what they are supposed to do.

The picture that emerges from this analysis is that RNs, case-mix, type of ownership, and urban or rural location are important factors in determining the probability that a facility will be a high- or low-quality facility. The influence of

TABLE 9 Logistic Regression Predicting High Quality Facilities; Predictors Re-Scaled for Clarity

Variable	Measurement Unit	Parameter Estimate	Standard Error	p	Odds Ratio	Lower Limit	Upper Limit
Intercept		5.07	0.59	0.0001			
Staff							
RN res/day	1/4 hour	0.55	0.12	0.0001	1.73	1.38	2.17
LPN res/day	1/4 hour	0.04	0.08	ns	1.04	0.89	1.22
NA res/day	1/4 hour	-0.01	0.04	ns	0.99	0.91	1.07
Medicaid	percent/10	-0.03	0.04	ns	0.97	0.90	1.05
Size							
< 60 beds	0–1	2.28	0.31	0.0001	9.74	5.25	18.05
61–120 beds	0–1	0.83	0.18	0.0001	2.28	1.60	3.27
≥ 120 beds	[reference group]						
Case-mix	3–19 scale	-0.42	0.05	0.0001	0.66	0.59	0.72
Ownership							
Non-profit	0–1	0.52	0.21	0.01	1.69	1.12	2.54
Government	0–1	1.95	0.63	0.002	7.02	2.05	24.04
For profit	0–1	0.48	0.20	0.02	1.62	1.09	2.41
For profit chain	[reference group]						
Location							
Rural	0–1	0.46	0.19	0.02	1.58	1.09	2.30
Urban	[reference group]						

Medicaid needs to be examined further. High-quality facilities had, in general, fewer Medicaid-covered residents except for the nonchain, for-profit facilities. Medicaid was not statistically significant in the logistic regression, however, probably due to colinearity with other variables such as size and RN, LPN, and NA staff, as evidenced in the bivariate analysis.

These data indicate the importance of RN staff in a nursing home. High-quality facilities not only staff at higher levels than the low-quality facilities, they also staff at levels higher than the national 1994 mean (0.42 compared to 0.34 hours per resident per day) for RNs, while low-quality facilities staff at less than the national mean (0.29 hours per resident per day). The match between services needed by residents and the capabilities of RNs is the likely explanation for the RN effect. While nursing homes of the past may have cared for a relatively stable, self-sufficient population, that no longer accurately describes the current set of residents. Residents have multiple, complicated needs demanding considerable clinical judgment and capability. In addition, the management skills of RNs may also be reflected in the better outcomes. Registered nurses may provide the necessary supervision needed in working with a predominantly nonprofessional staff in a difficult environment.

The finding that a low-quality facility would be nearly twice as likely to become a high-quality facility if it increased its RN staff by 15 minutes per resident per day (or 3.3 RN FTEs per day per 100 residents) has significant implications for staffing. A rough estimate of the cost of adding 3.3 RNs in the 210 low-quality facilities (assuming the average number of beds per facility is 100) would be approximately $22 million. This estimate is based on the national average salary of an RN in a nursing home being $31,298, and does not include fringe benefits or costs of recruitment. If the cost of staff required to bring the 14,000 facilities that fell into neither category into the high-quality category is considered, the total cost could well be in the hundreds of millions of dollars. The issues relating to the cost and quality trade-off are significant. State Medicaid budgets are already stretched beyond capacity, and additional RN time will cost additional dollars that currently are not available.

The importance of staffing based on case-mix is critical. Clearly, as case-mix increases so does the need for additional staff, particularly RNs to meet those needs. The low-quality facilities were trying to care for residents who were significantly more debilitated than those in the high-quality group, using the same number of LPN and NA staff but fewer RNs. This situation then produced facilities that had the highest number of pressure sores per number of bedbound residents, the greatest medication error rates, and the highest use of restraints. The ongoing work of HCFA in the Case-Mix Demonstration Project is very important to determining the levels of staff needed to achieve desired outcomes. As nursing homes care for increasingly debilitated residents, there is a need for sufficient staff both in numbers and capabilities.

The correlation between case-mix, percent Medicaid, occupancy, and total beds supports the notion that larger facilities take more Medicaid residents and residents who are more debilitated in order to fill their beds. The impact on facilities of additional Medicaid residents who are sicker may be the inability to afford increased numbers of staff, particularly if payment is not adjusted for case-mix. Smaller facilities can be more selective in taking less debilitated residents, given they have fewer beds to fill.

This study raises issues about the impact of ownership and quality. The for-profit facilities that are not chain owned fell into the high-quality category at as high a rate as nonprofit facilities while having substantially less staff and the highest proportion of Medicaid-covered residents. Exploring how these facilities manage to provide high-quality care under these circumstances could provide a better understanding of the influence that ownership exerts on care. These findings may reflect a direct commitment and oversight by the owners of nonchain, for-profit facilities that ultimately enhances care.

It should also be noted that chain-owned, for-profit facilities fell into the poor category at a higher rate than expected. This could be due to chain-owned facilities not having a direct accountability or to a management structure in some chain-owned facilities that does not provide effective oversight of quality of care. It should be noted, however, that facilities represented in the low-quality group could be clustered among a few nursing home chains and do not represent all for-profit-chain facilities.

Another important result in regard to type of ownership is that the not-for-profit group of facilities has the least percent of Medicaid residents, while the for-profit, nonchain facilities have the highest percent. One might assume that since the not-for-profit facilities receive some degree of public support though their tax status, not-for-profit facilities would have a greater commitment to providing a public good by taking more Medicaid-supported residents. This, however, is not the case. A possible, but unexplored, explanation may be that the not-for-profit facilities provide a greater amount of free care to residents and that residents simply don't apply for Medicaid assistance.

The finding that rural facilities are more than twice as likely to be a high-quality facility may be explained by several different dynamics. A rural facility may be more sensitive to its community's needs than an urban facility. The community sensitivity may be due to staff knowing the residents they care for and being concerned about the reputation of the facility. Even in rural areas, however, facilities that fell into the low-quality category had a higher percent of Medicaid residents, larger facility size, higher case-mix, and fewer RNs. It is also important to further examine different impacts on rural and urban facilities, since urban facilities in general staff at higher levels than rural facilities. A possible explanation for the higher staff levels is that the turnover rate is greater in urban areas because of numerous opportunities for jobs in the minimum wage category. Large turnover may require additional staff to provide continuity of care. Nursing staff in rural areas may be "locked in" to their jobs because of limited options in the rural community. There could also be a payment bias for higher staffing in urban areas. Finally, overall case-mix was somewhat higher in urban areas, which may account for some portion of the difference in staffing.

The consistent finding that high-quality facilities have fewer beds, after controlling for other variables, suggests that there may not be economies of scale for increasing the size of nursing facilities. The influence of large size may reflect the physical inaccessibility of staff to residents, inability of supervisory staff to effectively oversee care, or the difficulty of a facility in establishing a clear philosophy of caring. A larger facility may also have more difficulty recruiting and retaining competent staff.

Finally, the quality indicators used to select facilities relate solely to physical care. It is not at all clear that the high-quality facilities are those that also provide humane, time intensive end-of-life care or manage residents with behavioral problems well. The authors believe that much could be learned by further examining the high- and low-quality facilities extensively and systematically using qualitative as well as additional quantitative methods of investigation.

Limitations

The major potential limitation of this study is based on use of the OSCAR data for staffing information. Based on the authors' experience with the staffing data, the edits that were done to eliminate major errors produced staffing numbers that were within the range of staffing data reported in Medicaid and Medicare cost reports. In addition, the relationships that were found in this study were consistent with other studies. Another limitation is that quality was defined using physical parameters and not psychologic or social parameters, even though these may be very important to residents.

Conclusions

Based on information presented in both sections of this paper, the overview of nursing homes and the analysis of the high- and low-quality facilities, several important conclusions can be drawn. These include:

1. While the total staff time per resident per day was virtually the same for each category of care, after holding case-mix and other variables constant, the amount of RN time was very important. By increasing RN time by 15 minutes per resident per day, a facility in the low-quality category would have increased the probability nearly twofold that it would fall into the high-quality category. Given the relationship between RNs and quality of care, RN participation in care is very important. The federal requirement of one RN for 8 hours a day, 7 days a week, is not sufficient to ensure quality of care to residents.

2. Case-mix must be the basis for determining staffing needs. The low-

quality care facilities had a higher case-mix, the same level of total staffing, but fewer RNs. In order to provide adequate care, facilities must adjust staffing to accommodate residents who have a greater resource need. Increasing the number of RNs becomes very important as the case-mix index of a facility increases.

3. For all types of ownership, high-quality facilities had higher RN staff levels than the low-quality facilities. The not-for-profit and government-owned facilities, however, had higher RN levels for high-quality facilities than either category of for-profit high-quality facilities. It will be useful to examine the for-profit, nonchain group of facilities in that they staffed at lower levels than non-profit and government-owned facilities, yet had no higher than expected number of facilities in the poor care category.

4. Any discussion of staffing must take into account financing of staffing needs. Medicaid is the major payer for nursing home care, but Medicaid budgets are likely to decrease rather than increase. Data from this study indicate that low-quality facilities have a higher proportion of Medicaid residents. Given that Medicaid rates are usually lower than private pay rates, this may contribute to financial constraints in hiring additional staff. Policymakers are faced with an extremely tough choice with the trade-off between quality and cost. Considering that the population is aging and there is no cure for Alzheimer's and other chronic diseases, the demand for nursing home care will likely expand and funding mechanisms will need to ensure adequate staffing to meet the care needs of residents.

5. Additional research is needed to continue exploring the relationship between staffing inputs and resident outcomes. The case-mix project has gone a long way to examine resource needs and staffing needs. Yet the work of this project will not be complete until resident needs and staffing are linked to quality-of-care outcomes. In addition, a research agenda should be developed that focuses on qualitative aspects of nursing home care, including further study of resident and family needs and definitions of quality, and organizational characteristics affecting care. The categorization of high- and low-quality facilities was based on physical measures, which can at best provide only a partial examination of quality.

6. Given the importance of RN staff, it is necessary that educational programs prepare RNs for a leadership role in nursing facilities. If LPNs are to substitute for RNs and remain an important level of nursing staff, their capabilities in managing their role in nursing homes will need to be enhanced so that they can have a greater effect on positive resident outcomes.

REFERENCES

Abt Associates, Inc. Briefing Points on Preliminary Evaluation Requests. HCFA Leadership Conference, 1993.

American Health Care Association. *Facts and Trends: The Nursing Facility Sourcebook.* Washington, D.C.: The Association, 1994.

American Health Care Association. *Facts and Trends: The Nursing Facility Sourcebook.* Washington, D.C.: The Association, 1995.

Brandeis, G.H. Ooi, W.L., Hossain, M., et al. A Longitudinal Study of Risk Factors Associated with the Formation of Pressure Ulcers in Nursing Homes. *Journal of the American Geriatrics Society* 42:388–393, 1994.

Brooks, S., Warshaw, G., Hasse, L., and Kues, J.R. The Physician Decision-making Process in Transferring Nursing Home Patients to the Hospital. *Archives of Internal Medicine* 154:902–908, 1994.

Butler, P.A., and Schlenker, R.E. Case-mix Reimbursement for Nursing Homes: Objectives and Achievements. *Milbank Quarterly* 67:103–135, 1989.

Cherry, R. Agents of Nursing Home Quality of Care: Ombudsmen and Staff Ratios Revisited. *The Gerontologist* 31:302–308, 1991.

DeSisto, M. Residents Perspective of Nursing Home Care. Presentation at Maine Health Care Association meeting, 1994.

Fries, B.E., Schneider, D.P., Foley, W.J., et al. Refining a Case-Mix Measure for Nursing Homes: Resource Utilization Groups (RUG-III). *Medical Care* 32:668–685, 1994.

Hanson, H.A. Highlights of National Survey of Gerontological Nursing in the AND Curriculum. *The Community College–Nursing Home Partnership Newslink,* 1992.

Health Data Associates. *Nursing Home Yearbook.* Tacoma, Wash.: Health Data Associates, 1994.

Institute of Medicine. *Improving the Quality of Care in Nursing Homes.* Washington, D.C.: National Academy Press, 1986.

Johnson, J.Y. Curricular Trends in Accredited Generic Baccalaureate Nursing Programs Across the United States. *Journal of Nursing Education* 34:53–60, 1995.

Johnson-Pawlson, J. The Relationship Between Nursing Staff Variables and Quality of Care in Nursing Homes. UMI Dissertation Services. O.N. 9316112, 1993a.

Johnson-Pawlson, J. *Surveyor Performance Study.* Washington, D.C.: American Health Care Association, 1993b.

Karuza, and J., and Katz, P.R. Physician Staffing Patterns Correlates of Nursing Home Care: An Initial Inquiry and Consideration of Policy Implication. *Journal of the American Geriatrics Society* 42:787–793, 1994.

Lavizzo-Mourey, R.J., Zinn, J., and Taylor, L. Ability of Surrogates to Represent Satisfaction of Nursing Home Residents with Quality of Care. *Journal of the American Geriatrics Society* 40:39–47, 1992.

Mezey, M.D., and Lynaugh J.E. The Teaching Nursing Home Program. *Nursing Clinics of North America* 24:769–780, 1989.

Morrisey, M.A., Sloan, F.A., and Valvona, J. Medicare Prospective Payment and Posthospital Transfers to Subacute Care. *Medical Care* 26:685–698, 1988.

Moses, E. *The Registered Nurse Population. Findings from the National Sample Survey of Registered Nurses, March 1992.* Washington, D.C.: Division of Nursing, Bureau of Health Professions, Health Resources and Services Administration, U.S. Department of Health and Human Services, 1994.

Munroe, D.J. The Influence of Registered Nurse Staffing on the Quality of Nursing Home Care. *Research in Nursing and Health* 13:263–270, 1990.

National Center for Health Statistics. Characteristics of Registered Nurses in Nursing Homes: Preliminary Data from the 1985 Nursing Home Survey. *Advance Data from Vital and Health Statistics,* No. 152. Prepared by G. Strahan. Pub. no. (PHS) 88–1250. Hyattsville, Md.: National Center for Health Statistics, U.S Department of Health and Human Services, 1988.

National Citizen's Coalition for Nursing Home Reform. Quality of Care from a Nursing Home Resident Perspective. Washington, D.C.: The Coalition, 1986.

Office of Inspector General. States' Progress in Carrying Out Nursing Home Survey Reforms. Washington, D.C.: Department of Health and Human Services, 1993.

Rodman, D., Slater, E.J., Richardson, T.J., and Mattson, D.E. The Occurrence of Pressure Ulcers in Three Nursing Homes. *Journal of General Internal Medicine* 8:653–658, 1993.

Rodman, D., Bross, D., and Mattson, D.E. Clinical Indicators Derived from the Patient Assessment Instrument in the Long-Stay Residents of 69 VA Nursing Homes. *Journal of General Internal Medicine* 9:261–267, 1994.

Sager, M.A., Easterling, D.V., Kindig, D.A., and Anderson, O.W. Changes in the Location of Death After Passage of Medicare's Prospective Payment System. *New England Journal of Medicine* 320:433–439, 1989.

Schnelle, J.F., Newman, D.R., Fogarty, T.E., et al. Assessment and Quality Control of Incontinence Care in Long-term Nursing Facilities. *Journal of the American Geriatrics Society* 39(2)165–171, 1991.

Shaughnessy, P., and Kramer, A. The Increased Needs of Patients in Nursing Homes and Patients Receiving Home Health Care. *New England Journal of Medicine* 322:21–27, 1990.

Spector, W.D., and Takada, H. Characteristics of Nursing Homes that Affect Resident Outcomes. *Journal of Aging and Health* 3:427–454, 1991.

Weinberg, A.D., Pals, J.K., Levesque, P.G., et al. Dehydration and Death During Febrile Episodes in the Nursing Home. *Journal of the American Geriatrics Society* 42:968–971, 1994.

Weissert, W. and Musliner, M. *Access, Quality and Cost Consequences of Case-Mix Adjusted Reimbursement for Nursing Homes: A Critical Review of the Evidence.* Washington, D.C.: Public Policy Institute, American Association of Retired Persons, 1992.

Werner, P., Koroknay, V., Braun, J., and Cohen-Mansfield, J. Individualized Care Alternatives Used in the Process of Removing Physical Restraints in the Nursing Home. *Journal of the American Geriatric Society* 42:321–325, 1994.

Williams, B.C., Fries, B., Foley, W.J., et al. Activities of Daily Living and Costs in Nursing Homes. *Health Care Financing Review* 15:117–135, 1994.

Nursing Facility Quality, Staffing, and Economic Issues

Charlene A. Harrington, Ph.D.

Nursing facilities are an important component of a health industry that is increasingly complex. This paper examines the interrelationships of quality, staffing, costs, and ownership. The paper is divided into two sections. First, quality of care in nursing facilities (or nursing homes) is discussed including a review of how to measure quality. The quality of care continues to vary widely with some facilities known to provide exceptional care. On the other hand, two decades of studies have identified poor quality of care provided by some nursing facilities. Federal and state regulatory efforts have been initiated to improve quality but quality continues to be problematic.

Quality problems are closely associated with historic low registered nurse (RN) staffing levels in nursing facilities. Research on the relationship between staffing levels and quality is reviewed. A discussion of data on current staffing levels and appropriate staffing levels is presented along with discussion of current regulatory efforts to ensure adequate staffing.

Quality of care and staffing are intricately related to nursing home economics, discussed in Part II of this paper. The growing demand for nursing home care and the constrained supply of services form the context for examining these issues. Public reimbursement policies and industry resource allocation decisions have direct effects on both staffing levels and quality of care. Political and

Dr. Harrington is chair of the Department of Social and Behavioral Sciences, School of Nursing, University of California, San Francisco.

economic factors influence the feasibility of new policies to improve the care for nursing home residents.

PART I: QUALITY OF NURSING HOME CARE

Quality of care is the basic product of nursing facility care and the focus of providers, consumers, regulators, and public policymakers. Defining quality has been a difficult process. Traditionally, three types of indicators have been classified by Donabedian (1980) to define and measure the quality of care: structure, process, and outcomes. Structural measures include human, organizational, and material resources (e.g., size, ownership). Because such structural measures are the most objective, reliable, easily measured, and readily available, structural measures have historically formed the basis for quality indicators. Staffing is a structural measure that affects the processes and outcomes of care, but is considered in part to be determined by facility ownership and payment sources. Studies of nursing facilities generally consider the special characteristics of nursing home residents (physical, mental, and social) that could increase the difficulty of providing high quality of care.

Although structural measures assess the availability of resources as a necessary precondition for their use, process measures examine actual services or activities provided to residents. The process of care focuses on providing special care and treatments to prevent problems with outcomes such as cognition, communication and hearing, vision, physical functioning, continence, psychosocial functioning, mood and behavior, oral, nutritional, and dental care, skin condition, and medications (Morris et al., 1990). A number of studies of nursing home quality have examined process measures with nursing home quality (Zimmer, 1983, 1989; Zimmer et al., 1986). The most important approach to quality focuses on individual or group outcomes, but structure and process information are also needed (Kane, 1988; Kane and Kane, 1988).

Measuring Quality of Care

Over the past two decades, many efforts have been undertaken to refine the measures of nursing home quality. Simple unidimensional quantitative measures of quality have frequently been used in research, such as staff hours per patient day (Fottler et al., 1981; Greene and Monahan, 1981; Elwell, 1984), changes in physical functioning (Linn et al., 1977), mortality rates or hospital readmission rates (Lewis et al., 1985; GAO, 1988a,b; Spector and Takada, 1991), the number of deficiencies (Nyman, 1989b), and subjective measures (Hay, 1977).

Moos and Lemke (1984a,b) developed one of the early methods for conducting assessments of residential facilities on multidimensions: the Multiphasic Environmental Assessment Procedure (MEAP). The MEAP measures resources in terms of four conceptual domains: resident and staff characteristics, physical features, policies and services, and the social climate (Moos and Lemke, 1984a,b). The MEAP instruments are expensive to administer and are more appropriate for residential living arrangements than for skilled nursing facilities. Shaughnessy and his colleagues developed measures of nursing home processes of care. Using expert panels, 27 patient problems were categorized into 4 groups: nursing, medical, communicative, and psychosocial problems. Processes were measured through a comparison of the frequency and the provider type for each service rendered with preset standards for such services for each patient problem (Shaughnessy and Kramer, 1989; Shaughnessy et al., 1990).

Kane and colleagues (1983a,b) developed a multidimensional approach to measuring quality of care utilizing data from chart reviews, observations, and interviewer ratings. This approach was utilized in a longitudinal study of nursing home residents (Kane et al., 1983a,b). Gustafson and colleagues (1980, 1990) also constructed an instrument for measuring nursing home quality entitled the Quality Assessment Index (QAI). The QAI is a multidimensional instrument that used expert panels of judges to develop components of quality each with three to seven subcomponents. This instrument was used to measure quality in a 2-day nursing home visit. Zimmerman and colleagues (1985) used the QAI instrument to evaluate the state survey processes in three states for the Health Care Financing Administration (HCFA). The QAI also requires primary data collection that is costly to collect.

All of these instruments use primary data collection from individual residents. They are primarily designed to identify problems with quality for individuals and not to measure facility quality (except for the QAI instrument). Instruments for measuring quality that require primary data collection efforts on residents are costly to administer and impractical for use as a national approach to measuring quality (Harrington, 1990a). In spite of these many efforts, quality measures continue to be difficult to define and measure, especially for individuals with deteriorating conditions such as many of the residents of nursing facilities. Extensive research efforts continue to be needed in order to develop better process and outcome measures.

Variations in Quality of Care

A number of nursing facilities have been noted for providing high quality of care. The National Institute on Aging and the Robert Wood Johnson (RWJ) Foundation both initiated teaching nursing home programs to improve quality of care during the 1980s. The RWJ project was a 5-year program that ended in 1987 in 12 nursing facilities. These programs added geriatric and geropsychiatric nurse practitioners and clinicians to nursing facilities in collaboration with schools of nursing. The findings from the studies of these programs were that these nursing personnel were able to reduce hospitalization rates, bowel and urinary incontinence, and restraint use and to improve care (Mezey and Lynaugh, 1989,

1991). These programs were found to be successful and documented in a series of articles and books (Mezey et al., 1989; Shaughnessy and Kramer, 1989).

Poor Quality of Care

The quality of care provided in nursing facilities has long been a matter of great concern to consumers, health care professionals, and policymakers (NCCNHR, 1983). The Institute of Medicine (IOM) Committee on Nursing Home Regulation reported widespread quality-of-care problems (IOM, 1986). The problems were confirmed by the General Accounting Office (GAO, 1987) and the U.S. Senate (1986), which found that many of the nation's nursing facilities were operating at a substandard level by failing to meet minimum nursing home requirements considered to affect residents' health and safety.

A number of clinical practices have been associated with poor patient outcomes. Urethral catheterization may place residents at greater risk for urinary infection and hospitalization or other complications such as bladder and renal stones, abscesses, and renal failure (Ouslander et al., 1982; Ouslander and Kane, 1984; Ribeiro and Smith, 1985). Restraints have been under criticism because their use may cause decreased muscle tone, and increase the likelihood of falls, incontinence, pressure ulcers, depression, confusion, and mental deterioration (Evans and Strumpf, 1989; Libow and Starer, 1989; Burton et al., 1992; Phillips et al., 1993). A recent study by Phillips and colleagues (1993) suggests that the use of physical restraints continues to be a problem and the use of such restraints should require more nursing care and more nursing assistant time. They concluded that residents free of restraints are less costly to provide care to and that this could improve the quality of care and quality of life. Tube feedings also increase the risk of complications including lung infections, aspiration, misplacement of the tube, and pain (Libow and Starer, 1989). The improper use of psychotrophic drugs has been identified as a common problem in nursing facilities in numerous studies (Harrington et al., 1992b). Recent Senate hearings focused on the problems associated with the misuse and inappropriate use of chemical restraints, which the regulations of the 1990 Omnibus Budget Reconciliation Act were designed to reduce (U.S. Senate, 1991).

There are many negative outcomes in nursing facilities that have been identified in numerous studies (Zinn et al., 1993a,b). These include urinary incontinence, falls, weight loss, and infectious disease (Libow and Starer, 1989). Declines in physical functioning that could have been prevented are also important negative outcomes (Linn et al., 1977). Mortality rates or hospital readmission rates are simple outcome measures that are commonly used (Lewis et al., 1985; GAO, 1988a,b; Spector and Takada, 1991). Other common negative outcomes include accidents, behavioral and emotional problems, cognitive problems, psychotropic drugs reactions, and decubitus ulcers (Zinn et al., 1993a,b).

A recent analysis of the On-Line Survey Certification and Reporting (OS-

CAR) data showed that state surveyors continue to find problems with nursing home care. Data on all nursing facilities in the United States surveyed in 1993 found that 30 percent were given deficiencies for unsanitary food, 25 percent for inadequate care planning, 20 percent for inadequate sanitary environment, 20 percent for hazards in the environment, 19 percent for failure to maintain personal dignity, 18 percent for improper restraints, 16 percent for having no comprehensive assessment, 15 percent for inadequate infection control, 12 percent for inadequate treatment of incontinence, 12 percent for inadequate activities for residents, and other facilities received deficiencies for other problems (Harrington et al., 1995). (See Table 1.) The frequency of these deficiencies show that quality problems continue to exist in many nursing facilities.

In summary, probably no other type of health care organization has been demonstrated to have as many quality-of-care problems as nursing facilities. These problems have demonstrated the need for continued research and the development of public policies that could improve both the process and outcomes of care.

Regulatory Efforts

In order to participate in the Medicare or Medicaid programs, long-term-care facilities are required to meet federal certification requirements established by HCFA (42 CFR Part 843) under the Social Security Act. Long-term-care facilities include skilled nursing facilities (SNF) for Medicare (Title 18), nursing facilities (NF) for Medicaid (Title 19), and dually-certified facilities (for both Title 18 and 19). State survey agencies are authorized to determine whether SNFs and NFs meet the federal requirements. Surveyors conduct on-site inspections to observe care, review records, and determine compliance. These surveys are used as the basis for entering into, denying, or terminating a provider agreement with the facility.

In the early 1980s, the Reagan administration proposed deregulation of the nursing home industry. At the same time, Congress was concerned about quality-of-care problems in nursing facilities because of reports and complaints by consumer groups. Problems with the regulatory process had been identified in an evaluation of the state survey processes (Zimmerman et al., 1985). Because of the growing concern about nursing home quality, Congress requested a study by the IOM to examine the regulation of nursing facilities. The IOM Committee on Nursing Home Regulation documented quality-of-care problems and recommended revision and strengthening of the federal and state regulatory processes (IOM, 1986). Their recommendations, as well as the active efforts of many consumer advocacy and professional organizations, resulted in Congress passing the Omnibus Budget Reconciliation Act of 1987 (OBRA 87), a major reform of nursing home regulation (OBRA 87, 1987). This legislation was refined under subsequent legislation in 1988, 1989, and 1990.

TABLE 1 Deficiencies in Certified Nursing Facilities from the Federal On-Line Survey Certification and Reporting System, United States, 1993

Types of Deficiencies	Percent of Facilities with Deficiency
Process Deficiencies	
Unsanitary food (The facility must prepare and serve food under sanitary conditions; F377)	30
Inadequate care plan (The facility must develop a comprehensive care plan for each resident; F295)	25
Inadequate sanitary environment (The facility must provide housekeeping/ maintenance services for a sanitary environment; F261)	20
Hazards in the environment (The facility must ensure that the resident environment remains free of accident hazards; F329)	20
Improper restraints (Residents have the right to be free of physical restraints used for discipline or facility convenience; F221)	18
No comprehensive assessment (The facility must make a comprehensive assessment of resident needs; F271)	16
Inadequate infection control (The facility must investigate, control, and prevent infections; F441)	15
Inadequate activities (The facility must provide an ongoing program of activities to meet resident needs; F255)	12
No 24-hour nursing (The facility must provide sufficient numbers of personnel on a 24-hour basis; F354)	5
No RN on duty 7 days a week (The facility must have an RN on duty 8 hours a day for 7 days a week; F356)	5
Outcome deficiencies	
Failure to maintain dignity (The facility must promote care for residents that maintains dignity and respect; F241)	19
Inadequate treatment of incontinence (Incontinent residents must receive appropriate treatment; F322)	12
Failure to prevent pressure sores (The facility must ensure that residents without pressure sores do not develop them; F319)	9

TABLE 1 Continued

Types of Deficiencies	Percent of Facilities with Deficiency
Inadequate treatment of pressure sores (The facility must provide necessary treatment to residents with pressure sores; F320)	9
Poor nutrition (The facility must ensure that residents maintain acceptable levels of nutritional status; F331)	9
Abuse of residents (Residents have the right to be free of verbal, mental, and other abuse; F233)	2

NOTE: The relevant deficiency code follows the description of what the facility is obliged to provide.

SOURCE: Harrington et al., 1995.

The nursing home reform legislation in OBRA 87, which was implemented by HCFA regulations in October 1990, mandated a number of changes. First, the regulations eliminated the priority hierarchy of conditions, standards, and elements that were in the prior regulations. Second, the new 1990 regulations mandated comprehensive assessments of all nursing home residents using the new minimum data set (MDS) forms (Morris et al., 1990). Nursing facilities must complete the MDS forms for each resident within 14 days of admission and at least annually in order to assess the functional, cognitive, and affective levels of residents and must use the assessment in the care planning process. The federal survey procedures (conducted by state agencies) check the accuracy and appropriateness of the assessment and care planning process for a sample of residents. Third, more specific requirements for nursing, medical, and psychosocial services were designed to attain and maintain the highest practicable mental and physical functional status (Zimmerman, 1990).

These requirements were specified in new regulations and a detailed set of HCFA interpretive guidelines were developed for use by state surveyors in 1990. The state surveys were redesigned to be more outcome oriented than previously. Such outcome measures include residents' behavior, their functional and mental status, and conditions (e.g., incontinence, immobility, and decubitus ulcers). For example, the regulations established criteria for the use of antipsychotic drugs, prohibited their use without a specific indication of need, and required periodic review and dose reduction unless clinically contraindicated (Zimmerman, 1990). In addition, regulations detailing and protecting residents' rights were added.

One important recent advance was the development of the Nursing Home

Resident Assessment System. This system used the nursing home MDS for resident assessment and developed detailed protocols for resident assessment of specific problem areas to guide the care planning process (Morris et al., 1990). The MDS items were field-tested in 1990 and finalized with 15 domains: cognitive patterns, communication and hearing patterns, vision patterns, physical functioning and structural problems, continence, psychosocial well-being, mood and behavior patterns, activity pursuit patterns, disease diagnoses, health conditions, oral and nutritional status, oral and dental status, skin condition, medication use, and special treatments and procedures (Morris et al., 1990). Since October 1990, nursing facilities are required by HCFA to collect MDS data for every resident upon admission, when there are major changes in health status, and at least annually.

Zimmerman is currently developing Quality Indicators (QI) using the Minimum Data Set as a part of the National Nursing Home Case-Mix and Quality Demonstration study funded by HCFA. This effort builds upon his earlier work with the QAI to develop new QIs. Using MDS data on individual nursing home residents, a number of QIs have been developed: accidents, behavioral and emotional problems, cognitive problems, incontinence, psychotropic drugs, decubitus ulcers, physical restraints, weight problems, infections, and others. The QIs for individual residents and for facilities are compared to national norms, taking into account predisposing factors and case-mix factors related to each QI. Quality indicators that may indicate poor quality of care are identified and given to state surveyors to examine in the certification survey process. Using QI data, state surveyors are expected to determine whether or not the identified QIs are the result of, or are related to, poor care processes.

HCFA regulations are being proposed to require nursing facilities to computerize the MDS data, and then the QIs may be a valuable tool for monitoring the quality of nursing home care. The QIs will augment the nursing home survey process that collects and monitors quality of care for facilities for federal Medicare and Medicaid certification.

In November 1994, HCFA (1994a) released its final regulations for the survey, certification, and enforcement of skilled nursing facilities and nursing facilities (42 CFR Parts 401–498). The regulations made changes in the process of surveying and certifying facilities and developed procedures for enforcement. A number of alternative remedies instead of or in addition to termination may be imposed on facilities that do not comply with federal requirements. These include civil money penalties of up to $10,000, denial of payment for new admissions, state monitoring, temporary management, and other approaches. The extent and type of enforcement actions depend upon the scope (whether deficiencies are isolated, constitute a pattern, or are widespread) and severity of violations (whether there is harm or jeopardy to residents). The Health Care Financing Administration is also undertaking new efforts to train state surveyors in using the new survey, certification, and enforcement procedures.

Is Quality Improving?

One question is whether quality of care is improving as a result of increased efforts by the federal government to regulate quality. Consumer groups and anecdotal evidence from providers suggest there are improvements in nursing home care (Cotton, 1993). There are reports that a number of facilities have focused on reducing the inappropriate use of physical and chemical restraints and that the federal survey focus on resident problems represent substantial improvements in the survey process.

The U.S. Office of the Inspector General (1993) concluded that positive improvements are being made in the regulatory process. State budgets for regulation increased and state survey agencies were using the new resident outcome approach. Complaints about nursing facilities, however, were increasing on average by 74 percent, and state facilities expressed concern about their ability to respond to complaints quickly and effectively. The report concluded that work to improve the current survey process continues to be needed (U.S. Office of the Inspector General, 1993). A national evaluation of the survey process also identified a number of areas where improvement is needed in the survey process (Abt Associates and the Center for Health Policy Research, 1993). The recent release of the final federal enforcement regulations for skilled nursing facilities and nursing facilities should also improve the regulatory process (HCFA, 1994a).

It remains to be seen whether these extensive new regulatory efforts can make a substantial impact on improving the quality of care in nursing facilities. Deficiencies issued to facilities have actually declined since OBRA was implemented. The average deficiencies declined from 8.8 per facility in 1991 to 7.9 in 1993 (Harrington et al., 1995). Survey data also show that the percent of facilities without any deficiencies has increased slightly to 11.4 percent in 1993. Although the nursing facilities argue that this is an indication of improvements in quality of care, such declines could indicate problems with the enforcement process.

In summary, in spite of the recent possible improvements in nursing home quality and regulations, the quality of care provided by some nursing facilities is still problematic. The number and type of deficiencies and complaints reported by the state licensing agencies, consumer advocacy groups, families, and residents show poor quality in some facilities.

Nursing Home Staffing

Pre-OBRA Staffing Levels

Staffing is a critical structural factor that affects the processes and outcomes of nursing home care. Staffing levels in nursing facilities have been traditionally low and these are considered to affect quality of care directly. Of the 1.2 million full-time-equivalent (FTE) nursing home employees providing direct or indirect care, the National Nursing Home Survey indicates that about 7 percent were RNs in 1985 (Strahan, 1987). The ratios of nurses to residents has traditionally been substantially below the nurse-to-patient ratios in hospitals. In 1985, the national average was 1 RN per 49 patients in nursing facilities in contrast to a ratio of 1 RN for every 8 patients in hospitals (Jones et al., 1987; Strahan, 1987; Kanda and Mezey, 1991).

Another analysis of the National Nursing Home survey data reported an overall average of 6.3 RNs per 100 beds in 1985 (or 0.063 FTEs per bed). (FTEs can be converted to hours per resident day by multiplying by 35 hours per week for each nurse and dividing by 7 for each resident day.) Converting FTEs to resident hours showed that the average RN hours per resident day was 0.3 hours (19 minutes) in 1985 (Strahan, 1988). Of the total nursing staff in nursing facilities in 1985, 12 percent were RNs, 17 percent were licensed vocational nurses (LVN), and 71 percent were nurses assistants (NA). The total direct care staff was 0.43 FTEs per resident day, or 2.15 hours per resident day (Strahan, 1987).

Similar staffing ratios were identified in a study of 14,000 nursing facilities in 1987 using federal Medicare and Medicaid Automated Certification Survey (MMACS) data (now referred to as OSCAR data). Zinn (1993b) found that the average number of RNs per resident over 24 hours was 0.04 FTEs, licensed practical nurses (LPN) per resident was 0.09 FTEs, and aides per resident was 0.32 FTEs. The total direct care staffing per resident was an average of 0.45 FTEs per day. Zinn (1993a) found wide variations in nursing home staffing patterns in 10 standard metropolitan statistical areas, even after controlling for case-mix differences in residents using 1987 MMACS survey data. The number of RNs per resident over 24 hours varied from 0.01 FTEs in Oklahoma to 0.08 FTEs in Boston.

OBRA 87 Nurse Staffing Minimum Standards

The IOM Committee on Nursing Home Regulation recommended that nurse staffing standards be increased to improve the overall quality of nursing care (IOM, 1986). Following this recommendation, Congress increased the minimum standards for nursing home staffing in OBRA 87. This legislation was implemented in the 1990 Medicare and Medicaid regulations for SNFs and NFs, requiring a RN director of nursing, an RN on duty for 8 hours a day, 7 days a week, and a licensed nurse (either an RN, a licensed practical/vocational nurse, or both) on duty around the clock for nursing facilities (HCFA, 1991). OBRA 87 also required that nursing assistants must receive minimum training (75 hours) and be tested for competency. In addition, sufficient nursing staff were required to provide nursing and related services to attain or maintain the highest practicable level of physical, mental, and psychosocial well-being of each resident (HCFA, 1991).

Staffing regulations for Medicare skilled nursing facilities are the same as for Medicaid, where both are required to meet the actual care needs of clients. Because Medicare skilled nursing residents have higher care needs than Medicaid residents, Medicare has traditionally had higher staffing levels. Many Medicare certified beds are in acute care facilities where staffing levels have been higher than in freestanding facilities. Medicare payment rates are substantially higher than Medicaid rates to take these higher resident care and resource needs into account (Dor, 1989).

The OBRA 87 legislation allowed for waivers to the minimal nursing facility staffing requirements in areas where it may be difficult to hire RNs. Staffing waivers for Medicaid-only certified facilities (Title 19) can be granted by states, whereas staffing waivers for facilities with both Medicare and Medicaid certification (Title 18 and 19 facilities) or Medicare-only certified facilities (Title 18 only) must be granted by HCFA. The law allows the 24-hour licensed nursing coverage requirements and the 8 hours of RN coverage for 7 days a week to both be waived by states, but Medicare facilities are only allowed to have waivers for the 8 hours of RN coverage for 2 out of 7 days a week.

Recent data from HCFA (1994b) reported that 518 facilities in 13 states had been granted waivers for Medicaid-only facilities by states through 1994. These included 66 waivers for the 24-hour licensed nursing coverage and 490 waivers for the 8 hours of RN coverage. As of March 1994, only 16 waivers had been given to Medicare skilled nursing facilities (Title 18 and 19 or Title 18 only) for the 8 hours of RN coverage by HCFA. At this point, HCFA has not released guidelines to the states for issuing waivers. Perhaps the number of waivers will decline as the availability of RNs improves with recent layoffs of hospital nurses.

Mohler surveyed states regarding their staffing requirements for nursing facilities. She found that the majority of states had specific minimum staffing standards in addition to the federal standards for nursing facilities. These standards varied across states with some states specifying standards for RNs, others for nursing assistants, and still other states having standards for both (Mohler, 1993). Minnesota required a minimum of 2 hours of nursing care per resident day for all licensed nursing facilities but these were not required to be distributed evenly across the evening or night shifts (Chapin and Silloway, 1992). States are allowed to impose state penalties for facilities who have substandard staffing according to state regulations. Thus, the data demonstrate that minimum staffing standards for nursing facilities are considered necessary by most states, as well as by the federal government.

Staffing Levels After OBRA 87

Data from the 1991 National Health Provider Inventory identified 15,511 nursing facilities with 1,457,703 million residents (Moses, 1994a). For this group of residents, there was a national ratio of 0.069 RN FTEs per resident and a total of 0.55 direct care staff FTEs per resident (Moses, 1994a). When FTEs were converted to hours per resident day, the total RNs per resident day was 0.35 hours (21 minutes), and the total direct care staff was 2.75 hours per resident. This showed a slight increase in overall staff ratios over the 18 minutes of RNs time and 2.15 hours of total staff time per resident day reported above on the 1985 national nursing home survey (Strahan, 1988). These ratios do not, however, include vacation and sick time estimates. Moreover, the above estimates assume that staff are evenly distributed over 24 hours, which is not generally the situation. Most health facilities have fewer staff on evening and night shifts because there are somewhat fewer care activities than during the day. Staffing is usually lower on holidays and weekends, in terms of both licensed personnel ratios and total numbers of staff.

Detailed staffing data collected by state surveys were available from the federal OSCAR system. Staffing ratios from OSCAR were examined separately for Medicaid-only (Title 19) facilities and for Medicare-only (Title 18) or Medicare and Medicaid facilities (Title 18 and 19) surveyed during the calendar years of 1991, 1992, and 1993. These data were cleaned to eliminate facilities that appeared to be reporting erroneous data. This eliminated about 1 percent of facilities that reported low staffing levels and a little over 2 percent that reported high staffing levels (Harrington et al., 1995).

This analysis showed the ratio of RNs was 0.3 hours (18 minutes) per resident day, of LPN or LVN hours was 0.6, and of NA hours were 2.0 for a nursing total of 2.9 hours per resident day in about 12,000 Medicaid-only facilities for the 3-year period (Harrington et al., 1995). (See Table 2.) As expected, staffing levels for facilities with both Medicare and Medicaid certification were substantially higher, but this included only about 1,200 facilities. For these facilities the RN hours per resident day increased from 1.0 in 1991 to 1.4 in 1993 (84 minutes). The LPN or LVN hours per resident day increased from 1.2 in 1991 to 1.5 in 1993. The NA hours per resident day increased from 2.4 to 2.7 over the 3-year period. The total nursing hours per resident day increased from 4.4 in 1991 to 5.2 in 1993 (Harrington et al., 1995). Thus, staffing levels for all categories increased somewhat over the 3-year period for facilities with both Medicare and Medicaid certification, but essentially no change was observed for facilities with only Medicaid certification.

Data from OSCAR showed that there was a total of 56 facilities in 20 states in the United States that did not report any RN hours in 1991, 112 facilities in 1992, and 96 facilities in 1993 (Harrington et al., 1995). It was not known whether this was a result of reporting errors or represented an actual absence of RN staff. State surveyors did give nursing facilities deficiencies for failure to meet the minimum staffing levels. Five percent of facilities were given deficien-

TABLE 2 Nurse Staffing Levels for All Certified Nursing Facilities from the Federal On-Line Survey Certification and Reporting System, 1991–1993

Nurse Staffing Levels	Year		
	1991	1992	1993
Medicaid-Only Facilities			
Number of facilities	9,120	12,463	12,132
Hours per resident day			
RNs	0.3	0.3	0.3
LPNs	0.6	0.6	0.6
NAs	2.0	1.9	2.0
Total nurse hours[a]	2.9	2.8	2.9
Medicare/Medicaid and Medicare-Only Facilities			
Number of facilities	819	1,110	1,234
Hours per resident day			
RNs	1.0	1.2	1.4
LPNs	1.2	1.4	1.5
NAs	2.4	2.5	2.7
Total nurse hours[a]	4.4	4.8	5.2

NOTE: RN = registered nurse; LPN = licensed practical nurse; NA = nurse assistant.

[a]The columns do no necessarily add to the total nurse hours because the number of facilities is not the same in each category. The number represents the national average for facilities on which data are available.

SOURCE: Harrington et al., 1995.

cies for failure to have 24-hour nursing staff and 5 percent for failure to have RNs on duty 7 days a week in 1993 (Harrington et al., 1995).

As noted above, some reporting problems with the current OSCAR staffing data were identified (Harrington et al., 1995). Actual staffing levels in nursing facilities may be lower than the levels reported on OSCAR because of over-reporting, reporting errors, or both. Staffing data are reported to HCFA by facilities. Such data are not always audited nor confirmed by state surveyors. Moreover, HCFA guidelines for determining minimum staffing violations are not available.

Poor Nursing Compensation and its Consequences

Low compensation levels (salaries and benefits) have been a historic problem for nurses in nursing facilities compared with hospitals. The overall average annual earnings of RNs employed full-time in nursing facilities was $33,846 in 1992. This overall RN average was 14 percent lower in nursing facilities than in hospitals. Average staff nurses in nursing facilities had annual earnings 17 percent below average hospital staff nurses. This was especially low considering that RNs working in nursing facilities were more likely to be administrators (24 percent) than nurses in hospitals (3 percent). In fact, the average salary of nursing home nurses was lower than salaries in any other setting except for those in student health care services (Moses, 1994b).

In 1992, the average salary and benefits per FTE in nursing facilities (includes all nursing and nonnursing employees) were reported to be $20,238 by HCIA and Arthur Andersen (1994). This level was lower in investor-owned facilities ($19,961) and system-affiliated facilities ($20,642) and higher in non-profit facilities ($21,676). Salary levels were also lower in smaller facilities. The fact that many nursing facilities do not provide their employees with health benefits is also a problem. Recently, the American Health Care Association (AHCA) estimated that if mandatory national health insurance were adopted by Congress, nursing facility costs passed on to Medicaid would increase by $1 billion and costs to Medicare would increase by $100 million. The 1994 average health insurance costs for nursing facilities were estimated to be 3.9 to 5.9 percent of payroll. If all employees were provided health benefits, the health insurance costs would increase to 7.9 percent of payroll (AHCA, 1994).

Poor nursing home compensation encourages nurses to seek alternative employment in other health positions or outside the industry in better working environments. The traditionally high employee turnover rates in some facilities are directly related to low salaries and benefits (Harrington, 1990b). Nursing home nurses have had higher turnover rates than hospital nurses. Only 82 percent of the RNs reported working in a nursing home in the previous year compared with 92 percent for hospital nurses (Moses, 1994b). Munroe (1990) found turnover rates of over 100 percent in California nursing facilities in 1986. Where there is an adequate supply of nursing personnel some nursing facilities may encourage high turnover rates as a means of keeping average wage rates low (Harrington, 1990b). High turnover rates reduce the continuity of care and are expected to have a negative impact on quality of patient care (Harrington, 1990b). Munroe (1990) found that high RN turnover was associated with poor quality (in terms of the number of deficiencies given a facility) in a study of California nursing facilities.

Zinn (1993b) found that nursing facilities adjust staffing and care practices to local market conditions as would be expected. Her study of 14,000 nursing facilities in 1987 found that nursing facilities respond to local economic factors.

In areas where RN wages were higher, nursing facilities employed more nonprofessional nursing staff. Registered nurse staffing levels were higher in facilities with more private pay residents and nonprofit nursing facilities. Thus, controlling for resident characteristics, nursing facilities have economic incentives to hire fewer nursing personnel in high-cost market areas.

Inadequate Educational Training

There are many concerns about the adequacy of the education and training of nursing home personnel. The 1992 national survey of registered nurses estimated that 128,983 RNs were working in nursing facilities or extended care facilities (Moses, 1994b). Of those working in nursing facilities, nurses were more likely to have lower levels of educational preparation (45.5 percent of nursing home nurses had diplomas compared with only 27.5 percent in hospitals) and less likely to have a baccalaureate or master's degree. These lower education levels may be related to the low salaries and benefits in nursing facilities. In other situations, facilities may employ nurses with less education as a means of keeping salaries low. At the same time, nurses with higher education levels can be expected to seek employment in hospitals and other settings where they can receive higher wages and benefits, leaving nurses with less education for those facilities with lower salaries.

Another concern is the inadequate training that most nursing home personnel have had in geriatrics and gerontological nursing. A specialty area has developed in gerontological nursing with a strong knowledge base that argues for the necessity of geriatric training to improve the quality of care for the aged (Matteson and McConnell, 1988). The increased complexity of care required for nursing home residents (Shaughnessy et al., 1990) makes the need for specialty training even greater. Nursing facility directors of nursing and supervisors need advanced training in gerontology but few have such training.

Geriatric nurse practitioners (GNP) can improve the quality of care, including both nursing and primary care, for geriatric residents. Kane and colleagues (1988), in a study of GNPs employed in 30 nursing facilities, found that in spite of the difficulties in developing new roles for GNPs two-thirds of the facilities were enthusiastic about the program. Kane and colleagues (1989) in the same study also found modest improvements in the process of care but no consistent changes in health outcomes. Buchanan and colleagues (1990) found that the employment of GNPs does not adversely affect nursing home costs or profits, and that GNPs do reduce the use of hospital services. GNPs can provide special geriatric care to address common problems of nursing home residents and can provide geriatric training for staff. These studies used GNPs as consultants to the facilities, and not in primary care roles for patient management. Using GNPs in primary care roles, as substitutes for physician care, may be expected to have a greater beneficial effect than using GNPs as specialty nursing employees

(Buchanan et al., 1990). As noted above, the teaching nursing home programs have clearly demonstrated the value of using geriatrically trained nurses in improving patient care outcomes (Mezey and Lynaugh, 1989, 1991).

The level of training of nursing assistants has also been problematic. Even though OBRA 87 required 75 hours of training and competency testing, there is evidence that this is an inadequate level of training. California requires nursing assistants to have a minimum of 120 hours of training. Additional training could assist in improving the quality of care, especially if training is tied to problems of care identified in facilities. Improved training could also reduce turnover rates and reduce the number of injuries that staff sustain, which has been documented to be higher than in other types of health care organizations.

Staffing and Resident Characteristics

There is uniform agreement that there is a strong relationship between resident characteristics, nurse staffing time requirements, and nursing costs in nursing facilities. Numerous studies have examined these relationships and attempted to quantify the relationships (Weissert et al., 1983; Arling et al., 1989). Fries and Cooney (1985) studied resident characteristics were studied in terms of staffing resources in facilities judged to offer high quality of care in the development of the Resources Utilization Groups (RUG). Additional studies were used to create an updated RUGS-II (Schneider et al., 1988) and RUGS-III (Fries et al., 1994). RUGS-III was developed with 44 resident groups that were defined to explain 56 percent of the resource utilization variance (Fries et al., 1994). Thus, heavy-care residents have been shown to require more nursing staff time than other residents.

Staffing Levels and Quality of Care

Not surprisingly, higher staffing levels in nursing facilities have been associated with higher quality of care. One of the early studies that documented this relationship found that homes with more RN hours per patients were associated with patients being alive, having improved physically, and being discharged to home (Linn et al., 1977). Fottler and colleagues (1981) used RN hours and total nursing hours as the key indicator of quality of care in their study of profits. Nyman (1988b) found that higher nursing hours per resident were significantly and positively associated with three of eight quality measures in Iowa nursing facilities. Nyman and colleagues (1990) found in a study of nursing facilities that facilities with a higher percentage of nurse supervisory hours were more efficient and that the percentage of administrator hours was not related to efficiency. He also found that the quality of life in a nursing home was associated with the general staffing level. Nyman (1988b) showed that quality in nursing facilities is not associated with cost and that quality can be improved.

Gustafson and colleagues (1990) found a significant correlation between staffing and six measures of quality incorporated into the QAI index. Munroe's (1990) study of skilled nursing facilities found a positive relationship between nursing home quality (using number of health-related deficiencies received) and the number of RN and LVN nursing hours provided.

Spector and Takada (1991) examined 2,500 nursing home residents in 80 nursing facilities in Rhode Island and found that low staffing in homes with very dependent residents was associated with reduced likelihood of improvement. High rates of urinary catheter use, low rates of skin care, and low resident participation rates in organized activities were all associated with poor resident outcomes. Low RN turnover was also associated with an increased likelihood of functional improvement.

Zinn (1993a) found wide variations in nursing home staffing patterns in 10 standard metropolitan statistical areas, even after controlling for case-mix differences in residents using 1987 MMACS survey data. No consistent relationship was found between staffing levels and prevalence rates of poor outcomes (defined as the percentage of pressure ulcers, catheterized residents, residents not toileted, residents with tube feedings, and residents restrained).

Zinn (1993b) also conducted a study using data from 14,000 nursing facilities from the federal MMACS survey data in 1987. Using a weighted two-stage least squares regression model controlling for case-mix, she found that higher RN wages were associated with lower ratios of RN staff to residents employed by nursing facilities. Higher RN wages and fewer RNs were associated with higher use of urinary catheters, physical restraints, tube feedings, and with residents not being toileted. These negative resident conditions were also more likely to be associated with greater case-mix severity, lower private pay rates in a county, higher proprietary ownership, and less concentration of the nursing home market (each facility's market share of total beds). The results suggested that where there were incentives to hire less nursing staff, facilities used more labor-saving devices, such as catheters, that can cause poor outcomes for residents.

Another recent study of nursing facilities using the 1987 data from 449 freestanding nursing facilities in Pennsylvania found, after controlling for case-mix, that nonprofit nursing facilities provided significantly higher quality of care to Medicaid beneficiaries and to self-pay residents than did for-profit nursing facilities (Aaronson et al., 1994). Nonprofit facilities had higher staffing levels and fewer adverse outcomes from pressure sores controlling for case-mix, but no difference in restraint use was found.

As noted above, reductions in the levels of RN staffing because of recent controls on Medicaid reimbursement and prospective payment for hospitals and subsequent reductions in staffing levels are growing concerns for quality of care (Kanda and Mezey, 1991). The preponderance of evidence from a number of studies with different types of quality measures has shown a positive relationship between nursing staffing and quality of nursing home care. Thus, it can be concluded that lower staffing levels are related to poor process and outcome measures of nursing facility quality.

Appropriate Nurse Staffing Standards

Ideal nurse staffing standards are difficult to develop. In 1987, a panel of nurse experts from the Executive Committee of the Council on Nursing Administration of the American Nurses' Association proposed a minimum staffing approach for nursing facilities based on expert opinion (Turner, 1987). They recommended one full-time RN director of nursing and that at least one RN be on duty 24 hours a day, 7 days a week. In addition, facilities over 120 beds or more were recommended to have 2 additional RNs (one as an assistant director of nursing and one as an in-service education coordinator). The ratio of licensed nurses to residents was recommended at a minimum ratio of 1 to 30 during the day, 1 to 45 during the evening, and 1 to 60 at night. In addition, they recommended that direct caregivers ratios (including RNs, LVNs, and NAs) should be established at 1 to 8 during the day, 1 to 10 in the evening, and 1 to 15 at night. Mohler and Lessard (1991) reported that only 5 percent of the nursing facilities would have met this staffing standard in 1988, based on an analysis of staffing data from the MMACS/OSCAR system.

In order to develop a standard methodology for determining minimum staffing standards, the U.S. Army Headquarters (1990) conducted a workload management study of nursing services. This study recommended a minimum of one RN and one assistant for every nursing unit for every shift for hospitals. Additional staff requirements were developed based on patient characteristics and according to a standard methodology that was used for each unit and each shift. This system for determining nursing staff needs was adopted by the Department of Defense as a model for determining minimum standards for nursing facilities.

Another approach to appropriate staffing standards is to consider the current staffing patterns in Medicare certified facilities. As noted above, the average Medicare certified facility had 1.4 hours of RNs care per resident and a total of 5.2 hours of nursing care per resident. This level could be a target for Medicaid-only certified facilities.

Some nursing home association representatives have argued that current nursing staffing patterns are adequate. In contrast, many nursing experts and consumer groups have argued that the current minimum HCFA nursing standards are too low and should be increased (Mezey et al., 1989). Moreover, consumers suggest that the OBRA requirement for "sufficient staff" does not provide clear direction to nursing facilities and adequate protection of residents (NCCNHR, 1994). They suggest that HCFA expand and detail the minimum standards and develop guidelines for state survey agencies to determine whether or not facilities are complying with the staffing guidelines.

There are two basic approaches to improving nurse staffing levels. One is to mandate stricter staffing levels per resident through federal or state legislation and regulations. This would require changes in the current OBRA 87 legislation, or regulations, or state legislation. Another approach is to change reimbursement policies for nursing facilities or to change the economic incentives to increase staffing levels. Issues of economic and reimbursement policies are discussed in the following section.

PART II. ECONOMIC ISSUES:
NURSING HOME MARKET DEMAND

The demand for nursing home services is growing with the increasing numbers of individuals who are aged and chronically ill. In 1990, there were about 32 million Americans who were age 65 and older and this number is projected to increase to 64 million in 2030 (Zedlewski and McBride, 1992). As the population ages and develops chronic illnesses, the need for long-term-care services, including nursing home services, increases. The total risk for becoming a nursing home patient after age 65 is 43 percent and peaks at age 75 to 80 (Murtaugh et al., 1990). The number of elderly needing nursing home care is expected to increase from about 1.8 million in 1990 to 4.3–5.3 million in 2030, depending upon the projection assumptions (Zedlewski and McBride, 1992; Mendelson and Schwartz, 1993).

The demand for nursing facilities to provide more complex services is growing with the increased age and disability of the residents, shortened hospital stays, and early discharge programs. The degree of medical instability, impairment, and severity of illness in nursing home residents is increasing (Hing, 1989; Shaughnessy et al., 1990; Kanda and Mezey, 1991). Medical technology formerly used only in the hospital has been transferred to nursing facilities. The use of intravenous feedings and medication, ventilators, oxygen, special prosthetic equipment and devices, and other high technologies has made nursing home care more difficult and challenging (Harrington and Estes, 1989; Shaughnessy et al., 1990). Thus, changes in characteristics of nursing facility residents are placing greater demands on nursing care of residents. Nursing facility residents with greater levels of disability require greater professional care and supervision, evaluation, and resources than in the past.

Several federal policy changes in the 1980s have contributed to an increase in nursing home demand and government expenditures for nursing home services. The adoption of prospective payment systems (PPS) for hospitals by Medicare in 1983 resulted in shortened hospital stays and increased the number of referrals and admissions to nursing facilities (Guterman et al., 1988; Neu and Harrison, 1988; Latta and Keene, 1989; U.S. House of Representatives, 1990). In April 1988, HCFA issued new Medicare clarifying guidelines to the fiscal intermediaries regarding the administration of Medicare payments to nursing facilities that expanded coverage somewhat (U.S. House of Representatives, 1990). The

1988 Catastrophic Health Care legislation also expanded Medicare nursing home coverage, but this was repealed in 1989 with no overall increase. Legislation in 1988 established a minimum level of asset and income protection for spouses when determining Medicaid nursing home eligibility, which also contributed to an increase in Medicaid program costs (Letsch et al., 1992). These policy changes have all encouraged the demand for nursing home services and thereby the costs of Medicaid and Medicare.

States have also adopted policies to control Medicaid nursing home demand including Medicaid eligibility policies and preadmission screening programs (Ellwood and Burwell, 1990; HCFA, 1992a,b; Harrington et al., 1994c). These policies may have had a constraining effect on demand and consequently the growth in nursing home capacity.

Alternatives to or substitutes for nursing home care are expanding rapidly, which may reduce the demand for nursing home care. Federal Medicare policies expanded coverage for such services have dramatically increased during the past 5 years. The number of home care agencies and the volume of home care services have increased dramatically (Letsch et al., 1992; NAHC, 1993). In addition, states have attempted to expand alternatives to institutional care under the Medicaid home- and community-based waiver programs (Section 2176 of the Omnibus Budget Reconciliation Act of 1981, P.L. 97-35). Several legislative changes have further expanded Medicaid waivers (HCFA, 1992b; Gurny et al., 1993). These programs have increased the utilization of home- and community-based services during the past decade (Justice, 1988; Lipson and Laudicina, 1991; Miller, 1992; Folkemer, 1994). These types of programs may be reducing the demand for nursing facility care in some areas. On the other hand, these programs may be increasing as a response to the limited supply of nursing home beds in some areas.

Supply of Nursing Home Services

The capacity of long-term-care facilities to meet the demand for services has been strained during the past decade. The total number of licensed nursing facilities (including SNFs and NF that are both freestanding and hospital-based) was 16,959 in 1993 (DuNah et al., 1995). (See Table 3.) These nursing facilities had 1.74 million beds in 1993. In addition to these facilities, there was a total of 6,296 licensed intermediate care facilities for the mentally retarded (ICF-MR) with 136,697 beds in 1993. All states license some residential care (other than nursing facilities), depending upon each state law. These residential care facilities included board and care, personal care, foster care, and assisted living facilities. There were 39,080 licensed residential care facilities reported for the aged with 642,601 beds in 1993 (Harrington et al., 1994b). (See Table 3.) In addition, there were about 13,169 board and care facilities with 120,636 beds for the

TABLE 3 Licensed Long-term Care Providers, United States, 1992 and 1993

Provider Type	Providers in 1992	Providers in 1993	Percent Change
Nursing home facilities	16,800	16,959	1.0
Intermediate care facilities for the mentally retarded	5,894	6,296	6.8
Residential care[a] facilities	34,871	39,080	12.1
Home care agencies	8,117	10,084	24.2
Adult day care agencies	1,517	2,131	40.5

[a]Includes board and care, personal care, assisted living, and other categories of residential care for the aged that are licensed by states. Categories vary by state.

SOURCE: Harrington et al., in press.

mentally retarded in 1991 according to the national health provider inventory (Sirrocco, 1994).

Growth trends are useful to examine over time. The number of licensed nursing facilities increased by about 2 percent annually during the 1978 to 1993 period and 1 percent between 1992 and 1993 (DuNah et al., 1995). (See Table 3.) Based on past growth trends, future bed growth for nursing facilities can be expected to be only about 2 percent annually. The number of ICF-MR facilities (data on beds are unavailable) increased by 7 percent between 1992 and 1993 (Harrington et al., 1994b). The growth in residential care beds for the aged has been about 11 percent annually over the 1983 to 1993 period and 12 percent between 1992 and 1993 (Harrington et al., 1994c). In contrast, the number of licensed home health care agencies increased by 24 percent between 1992 and 1993 and licensed adult day care agencies increased by 41 percent. (See Table 3.)

One key concern is whether the growth in beds is keeping pace with the aging of the population. Previous studies have shown that growth has failed to meet the demand in some areas (Feder and Scanlon, 1980; Scanlon, 1980a,b; Nyman, 1985, 1989b, 1993; Bishop, 1988). The most recent data show that in 1993 the states on average had 53.0 licensed nursing facility beds per 1,000 people aged 65 plus (DuNah et al., 1995). The U.S. bed ratio for the aged 65 and over remained essentially flat over the past 16 years. On the other hand the population over age 85, who are the greatest users of nursing home services, was growing more rapidly than nursing home beds. The average number of nursing facility beds dropped from 610 per 1000 aged 85 and over in 1978 to 491 in 1993 (a 19.6 percent decline) (DuNah et al., 1995). (See Table 4.) Thus, the beds in most states are failing to keep pace with the growth in the oldest old population.

The variation in nursing facility bed ratios across states and regions is substantial. (See Table 4.) The north central region had the highest ratio (597

TABLE 4   Ratio of Licensed Nursing Home Beds per 1,000 Population Aged 85 and Over

	1978	1982	1986	1990	1993	Percent Growth 1978–1993
Alabama	597.8	538.2	488.0	430.7	398.2	−33.4
Alaska	1,426.6	998.8	833.0	677.8	578.7	−59.4
Arizona	308.9	305.0	460.4	416.6	350.2	13.4
Arkansas	752.7	689.3	689.0	611.3	597.1	−20.7
California	534.6	461.8	419.3	405.8	379.0	−29.1
Colorado	860.6	677.5	600.8	590.5	521.3	−39.4
Connecticut	706.9	652.0	638.3	609.1	595.3	−15.8
District of Columbia	257.2	237.1	303.1	330.7	321.0	24.8
Delaware	556.0	587.6	571.5	606.6	680.2	22.4
Florida	337.7	303.2	305.8	305.1	294.3	−12.9
Georgia	830.1	771.3	666.3	606.7	558.0	−32.8
Hawaii	478.7	403.7	353.7	323.2	288.9	−39.7
Idaho	571.5	505.9	477.2	476.8	438.9	−23.2
Illinois	785.0	699.0	661.8	639.4	622.0	−20.8
Indiana	807.0	853.4	790.2	806.2	758.2	−6.1
Iowa	707.9	655.3	639.7	593.3	612.5	−13.5
Kansas	809.4	720.5	677.7	704.2	636.0	−21.4
Kentucky	483.7	472.6	470.9	472.5	469.5	−2.9
Louisiana	695.9	666.0	741.1	714.0	662.0	−4.9
Maine	635.6	553.4	555.1	520.6	490.4	−22.8
Maryland	635.9	590.3	554.2	554.8	525.0	−17.4
Massachusetts	590.3	507.7	508.3	536.3	520.1	−11.9
Michigan	591.7	505.0	494.3	469.4	421.5	−28.8
Minnesota	794.0	714.6	696.1	640.9	601.7	−24.2
Mississippi	471.1	483.1	475.4	424.2	410.4	−12.9
Missouri	601.8	648.0	646.2	665.6	627.0	4.2
Montana	721.9	643.8	664.7	596.5	532.4	−26.2
Nebraska	809.6	707.6	667.6	663.8	621.6	−23.2
Nevada	621.4	500.4	436.2	397.2	359.6	−42.1
New Hampshire	646.8	603.3	539.2	492.2	461.1	−28.7
New Jersey	419.6	413.3	438.6	473.0	439.1	4.6
New Mexico	339.4	387.4	453.1	424.4	388.7	14.5
New York	457.2	410.4	397.7	390.2	387.3	−15.3
North Carolina	422.7	421.9	383.0	378.4	453.8	7.4
North Dakota	730.7	723.2	671.1	610.8	560.5	−23.3
Ohio	627.6	614.9	647.9	640.2	586.2	−6.6
Oklahoma	822.5	749.3	728.7	707.9	664.9	−19.2
Oregon	542.9	478.1	427.3	383.9	328.1	−39.6
Pennsylvania	530.5	521.7	523.8	495.0	468.6	−11.7
Rhode Island	722.8	653.6	664.0	628.2	603.0	−16.6

TABLE 4 Continued

	1978	1982	1986	1990	1993	Percent Growth 1978–1993
South Carolina	533.2	528.8	449.5	437.4	422.4	−20.8
South Dakota	733.2	667.5	623.4	607.1	577.4	−21.3
Tennessee	479.7	560.5	553.6	567.2	528.2	10.1
Texas	952.4	810.7	718.9	693.8	635.1	−33.3
Utah	683.0	539.2	538.8	517.2	438.2	−35.8
Vermont	487.2	448.6	467.2	465.0	427.0	−12.4
Virginia	420.7	450.7	411.1	447.1	435.9	3.6
Washington	719.1	598.2	516.7	508.4	449.1	−37.6
West Virginia	285.0	329.3	362.0	381.8	372.6	30.7
Wisconsin	955.8	840.4	779.8	662.0	603.6	−36.9
Wyoming	573.9	538.4	538.8	626.5	592.9	3.3
North Central	729.5	679.9	659.9	636.8	597.4	−18.1
North East	516.8	477.7	475.5	470.3	453.6	−12.2
South	594.5	552.9	520.7	504.2	455.1	−23.5
West	571.7	488.9	454.8	436.5	383.6	−32.9
United States	610.3	559.5	537.0	520.3	479.7	−21.4

SOURCE: DuNah et al., 1995.

nursing facility beds per 1,000 population aged 85 and over) and the west had the lowest (395 beds) in 1993 (DuNah et al., 1995). The beds per 85 and over aged population declined the most in the west (31 percent), the south (19 percent) and the north central regions (18 percent) (DuNah et al., 1995).

The average occupancy rates for U.S. nursing facilities was reported by states to be 91 percent (or about 1,582,000 residents) in 1992 and 1993 (DuNah et al., 1995). Average occupancy rates were higher (94 percent) for ICF-MR facilities. Although the occupancy rates were generally high for nursing facilities, states did show a wide range in rates. Occupancy rates were highest in the northeastern states (97 percent in 1993), about average in the southern and north central states, and lowest in the west (88 percent) in 1993. A recent survey of state officials reported that some states are considered to have an undersupply while others reported an oversupply of nursing facility beds (DuNah et al., 1995). Thus, some areas and states may have shortages of nursing home services and others may have an adequate or oversupply of nursing home beds (Swan and Harrington, 1986; Wallace, 1986; Harrington et al., 1992a, 1994a; Swan et al., 1993b; DuNah et al., 1995). Areas with shortages are of concern because they may limit access for those in need of services.

State Medicaid programs have undertaken a number of policy initiatives to control supply and reduce spending on nursing home care. This began in the early 1980s, when federal budget cuts to state Medicaid programs became standard features of the budget process (Bishop, 1988). The most important policies affecting the supply of long-term-care bed supply are state certificate-of-need (CON) programs.

The health planning and CON program established in 1974 (P.L. 94-641) gave states considerable authority and discretion to plan and control the capital expenditures for nursing facilities and other health facilities (Kosciesza, 1987). The effectiveness of CON policies in controlling bed supply has been widely debated and the policies opposed by many providers (Cohodes, 1982; Friedman, 1982; Swan and Harrington, 1990; Mendelson and Arnold, 1993). These controversies resulted in the federal repeal of the program in 1986 (Kosciesza, 1987).

Even after the federal repeal of the program, 44 states continued to use CON, moratoria policies, or both to regulate the growth in nursing facilities in 1993. In 1993, 31 states had CON, moratoriums, or both for ICF-MR facilities and 9 had CON for residential care. CON and moratoria policies for nursing facilities have been found to be associated with lower growth in bed ratios and higher occupancy rates (Harrington et al., 1994a). Other studies have shown that lower nursing home bed supply is associated with lower costs to the Medicaid program (Harrington and Swan, 1987; Nyman, 1988a). Thus, because of the cost pressures on states, we can expect most states to continue their efforts to limit the supply of nursing home beds even though their bed supply is not keeping pace with the aging of the population.

Market Competition Effects

Medicaid nursing home days of care account for a major proportion of all patient days (Levit et al., 1994). Nevertheless, most nursing facilities prefer private clients because facilities can generally charge private-paying residents higher daily rates than Medicaid (Scanlon, 1980a,b; Lee et al., 1983; Phillips and Hawes, 1988; Buchanan et al., 1991). Buchanan and colleagues (1991) estimated that private patient payment rates for nursing home care was 20 percent per day higher than Medicaid rates in 1987. Unfortunately, data on private pay rates for nursing facilities are generally unavailable.

Nursing facilities also tend to prefer those patients that are the least sick (unless they receive higher rates for sicker patients under case-mix reimbursement) or for whom they can provide the most cost efficient care (Holahan and Cohen, 1987; Kenney and Holahan, 1990; Falcone et al., 1991). When nursing facilities are selective in their admission policies, the access to care of those individuals with the greatest need may be limited. Where the supply of nursing home beds is limited, problems in gaining access to needed services may be exacerbated (Kenney and Holahan, 1990; Falcone et al., 1991). As noted above, nursing home bed capacity varies substantially across different states and regions in the United States (DuNah et al., 1995).

Access problems have been documented by waiting lists for nursing facilities, high nursing home occupancy rates, and delayed hospital discharges in some geographical areas (GAO, 1990). These access problems can have negative consequences for consumers and public payers. Kenney and Holahan (1990) found that limited nursing home bed supply in some areas is an important determinant of hospital discharge delays, which can add to the overall costs of hospital care. Nyman (1985, 1989b) argued that excess nursing home demand also can cause serious problems in the quality of nursing home care, especially for Medicaid nursing home residents. Nyman (1989b) found that nursing facilities had substantially fewer violations for poor quality of care in areas of Wisconsin where there were more available nursing home beds. In areas with an abundant supply of nursing home beds Medicaid recipients should have greater access to care, but this depends in part on the Medicaid reimbursement rates in relationship to the marginal costs of operation (Nyman, 1985, 1989b).

Nursing Home Expenditures and Sources of Payment

Nursing home services accounted for approximately $70 billion or 8 percent of the total health care expenditures in the United States in 1993 (Levit et al., 1994). The increase in nursing home expenditures was 6.3 percent between 1992 and 1993. Government comprises the largest payer of nursing home care. The Medicaid program paid for an estimated 52 percent of all the nation's nursing home expenditures in 1993 according to HCFA actuaries (Levit et al., 1994). (See Table 5.) Medicare paid for 9 percent and other government sources paid 2 percent of the total costs (Levit et al., 1994). Thirty-three percent was paid for directly out-of-pocket by consumers and 4 percent by private insurance and other private sources.

TABLE 5 National Expenditures by Source for Nursing Facilities, United States, 1993

	Percent of Total Expenditures for Nursing Facilities ($69.6 billion)
Medicaid	52
Medicare	9
Other public	2
Private insurance	4
Out-of-pocket	33

SOURCE: Levit et al., 1994.

TABLE 6 State Medicaid Nursing Facility
Reimbursement Methods and Rates, United
States, 1979 and 1993

Reimbursement Methods and Rates	1979	1993
Retrospective	13	1
Prospective		
Facility specific	16	17
Class	4	3
Combination	17	30
Total	50	51
Case-mix methods	3	19
Average Medicaid per diem rate	$28	$75

SOURCE: Swan et al., 1994.

Medicaid days of care were estimated to be 73.7 percent of the total free-standing nursing facility days of care, but Medicaid was estimated to pay for 55 percent of total free-standing facility expenditures in 1992 (HCIA and Arthur Andersen, 1994). Medicaid payments are lower than days of care because some Medicaid residents pay for a proportion of their care (under the state Medicaid spend-down requirements) and because private pay and Medicare payment rates are generally higher than Medicaid rates.

In 1993, the average Medicaid rate across states was $79.50 per day, which was about 4 percent higher than for 1992 (Swan et al., 1994). (See Table 6.) The national mean of 1993 rates, adjusted for the consumer price index, was unchanged from the previous year ($52.30 in 1993 compared to $52.16 in 1992). This increase is lower than in the 1989 to 1992 period, when rates were rising about 6 percent per year above inflation. It is also lower than the 1980 to 1989 period, when rate increases were approximately 2 percent per year above inflation. (Swan et al., 1994). Medicaid nursing home reimbursement rates vary widely across states in response to the varying methodologies used by states. Reimbursement rates increased on average about 4 percent between fiscal years 1992 and 1993, but when rates were adjusted for inflation they remained stable during that period. Thus, state Medicaid programs are bringing down the increases in reimbursement rates.

HCIA and Arthur Andersen (1994) reported a median net patient revenue of $67 per resident day for all free-standing nursing facilities in the United States in 1992 (total revenues divided by total resident days). The median total operating expenses per resident day was reported at $66.50. Revenues and expenses varied by the size of facility, the type of ownership, and other factors. Direct patient care costs were 35 percent of total expenses for all free-standing nursing facilities in the United States (HCIA and Arthur Andersen, 1994). These direct costs include nursing care, supervision, charting, and other resident services. Indirect patient care costs (laundry, housekeeping, dietary, and other costs) were reported to be 17 percent of total expenses, administrative and general costs were 28 percent, depreciation and interest were 9 percent, and ancillary costs were 2.5 percent in 1992. The increase in administrative costs and general expense was the largest of any of the 5 cost components (30 percent between 1990 and 1992) (HCIA and Arthur Andersen, 1994). These dramatic increases in administrative costs were not explained. Administrative and general expenses include telephone, billing, maintenance and repairs, operation of plant, personnel, employee benefits, and medical records. The current distribution of resources for nursing home should be evaluated to determine the extent to which is may contribute to poor quality of care in some facilities.

Medicaid Reimbursement

The rapidly increasing cost of nursing home care has been a major concern to state policymakers, especially because nursing facilities consumed 32 percent of the Medicaid budget in 1993 (Levit et al., 1994). Many state Medicaid programs have attempted to control the growth in nursing home reimbursement rates (Holahan and Cohen, 1987; Bishop, 1988; Nyman, 1988a; Holahan et al., 1993; Swan et al., 1993a,c). States have considerable discretion in developing Medicaid reimbursement methods and rates.

Until 1980, states were required to pay for Medicaid nursing home services on the basis of "reasonable costs" so that many states used retrospective reimbursement systems, paying the costs of care (GAO, 1986). The Omnibus Budget Reconciliation Act of 1980 gave states greater flexibility in developing reimbursement systems. This provision, known as the Boren amendment, allowed states to pay nursing facilities based upon what was "reasonable and adequate to meet the costs incurred by efficiently and economically operated nursing facilities in providing care." States began to change their reimbursement systems to gain greater control over costs.

Since 1980, there has been a pronounced shift away from retrospective reimbursement (one state in 1993) to prospective facility-specific methods (17 states in 1993) or combination or adjusted systems (30 states) (Swan et al., 1993a,c; Swan et al., 1994). (See Table 6.) Three states continued to use prospective class (or flat) rate systems in 1993. In addition, there has been a substantial increase in numbers of states with case-mix reimbursement (19 case-mix states in 1993). Four states were participating in the HCFA Case-Mix Demonstration project and two other states were implementing their case-mix systems in 1994 and 1995. Thus, by 1996, about half of all state Medicaid programs will be using case-mix reimbursement. (Swan et al., 1994). Most states included some ancillaries in their basic reimbursement rates, such as therapy services and prescription drugs. Capital reimbursement was largely based on historic costs (Swan et al., 1994). Medicaid nursing home per diem rates were the outcome of state reimbursement methods. Medicaid nursing home reimbursement rates varied widely across states in response to the varying methodologies used by states. In summary, state Medicaid reimbursement methods for nursing facilities are gradually changing to facility-specific methods and case-mix reimbursement systems.

Impact of Prospective Payment Systems

Several studies have been conducted to examine the effects of Medicaid payment systems for nursing facilities. Retrospective reimbursement has been widely criticized as resulting in higher costs and promoting inefficiency (Holahan and Cohen, 1987). Like retrospective systems, prospective systems with weak efficiency incentives, generous inflation adjustments, and low ceilings can have limited cost controls (Holahan, 1985). Most studies have found that prospective reimbursement systems lower Medicaid costs over retrospective systems (Ullmann, 1984; Swan et al., 1988, 1993c, 1994; Buchanan et al., 1991; Ohsfeldt et al., 1991; Coburn et al., 1993). The strong trend toward the conversion of Medicaid prospective systems reflects the noncontroversial nature of the cost savings findings.

Even though prospective payment systems control costs, a number of researchers have identified negative consequences of cost containment for access and quality, especially for Medicaid patients. In the long run, these may result in lower quality of care and fewer services provided to Medicaid recipients (Swan et al., 1988, 1993a,c; Buchanan et al., 1991; Coburn, et al., 1993). Lee and colleagues (1983) found that cost controls on nursing home rates appeared to have a negative impact on the access of public patients to nursing home care and also to result in reductions in service intensity and possibly in the quality of care. In Maine, after prospective payment was adopted by Medicaid, a decline in the Medicaid share of patient days occurred following the introduction of prospective payment (Coburn et al., 1993). Thus, the special incentives for increasing Medicaid's share of patients were ineffective in Maine. The findings also raised concerns about the financial viability over time of some facilities under prospective payment (Coburn et al., 1993).

Using a sample of 2,460 skilled nursing facilities in 1981, Cohen and Dubay (1990) also found that state Medicaid programs under prospective and flat rate systems are able to control costs, but these systems create access and quality problems. Facilities with these systems indicated they had less debilitated patients and some facilities reduced their staffing, which could lead to quality problems. They found that when reimbursement rates were lowered, nursing facilities responded by decreasing their resident case-mix and reducing staffing beyond the apparently appropriate level for the given case-mix (Cohen and Dubay, 1990).

Nyman (1988b) found that nursing facilities in Iowa with more private pay residents provided better quality of care (as measured by the number of deficiencies). Gertler (1989) also found a relationship between higher proportions of Medicaid patients and poorer quality of nursing home care. An increase in Medicaid reimbursement does increase access for Medicaid recipients, but this in turn lowers the quality of care (as measured by the nursing hours of care (Gertler, 1989). Spector and Takada (1991) were able to confirm that facilities with a low percentage of private residents were associated with poorer outcomes of care. Thus, a higher percentage of Medicare or private pay patients may be positively associated with higher quality and a higher percentage of Medicaid patients is negatively associated with higher quality of care (Nyman, 1988b, 1989a; Davis, 1993).

Hospital-based facilities with Medicare certification receive higher reimbursements than Medicaid facilities (Dor, 1989). Such facilities may have higher quality of care because they have higher staffing levels. Having accreditation may be positively associated with higher staffing levels and with higher quality of care. The existence of dedicated special care units, such as those for persons with Alzheimer's disease, may also be associated with higher quality of care because of higher staffing levels. Large size facilities may also be associated with higher quality although findings are mixed (Ullmann, 1981; Nyman, 1988b; Davis, 1991).

Regional variation can also impact on quality. Nyman (1988a) found that markets in Wisconsin with limited bed supply had less Medicaid reimbursement spent on patient care while the reverse was true when there was an excess supply. Higher quality for nursing facilities in Wisconsin was found in areas with greater competition for patients (Nyman, 1989b). Davis (1993) found that nursing home costs are lower in markets where beds are owned by fewer firms (less competitive markets) and higher in markets with more empty beds. In the same study in Kentucky, he found that for-profit facilities have lower costs and tend to operate in counties with higher market consideration. Ray and colleagues (1987) showed wide variations in the type of nursing home residents and their turnover rates across three states. Thus, the wide state variations in reimbursement methods and rates create major differences in facility revenues and the quality of care (Nyman, 1989a,b).

Policy Changes for Medicaid Reimbursement Policies

Many analysts have recommended that operating costs related to resident care should be separated from and treated differently than nonresident care costs (Holahan and Cohen, 1987; Lewin/ICF, 1991). These experts have strongly recommended that reimbursement controls on direct patient care costs should be minimal or nonexistent in order to encourage homes to maintain or expand care need in order to promote access and appropriate services for heavy-care patients. They recommended that strong efficiency incentives for cost containment should be placed on non-care-related operating costs. Efficiency incentives can allow nursing facilities to keep all or some of the difference between actual costs of care and a ceiling or target rate (Holahan, 1985; Holahan and Cohen, 1987).

Many states do not appear to be using this approach. Where limits on nursing are set at the minimum nursing staffing levels and average wages, this could encourage reductions in staffing rather than improvements in staffing. A survey of state Medicaid reimbursement methods in 1988 found that 23 states had ceilings imposed on administrative costs, 10 on profit rates, and 10 on capital reimbursement (Swan et al., 1993c). On the other hand, many states (19 states in 1988) used ceilings on nursing costs (Swan et al., 1993c). In a survey of 1993 Medicaid methods, 30 states reported using cost center limits for nursing or patient care costs and 18 had limits on general operating costs. Cost ceilings for direct patient care costs could have negative consequences for the staffing levels in nursing facilities and for quality of care (Swan et al., 1994). Some state reimbursement methods and rates may be more reflective of state budget resources than tied to the actual costs of providing nursing home care (Swan et al., 1993c). State reimbursement policies that discourage appropriate staffing levels should be reconsidered. Ceilings on direct resident care expenditures could have a negative impact on both staffing levels and quality of care. Most state reimbursement systems do not provide incentives to improve the quality of direct patient care.

The General Accounting Office (GAO, 1986) reviewed the state Medicaid reimbursement methods used by states for nursing facilities. This study concluded that HCFA had not established adequate guidelines for states and recommended a number of nursing home reimbursement changes that would ensure that states: disallow certain costs such as those for luxury items, use audited cost reports for computing rates, use inflation indices that reflect nursing facilities costs, perform more studies on subgroups of facilities and ceilings, do not use returns on equity for proprietary nursing facilities except in shortage areas, and limit sales and leases on property costs (GAO, 1986). It is not known to what extent these problems have been corrected. Continuing disputes between facilities and states over Medicaid reimbursement methods are shown by the many Boren amendment lawsuits filed by nursing facilities against state Medicaid agencies (Harrington et al., 1993; Weinberg et al., 1993). The varying state Medicaid reimbursement methods appear to be problematic, and may not ensure that the actual costs of providing direct resident care are covered.

Case-Mix Reimbursement

Case-mix reimbursement systems were developed for Medicaid as a means of making closer linkages between resident needs, payments, and costs and as a way for removing access barriers for heavy-care Medicaid patients (Schlenker et al., 1985; Schlenker, 1991a,b). As noted above, 19 states were using case-mix systems in 1993 (Swan et al., 1994). The most commonly used case-mix measure has been functional status (using Activities of Daily Living or ADL) although other disability scales have been used (Weissert and Musliner, 1992a,b). One of the best known approaches has been the RUGS methodology developed by Fries and Cooney (1985). This approach has been updated into a RUG-II and now a RUG-III version (Fries et al., 1994). Resident characteristics are typically examined for the amount of personnel resources needed to provide care to residents, which can be determined in different ways such as staff time and cost studies (Weissert et al., 1983; Fries and Cooney, 1985; Arling et al., 1987, 1989; Fries et al., 1989, 1994). Once costs are determined, they are tied to resident characteristics (Weissert and Musliner, 1992a,b). As Fries and colleagues (1994) pointed out, the development of classification systems and resource use groups is primarily a technical process, but the development and assignment of reimbursement categories is primarily a political process.

Several studies have been conducted of case-mix (Weissert et al., 1983; Cameron, 1985; Fries and Cooney, 1985; Arling et al., 1987, 1989; Schneider et al., 1988; Fries et al., 1994). Weissert and Musliner (1992a,b) have summarized the results of the many studies of case-mix reimbursement. These studies reported that most states that have used case-mix reimbursement have improved access for some heavy care residents (Ohio, Illinois, Maryland, and New York). On the other hand, there continued to be problems with access in some case-mix reimbursement states such as West Virginia (Holahan, 1984; Butler and Schlenker, 1988; Weissert and Musliner, 1992a,b). Access problems under case-mix have especially occurred in areas where there is a low supply of beds (Nyman, 1988b), where there are Medicaid processing delays (Weissert and Cready, 1988), and where reimbursement rates are low. Access problems occurred for those with low care needs and where community-based alternatives were not necessarily available (Butler and Schlenker, 1988; Feder and Scanlon, 1989).

In terms of the issue of costs, Weissert and Musliner (1992a,b) argued that case-mix may have distributed payments equitably among nursing facilities such as in New York. On the other hand, administrative costs tended to increase (Ohio costs tripled and Minnesota costs doubled) or remain neutral (e.g., Maryland and New York) depending on the system (Weissert and Musliner, 1992a,b).

Quality is a key issue with case-mix systems. For example, Weissert and Musliner (1992a,b) pointed out that New York and Minnesota payments for improved resident functioning did not produce an increase in restorative care. Ohio payment incentives for therapeutic services did not increase those services but Illinois payments for increases in services were effective (Butler and Schlenker, 1988). They also pointed out that when Maryland paid for extra turning and positioning services and Illinois paid for decubitus prevention, residents improvements did occur (Schlenker et al., 1988). On the other hand, higher payments for more care can lead to perverse incentives such as the extra payments in West Virginia for catheterized patients that resulted in increased urinary catheterization rates (Schlenker et al., 1988) or increased tube feeding and oxygen use in Maryland (Feder and Scanlon, 1989). Thus, some case-mix systems may have negative impacts on quality, while those that pay for special care services may improve the amount of care provided.

Case-mix reimbursement generally has not led to increases in nursing staff ratios. In Maryland, there was no evidence that extra nursing home payments were used to add more staff (Feder and Scanlon, 1989). New York also did not increase staff even though resident case-mix increased (Butler and Schlenker, 1988). Although West Virginia had some evidence of poor quality (e.g., increased catheterization), nursing resources did increase in the 1979 to 1981 period (Holahan and Cohen, 1987; Weissert and Musliner, 1992a,b). In the San Diego experiment where facilities were given financial incentives to take more heavy care residents, there was no evidence that extra payments were spent on extra care (Meiners et al., 1985). Of the six states systems reviewed by Weissert and Musliner (1992a,b), only Illinois was rated as having improved quality (Holahan, 1984; Butler and Schlenker, 1988).

HCFA is undertaking a demonstration project to introduce Medicaid case-mix in four states in 1994 to 1995. As Weissert and Musliner (1992b) have noted, it is not clear whether substantial new advances will be made in designing improved case-mix reimbursement systems in the demonstration project. An evaluation has been planned that will examine the outcomes of the demonstration on access, quality, and costs.

In summary, the support for case-mix reimbursement is mixed and has not been shown to improve quality. Weissert and Musliner (1992a,b) have concluded that the introduction of case-mix reimbursement may increase costs and will not improve quality. Case-mix reimbursement, therefore, may not increase the level of staffing or quality in nursing facilities unless new features are added to these Medicaid methodologies. New case-mix systems may be able to ensure that appropriate staffing levels are maintained and improved and that quality of care is maintained or enhanced.

Medicare Reimbursement

Medicare retrospective payments methods based on reasonable costs have been widely criticized as inflationary (Schieber et al., 1986; Holahan and Sulvetta, 1989). From 1982 to 1985, Congress made some minor changes in the nursing facility reimbursement methods to expand Medicare participation and to control costs (Schieber et al., 1986). One major advantage of Medicare reimbursement for nursing facilities is that its methodology is uniform across states and regions, unlike Medicaid reimbursement methods. Nevertheless, many nursing facilities have been reluctant to admit Medicare patients because of their traditionally higher costs and the low volume of residents eligible for such care. Staffing requirements for Medicare certified facilities are higher and residents must meet stringent need requirements under Medicare rules. Dor (1989) showed that Medicare-specific marginal costs were generally well above average Medicare long-term-care reimbursement rates. Thus, Medicare reimbursements are more attractive to long-term-care facilities that specialize in providing such care in order to gain economies of scale and scope (Dor, 1989).

Because prospective reimbursement systems have been shown to reduce costs, this approach is under consideration by HCFA. Congress has mandated that Medicare study prospective reimbursement as a means of controlling nursing facility costs. In response to Congress, HCFA is conducting a demonstration project to study prospective case-mix reimbursement for Medicare and for participating state Medicaid programs. If these new systems are adopted, Medicare may have some of the same problems that have resulted from the Medicaid prospective payment systems and case-mix reimbursement for nursing facilities. Other options could be developed for Medicare to address the goals of controlling costs while increasing access, providing care to resource-intensive residents, and improving quality (Holahan and Sulvetta, 1989; Weissert and Musliner, 1992a,b). Moreover, greater coordination is needed between the Medicare and Medicaid reimbursement policies and rates.

Ownership Structure and Profits

The majority of nursing facilities are proprietary and facilities are increasingly owned by investors. Of the total nursing facilities, 71 percent were reported as proprietary, 24 percent were nonprofit, and 5 percent were government owned in 1991 (Sirrocco, 1994). Although facilities can be classified by ownership, corporate goals differ within these ownership categories. Although nonprofit facilities generally have charitable goals, some nonprofit facilities may seek to maximize revenues. Proprietary facilities generally are oriented to maximizing profits and an increasing number of these facilities are publicly traded corporations.

Nursing facilities, like other segments of the health industry, are consolidating into large health care organizations. In 1984, there were 2,039 facilities and 234,478 beds owned or operated by investor-owned chains (Punch, 1985). Thus, 16 percent of the total beds were investor-owned (DuNah et al., 1995). In 1991, a survey identified 207 long-term-care systems that operated 4,073 facilities and 478,918 beds (Burns, 1992). This group had increased facilities by 3.7 percent and beds by 4.4 percent over the previous year. Of this group, 44 were Roman Catholic providers (23,973 beds) and 8 were public chains (3,154 beds). The largest chain was Beverly Enterprises, which reported 90,228 beds in 1991, and Hillhaven, which was second with 44,681 beds. The largest chains were reporting rapid growth although Beverly Enterprises and Hillhaven had both reduced their facilities and beds slightly over 1990. Thus, the chains had about 28 percent of the facilities and 29 percent of the total beds in 1991 (Burns, 1992). In contrast, the OSCAR system indicated that 48 percent of certified facilities surveyed in the calendar year of 1993 were chain facilities (Harrington et al., 1995).

HCIA and Arthur Andersen (1994) reported that 23 of the largest 25 nursing home chains in the United States were involved in acquisitions during 1993. They also reported that chains represent 34.5 percent of the total market and that the largest 20 chains operate 18 percent of the total beds. In addition, they reported that 16 nursing home companies have become public in the past 2 years, which gives these companies new sources of capital for growth and acquisitions.

Profit Margins

Profit margins reported for the nursing home industry have generally been good. Beverly Enterprises, the largest nursing home chain, reported revenue increases of 9 percent between 1990 and 1991 to $2.3 billion. Net income rose 126 percent to $29 million for 1991 over 1990 (1 percent profit) (Burns, 1992). Hillhaven, the second largest chain, had a net loss in 1991 of $7.3 million on revenues of $1.1 billion. Manor Care, the third largest nursing home chain, reported a net income of $71 million on $666 million in revenues (11 percent profit) (Burns, 1992; Abelson, 1993).

A 1991 study of profits in New York found that the average profit margin on facilities was 3 to 7 percent and the return on investment ranged from 15 to 26 percent. Less than 50 percent of the nonprofit facilities and 33 percent of the public facilities were reporting profits, so that most profits were made by proprietary facilities. At the same time, owners and their family members frequently received salaries from the facilities. In 1992, 8 facilities reported between $1 to $2 million in salaries to owners or family members (Rudder, 1994).

The total profit margin for the free-standing nursing home industry (calculated as the difference between total net revenue and total expenses divided by total net revenues reported from facility cost reports) was reported at 3.7 percent for 1992 (HCIA and Arthur Andersen, 1994). Profit margins were reported to have increased by 30 percent between 1990 and 1992. Profit margins were higher in investor-owned and system-affiliated facilities (4.15 percent in 1992) than in other types of facilities and in medium-sized facilities as compared to small facilities.

In 1994, Manor Care had a 18 percent return on equity for the latest 12 months and sales growth of 14 percent on $1.2 billion in revenue. (See Table 7.) The earnings per share increased by 16.5 percent and the profit margin was 6.9 percent. Hillhaven had a 25 percent return on equity for the latest 12 months and a 4 percent increase in sales growth on its $1.5 billion in revenues with a 4.2 percent profit margin (Walsh, 1995). Beverly Enterprises had a 9.6 return on equity for the past year and a sales growth of 4 percent on its $2.9 billion in revenues. Its overall profit margin was 2.5 percent for the year. National Medical had a deficit on return on equity over the past year and 5-year period. Health Care and Retirement Corporation had 12 percent return on equity and a 6.7 percent profit margin the past year. Real estate investment trusts are growing in importance for the ownership and operation of long-term-care facilities (Bowe, 1994). Health Trust is an organization with income-producing real estate. This corporation had a return on equity of 24.5 percent and a profit margin of 5.8 percent during the past year (See Table 7.)

Forbes reported that the all-industry medians for return on equity for 1 year was 12.6 percent and for 5 years was 11.4 percent in 1994 (Kichen, 1995). (See Table 7.) Manor Care, Health Trust, and Hillhaven exceeded the all-industry medians while Beverly was slightly lower. The all-industry profit margin for previous 12 months was 4.3 percent. Manor Care, Health Care and Retirement, and Health Trust exceeded the all-industry medians for-profit margin, Hillhaven was similar to the national industry medians, while Beverly fell below. Thus, most of these long-term-care firms were generally continuing to be profitable and some exceeded both the health medians and the all-industry medians for profitability (Walsh, 1995). The health care industry ranked first out of 21 industry groups for its 5-year return on equity.

Profit-making issues are complex and can not be fully developed in this paper. The issues of profits on investment, especially real estate investments, and hidden profits disguised as administrative or capital expenses must be more fully understood. Few studies of the industry have been conducted, especially studies that determine appropriate levels of expenditures for profits, administrative costs, and capital.

Historically, proprietary health facilities were paid a return on equity on their investment under the Medicare program, equivalent to earnings on investments in specified government securities. In 1985, the Combined Omnibus Budget Reconciliation Act eliminated this provision for hospitals. The 1993 OBRA eliminated this provision for Medicare skilled nursing facilities. Some states have also attempted to limit profits under the Medicaid program. For example, 10 states reported setting maximum cost limits on Medicaid profits and 23 states reported cost center limits for Medicaid administrative costs in 1988 (Swan et al., 1993c). Other states have disallowed any Medicaid payments for profits or return on equity. Payments for return on equity or profits for the Medicaid program and inadequate limits on administrative salaries and costs, especially to parties related to the owners, may be unnecessarily increasing Medicaid costs.

Ownership, Staffing, Costs, and Quality

Substantial differences in costs occur across facilities by ownership. Data for 1994 showed that nonprofit homes had the largest net patient revenue, prima-

TABLE 7   Profit Margins for the Nursing Home Industry, United States, 1994

| Company | Profitability (percent) | | | |
| | Return on Equity | | Return on Capital | |
	5-Year Average	Latest 12 Months	Latest 12 Months	Debt/Capital
Beverly Enterprises	2.0	9.6	7.5	45.0
Health Care and Retirement	NA	12.2	8.7	28.2
Health Trust	23.2[a]	24.5	14.0	60.9
Hillhaven	13.0[b]	25.2	9.8	60.9
Manor Care	20.5	18.0	11.0	32.9
National Medical	Deficit	Deficit	Deficit	13.4
Health median	18.6	17.6	11.0	32.1
All industry median	11.4	12.6	9.4	32.8

NOTE: D–P, deficit to profit; P–D, profit to deficit; NM, not meaningful; NA, not applicable.

[a]3-year average.
[b]4-year average.

SOURCE: Walsh, 1995.

rily because they had a higher proportion of private pay residents compared with other facilities (HCIA and Arthur Andersen, 1994). Nonprofit facilities had significantly higher median operating expenses and higher expenditures on direct patient care. The typical investor-owned facility had lower net revenues, lower expenditures, and fewer expenditures on direct patient care. Nonprofit facilities had higher median administrative and general expenses than investor-owned facilities, where investor-owned facilities had higher expenditures for capital (HCIA and Arthur Andersen, 1994). These relationships to ownership and costs are consistent with other studies (Lee et al., 1983; Cohen and Dubay, 1990; Arling et al., 1991).

The relationship of facility ownership to staffing, costs, and quality has been the subject of numerous studies and controversy. One of the major debates is whether the proprietary nature of the nursing home industry affects process and outcomes in terms of quality of care. A review of the research studies on ownership and quality shows a mixed picture in terms of the relationship (Koetting, 1980; Greene and Monahan, 1981; O'Brien et al., 1983; Hawes and Phillips, 1986; Nyman et al., 1990; Davis, 1991). Some researchers have found no difference in quality based on ownership or whether the facility is part of a chain (Cohen and Dubay, 1990). Ullmann (1987) also found that profit-making facilities had consistently lower costs when controlling for quality ratings and casemix.

Growth (percent)

Sales		Earning Per Share				Profit
5-Year Average	Latest 12 Months	5-Year Average	Latest 12 Months	Sales (in $ millions)	Net Income (in $ millions)	Margin (percent)
7.3	3.9	NM	D–P	2,937	74	2.5
10.8	10.6	NA	22.4	602	40	6.7
10.4	24.4	38.2[a]	22.0	2,970	173	5.8
7.1	4.0	NM	31.1	1,470	62	4.2
13.2	14.4	30.0	16.5	1,200	83	6.9
-3.3	-20.5	NM	P–D	2,858	-320	Deficit
23.6	13.0	10.8	22.3	1,237	51	4.0
5.5	6.3	-18.8	11.8	1,449	60	4.3

Recently, Nyman (1988b) found that nonprofit nursing facilities in Iowa were associated with higher quality of care. Davis (1993) found that for-profit and chain facilities in Kentucky had lower operating costs and lower quality (as measured by a composite index of the likelihood rates for decubitus ulcers, catheterization, physical restraints, chemical restraints, and drug error rates) even though they also had higher ratios of RN per resident and lower overall staffing levels. Fottler and colleagues (1981) found an inverse relationship between profitability and patient care quality (as measured by staffing hours). Elwell (1984) also found a strong relationship between nonprofit and government ownership and higher staffing.

Using a quality-adjusted methodology, Gertler and Waldman (1994) found that for-profits were more efficient (lower costs), but nonprofits had higher quality (about 4 percent). The nonprofits had higher costs related to producing the higher quality. Thus, proprietary ownership and chain ownership have been associated with lower staffing levels and poorer process and outcome measures. Davis (1991), in a comprehensive review of the studies of ownership and quality, concluded that findings were mixed, but other studies with composite measures of quality seemed to indicate higher quality within nonprofit facilities.

Reimbursement Policies and Quality Outcomes

Some studies have attempted to use reimbursement policies to provide incentives to improve quality in nursing facilities. Kane and colleagues (1983a,b), using a multidimensional approach to measuring quality of care from chart reviews, observations, and interviewer ratings, recommended that nursing facility outcomes be given incentive payments for high quality of care. Kane and colleagues (1983a) recommended that rewards could be based on aggregate outcomes for groups of facilities. Willemain (1980) also recommended quality outcomes incentives.

Nyman (1988b) argued that nurses are professionally trained and are motivated to meet professional standards. He found that incentive-oriented policies that are regulatory, such as requiring more professional nursing hours per patient day, would improve quality. Alternatively, the Medicaid reimbursement rate could be linked to the proportion of private patients in the home, in order to encourage quality competition for private pay patients. More research is needed on what incentives would be most effective.

Several states have experimented with quality-of-care incentives. The San Diego project, which provided incentives to take heavy care patients, did not result in more care being provided and provided no evidence that incentives improved outcomes (Weissert et al., 1983; Meiners et al., 1985). Connecticut developed a system that was later discontinued because the goals of the project were not obtained (Geron, 1991). A study of the Illinois quality incentive program (QUIP) found that positive incentives tied to reimbursement can result in improved patient care (Geron, 1991). The QUIP program distributed about $20 million in bonus payments in fiscal year 1989 to facilities that met any of six areas of quality improvement: structure and environment; resident participation and choice; community and family participation; resident satisfaction; care plans; and specialized intensive services. The facilities showed improvements in the measured areas, except that the resident satisfaction standard failed to discriminate among facilities. Unfortunately, the validity of the measures was not established (Geron, 1991). As noted above, the Maryland system of paying for facilities to turn and position patients to prevent decubitus ulcers and to pay for resident improvement in ADLs for 2 months have been rated as effective (Weissert and Musliner, 1992a,b). The effort in Michigan has not been evaluated (Lewin/ICF, 1991).

There are a number of difficulties in developing a model for financial incentives to improve quality outcomes. First, the complexities of defining, identifying, and measuring quality outcomes for individual residents are great (Chapin and Silloway, 1992). A second issue is determining which outcomes should be rewarded and how to weight these items based on perceived social value. Another issue is how to link the quality measures to payment (Chapin and Silloway,

1992). Another issue is the administrative costs of developing and managing this kind of system.

In a review of the use of reimbursement incentives for outcomes, Lewin/ICF (1991) concluded that this approach is yet not feasible because the technology to distinguish between outcomes attributable to "facility effort" and other random factors or patient deterioration is not adequate. Another problem is that outcome-based incentives could have some negative consequences. Such incentive could encourage facilities to select patients who may improve rather than more chronic patients. There is a lack of consensus about which outcomes to reward (Lewin/ICF, 1991). Incentives for improved staffing for special activities (such as the turning project) could be beneficial, but such an approach could take a number of years to develop.

In spite of the difficulty of instituting reimbursement incentives for quality, reimbursement incentives could be directed toward increasing staffing levels and educating and training staff in nursing facilities. The positive relationship between quality and nurse staffing ratios, cited earlier, suggests that improved reimbursement incentives focused on this relationship may be effective.

Political Barriers to Regulation

Several barriers exist to increasing the staffing requirements in nursing facilities. The first and most important one is economic. Since government pays for 61 percent of current nursing home expenditures (Levit et al., 1994), Congress has been reluctant to increase the staffing requirements even though some Congressional representatives have been sympathetic to the need for increased staffing levels. The small staffing increases under OBRA 87 required substantial new resources. These small increases were apparently based on the amount legislators considered to be financially and politically feasible, because most of the costs for increased staffing would be reflected in increases in the federal and state Medicaid budgets. The fact that staffing levels were increased by Congress during the poor economic climate of the 1980s and while there was a large federal budget deficit reflected a Congressional recognition of the need for the increases.

Since OBRA 87 was passed, federal legislation has been considered by selected Congressional representatives for increased staffing beyond the OBRA requirements, but such legislation has not had the political support to proceed. States have the authority to increase their Medicaid payment rates as a means of increasing staffing standards, but the economic problems facing the states because of the growing Medicaid budget make it unlikely that states will initiate increases in nursing home staffing requirements.

A major barrier to increased staffing requirements is that nursing facilities have not always used state Medicaid rate increases to improve resident care. In the past, Medicaid rate increases were not used to increase staffing and presumably were used by some facilities to improve profitability (Feder and Scanlon,

1989; Weissert and Musliner, 1992b). Thus, some public officials are unwilling to support additional profit making. Current Medicaid and Medicare reimbursement allocations could be used to redistribute existing payments toward resident care.

Another problem is the historic opposition of the nursing home industry to regulation, which represents a major political obstacle to regulatory reform. Although the nursing home industry supports financial incentives for higher quality, their opposition to further regulation may stifle reform efforts. In the current economic and political environment, consumer and professional organizational pressures for reform may not have the political power to counter the opposition of the nursing home industry to new regulation.

SUMMARY FINDINGS AND DISCUSSION

The nursing home market is being strained by a growing demand for services. The greater acuity of illness and disability of individuals needing long-term care is placing new demands on providers of care. The supply of nursing facility beds has not kept pace with the growth in the oldest old population. This has resulted in nursing facilities being able to be somewhat selective in their admission practices and has limited the access to care of some individuals who may have the greatest need for services. The limited supply in some areas also appears to have a negative impact on the quality of nursing home care delivered in those areas.

There are a number of high quality nursing home facilities in the United States. These facilities have demonstrated that they can provide high quality of care even under the current economic constraints. On the other hand, the quality provided by nursing facilities is variable. In spite of increased regulatory efforts resulting from the implementation of the Nursing Home Reform Act in OBRA 87, there are still many problems with quality identified by state surveyors, residents and family members, ombudsmen, advocates, and researchers. Process measures for nursing home quality have been well developed and are used as a part of the nursing home survey process. Quality outcomes measures continue to be difficult to define and measure, especially for individuals with deteriorating conditions. Nevertheless, new data systems and outcomes measures have been developed and advances are being made in outcome measurement and monitoring.

Direct patient care and nurse staffing are critical structural factors that impact on both the process and the outcomes of care. Nursing staffing levels in nursing facilities are low compared to hospitals, and this is particularly the case in proprietary nursing facilities. Low salaries and benefits contribute to quality-of-care problems and high staff turnover rates. Low staff educational levels in nursing facilities are associated with low salaries. Inadequate nurse staffing levels have been shown to be a major factor in poor quality of nursing home care.

Economic factors are major forces shaping nursing home quality and staffing. The primary source of all nursing home revenues is Medicaid, so state Medicaid reimbursement policies have a major impact on the nursing home industry. As most states have adopted Medicaid prospective payment systems and strict methods for controlling costs, major problems with access and quality have developed. Moreover, many state methods specifically limit spending for direct resident care, which can have a negative impact on quality. Case-mix reimbursement systems that link payment to resident characteristics are being widely adopted by Medicaid programs and are under consideration by Medicare. Goals of these systems are to encourage facilities to improve access for heavy care residents and to design a more rational approach to payment. Evaluations of case-mix systems suggest that this approach will not improve quality and may not improve either access or cost controls. In fact, depending upon the design, such systems may encourage poorer quality of care and put unnecessary limits on staffing expenditures. Case-mix systems require careful monitoring to ensure that staffing levels and quality are maintained. New and improved reimbursement approaches that provide incentives to improve quality and staffing levels are needed.

Nursing home facilities are primarily private, profit-making organizations that are increasingly part of multiorganizational systems and investor-owned corporations. Consequently, nursing facilities are oriented toward increasing profits. Profit margins for the industry are generally good and historically have been increased by government policies that have paid for a return on equity. New policies have eliminated such payments for Medicare and some states are attempting to eliminate reimbursement, limit profit margins, or do both. Reimbursement policies that allow facilities to make profits by lowering staffing levels and quality of care are problematic.

The regulation of nursing facility quality may have improved since the implementation of OBRA 87. Nevertheless, regulatory efforts to assure quality need to be improved. One approach is to establish stricter minimum staffing standards and to develop guidelines for determining staffing levels that both facilities and regulators monitoring facility staffing can use. Another approach is to regulate how facilities allocate reimbursement resources to ensure that sufficient resources are directed to resident care and to limit excess profit taking and administrative costs. Another approach is to remove reimbursement limitations on nurse staffing expenditures, while controlling reimbursement for other cost areas such as profits, administration, and capital. Finally, reimbursement incentive systems are another way to encourage higher staffing levels and higher quality of care.

One problem with increasing staffing requirements is that the increased costs would fall primarily on the Medicaid and Medicare programs. Government officials have been reluctant to adopt new policies that will increase federal and state costs. In the current climate of federal deficits and stalled economic growth, such new policies would be feasible only if strict cost controls were placed on other components of nursing home costs. There is some evidence that limiting profits, administrative costs, and capital costs could achieve a savings that could shift funds to improve the quality of direct resident care.

REFERENCES

Aaronson, W., Zinn, J.S., Rosko, M.D. Do For-Profit and Not-For-Profit Nursing Homes Behave Differently? *The Gerontologist* 34:775–786, 1994.

Abelson, R. Health. *Forbes* (January 4):162–167, 1993.

Abt Associates and the Center for Health Policy Research. Briefing Points on Preliminary Evaluation Results. Briefing for the HCFA Leadership Conference. Bethesda, Md.: Abt Associates, July 27, 1993.

AHCA (American Health Care Association). Costs of an Employer Health Care Mandate. *Provider* 20(5):8, 1994.

Arling, G., Nordquist, R.H., Brant, B.A., and Capitman, J.A. Nursing Home Case Mix. *Medical Care* 25:9–19, 1987.

Arling, G., Zimmerman, D., and Updike, L. Nursing Home Case Mix in Wisconsin. Findings and Implications. *Medical Care* 27:164–181, 1989.

Arling, G., Nordquist, R.H., and Capitman, J.A. Nursing Home Cost and Ownership Type: Evidence of Interaction Effects. *HSR (Health Services Research)* 22:255, 1991.

Bishop, C.E. Competition in the Market for Nursing Home Care. *Journal of Health Politics, Policy and Law* 13:341–361, 1988.

Bowe, J. Financing Climate Heats Up. *Provider* 20(1):41–42, 1994.

Buchanan, J.L., Bell, R.M., Arnold, S.B. et al. Assessing Cost Effects of Nursing-Home-Based Geriatric Nurse Practitioners. *Health Care Financing Review* 11(3):67–78, 1990.

Buchanan, R.J., Madel, R.P., and Persons, D. Medicaid Payment Policies for Nursing Home Care: A National Survey. *Health Care Financing Review* 13(1):55–72, 1991.

Burns, J. Long-Term-Care Chains Show Slight Growth. *Modern Healthcare* (May 18):81–94, 1992.

Burton, L.C., German, P.S., Rovner, B.W., et al. Mental Illness and the Use of Restraints in Nursing Homes. *The Gerontologist* 32:164–170, 1992.

Butler, P.A., and Schlenker, R.E. Administering Nursing Home Case Mix Reimbursement Systems: Issues of Assessment, Quality, Access, Equity, and Cost—An Analysis of Long-term Care Payment Systems. Final Report. Denver: Center for Health Services Research, University of Colorado, 1988.

Cameron, J.M. Case-Mix and Resource Use in Long Term Care. *Medical Care* 23:296–309, 1985.

Chapin, R., and Silloway, G. Incentive Payments to Nursing Homes Based on Quality-of-Care Outcomes. *Journal of Applied Gerontology* 11(2):131–145, 1992.

Coburn, A.F., Fortinsky, R., McGuire, C., and McDonald, T.P. Effect of Prospective Reimbursement on Nursing Home Costs. *HSR (Health Services Research)* 28:44–68, 1993.

Cohen, J.W., and Dubay, L.C. The Effects of Medicaid Reimbursement Method and Ownership on Nursing Home Costs, Case Mix, and Staffing. *Inquiry* 27:183–200, 1990.

Cohodes, D.R. What to Do About Capital? *Hospital & Health Services Administration* 27(5):67–89, 1982.

Cotton, P. Nursing Home Research Focus on Outcomes May Mean Playing Catch-up with Regulation. *Journal of the American Medical Association* 269:2337–2338, 1993.

Davis, M.A. Nursing Home Quality: A Review and Analysis. *Medical Care Review* 48:129, 1991.

Davis, M.A. Nursing Home Ownership Revisited: Market, Cost and Quality Relationships. *Medical Care* 31:1062–1068, 1993.

Donabedian, A. *Exploration in Quality Assessment and Monitoring, Volume 1: The Definition of*

Quality and Approaches to its Assessment. Ann Arbor, Mich.: Health Administration Press, 1980.

Dor, A. The Costs of Medicare Patients in Nursing Homes in the United States. *Journal of Health Economics* 8:253–270, 1989.

DuNah, R., Harrington, C., Bedney, B., and Carrillo, H. Variations and Trends in Licensed Nursing Home Capacity in the States, 1978–1993. Paper prepared for the Health Care Financing Administration. San Francisco: University of California, 1995.

Ellwood, M.R., and Burwell, B. Access to Medicaid and Medicare by the Low-Income Disabled. *Health Care Financing Review* Ann. Suppl.:133–148, 1990.

Elwell, F. The Effects of Ownership on Institutional Services. *The Gerontologist* 24:77–83, 1984.

Evans, L., and Strumpf, N. Tying Down the Elderly. *Journal of the American Geriatrics Society* 37:65–74, 1989.

Falcone, D., Bolda, E., and Leak, S.C. Waiting for Placement: An Exploratory Analysis of Determinants of Delayed Discharges of Elderly Hospital Patients. *HSR (Health Services Research)* 26:339–374, 1991.

Feder, J., and Scanlon, W. Regulating the Bed Supply in Nursing Homes. *Milbank Memorial Fund Quarterly/Health and Society* 58(1):54–88, 1980.

Feder, J., and Scanlon, W. Case-Mix Payment for Nursing Home Care: Lessons from Maryland. *Journal of Health Politics, Policy and Law* 14:523–547, 1989.

Folkemer, D. *State Use of Home and Community-Based Services for the Aged Under Medicaid: Waiver Programs, Personal Care, Frail Elderly Services and Home Health Services.* Washington, D.C.: Intergovernmental Health Policy Project, 1994.

Fottler, M.D., Smith, H.L., and James, W.L. Profits and Patient Care Quality in Nursing Homes: Are They Compatible? *The Gerontologist* 21:532–538, 1981.

Friedman, B. Economic Aspects of the Rationing of Nursing Home Beds. *Journal of Human Resources* 17:59–71, 1982.

Fries, B.E., and Cooney, L. Resources Utilization Groups: A Patient Classification System for Long-term Care. *Health Care Financing Review* 23(2):110–122, 1985.

Fries, B.E., Schneider, D., Foley, W., and Dowling, M. Case-Mix Classification of Medicare Residents in Skilled Nursing Facilities. *Medical Care* 9:843–858, 1989.

Fries, B.E., Schneider, D., Foley, W., et al. Refining a Case-Mix Measure for Nursing Homes: Resources Utilization Groups (RUGS-III). *Medical Care* 32:668–685, 1994.

GAO (U.S. General Accounting Office). *Medicaid: Methods for Setting Nursing Home Rates Should Be Improved.* Report to the U.S. Secretary of Health and Human Services. Pub. no. HRD-86-26. Washington, D.C.: GAO, 1986.

GAO. *Medicare and Medicaid: Stronger Enforcement of Nursing Home Requirements Needed.* Report to the Chairman, Subcommittee on Health and Long-term Care, Select Committee on Aging, U.S. House of Representatives. Washington, D.C.: GAO, 1987.

GAO. *Long-term Care for the Elderly: Issues of Need, Access, and Cost.* Report to the Chairman, Subcommittee on Health and Long-term Care, Select Committee on Aging, U.S. House of Representatives. Pub. no. HRD-89-4. Washington, D.C.: GAO, November, 1988a.

GAO. *Medicare: Improved Patient Outcome Analysis Could Enhance Quality Assessment.* Report to the Chairman, Subcommittee on Health and Long-term Care, Select Committee on Aging, U.S. House of Representatives. Washington, D.C.: GAO, 1988b.

GAO. *Nursing Homes: Admission Problems for Medicaid Recipients and Attempts to Solve Them.* Report to the Chairman, Subcommittee on Health and Long-term Care, Select Committee on Aging, U.S. House of Representatives. Pub. no. HRD-90-35. Washington, D.C.: GAO, 1990.

Geron, S.M. Regulating the Behavior of Nursing Homes Through Positive Incentives: An Analysis of Illinois' Quality Incentive Program (QUIP). *The Gerontologist* 31:292–301, 1991.

Gertler, P.J. Subsidies, Quality, and the Regulation of Nursing Homes. *Journal of Public Economics* 38:33–52, 1989.

Gertler, P.J., and Waldman, D.M. *Why Are Not-For-Profit Nursing Homes More Costly?* Pub. no. DRU–723–NIA. Santa Monica, Calif.: RAND, 1994.

Greene, V.L., and Monahan, D. Structure and Operational Factors Affecting Quality of Patient Care in Nursing Homes. *Public Policy* 29:399–415, 1981.

Gurny, P., Hirsch, M.B., and Gondek, K.E. Chapter 11: A Description of Medicaid-Covered Services. *Health Care Financing Review: 1992 Annual Supplement* pp. 227–234, 1993.

Gustafson, D.H., Fiss, C.J., Fryback, F.C., et al. Measuring the Quality of Care in Nursing Homes: A Pilot Study in Wisconsin. *Public Health Reports* 95(4):336–343, 1980.

Gustafson, D.H., Sainfor, F.C., Van Konigsveld, R., and Zimmerman, D.R. The Quality Assessment Index (QAI) for Measuring Nursing Home Quality. *HSR (Health Services Research)* 25:97–127, 1990.

Guterman, S., Eggers, P., Riley, G., et al. The First 3 Years of Medicare Prospective Payment: An Overview. *Health Care Financing Review* 9:67–77, 1988.

Harrington, C. Developing Information on Nursing Home Quality. *Journal of Aging and Social Policy* 3(1/2):127–146, 1990a.

Harrington, C. Wages and Benefits of Nursing Personnel in Nursing Homes: Correcting the Inequities. *Nursing Economic$* 8:378–385, 1990b.

Harrington, C., and Estes, C.L. Trends in Nursing Homes in the Post Medicare Prospective Payment Period. San Francisco, Calif.: Institute for Health and Aging, 1989.

Harrington, C., and Swan, J.H. The Impact of State Medicaid Nursing Home Policies on Utilization and Expenditures. *Inquiry* 24:157–172, 1987.

Harrington, C., Preston S., Grant, L.A., and Swan, J.H. Revised Trends in States' Nursing Home Capacity. *Health Affairs* 11(2):170–180, 1992a.

Harrington, C., Tompkins, C., Curtis, M., and Grant, L. Psychotropic Drug Use in Long Term Care Facilities: A Review of the Literature. *The Gerontologist* 32:822–833, 1992b.

Harrington, C., Weinberg, J., Stawder, K., and DuNah, R. *Nursing Home Litigation Under the Boren Amendment: Case Studies.* San Francisco: University of California, 1993.

Harrington, C., Curtis, M., and DuNah, R., Jr. Trends in State Regulation of the Supply of Long Term Care Services. Paper prepared for the Department of Housing and Urban Development and the Health Care Financing Administration. San Francisco: University of California, 1994a.

Harrington, C., DuNah, R., Jr., and Bedney, B. The Supply of Community-Based Long Term Care Services in 1992. Paper prepared for the Department of Housing and Urban Development and the Health Care Financing Administration. San Francisco: University of California, 1994b.

Harrington, C., DuNah, R., Jr., and Curtis, M. State Variations and Trends in Preadmission Screening. Paper prepared for the Department of Housing and Urban Development and the Health Care Financing Administration. San Francisco: University of California, 1994c.

Harrington, C., Thollaug, S.C., and Summers, P.R. Nursing Facilities, Staffing, Residents and Facility Deficiencies, 1991–93. Paper prepared for the Health Care Financing Administration. San Francisco: University of California, 1995.

Harrington et al. *1993 State Data Book on Long-term Care Programs and Market Characteristics.* Baltimore, Md.: Health Care Financing Administration, in press.

Hawes, C., and Phillips, C.D. The Changing Structure of the Nursing Home Industry and the Impact of Ownership on Quality, Cost, and Access. Pp. 492–538 in: Institute of Medicine. *For-Profit Enterprise in Health Care.* B.H. Gray, ed. Washington, D.C.: National Academy Press, 1986.

Hay, D.G. Health Care Services in 100 Superior Nursing Homes. *Long-term Care and Health Services Administration Quarterly* 1:300–313, 1977.

HCFA (Health Care Financing Administration). Medicare and Medicaid Requirements for Long Term Care Facilities. Final Rule. *Federal Register*, 1991.

HCFA. *Medicaid spDATA System. Characteristics of Medicaid State Programs. Volume 1. National Comparisons.* Pub. no. 02178. Washington, D.C.: Medicaid Bureau, HCFA, 1992a.

HCFA. *State Medicaid Manual. Part 2 State Organization and General Administration.* Transmittal No. 79. HCFA Pub. no. 45–2. Washington, D.C.: HFCA, 1992b.

HCFA. *Medicare and Medicaid Programs; Survey, Certification, and Enforcement of Skilled Nursing Facilities and Nursing Facilities.* Final Rule 42 CFR Parts 401–498. *Federal Register* 59(217):56116–56252, 1994a.

HCFA. *Report to Congress on Nursing Facility Staffing Requirements.* Washington, D.C.: Medicaid Bureau, HCFA, 1994b.

HCIA and Arthur Andersen. *The Guide to the Nursing Home Industry.* Baltimore, Md.: HCIA Inc., and Arthur Andersen and Company, 1994.

Hing, E. Effects of the Prospective Payment System on Nursing Homes. Pub. no. PHS-89-1759. Washington, D.C.: National Center for Health Statistics, 1989.

Holahan, J. *Nursing Home Care Under Alternative Patient-Related Reimbursement Systems.* Washington, D.C.: The Urban Institute, 1984.

Holahan, J. State Rate-Setting and Its Effects on the Cost of Nursing-Home Care. *Journal of Health Politics, Policy and Law* 9:647–667, 1985.

Holahan, J., and Cohen, J. Nursing Home Reimbursement: Implications for Cost Containment, Access, and Quality. *Milbank Quarterly* 65(1):112–147, 1987.

Holahan, J., and Sulvetta, M.B. Assessing Medicare Reimbursement Options for Skilled Nursing Facility Care. *Health Care Financing Review* 10(3):13–27, 1989.

Holahan, J., Rowland, D., Feder, J., and Heslam, D. DataWatch: Explaining the Recent Growth in Medicaid Spending. *Health Affairs* 12(3):177–193, 1993.

IOM (Institute of Medicine). *Improving the Quality of Care in Nursing Homes.* Washington, D.C.: National Academy Press, 1986.

Jones, D. Bonito, A., Gower, S., and Williams, R. *Analysis of the Environment for the Recruitment and Retention of Registered Nurses in Nursing Homes.* Washington, D.C.: U.S. Department of Health & Human Services, 1987.

Justice, D. *State Long Term Care Reform: Development of Community Care Systems in Six States.* Washington, D.C.: National Governors' Association, April, 1988.

Kanda, K., and Mezey, M. Registered Nurse Staffing in Pennsylvania Nursing Homes: Comparison Before and After Implementation of Medicare's Prospective Payment System. *The Gerontologist* 31:318–324, 1991.

Kane, R.A. Assessing Quality in Nursing Homes. *Clinics in Geriatric Medicine* 4:655–666, 1988.

Kane, R.A., and Kane, R.L. Long-term Care: Variations on a Quality Assurance Theme. *Inquiry* 25:132–146, 1988.

Kane, R.L., Bell, R., Riegler, S., et al. Assessing the Outcomes of Nursing Home Patients. *Journal of Gerontology* 38(4):385–393, 1983a.

Kane, R.L., Bell, R., Riegler, S., et al. Predicting the Outcomes of Nursing Home Patients. *The Gerontologist* 23:200–206, 1983b.

Kane, R.A., Kane, R.L., Arnold, S. et al. Geriatric Nurse Practitioners as Nursing Home Employees: Implementing the Role. *The Gerontologist* 28:469–477, 1988.

Kane, R.L., Garrard, J., Skay, C.L. et al. Effect of a Geriatric Nurse Practitioner on the Process and Outcomes of Nursing Home Care. *American Journal of Public Health* 79:1271–1277, 1989.

Kenney, G., and Holahan, J. The Nursing Home Market and Hospital Discharge Delays. *Inquiry* 27:73–85, Spring, 1990.

Kichen, S. Annual Report on American Industry. *Forbes* (January 2):122–125, 1995.

Koetting, M. *Nursing Home Organization and Efficiency.* Lexington, Mass.: Lexington Books, 1980.

Kosciesza, I. What's Ahead in the Post-Health Planning Era. *Health Policy Week Special Report* (June 1):1–5, 1987.

Latta, V.B., and Keene, R.E. Use and Cost of Skilled Nursing Facility Services Under Medicare, 1987. *Health Care Financing Review* 11(1):105–116, 1989.

Lee, A.J., Birnbaum, H., and Bishop, C. How Nursing Home Behave: A Multi-Equation Model of Nursing Home Behavior. *Social Science and Medicine* 17(23):1897–1906, 1983.

Letsch, S.W., Lazenby, H.C., Levit, L.R., and Cowan, C.A. National Health Expenditures, 1991. *Health Care Financing Review* 14(2):1–30, 1992.

Levit, K.R., Sensenig, A.L., Cowan, C.A. et al. National Health Expenditures 1993. *Health Care Financing Review* 16(1):247–294, 1994.

Lewin/ICF. *Synthesis of Medicaid Reimbursement Options for Nursing Home Care.* Submitted to the Health Care Financing Administration. Washington, D.C.: Lewin/ICF, 1991.

Lewis, M., Kane, R., Cretin, S., and Clark, V. The Immediate and Subsequent Outcomes of Nursing Home Care. *American Journal of Public Health* 75(7):758–762, 1985.

Libow, L., and Starer, P. Care of the Nursing Home Patient. *New England Journal of Medicine* 321:93–96, 1989.

Linn, M, Gurel, L., and Linn, B.A. Patient Outcome as a Measure of Quality of Nursing Home Care. *American Journal of Public Health* 67:337–344, 1977.

Lipson, L., and Laudicina, S. *State Home and Community-Based Services for the Aged Under Medicaid: Waiver Programs, Optional Services Under the Medicaid State Plan, and OBRA 1990 Provisions for a New Optional Benefit.* Washington, D.C.: American Association of Retired Persons, 1991.

Matteson, M., and McConnell, E.S. *Gerontological Nursing.* Philadelphia: W.B. Saunders, 1988.

Meiners, M., Thornburn, P., Roddy, P., and Jones, B. *Nursing Home Admissions: The Results of an Incentive Reimbursement Experiment.* Long Term Care Studies Program Research Report. Pub. no. PHS 86-3397. Rockville, Md.: National Center for Health Services Research and Health Care Technology Assessment, 1985.

Mendelson, D.N., and Arnold, J. Certificate of Need Revisited. *Spectrum* (Winter):36–44, 1993.

Mendelson, D.N., and Schwartz, W.B. The Effects of Aging and Population Growth on Health Care Costs. *Health Affairs* 12(1):119–125, 1993.

Mezey, M.D., and Lynaugh, J.E. The Teaching Nursing Home Program. *Nursing Clinics of North America* 24(3):769–780, 1989.

Mezey, M.D., and Lynaugh, J.E. Teaching Nursing Home Program: A Lesson in Quality. *Geriatric Nursing* (March/April):76–77, 1991.

Mezey, M.D., Lynaugh, J.E., and Cartier, M.M., eds. *Nursing Homes and Care: Lessons from Teaching Nursing Homes.* New York: Springer, 1989.

Miller, N.A. Medicaid 2176 Home and Community-Based Care Waivers: The First Ten Years. *Health Affairs* 11(4):162–171, 1992.

Mohler, M. Combined Federal and State Nursing Services Staffing Standards. Washington, D.C.: National Committee to Preserve Social Security and Medicare, 1993.

Mohler, M., and Lessard, W. Nursing Staff in Nursing Homes: Additional Staff Needed and Cost to Meet Requirements and Quality of OBRA 87. Testimony prepared for the U.S. House of Representatives, Select Committee on Aging. Washington, D.C.: U.S. House, 1991.

Moos, R.H., and Lemke, S. *Multiphasic Environmental Assessment Procedure Manual.* Palo Alto, Calif.: Social Ecology Laboratory, Veterans Administration and Stanford University Medical Center, 1984a.

Moos, R.H., and Lemke, S. Supportive Residential Settings for Older People. In: I. Altman, M.P. Lawton, and J.F. Wohlwill, eds. *Elderly People and the Environment.* New York: Plenum, 1984b.

Morris, J.N., Hawes, C., Fries, B.E., et al. Designing the National Resident Assessment Instrument for Nursing Homes. *The Gerontologist* 30:293–307, 1990.

Moses, E. 1991 National Employment Estimates of Selected Health Care Personnel in Home Health Care Agencies, Hospices, Nursing Homes, and Board and Care (Residential) Homes. Unpublished Data from the 1991 National Health Provider Inventory. Washington, D.C.: Division of Nursing, Bureau of Health Professions, Health Resources and Services Administration, 1994a.

Moses, E.B. *1992 The Registered Nurse Population: Findings from the National Sample Survey of Registered Nurses, March 1992.* Washington, D.C.: Division of Nursing, Bureau of Health Professions, Health Resources and Services Administration, 1994b.

Munroe, D.J. The Influence of Registered Nursing Staffing on the Quality of Nursing Home Care. *Research in Nursing and Health* 13(4):263–270, 1990.

Murtaugh, C.M., Kemper, P., and Spillman, B.C. The Risk of Nursing Home Use in Later Life. *Medical Care* 28:952–962, 1990.

NAHC (National Association for Home Care). *Basic Statistics about Home Care 1992.* Washington, D.C.: NAHC, 1993.

NCCNHR (National Citizens' Coalition for Nursing Home Reform). *Consumer Statement of Principles for the Nursing Home Regulatory System—State Licensure and Federal Certification Programs.* Washington, D.C.: NCCNHR, 1983.

NCCNHR. Advocates Urge IOM Panel to Back Nurse Staffing Standards. *Quality Care Advocate* 9(6):1,7,8, 1994.

Neu, C.R., and Harrison, S.C. *Posthospital Care Before and After the Medicare Prospective Payment System.* Health Care Financing Administration. Santa Monica, Calif.: RAND, 1988.

Nyman, J.A. Prospective and "Cost-Plus" Medicaid Reimbursement, Excess Medicaid Demand, and the Quality of Nursing Home Care. *Journal of Health Economics* 4:237–259, 1985.

Nyman, J.A. The Effect of Competition on Nursing Home Expenditures Under Prospective Reimbursement. *HSR (Health Services Research)* 23:555, 1988a.

Nyman, J.A. Improving the Quality of Nursing Home Outcomes: Are Adequacy- or Incentive-Oriented Policies More Effective? *Medical Care* 26:1158–1171, 1988b.

Nyman, J.A. Analysis of Nursing Home Use and Bed Supply, Wisconsin, 1983. *HSR (Health Services Research)* 24:511–538, 1989a.

Nyman, J.A. Excess Demand, Consumer Rationality, and the Quality of Care in Regulated Nursing Homes. *HSR (Health Services Research)* 24:105–127, 1989b.

Nyman, J.A. The Future of Nursing Home Policy: Should Policy Be Based on an Excess Demand Paradigm? *Advances in Health Economics and Health Services Research* 11:229–250, 1990.

Nyman, J.A. Testing for Excess Demand in Nursing Home Care Markets. *Medical Care* 31:680–693, 1993.

Nyman, J.A., Breaker, D.L., and Link, D. Technical Efficiency in Nursing Home. *Medical Care* 28:541–551, 1990.

O'Brien, J., Saxberg, B.O., and Smith, H.L. For Profit or Not-For-Profit Nursing Homes: Does It Matter? *The Gerontologist* 23:341–348, 1983.

Ohsfeldt, R.L., Antel, J.J., and Buchanan, R.J. *The Effect of Prospective Payment on Medicaid Payment Rates for Nursing Home Care.* Birmingham, Ala.: Lister Hill Center for Health Policy, pp. 54–64, 1991.

OBRA 87 (Omnibus Budget Reconciliation Act of 1987). Public Law 100–203, subtitle C: Nursing Home Reform. Signed by the President, Washington, D.C., December 22, 1987.

Ouslander, J., and Kane, R. The Costs of Urinary Incontinence in Nursing Homes. *Medical Care* 22:69–79, 1984.

Ouslander, J., Kane, R., and Abrass, A. Urinary Incontinence in Elderly Nursing Home Patients. *Journal of the American Medical Association* 248:1194–1198, 1982.

Phillips, C.D., and Hawes, C. *Discrimination by Nursing Homes Against Medicaid Recipients: The Potential Impact of Equal Access on the Industry's Profitability.* Research Triangle Park, N.C.: Research Triangle Institute, 1988.

Phillips, C.D., Hawes, C., and Fries, B.E. Reducing the Use of Physical Restraints in Nursing Homes: Will It Increase Costs? *American Journal of Public Health* 83:342–348, 1993.

Punch, L. Investor-Owned Chains Lead Increase in Beds. *Modern Healthcare* (June 7):126–136, 1985.

Ray, W.A., Federspiel, C.F., Baugh, D.K., and Dodds, S. Interstate Variation in Elderly Medicaid Nursing Home Populations. *Medical Care* 25:738–753, 1987.

Ribeiro, B.J., and Smith, S.R. Evaluation of Urinary Catheterization and Urinary Incontinence in a General Nursing Home Population. *Journal of the American Geriatrics Society* 33:479–482, 1985.

Rudder, C. *New York State's Nursing Home Industry: Profit, Losses, Expenditures and Quality.* New York, N.Y.: Nursing Home Community Coalition of New York State, 1994.

Scanlon, W.J. Nursing Home Utilization Patterns: Implications for Policy. *Journal of Health Politics, Policy and Law* 4(4):619–641, 1980a.

Scanlon, W.J. A Theory of the Nursing Home Market. *Inquiry* 17(1):25–41, 1980b.

Schieber, G., Wiener, J., Liu, K., and Doty, P. Prospective Payment for Medicare Skilled Nursing Facilities: Background and Issues. *Health Care Financing Review* 8(1):79–85, 1986.

Schlenker, R.E. Comparison of Medicaid Nursing Home Payment Systems. *Health Care Financing Review* 13(1):93–109, 1991a.

Schlenker, R.E. Nursing Home Costs, Medicaid Rates, and Profits Under Alternative Medicaid Payment Systems. *HSR (Health Services Research)* 26:623–649, 1991b.

Schlenker, R.E., Shaughnessy, P.W., and Yslas, I. Estimating Patient-Level Nursing Home Costs. *HSR (Health Services Research)* 20:103–128, 1985.

Schlenker, R.E., Stiles, J.D., Carlough, T., and DeVore, P.A. *A Multi-State Analysis of Medicaid Nursing Home Payment Systems: An Analysis of Long-term Care Payment Systems.* Final Report. Denver, Colo.: Center for Health Services Research, University of Colorado, 1988.

Schneider, D.P., Fries, B.E., Foley, W.J., et al. Case Mix for Nursing Home Payment: Resource Utilization Groups, Version II. *Health Care Financing Review* Ann. Suppl.:39–52, 1988.

Shaughnessy, P.W., and Kramer, A.M. Tradeoffs in Evaluating the Effectiveness of Nursing Home Care. In: M.D. Mezey, J.E. Lynaugh, and M.M. Cartier, eds. *Nursing Homes and Care: Lessons from Teaching Nursing Homes.* New York: Springer Publishing, 1989.

Shaughnessy, P.W., Schlenker, R.E., and Kramer, A.M. Quality of Long-term Care in Nursing Homes and Swing-Bed Hospitals. *HSR (Health Services Research)* 25:65–96, 1990.

Sirrocco, A. Nursing Homes and Board and Care Homes: Data From the 1991 National Health Provider Inventory. *Advance Data from Vital and Health Statistics.* No. 244. Pub. no. 94-1250. Hyattsville, Md.: National Center for Health Statistics, 1994.

Spector, W.D., and Takada, H.A. Characteristics of Nursing Homes That Affect Resident Outcomes. *Journal of Aging and Health* 3(4):427–454, 1991.

Strahan, G. Nursing Home Characteristics: Preliminary Data from the 1985 National Nursing Home Survey. *Advance Data from Vital and Health Statistics.* No. 131. Pub. no. (PHS)87-1250. Hyattsville, Md.: National Center for Health Statistics, 1987.

Strahan, G. Characteristics of Registered Nurses in Nursing Homes: Preliminary Data from the 1985 National Nursing Home Survey. *Advance Data from Vital and Health Statistics.* No. 152. Pub. no (PHS)88-1250. Hyattsville, Md.: National Center for Health Statistics, 1988.

Swan, J.H., and Harrington, C. Estimating Undersupply of Nursing Home Beds in States. *HSR (Health Services Research)* 21:57–83, 1986.

Swan, J.H., and Harrington, C. Certificate of Need and Nursing Home Bed Capacity in States. *Journal of Health and Social Policy* 2(2):87–105, 1990.

Swan, J.H., Harrington, C., and Grant. L.A. State Medicaid Reimbursement for Nursing Homes, 1978–1986. *Health Care Financing Review* 9(3):33–50, 1988.

Swan, J.H., Dewit, S., Pickard, R., et al. *Trends in State Medicaid Reimbursement for Nursing Homes, 1978–92.* Paper prepared for the U.S. Department of Housing and Urban Development and the U.S. Health Care Financing Administration. Wichita, Kans.: Wichita State University, 1993a.

Swan, J.H., Harrington, C., DuNah, R., et al. Estimating Adequacy of Nursing Home Bed Supply in the States. Paper prepared for the U.S. Department of Housing and Urban Development and the U.S. Health Care Financing Administration. Wichita, Kans.: Wichita State University, 1993b.

Swan, J.H., Harrington, C., and Grant, L.A. State Medicaid Reimbursement for Nursing Homes, 1978–88. *Health Care Financing Review* 14(4):111–131, 1993c.

Swan, J.H., Dewit, S., and Harrington, C. State Medicaid Reimbursement Methods and Rates for Nursing Homes, 1993. Paper prepared for the U.S. Department of Housing and Urban Development and the U.S. Health Care Financing Administration. Wichita, Kans.: Wichita State University, 1994.

Turner, T. Executive Committee of the Council on Nursing Administration. Letter on Nursing Staffing. Washington, D.C.: American Nurses Association, 1987.

U.S. Army Headquarters. *The Workload Management System for Nursing.* Pub. no. FM 8-501. Washington, D.C.: U.S. Department of Defense, 1990.

U.S. House of Representatives, Committee on Ways and Means. *Overview of Entitlement Programs, 1990 Green Book.* Washington, D.C.: U.S. Government Printing Office, p. 147–149, 1990.

U.S. Office of the Inspector General. *State Progress in Carrying Out the Nursing Home Survey Reforms.* Pub. no. OEI-01-91-01580. Washington, D.C.: The Office, 1993.

U.S. Senate, Special Committee on Aging. *Nursing Home Care: The Unfinished Agenda.* 1 (Special Hearing and Report), May 21, 1986. Washington, D.C.: U.S. Government Printing Office 1986.

U.S. Senate, Special Committee on Aging. *Reducing the Use of Chemical Restraints in Nursing Homes*: *Workshop Before the Special Committee.* Pub. no. SN 102-6. Washington, D.C.: U.S. Government Printing Office, 1991.

Ullmann, S.G. Assessment of Facility Quality and Its Relationship to Facility Size in the Long-term Health Care Industry. *The Gerontologist* 21:91–97, 1981.

Ullmann, S.G. Cost Analysis and Facility Reimbursement in the Long-term Health Care Industry. *HSR (Health Services Research)* 19:83–102, 1984.

Ullmann, S.G. Ownership, Regulation, Quality Assessment, and Performance in the Long-term Health Care Industry. *The Gerontologist* 27:233–239, 1987.

Wallace, C. Chains Plan Growth in Response to Rising Demand for Services. *Modern Healthcare* (June 6):116–126, 1986.

Walsh, M. Health. *Forbes* (January 2):180–182, 1995.

Weinberg, J., Harrington, C., Stawder, K., and DuNah, R. *Nursing Home Litigation Under the Boren Amendment: Issues and Analysis.* San Francisco: University of California, 1993.

Weissert, W.G., and Cready, C.M. Determinants of Hospital-to-Nursing Home Placement Delays: A Pilot Study. *HSR (Health Services Research)* 23:619–646, 1988.

Weissert, W.G., and Musliner, M.C. *Access, Quality, and Cost Consequences of Case-Mix Adjusted Reimbursement for Nursing Homes.* Pub. no. 9109. Washington, D.C.: American Association of Retired Persons, 1992a.

Weissert, W.G., and Musliner, M.C. Case Mix Adjusted Nursing-Home Reimbursement: A Critical Review of the Evidence. *Milbank Quarterly* 70(3):455–490, 1992b.

Weissert, W.G., Scanlon, W.J., Wan, T.T.H., and Skinner, D.E. Care for the Chronically Ill: Nursing Home Incentive Payment Experiment. *Health Care Financing Review* 5:41–49, 1983.

Willemain, T.R. A Comparison of Patient-Centered and Case Mix Reimbursement for Nursing Home Care. *HSR (Health Services Research)* 15:365–77, 1980.

Zedlewski, S.R., and McBride, T.D. The Changing Profile of the Elderly: Effects on Future Long-term Care Needs and Financing. *Milbank Quarterly* 70(2):247–275, 1992.

Zimmer, J.G. Quality of Care Assessment in Long-term Care Facilities. *Evaluation and the Health Professions* 6:339–344, 1983.

Zimmer, J.G. *Quality Assurance. Principles and Practice of Nursing Home Care.* P.R. Katz and E. Calkins, eds. New York: Springer Publishing, 1989.

Zimmer, J.G., Bentley, D.W., Valenti, W.M., and Watson, N.M. Systemic Antibiotic Use in Nursing Homes: A Quality Assessment. *Journal of American Geriatric Society* 34:703–710, 1986.

Zimmerman, D.R. *Impact of New Regulations and Data Sources on Nursing Home Quality of Care.* Madison, Wisc.: Center for Health Systems Research and Analysis, 1990.

Zimmerman, D.R., Egan, J.R., Gustafson, D. et al. *Evaluation of the State Demonstrations in Nursing Home Quality Assurance Processes.* Final Report to the Health Care Financing Administration. Madison, Wisc.: Mathematica Policy Research, 1985.

Zinn, J.S. Inter-SMSA Variation on Nursing Home Staffing and Management Practices. *Journal of Applied Gerontology* 12(2):206–224, 1993a.

Zinn, J.S. The Influence of Nurse Wage Differentials on Nursing Home Staffing and Resident Care Decisions. *The Gerontologist* 33:721–729, 1993b.

Zinn, J.S., Aaronson, W.A., and Rosko, D.M. The Use of Standardized Indicators as Quality Improvement Tools: An Application in Pennsylvania Nursing Homes. *American Journal of Medical Quality* 8:456–465, 1993a.

Zinn, J.S., Aaronson, W.A., and Rosko, D.M. Variations in Outcomes of Care Provided in Pennsylvania Nursing Homes: Facility and Environmental Correlates. *Medical Care* 31:475–487, 1993b.

Nursing Injury, Stress, and Nursing Care

Bonnie Rogers, Dr.P.H., C.O.H.N., F.A.A.N.

The health care industry is one of the largest employers in the United States, with more than 7 million employees in 1990 and with that number expected to increase to more than 10 million by the year 2000 (BLS, 1991). These health care environments are high-risk workplaces with a wide range of exposures and hazards (see Table 1) (Hudson, 1990; Rogers and Travers, 1991; Wilkinson et al., 1992). The U.S. Bureau of Labor Statistics (BLS) reports the incidence rate per 100 full-time workers for nonfatal occupational injuries and illnesses for 1993 was 11.8 for hospital establishments and 17.3 for nursing and personal care facilities. This compares to a private industry rate of 8.5 (BLS, 1994b). In addition, the Bureau reports that for 1992 the incidence of injuries and illnesses involving days away from work is greater for certain occupations than their proportion of total employment. These relatively hazardous occupations include male-dominated work, such as construction and transportation; female-dominated activities, such as nursing care and housekeeping services; and gender-shared activities, such as assembling products. Nurses' aides (NA) were second only to truck drivers in the total number of cases of disabling injury and illness, with an estimated 145,900 cases for truck drivers compared to 111,100 for NAs. For persons in all occupations working less than 1 year, NAs were reported as having the most injuries or illnesses (approximately 67,000), primarily sprains

Dr. Rogers is an associate professor of nursing and public health and director of the Occupational Health Nursing Program, University of North Carolina, Chapel Hill.

TABLE 1 Categories of Potential or Actual Occupational Hazards

Biologic-infectious hazards: Infectious-biologic agents, such as bacteria, viruses, fungi, or parasites, that may be transmitted via contact with infected patients or contaminated body secretions or fluids.

Chemical hazards: Various forms of chemicals that are potentially toxic or irritating to body systems, including medications, solutions, and gases.

Environmental-mechanical hazards: Factors encountered in work environments that cause or potentiate accidents, injuries, strain, or discomfort (e.g., poor equipment or lifting devices, slippery floors).

Physical hazards: Agents within work environments, such as radiation, electricity, extreme temperatures, and noise, that can cause tissue trauma.

Psychosocial hazards: Factors and situations encountered or associated with the job or work environment that create or potentiate stress, emotional strain, and interpersonal problems.

and strains, and they cited overexertion related to patient care as the primary cause.

The cost implications to health care providers of relatively high injury rates for their employees are especially troublesome down the road because, according to BLS estimates, the industry's work force is expected to grow at twice the rate for all nonfarm wage and salary workers between 1992 and 2005. In 1992, private sector health services employed 8.5 million workers, for whom nearly 700,000 work-related injuries and illnesses were reported that year.

Nursing personnel deliver care to individuals in a variety of settings including hospital-based and community-based environments. Only within recent years has any real attention been paid to the occupational risks and injuries of nurses. Also, there is evidence that stress related to work overload and staffing patterns, including shift work, can and does contribute to illness and injury in the nurse population (Jung, 1986; Phillips and Brown, 1992). Many factors such as the physical work environment, organizational and institutional characteristics, and personal work practice habits contribute to health care workers' occupational risk for hazard exposure and the resultant injury and stress that occurs (Rogers and Travers, 1991). The impact of these events is of concern not only in terms of the health risk to the worker, but also because of the effects on quality care and nursing.

In this paper, much of the research that is discussed describes the nature and severity of specific injuries of major concern in nursing and stress in nursing. The paper also provides some linkage, although less frequently, for the relationships of injury and stress to the quality of nursing care delivered and the impact of these factors on the nursing profession. Several investigations have reported various types of injuries, but back injuries and needlestick injuries are of most concern and therefore will be most examined. While the reporting of assaults on health care workers may be improved, violence toward this group seems to be rising and will be discussed as a serious emerging threat (Lanza, 1992; Lechky, 1994). In addition, stress continues to plague nurses resulting in burnout and high turnover. It is clear that factors influencing injury and stress, and interactions between and among them, are of significant importance.

INJURIES IN NURSING PRACTICE

Back Injuries

Although back injuries are considered the most expensive workers' compensation problem today (McAbee, 1988), the extent of low back pain and injury in nursing personnel is thought to be underestimated. A survey by Owen (1989) of 503 nurses found that only 34 percent of respondents with work-related low back pain filed an injury report, and 12 percent were contemplating leaving the profession because of the problem. Several studies indicate that tertiary care hospital staff have reported work-related back pain and injury and that they implicate lifting techniques, poor staffing, ergonomics, inadequate communication, and constitutional factors as contributory factors. Recommended approaches to reduce the incidence of occupational back injury include better mechanical lifting devices, improved staffing, improved training and education, and attention to worker-job capabilities. (Harber et al., 1985; Marchette and Marchette, 1985; Arad and Ryan, 1986; Jensen, 1987; Carney, 1993; Jorgensen et al., 1994).

Wilkinson and colleagues (1992) retrospectively investigated occupational injuries among 9,668 university health science center and hospital employees during a 32-month period. During this time, 1,513 injuries were reported with the most frequent being needlestick injuries (32.1 percent) followed by sprains and strains (17.2 percent); of the latter, 55 percent involved back injuries that were reportedly caused by lifting and twisting motions. Nearly 10 percent of those injured lost time from work. Out of 18 job classifications analyzed, nursing, which included NAs, ranked third highest in injury reports. In overall reporting, professional nurses reported the highest number of illnesses and injuries; within the total nursing group, however, NAs reported the highest injury attack rate after data were adjusted for the size of the population at risk. Workers' compensation costs were highest for back injuries, which equaled $171,957. Other types of injuries reported included lacerations and contusions.

Through survey and ergonomic analysis, including videotaping in a Wisconsin nursing home/long-term-care facility, Owen and Garg (1991) evaluated 38 nursing assistants with respect to factors associated with back injury. Tasks were categorized into 16 areas, and activities associated with transferring clients from one location to another (e.g., transfer from toilet to chair; bed to chair; tub to chair) were ranked highest (the top 6 out of the 16 categories).

In a related article, Garg and colleagues (1992) observed nursing assistants who worked in teams of 2 and performed 24 patient transfers per 8 hour shift by manually lifting and carrying patients. Assistive devices (e.g., hydraulic lift) were used less than 2 percent of the time. Patient safety and comfort, lack of accessibility, physical stresses associated with the devices, lack of skill, increased transfer time, and lack of staffing were some of the reasons cited for not using these assistive devices. The 2-person walking belt manual method for transferring was perceived to be the most comfortable, secure, and least stressful approach. Adequate numbers of effectively trained personnel, however, are needed to carry out this approach. In addition, environmental barriers (such as confined workplaces, an uneven floor surface, lack of adjustability of beds, stationary railings around the toilet) made the job more difficult. Nursing assistants had a high prevalence of low-back pain and 51 percent of nursing assistants reported visiting a health care provider in the past 3 years for work-related low-back pain.

Kaiser-Permanente Medical Centers in Portland, Oregon, found back injury rates from workers' compensation claims ranging from 10 percent to 30 percent on hospital units. As a result, a back injury prevention project was pilot tested (Feldstein et al., 1993). Divided into intervention and control groups, 55 nurses, NAs, and orderlies participated in the project. Instructional methods on body mechanics, transfer maneuvers, exercise, and stretching were provided to the intervention group. Prior to the intervention, information specific to back pain and injury was collected, resulting in the following data: 86 percent reported work-related back fatigue; 74 percent reported that back pain interfered with the quality of work performance; 55 percent reported lost work time; 32 percent reported lost time of more than 3 days related to the injury; 60 percent required medical intervention; and 91 percent reported that patient handling put them at risk. "New" nurses with less than 5 years of experience reported more frequent back pain, but veteran nurses considered their injuries more disabling. Body mass index and lack of flexibility were significantly associated with back pain and injury, while educational levels were inversely related. Age, height, weight, and job title showed no association. Although not statistically significant, scores used to measure back pain and fatigue were reduced after the intervention while no such reduction was seen in the control group. The intervention group had a 19 percent improvement in their average total score for the quality of patient transfers, a 17 percent improvement in preparation for transfer, a 15 percent improvement in the position for transfer, and a 26 percent improvement in the actual transfer. The control group did not show any significant improvement during the same time period. The study findings suggest that if new nurses are truly at higher risk, the need for aggressive new employee training is needed.

In a British study of work-related back pain, Newman and Callaghan (1993) analyzed data from 173 nurses and midwifery staff (the response rate was 65 percent). Of those responding, 76 percent had experienced pain in the past 2 years and 50 percent either took time off work or needed to recuperate on days off. The total number of days nurses were "unfit" to work totaled 2,769 or 2.63 days per nurse per year. An estimated cost for lost work time equaled $146,622. Only 6 percent of nurses indicated that they reported every back pain injury they suffered. Perceived risk factors for back injury included inadequate staffing and staffing patterns, heavy dependent patients, previous back injury, lack of equipment, working in confined spaces, and the type of uniform worn (the dress-type uniform created lifting and motion problems).

Based on a survey of 100 nurses who reported work-related back injuries and comparison with a control group of uninjured nurses, Garrett and colleagues (1992) found that nurses in the early phases of assignment on long-term-care units were at greatest risk of back injury. In addition, severity of injury was significantly related to the evening tour of duty and the weight of the nurse (greater than 200 pounds), with the latter always leading to lost work time. Forty percent of nurses in this category were ultimately disabled. Approximately three-fourths of the reported back injuries resulted in lost duty or light duty assignments compared to only 11 percent for other injuries reported. No differences were found among genders or nurse job classifications (registered nurse, licensed practical nurse, nurse assistant). The findings in this study related to lack of or limited work experience are consistent with those of McAbee (1988) who reported that 72.3 percent of study subjects with less than 3 years of experience suffered back injuries.

Cato and colleagues (1989) surveyed 53 orthopedic staff nurses in a large hospital regarding the incidence and severity of back pain and injury. Nearly two-thirds of respondents reported work-related back pain, with 90 percent indicating that patient handling was responsible for their most severe pain episode. While assistive devices were considered to be adequate, staffing levels were cited frequently as inadequate for lifting assistance. Better staffing and staff availability, improved body mechanics, and assistance with transfers were identified as the most helpful risk reduction strategies.

Several related studies have linked nurse-to-patient ratios and the incidence of back pain or injury. Larese and Fiorito (1994) compared musculoskeletal disorders in nurses working on general hospital (GH) and oncology department (OD) units. For nurses working on the GH unit, 48 percent reported work-related back pain and 19 percent had lost work time, compared to 33 percent and 9 percent of the OD nurses, respectively. The most important factor associated with back pain and injury was the nurse-to-patient ratio for assisting patients. The authors reported that an analysis of working conditions revealed that both groups of nurses were subject to frequent and heavy lifting, lowering, pushing-pulling, and so on. The nurse-to-patient ratio for GH nurses, however, was 0.57 nurses for every 1 patient, compared to 1.27 for OD unit nurses. A better ratio between nurses and patients and work distribution, as well as specific ergonomic training, was recommended.

Rodgers (1985) reports that in a study of 95 back-injured nurses, many nurses were forced to lift alone when assistance was not immediately available. Nurses reportedly felt pressure to complete the task even though they knew the procedure was dangerous. The author indicated that management must be more responsive to establishing better staffing levels that could assist in the prevention of both the initial injury and reinjury to the back.

Greenwood (1986) completed a retrospective study of 4,000 back injury reports of hospital employees, including dietary staff, housekeepers, registered nurses (RN), licensed practical nurses (LPN), and NAs. Forty percent of the back injury cases were represented by NAs. Influencing factors included employment for less than 1 year and long working hours. Nearly 40 percent of the cases resulted in lost work time. In another report, Venning and colleagues (1987) surveyed and observed RNs, NAs, and orderlies and found several factors as significant predictors: jobs with patient lifting; frequency of lifting; job category (i.e., NAs and orderlies were nearly twice as likely to sustain an injury); and history of previous back injury.

Because of a high proportion of workers' compensation claims among hospital medical center employees (twice the rate of all state employees), Neuberger and colleagues (1988) conducted a descriptive study to investigate occupational injuries in this population. An analysis of workers' compensation claims for the 1-year period indicated that 855 injury events were reported, resulting in 4,825 lost work days and $326,886 in medical care and disability claims costs. The overall annual reporting rate was nearly 20 per 100 full-time-equivalent workers and occurred more often in women employees under 30 years of age. In fact, the rate in younger employees was 77 percent higher than in older employees. Those with repeat injuries had nearly twice as many lost work days and accounted for nearly one-fifth of those injured, one-third of the reported incidents, and one-half of the claims costs.

The Royal College of Nursing in Great Britain estimates that as many as 3,600 nurses leave the profession each year as a result of back injury, which incurs a replacement cost of approximately $90 million and more than $100 million in health care costs. In addition, other national findings suggest that a high proportion of back injuries in nurses and nursing assistants go unreported, that mechanical aides are inadequate, that reports are not investigated, and that back injuries may be thought of as acceptable risks (*Nursing Times,* 1992).

Evidence is clear that back pain and injury are a major problem in nursing, and they affect all practitioners who handle patients. The effect of these injuries can be measured in worker pain and suffering, disability, lost work time, absenteeism, medical care costs, personnel replacement costs, decreased productivity, and anger and confusion. Several authors implicate poor staffing, working conditions, and equipment design as factors contributing to decreased productivity, fatigue, and absenteeism, which then affect the quality of nursing care delivered and available. Clearly, more research is needed to validate these propositions.

Needlestick Injuries and Exposure Risk

A new era of concern about occupational hazards for health care workers began in 1984 when the first case of human immunodeficiency virus (HIV) transmitted by needlestick injury was reported in *The Lancet* (Jagger, 1994a). This has heightened the awareness in the health care community that numerous biological agents may be transmitted via needlestick and that exposure to blood-borne pathogens, including hepatitis B and C viruses (HBV and HCV) and other potentially infectious materials, need to be considered a major threat (CDC, 1992; Editorial, 1993). Marcus and colleagues (1991) report that needlestick exposure to HBV carries a 30 percent risk of infection while HIV needlestick contact carries less than a 1 percent chance of seroconversion. In a more recent review of the literature on HBV, HIV, and HCV exposure, however, Gerberding (1995) reports that the risk of transmission of HBV and HIV after needlestick injury seems to be related to the level of viral titer in the contaminant and, for HBV, correlates with the presence or absence of hepatitis B e antigen (HBeAg). The author reports on estimates of HBV infectivity ranging from 2 percent (HBeAg absent) to 40 percent (HBeAg present) and ranging for HIV from 0.2 to 0.5 percent. Estimates for HCV transmission are not well documented, but range from 3 to 10 percent. Although studies have indicated that the risk of HIV transmission is substantially lower than that for HBV, the fear of HIV acquisition is greater (Becker et al., 1989; Moore and Kaczmarek, 1990).

Occupational exposure may occur from a needlestick injury or other "sharps" injury, or from mucous membrane contact with contaminated blood or body fluid. Needlestick injury is the principal exposure route accounting for 80 percent of the occupational HIV exposure (Marcus et al., 1991). Numerous studies have found that nurses are the primary target of needlestick injuries (McEvoy et al., 1987; Wilkinson, 1987; Henderson et al., 1990; Marcus et al., 1991; Doan-Johnson, 1992). Several studies have reported incidence rates for needlestick injuries ranging from 10 percent to 34 percent (Jackson et al., 1986; Willy et al., 1990; Linnemann et al., 1991). These figures may be seriously underestimated, however, as studies also indicate estimates ranging from 30 percent to 60 percent for nurses' failure to report needlestick incidents (Hamory, 1983; Jackson et al., 1986; AHC, 1990; Moorhouse et al., 1994).

Work practice behaviors may lend themselves to increased risk of injury. Results of a national survey of certified nurse midwives indicated that 36 percent of respondents reported breaking needles and 63 percent (453 of 721) continued to cap needles (Willy et al., 1990), even though evidence is clear that recapping is the cause of one-third of all needlestick injuries (Jagger et al., 1988). Another study of 4 Michigan hospitals found, upon inspection of sharps disposal containers, that up to 60 percent of needles were capped (Becker et al., 1990). The effectiveness of work practice controls is of concern and the use of engineering controls would be more effective (Kopfer and McGovern, 1993).

English (1992) reported findings of a study on needlestick injuries conducted for a 1-month period in 17 hospitals in Washington, D.C. Of the 72 injuries reported, 46 percent were from RNs and recapping was most associated with needlestick injuries (14 percent). Eighteen injuries (25 percent) were to "downstream" housekeepers and aides who did not use such devices in their practice. Mallon and colleagues (1992) reported similar findings in a study of 332 reports of occupational blood and body fluid exposure. During a 9-month period needlestick and other sharps injuries accounted for 83.4 percent of all reports. In addition, failure to use universal precautions was cited in 34 percent of the reports.

Much of the concern related to needlestick injuries is related to the possible consequences of contracting AIDS. As of December, 1991, in the United States alone, 218,301 persons had been diagnosed with AIDS. The Centers for Disease Control and Prevention (CDC) reports that this figure may be 50 percent lower than the actual figure, due to inadequate diagnoses and non-diagnosis due to individual fear of positive test results. In addition, as of December 1993 the CDC has identified 123 documented or possible cases of occupationally acquired HIV (CDC, 1994), which represents two-thirds of the 176 documented cases worldwide (Jagger et al., 1994). Nurses and clinical laboratory workers, primarily phlebotomists, ranked first among HIV infected workers, with each group accounting for 24 percent of the 123 cases.

Jagger (1994b) reports surveillance data on percutaneous injuries for a 1-year period (1992–1993) from 58 participating hospitals. Of all the cases reported (n = 471), nurses and phlebotomists each accounted for 157 and 150 injuries (33.3 percent and 31.8 percent) respectively, with two-thirds of the injuries occurring in patient rooms (53.3 percent) and in the emergency department (14.0 percent). Recapping needles has been identified as a continual source of worker exposure (Ribner et al., 1987), and many of these injuries are considered to be preventable through use of safer devices, procedures, and work practices. In another study by Neuberger and colleagues (1988) of RNs and LPNs, needlestick injuries were the most frequently reported (69 percent and 50 percent respectively) and lifting injuries accounted for the most lost work time. Neuberger compared the needlestick injury findings to an earlier study of needlestick injuries (Neuberger et al., 1984) in the same population and found significant reductions (74 percent) in needlestick injury rates. Neuberger contributes these reductions to improved staffing and equipment and to employee education.

Several studies have found that nurses and other health care workers have expressed fear of contagion for self and family members with respect to caring for AIDS patients (Barrick, 1988; Baer and Longo, 1989; Boland, 1990). Based on a statewide survey of 243 Florida hospital nurse administrators, Nagelkerk

(1994) discusses in detail the impact of AIDS on recruitment and retention in hospitals, and notes that AIDS patient care is resource and manpower intensive and that nurses have a significant fear of exposure. For example, the author states:

> Not only did nurse administrators report that their staff feared caring for those with AIDS, but patients also had fears and requested room or unit transfers. Many administrators resorted to assigning private rooms for AIDS patients. The nurses feared contagion and death. One nurse administrator wrote, "It's not like other communicable diseases; AIDS carries a death sentence." While there was empathy for nurses' concerns and fears, most reported setting one firm rule: Nobody refuses care for assigned patients regardless of diagnoses. Many reported confrontations with individual nurses, which ultimately ended in voluntary resignation, dismissal, or the nurses's agreement to care for the assigned AIDS patient. After one incident, the informal network or grapevine worked well and others did not openly challenge the rule (p. 32).

Nurse administrators also reported several findings:

- staff were frequently physically and mentally exhausted;
- universal precautions were seen as cumbersome and time-consuming and often were not used;
- staff nurses distanced themselves from patients, providing care quickly and limiting interactions (seen as both an emotionally protective and an exposure control measure).

In addition, nurse administrators feared shortages in qualified personnel caring for AIDS patients, as some staff nurses indicated they would not personally work on an AIDS unit and that they might get out of nursing altogether.

In a somewhat contrasting study, van Servellen and Leake (1994) conducted a convenience sample survey of 153 hospital nurses from 7 California-based hospitals who provided nursing care to AIDS patients. While nurses reported some degree of emotional exhaustion and somatic complaints, no significant associations were found between emotional distress and care involvement, perceived risk and fear of contracting AIDS, and willingness to and satisfaction with care for AIDS patients. This can partly be attributed to a better understanding of the transmission and disease processes. Nurses who expressed more fear of contracting AIDS, however, also tended to report significantly higher levels of discomfort. The authors point out that other job correlates such as job tension, workload demands, and shift work are also contributors that should be explored in future research.

A pilot study was conducted by van Wissen and Siebers (1993) to determine nurses' attitudes with respect to HIV and AIDS exposure. Of 286 nurses surveyed who handled blood, 132 (49.4 percent) always wore gloves, and only half of the respondents (n = 148, or 51 percent) treated all body fluids as potentially HIV positive. The possible attrition rate from nursing positions in the canvassed hospital was 2.8 percent, with a further 43 (15 percent) undecided about resigning from their post. This study demonstrates that further safety and education needs should be attended to or reinforced.

Baker (1993) reported survey results from studies conducted in 1986 and again in 1990 in New York on 2 separate samples of nearly 600 nurses. About half the nurses in each study stated they feared contagion. The number of nurses indicating they had the right to refuse to care for AIDS patients declined by 12 percent, even though 35 percent of the nurses maintained this position (which could have an impact on developing a therapeutic relationship). The change in attitude is attributed to education about AIDS.

Managing needlestick injuries in the health care setting is vitally important in order to reduce exposure to bloodborne pathogens such as HIV and hepatitis. As needlestick injuries occur for a variety of reasons, several approaches must be utilized to combat the problem. In addition, health care providers' attitudes and fears of contagion need to be explored further, as all of these factors impact quality of care, turnover, and outright leaving of the nursing profession. These include instituting appropriate and effective engineering controls, ensuring compliance with regulatory mandates and work practice policies and guidelines, conducting surveillance programs, and providing useful educational instruction. Adequate evaluation of injury prevention programs is essential in order to determine the effectiveness of interventions, and continued research is critical to measure outcomes in terms of increased injury rates, attitudes and behavior, and intervention effectiveness.

VIOLENCE TOWARD HEALTH CARE WORKERS

An emerging occupational health concern related to both injury and stress in the workplace is the risk of violence in general and toward health care workers. Homicides in the general workplace have gained prominence in recent years, and the Bureau of Labor Statistics counted 1,063 work-related homicides in 1993, most related to robbery (BLS, 1994a). In addition, the BLS recently began surveying the number of nonfatal assaults and acts of violence in private workplaces that required injured wage and salary workers to take off a workday or more. In 1992, about 22,400 such incidents were reported, each requiring, on average, about 5 days away from work to recuperate. A sizable proportion of the victims of nonfatal violence were care givers in nursing homes and hospitals. Ironically, some of these workers were injured by intransigent patients who resisted their assistance; others were assaulted by patients prone to violence. Most of these care givers were female nurses and their aides, and typically they required about 3 to 5 days away from work to recuperate from their injuries (BLS, 1994a).

There are various definitions of violence ranging from verbal threat, feelings of being threatened, to actual injury from assault (Aiken, 1984; Jones, 1985; Carmel and Hunter, 1989; Greenfield et al., 1989; Morrison, 1989). The lack of a standardized definition or a vagueness in definition makes it difficult to truly assess the problem and contributes to the underestimation of the scope of the problem (Lanza, 1991; Lipscomb and Love, 1992). In fact, Lion and colleagues (1981) reported that staff assaults by patients in a state psychiatric facility were underreported fivefold, which may reflect institutional policies and staff tolerance (Haller and DeLuty, 1988).

To date, the problem of violence in health care settings has focused mainly on psychiatric settings (Bernstein, 1981; Rix, 1987; Lanza, 1988). Poster and Ryan (1989) surveyed 154 psychiatric nurses and found that 74 percent of those responding indicated that staff members working with mentally ill patients could expect to be assaulted during their careers, and in fact 73 percent had already been assaulted. Lanza (1983) reports that staff assaults by patients in mental health facilities is as high as 80 percent.

In a study of 600 patients in a British psychiatric hospital, Larkin and colleagues (1988) found that more than 200 patients engaged in assaultive behavior. In another study, Lanza (1983) found that 40 psychiatric nurses in a VA hospital reported being assaulted an average of 7 times in their career (mean years of psychiatric experience was 6). Assaults were described as being grabbed, hit, choked, knocked out, and thrown about.

Using the Occupational Safety and Health (OSHA) definition of injury, Carmel and Hunter (1989) conducted a 1-year study of injuries in a 973-bed California maximum security hospital and found that injuries to staff occurred at a rate of 16 per 100 staff. In contrast, the rate for work-related injuries reported to OSHA in 1989 for all industries combined was 8.3 per 100 full-time workers (BLS, 1991).

Violence toward all health care workers appears to be on the rise (Lanza, 1992; Lipscomb and Love, 1992). Some have speculated about the cause for the increased violence in hospitals. Increased violence in the general population as a means of solving problems, increased use of mind-altering drugs and alcohol abuse, and the increased availability of weapons may all contribute to the problem of violence in the health care setting. Jones (1985) reported that in a VA the nursing assistants, followed by the nurses and physicians, were most likely to be assaulted. Lavoie and colleagues (1988) reported on results of a survey of 127 emergency room medical directors. Forty-three percent of the sample indicated at least one physical attack on a medical staff person per month, which included violent acts that resulted in death.

McCulloch and colleagues (1986) report that weapon carrying in psychiatric facilities and emergency rooms is not uncommon and that staff are usually unable to predict who the weapon carriers are. Several additional studies have reported on the issue of weapons in hospital settings. Wasserberger and colleagues (1989) reported that over a 9-year period nearly 5,000 weapons were confiscated from 21,456 patients at a Los Angeles trauma center. In Lavoie and colleagues' (1988) study of emergency room medical directors, nearly 20 percent of the respondents reported at least 1 threat with a weapon per month and nearly 50 percent of the hospitals had confiscated weapons. Goetz and colleagues (1991) reported that 11 percent of psychiatric patients admitted to an emergency department during a 20-month period and 0.4 percent of all medical patients were searched for weapons, with 17.3 percent and 15.7 percent found to be carrying weapons, respectively.

Several environmental or administrative factors are thought to contribute to violence against health care workers. These include limited training in the management of assaultive behavior or in containing or restraining an assailant; short staffing and use of agency staff; and the day shift tour of duty, when there are generally increased levels of activity on the wards (Infantino and Musingo, 1985; Jones, 1985; Carmel and Hunter, 1990).

As the number of elders in the general population increases, the number of nursing home patients is also likely to increase with a concomitant rise in staff. The largest proportion of staff in nursing homes are NAs; only one study, however, has been reported on violence in this population. Lusk (1992) reported on results of focus groups with NAs in seven nursing homes. Aides indicated "they get hurt everyday, . . . and that patients hit, scratch, pull hair, kick, bite and pinch" (p. 239). In addition, aides expressed concern about the lack of protection afforded them.

The actual costs of violence toward health care workers have not been widely studied; Carmel and Hunter (1989) reported, however, that of 121 staff injuries, 43 percent of those injured lost time from work with 13 percent of those injured absent more than 21 days. Lanza and Milner (1989) reported that for 99 staff assaults nearly 40 percent resulted in lost work time with 12 percent requiring more than a month off duty for full recovery. The actual dollar costs were not reported.

The study of violence toward health care workers as an occupational hazard is relatively new. The emphasis in the studies reported is primarily on reporting data relative to incidence and prevalence. More emphasis must be placed on identifying root causes of violence in these settings and prevention strategies to reduce health care worker risk. Risk factors such as poor staffing patterns, reduced staffing levels, and violence containment issues must be addressed by management in order to afford a safe work environment and reduce the emotional impact of this type of violence on workers.

STRESS AND NURSING

Packard and Motowidlo (1987) have stated that:

When patients require bodily care, understanding, empathy and full, unconditional acceptance, or when many complex tasks are required unexpectedly, hospital nurses find practical, tangible evidence of the worth of their talents, skills, and commitment to people. But when nurses recognize that their work is undervalued, underappreciated, disparaged, taken for granted and when in addition they are treated discourteously or even pitted against one another for the meager rewards of their jobs, then nurses properly regard such stressors as undesirable.

The authors purport that when this happens job performance is poorer.

It is well documented in the literature that nursing work results in significant amounts of stress leading to a variety of work-related problems such as absenteeism, staff conflict, staff turnover, decreased morale, and decreased practice effectiveness (MacNeil and Weisz, 1987; Doering, 1990; Hiscott and Connop, 1990; Rees and Cooper, 1992; Fielding and Weaver, 1994). The review of the literature that follows examines the relationship between nursing work and stress and related outcomes, emphasizing the impact on work and performance.

In an early study, Gentry and colleagues (1972) examined the psychological responses of 34 RNs working in various intensive care units (ICU) and non-ICU settings within a Medical Center–Veterans Administration hospital (VAH) complex. A battery of standardized psychological test measures was used. Medical Center ICU (MC-ICU) nurses reported more depression, hostility, and anxiety then did non-ICU nurses and nurses in the VAH critical care units (CCU).

The MC-ICU settings produced more complaints and ones concerned with an overwhelming workload, limited facilities and space, inadequate help for proper patient care, too much responsibility, too little continuing education, poor organization, excessive paperwork, inadequate communication with physicians, transition of personnel, and intrastaff tension. The authors contend that:

> the finding that MC- and VAH-CCU nurses differed rather markedly both in their levels of affect and their likes/dislikes about their work was indeed interesting, since both groups perform essentially the same duties with the same type of patients in virtually identical physical surroundings. What it suggests is that the CCU setting as such is not intrinsically stressful, but rather becomes so when adequate help is not available to care for the patients properly, when nurses are not provided with necessary continuing education, and when a deliberate effort is not made to instill a feeling of pride and "team spirit" within the staff as a whole.

Packard and Motowidlo (1987) conducted a survey study for 5 hospitals to assess the relationship between subjective stress, job satisfaction, and job performance in 366 hospital RNs and LPNs. A second survey instrument was sent to the supervisor and a coworker of the primary nurse subject (n = 165 and 139, respectively) asking about the nurse's work performance. Increased stress encounters diminished both job satisfaction and job performance and increased episodes of depression. Job satisfaction was not related to job performance, but depressed and hostile nurses had lower job performances than did nurses with little or no depression or personal hostility.

Early studies have purported that critical care and intensive care nurses experience more stress than nurses in other areas. Research has not consistently validated this concept, however. MacNeil and Weisz (1987) measured the level of psychological distress experienced by critical care nurses (n = 80) and non-critical-care nurses (n = 106) employed in a large acute care hospital, and its relationship to absenteeism. Non-critical-care nurses reported significantly higher psychological distress scores than did the critical nursing group and nearly twice the rate of absenteeism. These results may indicate better staffing or orientation in critical care nursing. Alterations in the work environment and conditions and stress management programs are needed to reduce nurses' distress.

Foxall and colleagues (1990) surveyed 138 nurses including 35 ICU nurses, 30 hospice nurses, and 73 medical-surgical nurses to determine differences in stress levels among the groups. While there were no overall significant differences among the groups with respect to stress levels, significant differences did occur for subscales: ICU and hospice nurses perceived significantly more stress related to death and dying than did medical-surgical nurses; ICU and medical-surgical nurses perceived significantly more stress related to floating than did hospice nurses; and medical-surgical nurses perceived significantly more stress related to work-overload and staffing than did ICU and hospice nurses. While the effects of job stress on the quality of patient and family care were not specifically addressed, stress management programs were encouraged, particularly in the area of death and dying, to alleviate burnout and facilitate more effective care. In addition, work environment issues such as increased staffing levels and decreased floating were encouraged to minimize work overload and the potential for reduced quality of care. Similar findings were reported by Boumans and Landeweerd (1994) who studied 561 ICU and non-ICU nurses from 36 units in 16 hospitals. Non-ICU nurses had more work pressure, absenteeism, and health complaints than did the ICU nurses.

Yu and colleagues (1989) surveyed a random sample of 952 RNs obtained through a statewide nurses association membership list to identify specific job stressors across 10 clinical specialties. Results indicated that stress seems to arise from the overall complexity of nurses' work rather than specific tasks. Stressors were uniform across specialty areas, with the greatest levels reported in administration, cardiology, medical-surgical, and emergency room nursing.

Several studies have examined stress in other types of nursing fields. Jennings (1990) found that among 300 U.S. Army head nurses in 37 different army hospitals, stress resulted in psychological symptoms as measured by the Brief Symptom Inventory. Of particular importance is the notion that managers bear the responsibility for attenuating the stress experienced by staff. The question raised is: Can managers who are experiencing psychological distress themselves adequately intercede to reduce staff stress, as well as manage their units efficiently and effectively?

Using several instruments, Power and Sharp (1988) compared stress and job satisfaction among 181 nurses at a mentally handicapped hospital and 24 hospice nurses. Hospice nurses characteristically reported stress as primarily associated with death and dying and with inadequate preparation to meet the emotional needs of patients and families, but did not report significantly high workload stress as had been observed in other studies. This may be due partly to the relatively high staff-to-patient ratio in a hospice setting. Conversely, nurses working with mental handicapped patients reported significantly more stress associated with workload, conflict with other nurses, and the nursing environment.

In a study of neurosurgical nurses, the authors interviewed several nurses about aspects of neurosurgical nursing that were perceived as stressful by staff. Findings suggest that being exposed to life-and-death situations among young children, being short of essential resources, being on duty with too few staff, and dealing with aggressive relatives constituted major stressful events. Comments made by staff suggested that performance at work is adversely influenced by stress (Snape and Cavanagh, 1993). These findings were echoed in a study of dialysis nurses who also indicated that work load is a major contributing factor not only to overall stress and work performance, but to burnout as well (Lewis et al., 1992). In addition, a sample of 155 members of the Association of Pediatric Oncology Nurses reported that the relapse or sudden death of a favorite patient was their greatest source of stress. The second most common stressor was a workload perceived as too great to give quality patient care (Emery, 1993).

Hawley (1992) surveyed 69 emergency room nurses to identify sources of stress and effective strategies for addressing them. Repeatedly, nurses described inadequate staffing and resources, too many non-nursing tasks, changing trends in emergency department use, and patient transfer problems as having considerable impact on their ability to provide quality patient care. Nurses were also stressed by continual confrontations with patients and families who exhibit crisis behavior. Staff also reported that a shortage of nursing staff, especially during busy periods and at night, was particularly stressful and that because of these shortages they were unable to give adequate care to patients. Adding untrained relief staff compounded the stress burden.

In order to compare sources and outcomes of stress among hospital pharmacists and nurses, Wolfgang and colleagues (1988) randomly surveyed 1,002 RNs and 1,006 pharmacists using national mailing lists. While 462 (46 percent) nurses and 465 (46 percent) pharmacists returned surveys, only 263 (69.4 percent of respondents) and 107 (27.6 percent of respondents) were hospital-based and therefore useable. All subjects completed the Health Professions Stress Inventory and moderate stress levels were found for both groups with significant differences noted. Interruptions, poor opportunities for advancement, inadequate staffing, excessive workload, and inadequate pay were considered to be very stressful by both groups. The pharmacists considered a lack of challenge in their work to be more stressful than did the nurses. Situations relating to patient care, such as being uncertain about what to tell a patient or family members about the patient's condition or treatment and caring for terminally ill patients, were perceived by nurses as being more stressful than they were perceived by the pharmacists. Forty-eight of 106 pharmacists and 95 of 259 nurses said that they would probably not pursue the same career if they started over again. While some stressful situations are similar for both groups, sources of stress for nurses tend to be more patient-care related than for pharmacists.

Gordon and colleagues (1993) surveyed all nurses in the Haemophilia Nursing Network Directory, compiled by the National Haemophilia Foundation, to investigate distress in this group of nursing practitioners. Questionnaires were returned by 75 percent (136 of 181) of those surveyed. Areas associated with the greatest distress were: (1) failure of patients to take steps to prevent transmission of HIV; (2) fear of getting infected; and (3) the repeated loss experienced as patients died from infection. Nurses working with haemophiliacs for 11 to 15 years were particularly vulnerable to feelings of guilt for having participated in the treatment that resulted in HIV infection. Looking for a new job was related to all major sources of distress.

Cull (1991) and van Servellen and Leake (1994) describe oncology nurses as having significant amounts of stress associated with their practice and that absenteeism, high staff turnover, poor quality-control of work, poor industrial relations, and emotional exhaustion are likely results. Recommendations include reviewing institutional policies and work conditions to reduce stressors as well as utilizing support groups.

Scalzi (1990) surveyed 75 top level nurse executives in all hospitals in a large metropolitan city to examine the relationships between role conflict, ambiguity, and depression and job satisfaction and stress. Three predominant job stressors were examined and designated respectively as: the *overload stressor,* because it was composed of items that dealt primarily with conflict and overload due to too many expectations; the *quality concern stressor,* which included stress generated by poor quality of nursing staff, medical staff, and patient care; and the *lack of support stressor,* which included stress items measuring lack of support from hospital administration and from immediate subordinates, and difficult relationships with other departments.

These executives perceived high role conflict, moderately high role ambiguity, and moderately high levels of depression symptoms. Both role conflict and role ambiguity were positively and significantly correlated with depressive symptoms, and higher levels of depressive symptoms were significantly associated with both lower levels of job satisfaction and higher levels of quality concern stress. Role conflict was positively correlated with role ambiguity and stress from quality concerns and role conflict was negatively correlated with job satisfaction.

The quality concern stressor was the source of the most severe job stress and had strong associations with increased depressive symptomatology, increased role conflict, and decreased job satisfaction. The author states that this particular job-related stress is specific to the health care industry and involves both ethical and professional responsibilities to provide safe (quality) care.

Research studies on shift work have reported adverse effects on workers' health, performance, and mental and physical fitness (Jung, 1986; Gold et al., 1992; Todd et al., 1993). Shift workers have reported a lower sense of well-being with lower participation rates in social organizations, engagement in more solitary activities, higher incidences of family and sexual problems, higher rates of divorce than day workers, and decreased work performance. Gold and colleagues (1992) conducted a hospital-based survey on shift work, sleep, and accidents among 635 Massachusetts nurses. In comparison to nurses who worked only day and evening shifts, rotators had more sleep-wake cycle disruption and nodded off more at work. Rotators had twice the odds of nodding off while driving to or from work and twice the odds of a reported accident or error related to sleepiness. Factors that affect adjustments to shift work include the type of shift work schedule, the frequency of the schedule changes, the degree to which workers adjust their social, dietary, and sleeping habits to coincide with their shift work schedule, and the age of the worker. Research has shown that workers who rotate shifts have more difficulty adjusting to schedules that change more frequently than once every 2 to 3 weeks. Periods of less than 2 to 3 weeks do not allow sufficient time for workers' circadian rhythms to resynchronize to a new shift assignment. Rotating shifts work better if they change clockwise, from day to evening to night, instead of from day to night and then evening shifts (Jung, 1986). Application of circadian principles to the design of hospital work schedules may result in improved health and safety for nurses and patients.

In a study related to working hours, Todd and colleagues (1993) surveyed nurses who worked 12-hour shift rotations and who reported decreased satisfaction with their jobs, conditions of work, and patient care, and problems with domestic and social arrangements. The vast majority (83 percent) reported that they did not want to go on working the shift and there was support for the view that recruitment to nursing would be adversely affected by the shift. A further discussion of shift work as it relates to burnout is presented later.

Burnout in Nurses

Berland (1990) discusses the issue of burnout in nurses at Vancouver General Hospital and factors that influence burnout, including increasing patient activity, greater family needs, higher professional standards, and static hospital budgets that often result in staff shortages and reduced quality of care. To address the problem, the hospital administration empowered head nurses to restrict patient admission to their unit to protect staff nurses from burnout. After 18 months, evaluation of the new policy indicated that staff nurses felt more in control of their workload and could better shape and improve quality of care for patients.

Beard (1994) reported findings from studying stress and "floating" in 42 nurses in a community hospital. The nurses served as their own controls when they were not floating. Using the Derogates Stress Profile, results showed significant stress levels were produced when the nurses floated. The resultant impact was increased turnover, reduced patient and physician satisfaction, and decreased productivity.

Using the Maslach Burnout Inventory, Kandolin (1993) studied 286 Finnish nurses to determine if burnout was more common among those who experienced shift work compared to those who did not. It was reported that more than one-third of the nurses often experienced high levels of time pressure in their work, and 10 percent of the nurses reported working at a workplace with a tense social atmosphere. Female nurses in 3-shift work had significantly more stress symptoms and ceased to enjoy their work more often than women in 2-shift work, which relates to loss of enthusiasm, efficiency, value placed on work, and work positivity. There were no gender differences in burnout.

Keim and Robinson (1992) also report increased levels of stress, described by third-shift nurses as being related to lack of supervisor support, work involvement, and peer cohesion. The authors point out that nursing shortages and increased vulnerability to stress may result in many nurses leaving their jobs to relieve stress and eventual burnout.

Pines and Maslach (1978) have defined burnout as "a syndrome of physical and emotional exhaustion involving the development of a negative self-concept, negative job attitude and loss of concern and feeling for clients" (p. 236). Husted and colleagues (1989) state that the nurse who is experiencing burnout often is disgruntled, unhappy, complaining, fatigued, impatient with self, short with patients and their families, rigid, distant from coworkers, quick to anger and, in general, unpleasant to be around. Fortunately, when a cluster of these symptoms occurs, the nurse is not around too often or too long. Absenteeism increases and turnover results. A ripple effect becomes operational and observable. The unhappy nurse seeks coworkers who will listen and sympathize. As absenteeism increases, the workload of coworkers increases proportionately, which contributes to the spread of burnout.

With increasingly successful technology, younger and smaller neonates are surviving to become chronically ill with the need for many months of intensive care (Oehler et al., 1991). Thus, neonatal nurses are reported to be victims of stress and subsequent burnout and the authors sought to study this phenomenon. Specific stressors within the neonatal intensive care unit (NICU) are (1) ethical dilemmas surrounding life-and-death situations of critically ill neonates; (2) death of an infant; (3) demands on the family of a high-risk infant; (4) challenging and constantly changing technology in neonatal nursing; and (5) conflicts of under-staffing in a busy NICU (Marshall and Kasmen, 1980).

Oehler and colleagues (1991) surveyed 49 RNs and LPNs working in a neonatal intensive care unit of a large major medical center using the Maslach Burnout Inventory, State-Trait Anxiety Inventory, and social support measures. On the Maslach Burnout Inventory, subjects scored in a moderate range of burn-out for emotional exhaustion and depersonalization and in a high range of burn-out for sense of personal accomplishment. Stepwise regression analyses revealed that higher job stress scores, higher anxiety scores, perception of less supervisor (head nurse) support, and less experience were associated with higher burnout sub-scale scores. This type of nursing, wherein the needs of the patients and family are high, can be very emotionally fatiguing. Supervisory support and ongoing information about coping strategies are essential.

Because of the nature of nursing work, the nursing profession may be the helping profession most at risk of burnout (Johnson, 1992). Duquette and colleagues (1994) describe burnout as having psychological, physical, and behavioral components:

> Often the first symptoms that appear are the sensations of emotional exhaustion and extreme tiredness. The person lacks energy; is irritable, anxious, and angry; and has feelings of helplessness and hopelessness. The person often complains of various manifestations of a physical nature such as headaches, backaches, and gastrointestinal disorders. The emotionally exhausted person develops negative attitudes and feelings toward patients and may become indifferent, cold, and cynical. The person feels frustrated with his or her work, may develop feelings of guilt and failure, and may have a negative self-image as well as a tendency to be absent often from work and may seek other employment (p. 337).

The authors indicated that organizational stressors influence the development of burnout, particularly role ambiguity, staffing, and workload; age, with younger nurses being more susceptible to seeing their role as more ambiguous and their workload heavier; and buffering factors including hardiness, social support, and coping.

In another study by Dolan (1987) that comprised each of 30 psychiatric, general duty, and administrative nurses, the study subjects completed the Maslach Burnout Inventory and job satisfaction questionnaire. Job satisfaction was inversely related to burnout in a descending order from general duty, to psychiatric, to administrative nurses. The rapid turnover of patients in general hospitals, compared to psychiatric hospitals, was cited as increasing the workload for the general nurse. Nurses felt that having to treat too many patients in too short a time restricts their need to meet their own professional standards and to attend fully to the psychological as well as the physical needs of the patient.

Turnover

Eriksen and colleagues (1992) describe two potentially negative consequences of consistently high workloads in an understaffed situation: decreased quality of care and lower job satisfaction, which may lead to increased nurse turnover. An RN-LPN nurse partnership model of care was implemented in the critical care setting to prevent these potential consequences. The purpose of the model program was to develop "qualified extenders" for the critical care staff nurse so as to reduce workload and thereby affect the quality of care given. In this model, vocational nurses were given an 8-week education and orientation program termed the "licensed vocational nurse critical care specialty program." Certain aspects of direct and indirect nursing care were taught that were then to be considered tasks delegated to the licensed vocational nurse extenders. Evaluation of the program revealed statistically significant increases in nurse job satisfaction; perceptions of reduced workload and stress; a perception by RNs and physicians of increased nursing care quality; decreased RN turnover and sick time; and a positive perception of the role of the LPN in the critical care unit.

Mann and Jefferson (1988) describe many reasons for high turnover rates on medical intensive care units (MICU) including heavy workloads, lack of recognition, and lack of administrative support and leadership that can lead to stress. The authors surveyed 47 nurses in the MICU and found that understaffing and workload were the most stressful problems that influenced the quality of care. Proactive measures were implemented to reduce problems.

Hinshaw and colleagues (1987) examined retention strategies of nursing staff, as turnover is considered detrimental to maintaining quality of care and containing health care costs. The investigators analyzed questionnaire data from 1,597 nursing staff members (RNs, LPNs, NAs) in both urban and rural settings, and diverse clinical areas. In general, the study results emphasized that job stress is buffered by satisfaction that in turn leads to less anticipated turnover. The satisfiers can be converted into organizational strategies for retaining nursing staff. The major stressors to be buffered were lack of team respect and feelings of incompetence, while the primary satisfiers were professional status and general enjoyment in one's position, which correlated significantly with the ability to deliver quality nursing care.

Ackerman (1993) notes the importance of retaining pediatric intensive care unit staff and points out that high rates of turnover result in insufficiency in meeting patient care needs and compromised care. The author stipulated that perhaps the most important retention strategy is the initial recruitment of individuals who are most likely to fit in with the established goals of the unit. Once the best possible candidate has been hired, retention depends on maintaining the individual's job satisfaction, which may be accomplished via mechanisms such as: (1) providing a reasonable workload; (2) providing effective communication between the manager and the staff; (3) having a manager with an effective management style; (4) ongoing and meaningful nurse–physician collaboration; and (5) reasonable compensation for work being done. In addition, reasonable workload must assume that patient care assignments are such that the staff can take pride in the quality of the job done, while delivering safe, consistent bedside care without the addition of excessive overtime hours. When unpredicted shortages occur, based on increased patient acuity or census or decreased staff availability, these shortages must be managed in ways that preserve the functioning of the unit and the morale of the remaining staff. Possible responses include the use of "floaters," agency nurses, or even closing beds for the short term.

Shanahan (1993) compares and contrasts factors that affect recruitment and retention of physical therapists and RNs. The author points out that professional staff shortages in hospital settings can drastically increase operating costs and compromise the quality of care. Lower quality of care can limit the ability of the hospital to attract customers and staff, and can increase the hospital length of stay with a concomitant increase in costs. While salary and compensation are considered important incentive factors in retention, other factors such as image and job satisfaction remain important considerations. A disturbing finding by Porter and colleagues (1989), however, is that only 72 percent of nurses have a positive image about their profession. This was a lower perception than that of the general public (84 percent) or of physicians (100 percent). Hospital chief executive officers ranked nursing as the most significant factor contributing to quality health care (97.3 percent). Hospital management must address issues related to turnover in order to fully reach quality-of-care demands.

Dolan and colleagues (1992) discuss issues surrounding the propensity of nursing staff to quit, which has been acknowledged as the best predictor of turnover. Behaviors related to stress, burnout, and depression are notable and can have a subsequent impact on quality of care and turnover. The cost for a single nurse replacement is estimated at about $2,000. The investigators surveyed 1,237 staff who worked in 30 Quebec hospital emergency rooms and intensive care units about 14 job demands (the response rate was 84 percent). Results indicated that lack of professional latitude (which included restricted autonomy, skill underutilization, and lack of participation in clinical decision making), clinical demands, role difficulties, and workload problems all contributed to the propensity to quit. The authors suggested that interventions aimed at improving the quality of work and the general work-related quality of life should be implemented to enhance employee mental health, reduce rates of turnover, and curb costs.

The work of nurses is repeatedly cited as being highly stressful for its practitioners and can result in burnout. While inadequate staffing levels are considered the major cause of stress for nurses, other factors such as the dying and death of patients, work overload, shift work, decreased job satisfaction, inadequate resources, replacement orientation, role conflict, and lack of management support are frequently implicated as significant causes of stress and burnout in nursing.

Many authors indicate that the quality of nursing care is seriously jeopardized and that nurses often leave nursing as a result of the burnout syndrome they suffer (Anonymous, 1986; Masterson-Allen et al., 1987; Lucas et al., 1993).

Many organizational factors have been cited that influence nursing stress, burnout, and productivity in nursing care, and that may result in short-term or long-term absenteeism. Other than personal illness, however, child care problems are the primary personal factors that contribute to absenteeism (Miller and Norton, 1986; Bourbonnais et al., 1992). Although it is unclear if this problem is consistent across occupations, available data indicate that handling child care issues falls primarily to the mother (Roberts and McGovern, 1993). As nursing and nursing-related work is performed mostly by women, this clearly becomes an issue in the nursing work force. Because of a nearly $1 million cost associated with nursing absenteeism and concern about loss of productivity, quality of patient care, and decreased morale, an analysis of absenteeism was conducted in a 3-hospital system in the mid-southern region of the United States. A total of 865 RNs, LPNs, unit secretaries, and medical attendants were surveyed, with 90 percent women responders. Results indicated that issues related to child care were the major contributor to absenteeism with 87 percent of those surveyed indicating that they missed work due to child illness. Other important findings included significant conflict between parent and employee roles (e.g., leaving sick child at home or leaving children at home unsupervised); staffing and scheduling difficulties resulting in employees admitting to missing work (e.g., too long stretches of work days and inadequate staffing); and indifferent attitudes about sick leave (e.g., administrators should not complain if employees were absent without pay). Attitudes of professional and nonprofessional staff were similar. Findings raised serious concern about productivity, lack of continuity of care, and resultant implications for quality of patient care.

Hospitals are plagued with high rates of turnover and absenteeism as many nurses trying to cope with stress move from hospital to hospital (Gelfant, 1990). While staffing levels are reduced, the number of patients stay the same, the complexity of the work increases, and the work is expected to be done with the same level of quality. Consequently stress, guilt, and burnout ensue (Lees and Ellis, 1990).

Health care administrators must address the issues of the impact of organizational stressors on nurses if there is to be any hope of resolving the problem (Whitley and Putzier, 1994). New approaches to staff selection and recruitment, flexibility in staffing, increased resources, and increased decision making by nurses is essential.

GENERAL CRITIQUE OF STUDIES

The studies discussed provide valuable information on the problem of injury and stress in nursing and the relationship of this problem on nursing care. Figure 1

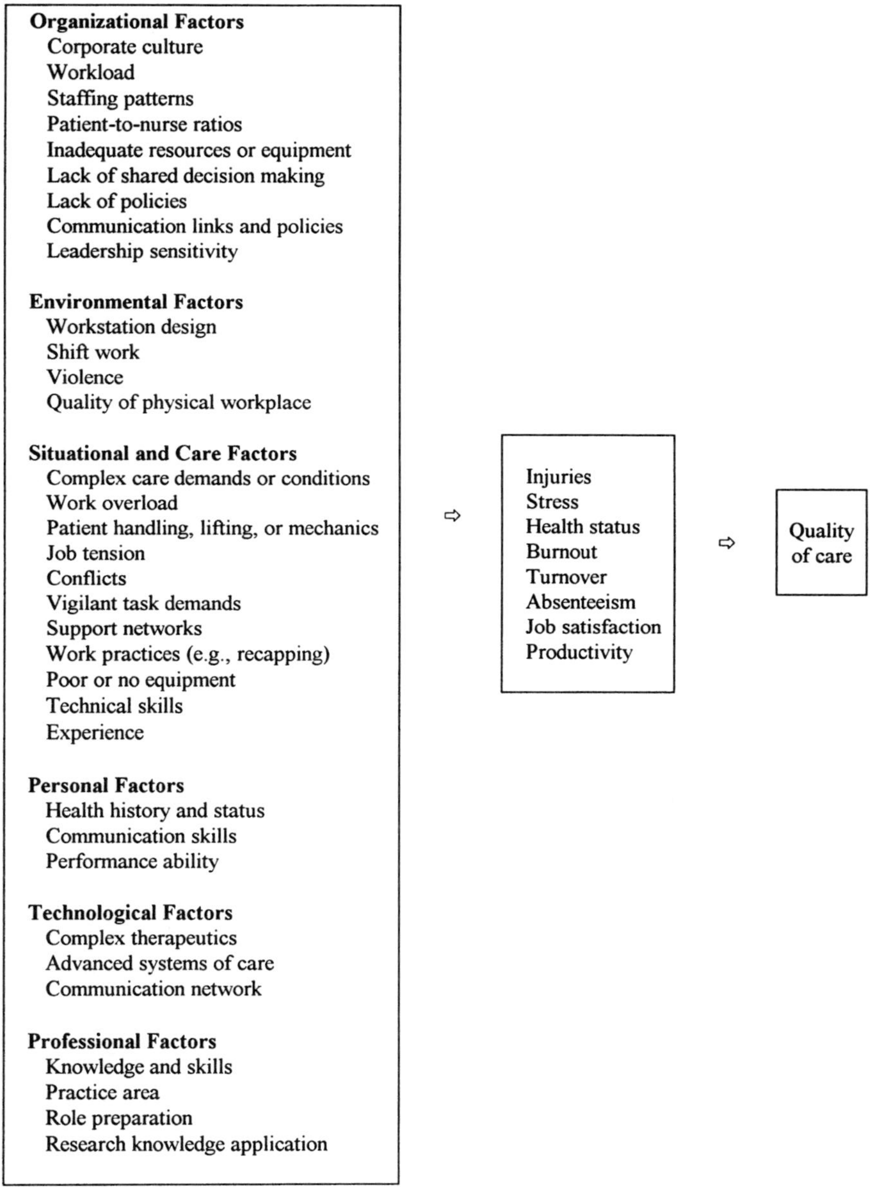

Organizational Factors
    Corporate culture
    Workload
    Staffing patterns
    Patient-to-nurse ratios
    Inadequate resources or equipment
    Lack of shared decision making
    Lack of policies
    Communication links and policies
    Leadership sensitivity

Environmental Factors
    Workstation design
    Shift work
    Violence
    Quality of physical workplace

Situational and Care Factors
    Complex care demands or conditions
    Work overload
    Patient handling, lifting, or mechanics
    Job tension
    Conflicts
    Vigilant task demands
    Support networks
    Work practices (e.g., recapping)
    Poor or no equipment
    Technical skills
    Experience

Personal Factors
    Health history and status
    Communication skills
    Performance ability

Technological Factors
    Complex therapeutics
    Advanced systems of care
    Communication network

Professional Factors
    Knowledge and skills
    Practice area
    Role preparation
    Research knowledge application

⇨

Injuries
Stress
Health status
Burnout
Turnover
Absenteeism
Job satisfaction
Productivity

⇨

Quality
of care

FIGURE 1 Examples of factors affecting nursing and practice.

summarizes these points. The studies purport that inadequate staffing, staffing patterns, excessive patient-to-nurse ratios, clinical issues (e.g., patient deaths), poorly designed equipment, lack of administrative support, lack of decision making authority, lack of resources, training and education, poor body mechanics, and pressure to work in at-risk conditions are significant contributors to the problem. The data provided are somewhat limited, however, due to lack of replication and little evidence of causality with respect to quality care outcomes. In addition, sample sizes and sampling procedures are of concern particularly in terms of the generalizability of findings.

Many of the studies are descriptive, cross-sectional, and retrospective in design, and report anecdotal findings. To have a full meaning of outcomes measurement, experimental and cohort studies should be conducted. Not enough evidence is presented on the effectiveness of equipment design and other types of intervention strategies (e.g., improved staffing, child day care availability) that may improve working conditions. In addition, few data are available on the costs related to the impact of nursing injury and stress, particularly as they relate to quality and patient care. In conclusion, many challenges exist to effectively manage and alleviate injury and stress in the nursing workplace environment. Risk reduction is of prominent importance but research in the relevant areas is sorely lacking.

REFERENCES

Ackerman, A.D. Retention of Critical Care Staff. *Critical Care Medicine* 21(9 Suppl):S394–S395, 1993.

Aiken, G.J.M. Assaults on Staff in a Locked Ward: Prediction and Consequences. *Medicine, Science and the Law* 24(3):199–207, 1984.

AHC (American Health Consultants). One Third of Needlesticks Go Unreported at Hospital. *Hospital Infection Control* 17(18):107, 1990.

Anonymous. What Really Makes Nurses Angry. *RN* 49(1):55–60, 1986.

Arad, D., and Ryan, M. The Incidence and Prevalence in Nurses of Low Back Pain: A Definitive Survey Exposes the Hazards. *Australian Nurse Journal* 16:44–48, 1986.

Baer, C., and Longo, M.S. Talking About It: Allaying Staff Concerns About AIDS Patients. *Journal of Psychosocial Nursing* 27(10):30–32, 1989.

Baker, L. Half of Nurses Fear Contracting AIDS. *Journal of Psychosocial Nursing* 31(6):40–41, 1993.

Barrick, B. The Willingness of Nursing Personnel to Care for Patients with Acquired Immune Deficiency Syndrome: A Survey Study and Recommendations. *Journal of Professional Nursing* 4(5):366–372, 1988.

Beard, E.L. Stop Floating—The Next Paradigm Shift? *Journal of Nursing Administration* 24(3):4, 1994.

Becker, C, Cone, J., and Gerberding, J. Occupational Infection with Human Immunodeficiency Virus: Risks and Risk Reductions. *Annals of Internal Medicine* 110(8):653–656, 1989.

Becker, M.H., Janz, N.K., Band, J., Bartley, J., Snyder, M.B., and Gaynes, R.P. Noncompliance with Universal Precautions Policy: Why Do Physicians and Nurses Recap Needles? *American Journal of Infection Control* 17(46):232–239, 1990.

Berland, A. Controlling Workload. *Canadian Nurse* 86(5):36–38, 1990.

Bernstein, H.A. Survey of Threats and Assaults Directed Toward Psychotherapists. *American Journal of Psychotherapy* 35(4):542–549, 1981.

BLS (Bureau of Labor Statistics, U.S. Department of Labor). *Occupational Injuries and Illnesses in the United States by Industry, 1989.* Bulletin 2379, 1991.

BLS. *Issues in Labor Statistics. Violence in the Workplace Comes Under Closer Scrutiny.* Summary 94-10. August, 1994a.

BLS. *Issues in Labor Statistics. Worker Safety Problems Spotlighted in Health Care Industries.* Summary 94-6. June, 1994b.

Boland, B. Fear of AIDS in Nursing Staff. *Nursing Management* 21(8):40–44, 1990.

Boumans, N.P., and Landeweerd, J.A. Working in an Intensive or Non-Intensive Care Unit: Does it Make Any Difference? *Heart and Lung* 23(1):71–79, 1994.

Bourbonnais, R., Vinet, A., Meyer, F., and Goldberg, M. Certified Sick Leave and Work Load. A Case Referent Study Among Nurses. *Journal of Occupational Medicine* 34(1):69–74, 1992.

Carmel, H., and Hunter, M. Staff Injuries from Inpatient Violence. *Hospital and Community Psychiatry* 40(1):41–46, 1989.

Carmel, H., and Hunter, M. Compliance with Training in Managing Assaultive Behavior and Injuries from Inpatient Violence. *Hospital and Community Psychiatry* 41(5):558–560, 1990.

Carney, R.M. Protect your Nursing Athletes! *Nursing Management* 24(3):69–71, 1993.

Cato, C., Olson, K., and Studer, M. Incidence, Prevalence and Variables Associated with Low Back Pain in Staff Nurses. *AAOHN (American Association of Occupational Health Nurses) Journal* 321–327, 1989.

CDC (Centers for Disease Control). The Second 100,000 Cases of Acquired Immunodeficiency Syndrome—United States, June 1981–December 1991. *Morbidity and Mortality Weekly Report* 41(2):28–29, 1992.

CDC (Centers for Disease Control and Prevention). *HIV/AIDS Surveillance Report* 5(19), 1994.

Cull, A.M. Studying Stress in Care Givers: Art or Science? *British Journal of Cancer* 64(6):981–984, 1991.

Doan-Johnson, S. Taking a Closer Look at Needle Sticks. *Nursing92* 22(8):24, 27, 1992.

Doering, L. Recruitment and Retention: Successful Strategies in Critical Care. *Heart and Lung* 19(3):220–224, 1990.

Dolan, N. The Relationship Between Burnout and Job Satisfaction in Nurses. *Journal of Advanced Nursing* 12(1):3–12, 1987.

Dolan, S.L., Van-Ameringen, M.R., Corbin, S., and Arsenault, A. Lack of Professional Latitude and Role Problems as Correlates of Propensity to Quit Amongst Nursing Staff. *Journal of Advanced Nursing* 17(12):1455–1459, 1992.

Duquette, A., Kerouac, S., Sandhu, B.K., and Beaudet, L. Factors Related to Nursing Burnout: A Review of Empirical Knowledge. *Issues in Mental Health Nursing* 15:337–358, 1994.

Editorial. Transmission of Hepatitis C via Blood Splash into Conjunctiva. *Scandinavian Journal of Infectious Diseases* 25:270–271, 1993.

Emery, J.E. Perceived Sources of Stress Among Pediatric Oncology Nurses. *Journal of Pediatric Oncology Nursing* 10(3):87–92, 1993.

English, J.F. Reported Hospital Needlestick Injuries in Relation to Knowledge/Skill, Design, and Management Problems. *Infection Control and Hospital Epidemiology* 13(5):259–264, 1992.

Eriksen, L.R., Quandt, B., Teinert, D., et al. A Registered Nurse–Licensed Vocational Nurse Partnership Model for Critical Care Nursing. *Journal of Nursing Administration* 22(12):28–38, 1992.

Feldstein, A., Valanis, B., Vollmer, W., et al. The Back Injury Prevention Project Pilot Study: Assessing the Effectiveness of Back Attack, an Injury Prevention Program Among Nurses, Aides, and Orderlies. *Journal of Occupational Medicine* 35(2):114–120, 1993.

Fielding, J., and Weaver, S.M. A Comparison of Hospital- and Community-based Mental Health Nurses: Perceptions of their Work Environment and Psychological Health. *Journal of Advanced Nursing* 19(6):1196–1204, 1994.

Foxall, M.J., Zimmerman, L., Standley, R., and Bene, B. A Comparison of Frequency and Sources of Nursing Job Stress Perceived by Intensive Care, Hospice and Medical-Surgical Nurses. *Journal of Advanced Nursing* 15(5):577–584, 1990.

Garg, A., Owen, B.D., and Carlson, B. An Ergonomic Evaluation of Nursing Assistants' Job in a Nursing Home. *Ergonomics* 35(9):979–995, 1992.

Garrett, B., Singiser, D., and Banks, S.M. Back Injuries Among Nursing Personnel: The Relationship of Personal Characteristics, Risk Factors, and Nursing Practices. *AAOHN (American Association of Occupational Health Nurses) Journal* 40(11):510–516, 1992.

Gelfant, B.B. How the Environment Affects Turnover. *Journal of Practical Nursing* 40(1):33, 51, 1990.

Gentry, W.D., Foster, S.B., and Froehling, S. Psychologic Response to Situational Stress in Intensive and Nonintensive Nursing. *Heart and Lung* 1(6):793–796, 1972.

Gerberding, J.L. Management of Occupational Exposures to Blood-borne Viruses. *New England Journal of Medicine* 332(7):444–449, 1995.

Goetz, R.R., Bloom, J.D., Chenell, S.L., and Moorhead, J.C. Weapons Possession by Patients in a University Emergency Department. *Annals of Emergency Medicine* 20(1):8–10, 1991.

Gold, D.R., Rogacz, S., Bock, N., et al. Rotating Shift Work, Sleep, and Accidents Related to Sleepiness in Hospital Nurses. *American Journal of Public Health* 82(7):1011–1014, 1992.

Gordon, J.H., Ulrich, C., Feeley, M., and Pollack, S. Staff Distress Among Haemophilia Nurses. *AIDS Care* 5(3):359–367, 1993.

Greenfield, T.K., McNeil, D.E., and Binder, R.L. Violent Behavior and Length of Psychiatric Hospitalization. *Hospital and Community Psychiatry* 40(8):809–814, 1989.

Greenwood, J.G. Back Injuries Can Be Reduced with Worker Training, Reinforcement. *Occupational Health and Safety* 55(5):26–29, 1986.

Haller, R.M., and DeLuty, R.H. Assaults on Staff by Psychiatric Inpatients: A Critical Review. *British Journal of Psychiatry* 152:174–179, 1988.

Hamory, B.H. Underreporting of Needlestick Injuries in a University Hospital. *American Journal of Infection Control* 11(5):174–177, 1983.

Harber, P., Billet, E., Gutowski, M., et al. Occupational Low Back Pain in Hospital Nurses. *Journal of Occupational Medicine* 27(7):518–524, 1985.

Hawley, M.P. Sources of Stress for Emergency Nurses in Four Urban Canadian Emergency Departments. *Journal of Emergency Nursing* 18(3):211–216, 1992.

Henderson, D.K., Fahey, B.J., Willy, M., et al. Risk for Occupational Transmission of Human Immunodeficiency Virus Type 1 (HIV-1) Associated with Clinical Exposures. *Annals of Internal Medicine* 113(10):740–746, 1990.

Hinshaw, A.S., Smeltzer, C.H., and Atwood, J.R. Innovative Retention Strategies for Nursing Staff. *Journal of Nursing Administration* 17(6):8–16, 1987.

Hiscott, R.D., and Connop, P.J. The Health and Well-Being of Mental Health Professionals. *Canadian Journal of Public Health* 81(6):422–426, 1990.

Hudson, G. The Toxic Ecology of Work: Are the Carers Taking Care? *Australian Nurse Journal* 19(10):17, 1990.

Husted, G.L., Miller, M.C., and Wilczynski, E.M. Retention is the Goal: Extinguish Burnout with Self-Esteem Enhancement. *Journal of Continuing Education in Nursing* 20(6):244–248, 1989.

Infantino, J.A., and Musingo, S.Y. Assault and Injuries Among Staff With and Without Training in Aggression Control Techniques. *Hospital and Community Psychiatry* 36(12):1312–1314, 1985.

Jackson, M.M., Dechairo, D.C., and Gardner, D.F. Perceptions and Beliefs of Nursing and Medical Personnel About Needle-Handling Practices and Needlestick Injuries. *American Journal of Infection Control* 14(1):1–10, 1986.

Jagger, J. A New Opportunity to Make the Health Care Workplace Safer. *Advances in Exposure Prevention* 1(1):1–2, 1994a.

Jagger, J. Report on Blood Drawing: Risky Procedures, Risky Devices, Risky Job. *Advances in Exposure Prevention* 1(1):4–9, 1994b.

Jagger, J., Hunt, E.H., Brand-Elnagger, J., and Pearson, R.D. Rates of Needlestick Injury Caused by Various Devices in a University Hospital. *New England Journal of Medicine* 5:284–288, 1988.

Jagger, J., Cohen, M., and Blackwell, B. EPINet: A Tool for Surveillance of Blood Exposures in Health Care Settings. *Essentials of Modern Hospital Safety* 3:223–239, 1994.

Jennings, B.M. Stress, Locus of Control, Social Support, and Psychological Symptoms Among Head Nurses. *Research in Nursing and Health* 13(6):393–401, 1990.

Jensen, R.C. Back Injuries Among Nursing Personnel: Research Needs and Justifications. *Research in Nursing and Health* 10:29–38, 1987.

Johnson, C. Coping with Compassion Fatigue. *Nursing* 22(4):116–119, 1992.

Jones, M.K. Patient Violence Report of 200 Incidents. *Journal of Psychosocial Nursing and Mental Health Services* 23(6):12–17, 1985.

Jorgensen, S., Hein, H.O., and Gyntelberg, F. Heavy Lifting at Work and Risk of Genital Prolapse and Herniated Lumbar Disc in Assistant Nurses. *Occupational Medicine* 44(1):47–49, 1994.

Jung, F. Shiftwork: Its Effect on Health Performance and Well-Being. *AAOHN (American Association of Occupational Health Nurses) Journal* 34(4):161–164, 1986.

Kandolin, I. Burnout of Female and Male Nurses in Shiftwork. *Ergonomics* 36(1–3):141–147, 1993.

Keim, J., and Robinson, S. Work Environment Factors Influencing Burnout Among Third Shift Nurses. *Journal of Nursing Administration* 22(11):52, 56, 1992.

Kopfer, A.M., and McGovern, P.M. Transmission of HIV via a Needlestick Injury: Practice Recommendations and Research Implications. *AAOHN (American Association of Occupational Health Nurses) Journal* 41:374–381, 1993.

Lanza, M.L. The Reactions of Nursing Staff to Physical Assault by a Patient. *Hospital and Community Psychiatry* 34(1):44–47, 1983.

Lanza, M.L. Factors Relevant to Patient Assault. *Issues in Mental Health Nursing* 9:239–257, 1988.

Lanza, M.L. Patient Assaults: A Comparison Study of Reporting Methods. *Journal of Nursing Quality Assurance* 5(4):60–68, 1991.

Lanza, M.L. Nurses as Patient Assault Victims: An Update, Synthesis, and Recommendations. *Archives of Psychiatric Nursing* VI(3):163–171, 1992.

Lanza, M.L., and Milner, J. The Dollar Cost of Patient Assault. *Hospital and Community Psychiatry* 40(12):1227–1229, 1989.

Larese, F., and Fiorito, A. Musculoskeletal Disorders in Hospital Nurses: A Comparison Between Two Hospitals. *Ergonomics* 37(7):1205–1211, 1994.

Larkin, E., Murtagh, S., and Jones, S. A Preliminary Study of Violent Incidents in a Special Hospital (Rampton). *British Journal of Psychiatry* 153:226–231, 1988.

Lavoie, F., Carter, G.L., Danzl, D.F., and Berg, R.L. Emergency Department Violence in United States Teaching Hospitals. *Annals of Emergency Medicine* 17(11):1227–1233, 1988.

Lechky, O. Nurses Face Widespread Abuse at Work, Research Team Says. *Canadian Medical Association Journal* 150(5):737–742, 1994.

Lees, S., and Ellis, N. The Design of a Stress-Management Programme for Nursing Personnel. *Journal of Advanced Nursing* 15(8):946–961, 1990.

Lewis, S.L., Campbell, M.A., Becktell, P.J., et al. Work Stress, Burnout, and Sense of Coherence Among Dialysis Nurses. *ANNA (American Nephrology Nurses' Association) Journal* 19(6):545–553, 1992.

Linnemann, C.C., Cannon, C., DeRonde, M., and Lanphear, B. Effect of Educational Programs, Rigid Sharps Containers, and Universal Precautions on Reported Needlestick Injuries in Health Care Workers. *Infection Control and Hospital Epidemiology* 12(4):214–219, 1991.

Lion, J.R., Snyder, W., and Merrill, G.L. Brief Reports: Understanding of Assaults of Staff in a State Hospital. *Hospital & Community Psychiatry* 322(7):497–498, 1981.

Lipscomb, J.A., and Love, C.C. Violence Toward Health Care Workers: An Emerging Occupational Hazard. *AAOHN (American Association of Occupational Health Nurses) Journal* 40(5):219–226, 1992.

Lucas, M.D., Atwood, J.R., and Hagaman, R. Replication and Validation of Anticipated Turnover Model for Urban Registered Nurses. *Nursing Research* 42(1):29–35, 1993.

Lusk, S.L. Violence Experienced by Nurses' Aides in Nursing Homes: An Exploratory Study. *AAOHN (American Association of Occupational Health Nurses) Journal* 40(5):237–242, 1992.

MacNeil, J.M., and Weisz, G.M. Critical Care Nursing Stress: Another Look. *Heart and Lung* 16(3):274–277, 1987.

Mallon, D.F., Shearwood, W., Mallal, S.A., et al. Exposure to Blood Borne Infections in Health Care Workers. *Medical Journal of Australia* 157(9):592–595, 1992.

Mann, E.E., and Jefferson, K.J. Retaining Staff: Using Turnover Indices and Surveys. *Journal of Nursing Administration* 18(7–8):17–23, 1988.

Marchette, L., and Marchette, B. Back Injury: A Preventable Occupational Hazard. *Orthopaedic Nursing* 4(6):25–29, 1985.

Marcus, R.A., Tokars, J.I., Culver, P.S., and McKibben, D.M. Zidovudine Use After Occupational Exposure to HIV-infected Blood. Abstract no. 979. Presented by R.A. Marcus at the 1991 31st Interscience Conference on Antimicrobial Agents and Chemotherapy (ICAAC), Chicago, 1991.

Marshall, R.E., and Kasmen, C. Burnout in the Neonatal Intensive Care Unit. *Pediatrics* 65:1161–1165, 1980.

Masterson-Allen, S., Mor, V., and Laliberte, L. Turnover in National Hospice Study Sites: A Reflection of Organizational Growth. *Hospital Journal* 3(2–3):147–164, 1987.

McAbee, R. Nursing and Back Injuries. *AAOHN (American Association of Occupational Health Nurses) Journal* 36:200–209, 1988.

McAbee, R.R., and Wilkinson, W.E. Back Injuries and Registered Nurses. *AAOHN (American Journal of Occupational Health Nurses) Journal* 36(3):106–112, 1988.

McCulloch, L.E., McNeil, D.E., Binder, R.L., and Hatcher, C. Effects of a Weapon Screening Procedure in a Psychiatric Emergency Room. *Hospital and Community Psychiatry* 37:837–838, 1986.

McEvoy, M., Porter, K., Mortimer, P., et al. Prospective Study of Clinical, Laboratory, and Ancillary Staff with Accidental Exposures to Blood or Body Fluids from Patients Infected with HIV. *British Medical Journal* 294:1595–1598, 1987.

Miller, D.S., and Norton, V.M. Absenteeism. Nursing Service's Albatross. *Journal of Nursing Administration* 16(3):38–42, 1986.

Moore, R., and Kaczmarek, R. Occupational Hazards to Health Care Workers: Diverse, Ill-Defined, and Not Fully Appreciated. *American Journal of Infection Control* 18(5):316–327, 1990.

Moorhouse, A., Bolen, R., Evans, J., et al. Needlestick Injuries: The Shock and the Reality. *CINA: Official Journal of the Canadian Intravenous Nurses Association* 10(1):14–18, 1994.

Morrison, E.F. Theoretical Modeling to Predict Violence in Hospitalized Psychiatric Patients. *Research in Nursing and Health* 12:31–40, 1989.

Nagelkerk, J. The Impact of AIDS on Recruitment and Retention in Hospitals. *Nursing Administration Quarterly* 18(2):30–35, 1994.

Neuberger, J., Harris, J., Kundin, W., et al. Incidence of Needlestick Injuries in Hospital Personnel: Implications for Prevention. *American Journal of Infection Control* 12:171–176, 1984.

Neuberger, J.S., Kammerdiener, A.M., and Wood, C. Traumatic Injuries Among Medical Center Employees. *AAOHN (American Association of Occupational Health Nurses) Journal* 36(8):318–325, 1988.

Newman, S., and Callaghan, C. Work-related Back Pain. *Occupational Health* 45:201–205, 1993.

Nursing Times. The Hidden Scandal. 88(41):25–29, 1992.

Oehler, J.M., Davidson, M.G., Starr, L.E., and Lee, D.A. Burnout, Job Stress, Anxiety, and Perceived Social Support in Neonatal Nurses. *Heart and Lung* 20(5):500–505, 1991.

Owen, B.D. The Magnitude of Low-Back Problems in Nursing. *Western Journal of Nursing Research* 11(2):234–242, 1989.

Owen, B.D., and Garg, A. Reducing Risk for Back Injury in Nursing Personnel. *AAOHN (American Association of Occupational Health Nurses) Journal* 39(1):24–33, 1991.

Packard, J.S., and Motowidlo, S.J. Subjective Stress, Job Satisfaction, and Job Performance of Hospital Nurses. *Research in Nursing and Health* 10(4):253–261, 1987.

Phillips, J.A., and Brown, K.C. Industrial Workers on a Rotating Shift Pattern: Adaptation and Injury Status. *AAOHN (American Association of Occupational Health Nurses) Journal* 40(10):468–476, 1992.

Pines, A., and Maslach, C. Characteristics of Staff Burnout in Mental Health Settings. *Hospital and Community Psychiatry* 29:233–237, 1978.

Porter, R.T., Porter, M.J., and Lower, M.S. Enhancing the Image of Nursing. *Journal of Nursing Administration* 19(2):36–40, 1989.

Poster, E.C., and Ryan, J.A. Nurses Attitudes Toward Physical Assaults by Patients. *Archives of Psychiatric Nursing* 3(6):315–322, 1989.

Power, K.G., and Sharp, G.R. A Comparison of Sources of Nursing Stress and Job Satisfaction Among Mental Handicap and Hospice Nursing Staff. *Journal of Advanced Nursing* 13(6):726–732, 1988.

Rees, D.W., and Cooper, C.L. Occupational Stress in Health Service Workers in the UK. *Stress Medicine* 8(2):79–90, 1992.

Ribner, B.S., Landry, M.N., Gholson, G.L., and Linden, L.L. Impact of a Rigid, Puncture Resistant Container System upon Needlestick Injuries. *Infection Control* 8(2):63–66, 1987.

Rix, G. Staff Sickness and its Relationships to Violent Incidents on a Regional Secure Psychiatric Unit. *Journal of Advanced Nursing* 12(2):223–228, 1987.

Roberts, C.R., and McGovern, P. Working Mothers and Infant Care: A Review of the Literature. *AAOHN (American Association of Occupational Health Nurses) Journal* 41(11):541–546, 1993.

Rodgers, S. Back Pain Four: Positive Lifting. *Nursing Times* 81:43–45, 1985.

Rogers, B., and Travers, P. Occupational Hazards of Critical Care Nursing: Overview of Work-related Hazards in Nursing: Health and Safety Issues. *Heart and Lung* 20(5):486–499, 1991.

Scalzi, C.C. Role Stress in Top-Level Nurse Executives. *Western Journal of Nursing Research* 12(1):85–94, 1990.

Shanahan, M.M. A Comparative Analysis of Recruitment and Retention of Health Care Professionals. *Health Care Management Review* 18(3):41–51, 1993.

Snape, J., and Cavanagh, S.J. Occupational Stress in Neurosurgical Nursing. *Intensive and Critical Care Nursing* 9(3):162–170, 1993.

Todd, C., Robinson, G., and Reid, N. 12-Hour Shifts: Job Satisfaction of Nurses. *Journal of Nursing Management* 1(5):215–220, 1993.

van Servellen, G., and Leake, B. Emotional Exhaustion and Distress Among Nurses: How Important Are AIDS-Care Specific Factors? *Journal of the Association of Nurses in AIDS Care* 5(2):11–19, 1994.

van Wissen, K.A., and Siebers, R.W. Nurses' Attitudes and Concerns Pertaining to HIV and AIDS. *Journal of Advanced Nursing* 18(6):912–917, 1993.

Venning, P.J., Walter, S.D., and Stitt, L.W. Personal and Job-related Factors as Determinants of Incidence of Back Injuries Among Nursing Personnel. *Journal of Occupational Medicine* 28(10):820–825, 1987.

Wasserberger, J., Ordog, G.J., Kolodny, M., and Allen, K. Violence in a Community Emergency Room. *Archives of Emergency Medicine* 6:266–269, 1989.

Whitley, M.P., and Putzier, D.J. Measuring Nurses' Satisfaction with the Quality of their Work and Work Environment. *Journal of Nursing Care Quality* 8(3):43–51, 1994.

Wilkinson, W. Occupational Injury at a Midwestern Health Science Center and Teaching Hospital. *AAOHN (American Association of Occupational Health Nurses) Journal* 35(8):367–376, 1987.

Wilkinson, W.E., Salazar, M.K., Uhl, J.E., et al. Occupational Injuries: A Study of Health Care Workers at a Northwestern Health Science Center and Teaching Hospital. *AAOHN (American Association of Occupational Health Nurses) Journal* 40(6):287–293, 1992.

Willy, M.E., Dhillon, G.L., Loewen, N.L., et al. Adverse Exposures and Universal Precautions Practices Among a Group of Highly Exposed Health Professionals. *Infection Control and Hospital Epidemiology* 11(7):351–356, 1990.

Wolfgang, A.P., Perri, M., and Wolfgang, C.F. Job-related Stress Experienced by Hospital Pharmacists and Nurses. *American Journal of Hospital Pharmacy* 45(6):1342–1345, 1988.

Yu, L.C., Mansfield, P.K., Packard, J.S., et al. Occupational Stress Among Nurses in Hospital Settings. *AAOHN (American Association of Occupational Health Nurses) Journal* 37(4):121–128, 1989.

Index

A

Abuse and violence
  in hospitals, 178-179
  in nursing homes, 179-183, 375-377
  toward patients, 170, 180-183, 185-186, 375-376, 377
  toward staff, 15-16, 170, 177-183, 187-188, 376-377, 512-514
Access to care, 36, 353
  in nursing homes, 59, 164, 377-378, 476-477
Acquisitions, 53, 64
Activities of daily living (ADL), 39, 40, 131, 378
Acuity, *see* Case-mix acuity
Acute care, *see* Hospitals
Admissions to hospitals, 53, 54, 55, 279-280, 292
Advanced practice nurses (APN), 17, 97-100, 248, 342
  barriers to practice, 7, 100, 325, 348, 353
  education, 90, 336, 340, 342, 347, 348, 349

see Clinical nurse specialists; Geriatric and gerontological nursing; Nurse practitioners
Adverse incidents, 319-320
Age, of nurses, 72-74, 340, 350-351, *see also* Elderly population
Agency for Health Care Policy Research (AHCPR), 17, 122, 352
AIDS
  in nursing home case mix, 379
  special care units, 58, 120
  staff attitudes toward patients, 510-512
  see HIV transmission
Almshouses, 362
Alzheimer's disease and other dementia, 39, 363-364, 366
  special care units (SCU) for, 65, 184-185, 380
  staff problems with, 179-180, 184, 389
Ambulatory care, 51, 55-56, 70, 81
American Board of Nursing Specialities, 342, 349
American Indians, 373-374

American Nurses Association (ANA), 10-11, 122, 123, 124, 309, 381

Ancillary personnel, *see* Nurse assistants (NA) and ancillary nursing personnel

Antipsychotic drugs, 131, 135, 139, 363, 381

Asian and Pacific Islander population, 34, 35, 374

Assault, 178, 513-514

Assisted living services, 39, 40, 65, 131, 365-366, 368, 378

Assistive lifting devices, 18, 174, 175, 177, 506, 507

Associate degree (AD) programs, 74, 75, 76, 83, 300-301, 302, 335-342 *passim*, 350

Autonomy and control, 88, 91, 117, 120, 315-316

B

Baccalaureate programs, 74-75, 76, 87, 300-301, 302, 334-342 *passim*, 349, 351

Background checks, 18, 181, 182

Back injuries and pain, 173-175, 505-509

Barriers to practice, 7, 100, 325, 348, 353

Black population, 34, 35, 38
in nursing homes, 78, 373

Blood and body fluids handling, 511-512

Board and care facilities, 63, 364-365

Boren Amendment, 61, 479

Bureau of Health Professions, Division of Nursing, 106, 122

Burnout, 183, 184, 185-186, 347, 388-389, 519-521, 523, 524

C

Career development and mobility, 106, 340, 345, 354

Care planning, 96, 316
in nursing homes, 131, 134, 146

Care teams, 1-2, 89, 95, 96, 101, 322-323, 352, 363-364

Case management, 6, 89, 95, 96-97, 321, 434

Case-mix acuity, 261
hospitals, 54-55, 79, 84-85, 93
nursing homes, 58, 129, 131-132, 147, 363, 366, 378-379, 434-435

Case-mix reimbursement, 61-62, 368, 400-401
under Medicaid, 163-165, 479-480, 482-484

Certificate of Need (CON) program, 43, 61, 476

Certification, *see* Licensing and certification

Chronic conditions, 38-39, 40, 58

Clinical nurse specialists, 97-99, 249, 342

Closures, of hospitals, 52, 53

Collaboration, *see* Care teams

Community college programs, 77, 87-88, 335, 340, 350

Community-oriented care, 89-90, 261, 345, 351-352, 354

Competencies
in graduate programs, 342, 351-352
of nurse assistants (NA), 17, 70, 102-103

Complication rates, 318-319

Computer skills, 345, 352

Conditions of Participation, 11, 125

Conflict resolution, 183

Continuing education (CE), 342-343, 353, 434

Continuous quality improvement (CQI), 94-95, 104, 384

Continuum of care, 51, 55-58, 66, 96-97, 343

Cost containment and cost reduction, 19, 27-28, 43-44, 343
through cuts in nursing staff, 85-86, 90, 94, 103, 261-262, 347, 409

through hospital restructuring, 1-2, 51, 52, 53, 94

through shifting of care, 55-56, 66

Council on Performance Measurement, 126

Culturally sensitive care, 7, 17, 18, 35-36, 102, 103, 158, 351, 372-373

D

Data bases and data management systems, 347, 352

administrative, 112, 145

nursing home assessments, 135-136, 145

patient records, 112-113, 408-409

Dementia, see Alzheimer's disease and other dementia

Department of Education, 350

Diagnosis-related groups (DRG), 44, 114, 435

Differentiated practice, 69, 90-91, 337, 340-342, 344-345, 349-350

Diploma programs, 74, 75, 76, 83, 300-301, 302, 334, 335, 336, 350, 433

Directors of nursing, 14-15, 18, 83, 141, 158-159, 348, 391, 397

education, 18, 158-159, 391, 397

Discharge planning, 39-40, 97, 98

Discharges from hospitals, 54, 114-115, 282

Diversity, see Racial and ethnic groups

Doctoral degree programs, 335, 336, 337, 338, 339, 341, 342, 348

Downsizing and layoffs, 2, 82, 83, 92, 93, 103, 105-106, 246, 347, 354

E

Education and training, 86, 88-91, 256-257, 271-272, 333-354

of advanced practice nurses (APN), 90, 336, 340, 342, 347, 348, 349

for alternative settings, 89-90

in conflict management, 17, 18, 102, 158, 183

continuing (CE), 342-343, 353, 434

differentiated practice, 90-91, 337, 340-342, 349-350

of directors of nursing, 18, 158-159, 391, 397

in interdisciplinary team care, 89, 352

of licensed practical nurses (LPN), 76-77, 303, 335, 338, 432-433

of nurse assistants (NA), 7, 18, 70, 78, 100-101, 102, 157-158, 181, 391, 432, 468

in occupational safety, 15, 17, 18, 102, 158, 174, 175, 177, 506

of registered nurses (RN), 69, 73-76, 83, 87-88, 300-302, 335, 338, 339, 350-351, 433

in research skills, 336, 337, 342, 346, 349, 352-353

teaching and faculties, 345, 349, 351

Elderly population, 2, 20, 31, 32-41

abuse of, 180, 374-375

aged 85 and over, 32, 33, 34, 38, 40, 58, 59, 366

health and disability status, 38-39

home health services use, 63

hospital use, 39-40, 54, 282-283, 292

nursing home demand and use, 38, 39, 40, 41, 58, 59, 366, 378-379

see Geriatric and gerontological nursing

Emergency rooms, stress and violence in, 178, 184, 513-514

Employment in health occupations, 4, 69, 72, 304-305

registered nurses (RN), 71-72, 93, 304-305

Enrollments in nursing programs, 75, 76, 301, 302, 303

Ethnic groups, see Racial and ethnic groups

Evaluation research, 17, 106, 342, 345, 352-353

F

Falls, 170, 171
Families, 36-37
  role in nursing home care, 131,
    165-167, 268, 384-386, 410-
    411, 413
Fatigue, 169
Fee-for-service (FFS) system, 47, 48, 49
Functional status, 109, 131, 378-379

G

Gender, *see* Men; Women
Generic screens, 112-113
Geriatric and gerontological nursing,
    321, 350, 379
Graduate degree programs, 335-336,
    342, 350, *see also* Advanced
    practice nurses (APN)
Graduations from nursing programs, 73,
    75-76, 301, 302, 303, 337, 350

H

Health Care Financing Administration
    (HCFA), 112, 122
  hospital regulation, 125
  nursing home regulation, 13, 133,
    134-135, 136, 402, 457, 459-
    460, 462-463
Health maintenance organizations
    (HMO), 43, 45, 47, 48, 49, 125,
    290
Health promotion, 343, 352
Hepatitis transmission, 175, 176, 509
Hispanic population, 34, 35, 38, 374
  in nursing homes, 351, 374
HIV transmission, 175, 176, 509, 510
Home health care, 54, 63-64, 70, 365
Home health services, of hospitals, 56,
    57, 58, 287
Hospices, 56, 57, 58, 288-289
Hospitals, 22, 51-58, 79-81, 83-85
  abuse and violence in, 178-179,
    184, 513-514

beds, 54, 55, 79, 284-286, 292
  case mix, 54-55, 79, 84-85, 93
  closures, 52, 53
  continuum of care, 51, 55-58, 96-
    97
  discharge planning, 39-40, 97, 98
  home health services offered, 56,
    57, 58, 287
  hospice services offered, 56, 57,
    58, 288-289
  injuries among staff, 170, 171,
    175, 503
  inpatient activity, 1, 53-55, 279-
    283, 292
  licensed practical nurses (LPN) in,
    77, 78, 93, 106, 294-297
  mergers, 53
  nurse assistants (NA) in, 17, 78,
    95, 100-103
  outpatient care, 55, 56-57, 99, 289,
    292
  registered nurses (RN) in, 4, 6-7,
    44, 45, 79-84, 93, 95, 293-299
  regulation of, 11, 102-103, 124-
    126
  restructuring, 1-2, 5-6, 51, 52, 53,
    94-106, 113
  skilled nursing units, 56, 57-58,
    287-288
  special care units, 55, 57, 58
  staffing levels and mix, 9-12, 44,
    45, 68, 70, 79-81, 113, 116-122,
    262-263, 294-299
  staffing regulations, 11, 125
  see Intensive care units (ICU);
    Quality of hospital care

I

Income, 38
  and Medicaid eligibility, 60, 377-378
Incontinence, 131, 133, 140, 366
Independence, of nursing home
    residents, 138
Independent practice associations
    (IPA), 47, 49, 52

Indian Health Service (IHS), 373-374
Informatics, 352
Injuries and illness among staff, 15,
  169-172, 246, 248, 503-505
  back injuries and pain, 173-175,
    505-509
  needlesticks, 18, 175-177, 505,
    509-512
  relation to staffing levels, 15, 173-
    177, 187
  research needs, 18, 175
  safety training, 15, 17, 18, 102,
    158, 174, 175, 177, 506
Inpatient activity, 1, 53-55, 279-283, 292
  impacts on hospital staffing, 79,
    84, 93
Instrumental activities of daily living
  (IADL), 40, 378
Insurance, 46-47, 51, 125
Integrated systems, 51-52, 64, 99
Intensive care units (ICU), 55, 79, 93,
  286, 515, 516, 522

J

Job satisfaction, 315-316, 323-324, 325,
  515-516
  among nursing home staff, 159-160
Job security, 86, 92, 345, 354
Joint Commission on Accreditation of
  Healthcare Organizations
  (JCAHO)
  and hospitals, 11, 125-126
  subacute care unit standards, 66, 380

K

Kerr-Mills Medical Assistance to the
  Aged Act, 362

L

Language skills and barriers, 36, 351,
  372-373
Layoffs, *see* Downsizing and layoffs
Legislation, *see* Nursing Home Reform

Act; Omnibus Budget
  Reconciliation Act (OBRA);
  Social Security Act; Tax Equity
  and Fiscal Responsibility Act
  (TEFRA)
Length of hospital stay, 53, 54, 55,
  280-281, 282-283, 292
Licensed practical nurses (LPN), 69,
  72, 73, 76-78, 80, 304-305
  education, 76-77, 303, 335, 338,
    432-433
  in hospitals, 77, 78, 93, 106, 294-
    297
  injuries among, 172
  in nursing homes, 18, 70, 77, 78,
    143, 144, 149-154, 158, 430-433
Licensing and certification
  of advanced practice nurses, 100,
    342, 349
  of health care providers, 11, 125
  of licensed practical nurses (LPN),
    69
  of nurse assistants, 17, 70, 102,
    181-182
  of nursing homes, 133, 136, 460
  of registered nurses (RN), 69, 71,
    337
Life expectancy, 32, 34
Lifting injuries, 15, 18, 171, 174, 175,
  177, 505, 507-508
Living arrangements, 36-37
Long-term care, *see* Assisted living
  services; Nursing homes

M

Managed care, 1, 19, 45, 47-49, 52, 96,
  261-262, 348
Master's degree programs, 83, 335-336,
  337, 338, 339, 341, 351, *see also*
  Advanced practice nurses (APN)
Medicaid, 23, 38, 46, 51, 60, 61-62,
  133, 163-165, 353, 362, 377-
  378, 463, 475-484 *passim*
  case-mix reimbursement, 163-165,
  479-480, 482-484

and cost containment for nursing
  homes, 61-62, 385
income and asset eligibility, 60,
  377-378
prospective payment system, 61,
  62, 163, 479, 480-481
Medicare, 38, 46, 51, 113, 126, 350, 353
home health service coverage, 57
and nursing homes, 46, 60, 62,
  133, 362, 363, 377, 484-485
prospective payment system (PPS),
  43-44, 62, 79, 114
Men
  elderly, 36
  in nursing, 72, 345, 351
Mergers and acquisitions, 53, 64
Minimum data set (MDS), 13, 134, 135,
  145-146, 383, 415, 460
Minority groups, *see* Racial and ethnic
  groups
Mortality rates, 109, 112, 114
  in nursing homes, 131, 133
  relation to staffing ratios, 9, 112,
    117-120, 317-318, 348
Multistate Nursing Home Case-mix and
  Quality Demonstration Project,
  147, 402

N

National Center for Health Statistics,
  106, 122
National Institute of Nursing Research
  (NINR), 17, 106, 122, 336, 352
National League of Nursing (NLN),
  334, 348
Needlestick injuries, 18, 175-177, 505,
  509-512
Neonatal intensive care units (NICU),
  520-521
Nurse anesthetists, 85, 100
Nurse assistants (NA) and ancillary
  nursing personnel, 2*n*, 69-70,
  72, 73, 78, 304-305, 347-348
  abuse and violence involvement,
    16, 18, 180-182, 376, 514

competencies, 17, 70, 102-103
conflict management training, 17,
  18, 102, 158
and culturally sensitive care, 17,
  18, 102, 103, 158, 372-373
in hospitals, 7, 17, 70, 100-103,
  294-297
injuries among, 15, 171, 172, 174,
  503-504, 505-506
occupational safety training, 15,
  17, 18, 102, 158
training, 7, 18, 70, 78, 100-101,
  102, 157-158, 181, 391, 432,
  468
wages, 156, 160, 370, 371
Nurse midwives, 85, 100
Nurse practitioners, 85, 97, 99-100,
  342, 347, 350
Nursing Home Reform Act, 68, 83
Nursing Home Resident Assessment
  System, 135, 459-460
Nursing homes, 58-66, 362-366, 426-
  429, 471-473, 477-479
  abuse and violence in, 179-183,
    374-377
  access issues, 59, 164, 377-378,
    476-477
  alternative services, 40, 42-43, 64-
    65, 365-366, 472
  bed supply and occupancy, 58-59,
    472-476
  case mix, 58, 129, 131-132, 147,
    363, 366, 378-379, 434-435
  complex technologies in, 59, 65
  conflict management, 183
  cultural issues, 372-374, 411, 413-
    414
  directors of nursing in, 14-15, 18,
    141, 158-159, 391, 397
  injuries among staff, 170, 171,
    173-174, 269, 503
  and Medicaid, 23, 46, 60, 61-62,
    133, 163-165, 362, 377-378,
    463, 475-484 *passim*
  and Medicare, 46, 60, 62, 133,
    362, 363, 377, 484-485
  mergers and acquisitions, 64

nurse assistants (NA) in, 13-14, 18, 70, 78, 143, 144, 149-154, 156-158, 160, 252-253, 263-265, 369, 370-371, 381, 399, 432
ownership, 50, 162, 364, 403, 485-489
profits, 486-487, 488
registered nurse (RN) in, 13-14, 83, 141, 142, 143, 144, 148-154, 160, 161, 199-204, 371, 381, 391, 430-432, 462-463
regulation of, 133-136, 141-142, 367-368, 381-382, 457, 459-461
reimbursement mechanisms, 46, 61-62, 162-165, 270-271, 368, 385, 479-485
restructuring, 64-66
salaries, 160-161, 369, 371-372, 466-467
shift to rehabilitative care, 42-43, 64-65, 134, 367, 379, 412-413
special care units (SCU), 65, 379, 380
staff education and training, 83, 411-412, 432-434
staffing levels and mix, 4-5, 12-13, 18, 68, 129, 141-144, 146-158, 167-168, 190-191, 368-370, 393-399, 429-430, 435-436, 437-450, 461-465, 468-470
staffing needs and demand factors, 13, 22-23, 59, 83, 381, 434-435
staffing regulation, 141-142, 167-168, 253, 369-370, 381-382, 427, 462-463, 470-471, 491-492
staff turnover, 263, 430
subacute care units, 5, 65-66, 366, 379-380
24-hour registered nurse (RN) presence, 18, 83, 141-142, 153-155, 162, 199-204, 369, 381, 403
see Quality of nursing home care
Nursing shortage, 71, 353, 371
educational component, 349
and nursing homes, 141

O

Occupational health, *see* Injuries and illness among staff; Stress
Older persons, *see* Elderly population
Ombudsmen, 167, 250*n*, 394
Omnibus Budget Reconciliation Act (OBRA), 12, 61, 62, 133-134, 168, 181-182, 364, 367-368, 381, 383, 457, 459
implementation, 140-141
nursing coverage requirements, 12, 141-142, 383-384, 462-463
waivers, 141-142, 369, 381-382, 382
Oncology clinical nurse specialists, 98
Organizational factors, 17, 118, 121, 122, 308-309, 314
Outcome measures, 23-24, 344, 345, 346
hospitals, 108-109, 111, 123-124, 313-315, 325-328
nursing homes, 130, 131, 383, 456
Outpatient care, 55, 56-57, 99, 289, 292
Overexertion, 170, 171, 174
Ownership of facilities, 50, 247
nursing homes, 50, 162, 364, 403, 485-489

P

Partners-in-practice models, 101-102, 344
Patient-centered care, 94-95, 101
Patient satisfaction, 322-323, 325
with managed care, 48, 49
with nursing homes, 131
and restructuring, 17, 106
Peer Review Organizations (PRO), 113
Perkins Act programs, 350
Personal care activities of daily living (ADL), 40, 378
Population, growth rate, 32-34, *see also* Elderly population; Racial and ethnic groups
Postdoctoral training, 337, 339
Poverty status, 38

Preferred provider organizations (PPO), 45, 291

Pressure sores and decubitis, 131, 133, 157

Preventive medicine, 343

Primary care, 97, 342, 343, 344

Process of care indicators, 108, 110-111
  for nursing homes, 129, 130, 131, 456-457

Professional practice models, 118, 258, 310-311, 313, 315-316, 324, 405-407

Profit margins, 50

Prospective payment system (PPS), 60
  impacts on staffing, 44, 79
  under Medicaid, 61, 62, 163, 479, 480-481
  under Medicare, 43-44, 62, 79, 114

Psychiatric clinical nurse specialists, 342, 348

Public health nursing, 90

Q

Quality assurance and quality improvement (QA/QI), 10-11, 104, 107
  in nursing home assessment, 135-136, 460

Quality of hospital care, 28, 113-116, 245-250, 265-267
  advanced practice nurses role in, 17, 97-100
  and ancillary nursing personnel, 17, 100-103
  elements of, 107-109, 110-111
  legislation and regulation, 11, 102-103, 124-126
  measurement of, 8-9, 106-113, 325-328
  and organizational restructuring, 5-6, 94-106, 113
  performance indicators and standards, 122-124
  prospective payment system impacts, 9, 114-115

research needs, 8, 10-11, 17, 106, 116, 121-122, 127
  and staffing level and mix, 9-12, 113, 116-122

Quality of nursing home care, 12, 28, 132-146, 250-256, 267-269, 456-457
  elements of, 129-131
  families' roles in, 131, 165-167, 268, 384-386, 410-411, 413
  and geriatric specialists, 18, 155-156, 381-382, 396-398, 414-415, 467-468
  and job satisfaction, 386-387, 399
  and job stress, 387-390
  legislation and regulation, 133-136, 141-142, 367-368, 381-382, 457, 459-461
  management issues, 18, 158-159, 403-405
  measurement of, 129-132, 382-385, 407-409, 454-457
  and nurse assistants (NA), 18, 156-158, 399
  ombudsmen's role in, 167, 394
  outcomes-based incentives, 165, 490-491
  and ownership, 162, 403, 487-489
  and patient mix, 131-132
  and reimbursement mechanisms, 15, 385, 400-403, 412, 490-491
  research needs, 18, 407-411
  resident assessment tools, 135-136
  and staffing levels and mix, 12-13, 18, 146-158, 167-168, 190-191, 393-399, 435-436, 437-450, 468-470
  and staff training, 390-392, 467-468
  and staff turnover, 159-160, 386-387, 394, 399-400
  24-hour registered nuse (RN) presence, 18, 141-142, 153-155, 199-204, 381
  volunteers and, 166

R

Racial and ethnic groups, 34
  elderly population, 32, 34-36, 38, 373-374
  in nursing, 249, 345, 351
  nursing home residents, 374
  nursing home staff, 372-373
  see American Indians; Asian and Pacific Islander population; Black population; Culturally sensitive care; Hispanic population; White population
Record review, 112-113
Registered nurses (RN), 4, 69, 70, 304-305, 350-351
  autonomy and control, 88, 117, 120
  differentiated practice, 69, 90-91
  education, 69, 73-76, 83, 87-88, 300-302, 335, 338, 339, 350-351, 433
  in hospitals, 4, 6-7, 44, 45, 79-84, 93, 95, 293-299
  injuries among, 172
  in nursing homes, 13-14, 83, 141, 142, 143, 144, 148-154, 160, 161, 199-204, 371, 381, 391, 430-432, 462-463
  salaries, 80, 85-86, 160, 161, 337, 369, 371
  shifts in service settings, 81-82
  supervisory duties, 13-14, 95, 347
  see Advanced practice nurses (APN)
Registries, 181-182
Regulation
  of hospital operations, 11, 102-103, 124-126
  of hospital staffing, 11, 125
  of nursing home operations, 133-136, 141-142, 367-368, 381-382, 457, 459-461
  of nursing home staffing, 141-142, 167-168, 253, 369-370, 381-382, 427, 462-463, 470-471, 491-492

Rehabilitative care, 42-43, 64-65, 134, 367, 379, 412-413
Rehospitalization rates, 131, 133
Reimbursement mechanisms, 43-44, *see also* Case-mix reimbursement; Prospective payment system (PPS)
Report cards, 122-124
Research needs, 192
  for quality of hospital care, 8, 10-11, 17, 106, 116, 121-122, 127
  for quality of nursing home care, 18, 407-411
Resident assessment instrument (RAI), 134, 135-136
Resident assessment protocols (RAP), 134, 135
Resident assistants, 157
Residential facilities, 63, 64
Resource constraints, 107, 129
Resource utilization groups (RUGS), 147, 163, 401, 402-403, 434-435
Respect, of nursing home residents, 138
Restraints, 131, 135, 138-139, 381
Restructuring, 19, 343-345, 347-349
  monitoring effects of, 17, 105-106
  and staffing patterns, 95-97
  staff involvement in, 17, 103-105, 265-267, 348
RUGS, *see* Resource utilization groups (RUGS)

S

Salaries and compensation
  nurse assistants (NA), 156, 160, 370, 371
  nursing home staff, 160-161, 369, 371-372, 466-467
  registered nurses (RN), 80, 85-86, 160, 161, 337, 369, 371
Satisfaction, *see* Job satisfaction; Patient satisfaction
Security measures, 65, 180
Service learning, 346, 348

Service utilization, 320-322
Sharp objects, 176, 509-510
Shift work, 519-520
Sigma Theta Tau, 334
Social Security Act, 125, 133, 141, 362, 457
Special care units (SCU), 55, 57, 58
    for AIDS, 58, 120
    for Alzheimer's disease, 65, 184-185, 380
    in nursing homes, 65, 379, 380
Specialization, 120
State boards of nursing, 7, 100, 257
State-level associations, 122, 247-249
State regulation, of nursing homes, 142
State surveyors, 133, 135, 140, 367-368, 413, 460, 461
Stress, 169, 183-187, 246, 248, 514-521
    and turnover, 185-186, 522-524
Structural measures of care, 108, 110, 118
    in nursing homes, 129, 130, 383
Subacute care units, 5, 65-66, 366, 379-380
Substitutions of staff, 85-86, 92, 246, 248, 343, 348, 385
Supply of nursing personnel, 4, 69-78, 87-91, 304-305, 342
Support networks, 187, 389-390

T

Tax Equity and Fiscal Responsibility Act (TEFRA), 43-44
Team care, 1-2, 89, 95, 96, 101, 322-323, 352, 363-364
Telecommunications, 352
Total quality management, 94-95, 104
Tube feedings, 133, 166
Turning patients in bed, 157
Turnover and retention
    of directors of nursing, 158
    of nursing home staff, 159-160, 263, 386-387, 394, 399-400, 430
    relation to stress, 185-186, 522-524

24-hour registered nurse (RN) presence, 18, 83, 141-142, 153-155, 162, 199-204, 369, 381, 403

U

Undergraduate programs, see Associate degree (AD) programs; Baccalaureate programs
Unemployment in nursing, 72, 73, 78, 105
Unions, 245-248, 251-252
University programs, 340, 345-347, 348-349, 350
Urethral catheterization, 132, 140

V

Ventilator care, 57, 59, 65
Violence, see Abuse and violence
Volunteers, 166, 191

W

Wages, see Salaries and compensation
Waivers
    home- and community-based care, 63
    nursing home staff requirements, 14, 141-142, 154, 200, 202-203, 369-370, 381-382
Weapons, 178-179, 513-514
White population, 34
    elderly, 34, 35, 38, 373
Women
    elderly, 36, 38, 375
    home health services use, 63
    as informal caregivers, 37
    in nursing, 72, 156
    occupational injuries among, 171, 172
    and violence, 178, 375
Workplace hazards, see Injuries and illness among staff; Stress